Language Development
An Introduction

FIFTH EDITION

Robert E. Owens, Jr.
State University of New York
Geneseo, New York

Allyn and Bacon

Boston London Toronto Sydney Tokyo Singapore

Executive Editor: Stephen D. Dragin
Editorial Assistant: Barbara Strickland
Senior Editorial-Production Administrator: Joe Sweeney
Editorial-Production Service: Walsh & Associates, Inc.
Composition Buyer: Linda Cox
Manufacturing Buyer: Chris Marson
Cover Administrator: Brian Gogolin

Library of Congress Cataloging-in-Publication Data

Owens, Robert E.
    Language development : an introduction / Robert E. Owens, Jr.—5th ed.
        p.   cm.
    Includes bibliographical references and indexes.
    ISBN 0-205-31926-2
    1. Language acquisition.   II. Title.
    P118.O93   2000
    401′.93—dc21   00–028848

Printed in the United States of America

10   9   8   7   6   5   4   3   2   1   04   03   02   01   00

Photo Credits: p. 2, Tony Freeman; p. 24, Gallaudet University; p. 30, Robert Harbison; p. 57, Will
Faller; p. 66, David Young-Wolff/Photo Edit; p. 99, Elizabeth Crews; p. 108, Deborah Davis/Photo
Edit; p. 116, Elizabeth Crews; p. 128, Hazel Hankin/Stock Boston; p. 137, Nita Winter/The Image
Works; p. 156, Dion Ogust/The Image Works; p. 188, Elizabeth Crews; p. 196, Laura Dwight/Photo
Edit; p. 224, Robert Brenner/Photo Edit; p. 236 & p. 240, Elizabeth Crews; p. 274, Jeff Greenberg/
Photo Edit; p. 297, Myrleen Ferguson/Photo Edit; p. 304 & p. 337, Elizabeth Crews; p. 348, Don
Smetzer/Stone; p. 368, Nancy Richmond/The Image Works; p. 380, Robin Sachs/Photo Edit;
p. 400, Myrleen Ferguson/Photo Edit; p. 408, Louise Gubb/The Image Works; p. 416, Tony
Freeman/Photo Edit; p. 438, Steve Dunwell/The Image Bank; p. 447, Judy Gelles/Stock Boston;
p. 456, David Young-Wolff/Photo Edit; p. 459, Elizabeth Crews.

"Say that again. I didn't hear you. I was listening to my toast."
Jessica Owens, age four

To my granddaughter Cassidy,
who has only just begun this wonderful journey,
and to my daughter Jessica,
her wonderful teacher along the way.

Contents

7 Language-Learning Processes in Young Children   196

8 A First Language   236

Preface

There is no single way in which children learn to communicate. Each child follows an individual developmental pattern. Still, it is possible to describe a pattern of general communication development and of English specifically. This text attempts such descriptions and generalizations but emphasizes individual patterns.

In recognition of the tremendous variation across children and languages, the fifth edition of *Language Development* devotes much more space to individual developmental differences and cultural differences. Discussion of other cultures has been included in the text wherever possible. In addition, the sections on bidialectism and bilingualism have been expanded to reflect more accurately the realities of everyday life in the United States.

In an attempt to make the text more readable, I have rewritten and updated it throughout. Many quotations have been removed, reworded, or shortened to make the flow more even. Each chapter ends with a discussion in an attempt to add relevance and to answer the question "So what?" In addition, Chapter 5, Cognitive and Perceptual Bases of Early Language, has been reorganized and placed in a more logical fashion.

Those students who will one day become parents should appreciate the value of this text as a guideline to development. Students who plan to work with children with disabilities and without will find that normal development can provide a model for evaluation and intervention. The developmental rationale can be used to decide on targets for training and to determine the overall remediation approach.

In recognition of the importance of the developmental rationale as a tool and of the changing perspectives in child language development, the fifth edition offers expanded coverage of preschool and school-age language development. Pragmatics receives increased attention, as does the conversational context within which most language development occurs. Prospective speech-language pathologists will find these developmental progressions valuable when making decisions concerning materials to use with children with speech and language impairments. As consumers of educational and therapeutic products, educators and speech-language pathologists must be especially sensitive to the philosophy that governs the organization of such materials. Many materials claim to be developmental in design but are not. I recall opening one such book to find *please* and *thank you* as the first two utterances to be taught to a child with deafness. These words violate many of the characteristics of first words.

The experienced teacher, psychologist, or speech-language pathologist need not rely on such prepackaged materials if she or he has a good base in communication development. An understanding of the developmental process and the use of a problem-solving approach can be a powerful combination in the hands of a creative clinician.

With these considerations in mind, I have created what I hope to be a useful test for future parents, educators, psychologists, and speech-language pathologists.

ACKNOWLEDGMENTS

A volume of this scope must be the combined effort of many people fulfilling many roles, and this one is no exception.

My first thanks go to all those professionals and students, too numerous to mention, who have corresponded or conversed with me and offered criticism or suggestions for this edition. The overall organization of this text reflects the general organization of my own communication development course and that of professionals with whom I have been in contact.

The professional assistance of Addie Haas, Kathy Jones, Linda House, and Linda Deats has been a godsend. Dr. Haas, professor in the Communication Disorders Department at State University of New York at New Paltz, is a dear friend; a trusted confident; a good buddy; a fellow hiker; a skilled clinician; a source of information, ideas, and inspiration; and a helluva lot of fun. Dr. Kathy Jones' expertise and, more importantly, her warmth have been a welcome source of encouragement. My department chair, Dr. Linda House, has created an environment at SUNY Geneseo in which I enjoy working. Finally, Linda Deats is always available to listen to my hare-brained, half-baked ideas and to laugh with me at the many ridiculous things I do. For her I wish a lifetime supply of lipstick and faux fur.

I would be remiss if I did not offer my heartfelt thanks to Dr. Christopher Dahl, President of SUNY Geneseo, for his encouragement and his warm supportive letters and e-mails. Through his efforts, our college has become a rich academic environment and a welcoming place in which to work.

I have also enjoyed the assistance of two able and distinguished reviewers: Kenyatta O. Rivers, University of Central Florida, and Michael W. Casby, Michigan State University.

Several friends also offered encouragement and support. They are Peggy Meeker, Marie Gibson, Harriet Smith, Irene Belyakov, Dr. Robin Goodman, Michael Deats, Bohdhan Jejna, and Jeff Pernell. Thanks so much. I love you all.

I would like to express my love and appreciation to my children, Jason, Todd, and Jessica, who are as beautiful as young adults as they were as youngsters; and to Tom, my life partner, who has had to endure the frustrations of having a temperamental author in the house. His encouragement, patience, kindness, and love, not to mention faithful doing of chores when I'm busy, are greatly appreciated. I love all four of you.

Finally, I am extremely grateful to those individuals who helped in the preparation of the CD that accompanies this text. Kelly Kennedy and Enrico Coloccia were responsible for the collection of samples and preparation of the disk. This was a time-consuming process and they performed very well. The parents and children featured include Anna M. Kowalchuk and K. Callaghan Cylke, Beverly Henke-Lofquist and Sam T. H. and Caysey J. H. Lofquist, Jessica B. Poe and Cassidy B. Poe, and Margaret S. Post and Henry and Samuel Post. The dialectal speakers are Irene K. Belyakov, Robyn S. Goodman, Linda I. House, Robert E. Owens, Jr., Patricia Marcelle Samson, and Edna Carter Young.

Language Development

1

The Territory

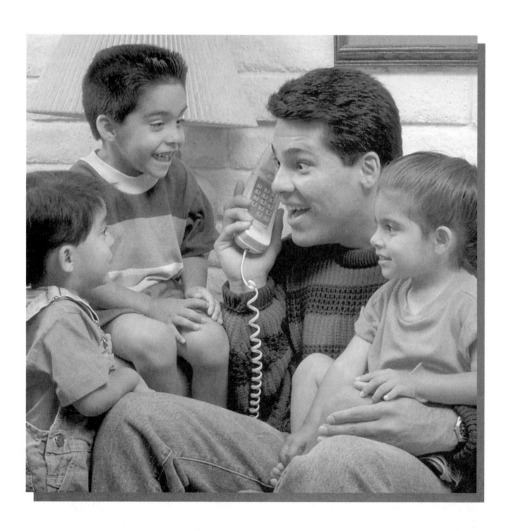

CHAPTER OBJECTIVES

Before we can discuss language development, we need to agree on a definition of language —what it is and what it is not. As a user of language, you already know a great deal about it. This chapter will organize your knowledge and provide some labels for the many aspects of language you know. When you have completed this chapter, you should understand

- the difference between speech, language, and communication.
- the difference between nonlinguistic, paralinguistic, and metalinguistic aspects of communication.
- the main properties of language.
- the five components of language and their descriptions.
- terms that will be useful later in the text:

antonyms	phoneme
bound morphemes	phonology
communication	pragmatics
communicative competence	psycholinguistics
dialects	selection restrictions
free morphemes	semantic features
grammars	semantics
intonation	sociolinguistics
language	speech
linguistic competence	speech act
linguistic performance	stress
metalinguistic cues	suprasegmental devices
morpheme	synonyms
morphology	syntax
nonlinguistic cues	word knowledge
paralinguistic codes	world knowledge

Don't panic, introductory chapters usually contain a lot of terminology so that we can all "speak the same language" throughout the text.

Language and the linguistic process are so complex that specialists devote their lives to investigating them. These specialists, called *linguists,* try to determine the language rules that individual people use to communicate. The linguist deduces the rules of language from the regularities or patterns demonstrated when we, as users of the language, communicate with one another. As a result, linguists attempt to develop theories that characterize particular languages or to describe cross-language phenomena. Two specialized areas of linguistics or the scientific study of language—psycholinguistics and sociolinguistics—combine the study of language with other disciplines. *Psycholinguistics* is the study of the way people acquire and process language. *Sociolinguistics* is the study of language and cultural and situational influences. In developmental studies the sociolinguist focuses on caregiver-child interactions and on the early social uses of language.

In a sense, each child is a linguist who must deduce the rules of his or her own native language. Unlike the linguist, however, the child does not yet have a mature language base to use in understanding another person.

To understand some of the complexity of the language system, let's reverse the linguist's procedure for a moment. Assume that you've been commissioned to create a large force of humanlike computers for interplanetary exploration. These humanoids must communicate using American English. As you imagine writing the computer program, you may begin to appreciate the intricate process that underlies language use. First, the computer must be able to encode and decode almost instantaneously. Some method of transmission must be found. If you choose speech transmission, you must program all possible English sounds. Once the sounds are programmed, each must be modified to accommodate the minute variations that are the result of sound combinations. And you must determine which sounds go together in English and which ones can never be used in combination. No English words begin with *bn*, for example.

Second, you must create a storage bank of words that can be produced by using the sounds and sound combinations already programmed. To produce smooth, efficient, humanlike speech, you will have to program intonation and stress patterns, too. In addition, each word must be stored under the appropriate category for easy reference and retrieval. Definitions must be programmed for each word. Categories can be appreciated best by examining some of the simple rules for combining words.

Third, you must program word combinations with rules such as the following:

Sentence = Noun + Verb

No one would argue with this rule. Examples are as follows:

Girl run. Boy eat.

Unfortunately, the **sentences** seem awkward. You must modify your rule slightly so that with singular nouns, such as *girl* or *boy*, an *s* is added at the end of the verb to form *runs* and *eats*, and with plural nouns, such as *girls* or *boys*, an *s* is added to the noun but not to the verb. What would you do with a sentence such as "Chair jumps"? It's a meaningless sentence. How could you avoid the creation of such sentences as "Chair jumps," "Desk walks," and "House flies"? You could write your program to delete all possible nonsense combinations, but this process would be very time-consuming. It would be more efficient to write a rule, but what rule could you write that would encompass all possibilities? Consider all the rules you would need to create for other categories, such as articles, adjectives, and adverbs, and for verb tenses, plurals, possessives, questions, imperatives, and so on. It might be easier to dismember your humanoid force, bid family and friends farewell, and explore the solar system yourself.

Our little experiment may seem trivial or overly tedious. You may even think it's unfair to ask you to state the rules of American English, especially in the first few pages of a language development textbook. You might claim that you don't know the rules—or at least not all of them. I'll let you in on a secret: Neither do linguists. Their task, like that of the very young child, is to deduce the language rules from the language used around them. Yet the linguist, the child, you, and I, as users of American English, demonstrate daily that we clearly know what the rules are.

Forcing you to think about the rules is not unfair; expecting you to program a humanoid for human communication is. In fact, even with linguists' knowledge, no one has been able to create a computerized spoken version of American English that has the complexity, the richness, or the flow of human communication. This puzzle is all the more interesting when we realize that most four-year-old children have deciphered American English and have well-developed speech, language, and communication skills. This feat is truly remarkable, given the complexity of the task.

You probably recall little of your own language-acquisition process. One statement is probably true: Unless you experienced difficulty, there was no formal instruction. Congratulations are in order because you probably did most of it on your own.

To appreciate the task involved in language learning, you need to be familiar with some of the terminology that is commonly used in the field. All the terms introduced in this chapter and throughout the text are summarized for you in the Glossary. The remainder of this chapter is devoted to an explanation of these terms. First, we discuss this text in general. Then we distinguish three often confused terms—*speech, language*, and *communication*—and look at some special qualities of language itself.

THIS TEXT AND YOU

Although the full title of this text is *Language Development: An Introduction*, it is not a watered-down or cursory treatment of the topic. I have attempted to cover every timely, relevant, and important aspect of language development that might be of interest to the future speech-language pathologist, educator, psychologist, child development specialist, or parent. Of necessity, the material is complex and specific as is the topic.

No doubt you've at least thumbed through this book. It may look overwhelming. It's not. I tell my students that things are never as bleak as they seem at the beginning of the semester. Over the last twenty years, I have taken 4,000 of my own students through this same material with a nearly 100 percent success rate. Let me try to help you find this material as rewarding to learn as it is to teach.

First, the text is organized into three overall sections. The first four chapters provide a background that includes terms, theories, overall development, and the brain and language. It's difficult to have to read this material when you really want to get to the development material, but all this background is necessary. The main topics of development are contained in Chapters 5 through 13, which are organized sequentially from newborns through adults with a separate chapter for language differences. Finally, the last two chapters cover research and the relationship between development and disorders, or a chance to answer the "so what?" question. Your professor may or may not follow this order.

As with any text, there are a few simple rules that can make the learning experience more fruitful.

- Note the chapter objectives prior to reading the chapter and be alert for this information as you read.
- Read each chapter in small doses then let it sink in for a while.
- Find the chapter organization described at the end of each chapter's introduction. This will help you follow me through the material.
- Take brief notes as you read. Don't try to write everything down. Stop at natural divisions in the content and ask yourself what was most important. Visual learners may be helped by the process of writing.
- Review your notes when you stop reading and before you begin again the next time. This process will provide a review and some continuity.
- Try to read a little every day or every other day rather than neglecting the text until the night before the test.
- Note the terms in the chapter objectives and try to define them as you read. Each one is printed in boldface in the body of the chapter. Please don't just thumb through or turn to the Glossary for a dictionary definition. The terms are relatively meaningless out of context. They need the structure of the other information. Context is very important.
- Try to answer the questions at the end of each chapter and at our website, abacon.com, from your notes or from your memory.
- I have tried to deemphasize linguists, authors, and researchers by placing all citations in parentheses. Unless your professor calls your attention to a specific person, she or he may not wish to emphasize these individuals either. It may be a waste of time to try to remember who said what about language development. "He said-she said" memorization can be very tedious. The exceptions, of course, are individuals mentioned specifically by name in lecture and in the text.
- Don't concentrate on who said what.
- Use the accompanying audio CD to supplement your reading. It contains audio samples of children's language at different ages in addition to examples of different dialectal speakers. Your professor has a script that accompanies the CD.

I hope that these suggestions will help, although none is a guarantee.

Roll up your sleeves, set aside adequate time, and be prepared to be challenged. Actually, your task is relatively simple when compared to the toddler faced with deciphering the language she or he hears.

SPEECH, LANGUAGE, AND COMMUNICATION

Child development professionals study the changes that occur in speech, language, and communication as children grow and develop. To the nonprofessional, these three terms are often interpreted as having similar meanings or as being identical. Actually, the terms are very different and denote different aspects of development and use.

Speech

Speech[1] is a verbal means of communicating or conveying meaning. Other ways of communicating include writing, drawing, and manual signing. The result of planning and executing specific motor sequences, speech is a process that requires very precise neuromuscular coordination. Each spoken language has specific sounds, or **phonemes**, and sound combinations that are characteristic of that language. In addition, speech involves other components, such as voice quality, intonation, and rate. These components enhance the meaning of the message. Speech is not the only means of human communication. We also use gestures, facial expressions, and body posture to send messages. When speaking on the phone, we rely on the speech modality to carry our message. In face-to-face conversation, more emphasis is placed on nonvocal means. It has been estimated that up to 60 percent of the information in face-to-face conversations may be transmitted through nonspeech means.

Humans are not the only animals to make sounds, although no other species can match the variety and complexity of human speech sounds. These qualities are the result of the unique structures of the human vocal tract, a mechanism that is functional months before the first words are spoken. Children spend much of their first year experimenting with the vocal mechanism and producing a variety of sounds. Gradually, these sounds come to reflect the language of the child's environment. Meaningful speech, however, must await the development of some linguistic rules.

Language

Without attached meaning, speech sounds are only grunts and groans or meaningless strings of sounds. The relationship between all the linguistic forms—individual sounds, meaningful units, and the combination of these units—is specified by the rules of language. **Language** can be defined as a socially shared code or conventional system for representing concepts through the use of arbitrary symbols and rule-governed combinations of those symbols. English is a language, as is Spanish or Navajo. Each has its own unique symbols and rules for symbol combination. **Dialects**[2] are subcategories of the parent language that use similar but not identical rules. All users of a language follow certain dialectal rules that differ from an idealized standard. For example, I sometimes find myself reverting to former dialectal usage in saying "*acrost* the street" and "open your *umbrella*." Note the dialectal speakers on the first track of the accompanying CD.

Languages are neither monolithic nor unchanging. Interactions between languages naturally occur in bilingual communities. Under certain circumstances, language mixing may result in a new form of both blended languages being used in that community (Backus, 1999).

---

[1]Words found in boldface in the text are defined in the Glossary at the end of the book.

[2]Dialects and bilingualism are discussed in more detail in Chapter 13.

Languages evolve; they grow and change. Those that do not become obsolete. Sometimes, for reasons other than linguistic ones, languages either flourish or wither. At present, for example, fewer than 100 individuals fluently speak Seneca, a western New York Native American language. The death of languages is not a rare event in the modern world. Languages face extinction as surely as plants and animals. When Kuzakura, an aged woman, died in western Brazil in 1988, the Umutina language died with her. It is estimated that as many as half the world's 6,000 languages are no longer learned by children. Many others are endangered. Most of these have less than a few thousand users. Only strong cultural and religious ties keep languages such as Yiddish and Pennsylvania Dutch viable.

The next century may see the eradication of most languages. This process is the result of government policy, dwindling indigenous populations and the movements of populations to cities, mass media, and noneducation of the young in a push for modernity. The Internet is also a culprit in the demise of some languages. The need to converse in one language is fostering increasing use of English.

Each language is a unique vehicle for thought. When we lose a language, we lose an essential part of the human fabric with its own unique perspective. A culture and thousands of years of communication die with that language (Diamond, 1993). Study of that one language or many such languages may have unlocked secrets about universal language features or about the very origins of language or the nature of thought.

The death of a language is more than an intellectual or academic curiosity. After a week's immersion in Seneca, Mohawk, Onondaga, and other Iroquois languages, one man concluded:

> In the native world, these languages are more than collectible oddities, pressed flowers to be pulled from musty scrapbooks.
> These languages are the music that breathes life into our dances, the overflowing vessels that hold our culture and traditions. And most important, these languages are the conduits that carry our prayers to the Creator. . . .
> [W]e are struggling to reclaim what was stolen from us. Our languages are central to who we are a native people.

"Come visit sometime," he offers. "I will bid you 'oolihelisdi.'" (Coulson, 1999, p. 8A)

Languages also grow as their respective cultures change. English has proven very adaptive, changing slowly through the addition of new words. Already the language with the largest number of words—approximately 700,000—English adds an estimated half dozen words per day. While many of these are scientific terms, they also include words popular on college campuses, such as *phat* (very cool), *herb* (geek), *cholo* (macho), and *dis* (scorn). English dictionaries have just recently added the following words: *bubba, 4x4, headbanger, pumped (up), megaplex, racial profiling, slamming, brownfield, body-piercing, homeschool, netiquette,* and *soft money*. These words tell us much about our modern world.

Although all the languages noted so far can be transmitted via speech, speech is not an essential feature of language. American Sign Language, which is transmitted via a manual or signing mode, is not a mirror of American English but is a separate language with its own rules for symbol combinations. As in spoken languages, individually meaningless units are combined following linguistic rules, although with signing, the units are hand and body movements. Approximately fifty sign languages are used worldwide. To some extent, the means of transmission of such visual-spatial languages influences their processing and learning, although underlying concepts may be similar to spoken languages (Emmorey, 1993; Lillo-Martin, 1991).

Mathematics is another language, but a more precise one than those previously mentioned. Mathematical symbols have exact values and represent specific quantities and relationships. For example, 8 is greater than 2, and the relationship between 8 and 2 can be stated in a variety of ways:

$$8 = 4(2) \qquad 8 = 4 \times 2 \qquad 8 = 2^3 \qquad 8 = 6 + 2$$

The two numbers represent definite quantities. Compare this precision to that of the English word *group*. In *group*, quantity is inherent but not specified. How many people or things form a group? Most users of English would recognize *group* as more than *couple* but less than *crowd*. The word *women* represents more quantity than *woman* but could refer to any quantity of more than one.

Following is the American Speech-Language-Hearing Association definition of *language* (Committee on Language, 1983). Like the proverbial camel who is the result of a committee trying to design a horse, this definition has a little of everything, but it also is very thorough.

Language is a complex and dynamic system of conventional symbols that is used in various modes for thought and communication.

- Language evolves within specific historical, social and cultural contexts;
- Language, as rule-governed behavior, is described by at least five parameters—phonologic, morphologic, syntactic, semantic, and pragmatic;
- Language learning and use are determined by the intervention of biological, cognitive, psychosocial, and environmental factors;
- Effective use of language for communication requires a broad understanding of human interaction including such associated factors as nonverbal cues, motivation, and sociocultural roles.

Languages exist because users have agreed on the symbols to be used and the rules to be followed. This agreement is demonstrated through language usage. Thus, languages exist by virtue of social agreement or convention. Just as users agree to follow the rules of a language system, they can agree to change the rules. For example, the *th* found as an ending on English verbs (ask*eth*) in the King James Version of the Bible has disappeared from use. New words can be added to a language; others fall into disuse. For example, we are adding new scientific terminology almost daily; such words as *compact disc* and *byte* were uncommon just a few years ago. In addition, users of one language can borrow words from another. For instance, despite the best efforts of the French government, its citizens seem to prefer the English word *jet* to the more difficult, though lyrical, *avion de reaction*. American English also incorporates words from other languages, such as *tsunami, barrio, jihad, sushi,* and *kvetch*.

The conventional or socially shared code of language allows the listener and speaker or writer and reader of the same language to exchange information. Internally, each uses the same code. The shared code is a device that enables each to represent an object, event or relationship. Let's see how this is done. Close your eyes for a few seconds and concentrate on the word *ocean*. While your eyes were closed, you may have had a visual image of surf and sand. The concept was transmitted to you and decoded without your having to be transported physically to the coast. In a conversation, listener and speaker switch from encoding to decoding and back again without difficulty. Words, such as *ocean*, represent concepts stored in our brains.

Each user encodes and decodes according to his concept of a given object, event, or relationship; the actual object, event, or relationship does not need to be present. Let's assume that you encounter a priest. From past experience, you recognize his social role. Common elements of these experiences are *Catholic*, *male*, and *clergy*. As you pass, you draw on the appropriate symbol and encode, "Morning, Father." This representational process is presented in Figure 1.1. Although the common word *father* may denote a male family member to both speaker and listener, the word may also connote or suggest a very different meaning, depending upon the experiences of each party. Let's assume for a moment that your biological father is an Episcopal minister. You see him on the street in clerical garb and say, "Good morning, father." A passerby, unaware of your relationship, will assume something very different from the meaning that you and your father share. Coding is a factor of the speaker's and listener's shared meanings, the linguistic skills of each, and the context in which the exchange takes place.

Individual linguistic units communicate little in isolation. Most of the meaning or information is contained in the way symbols are combined. For example, "Teacher Jim a is"

FIGURE 1.1 Symbol-Referent Relationship

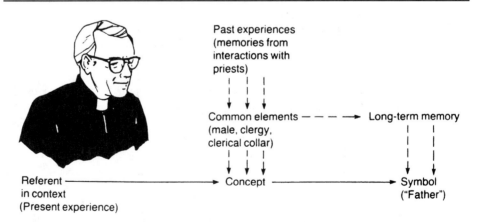

The concept is formed from the common elements of past experiences. The common elements of these experiences form the core of the concept. When a referent is experienced, it is interpreted in terms of the concept and the appropriate symbol applied.

seems a meaningless jumble of words. By shifting a few words, however, we can create "Jim is a teacher." Another modification could produce, "Is Jim a teacher?"—a very different sentence. Language rules specify a system of relationships among the parts. The rules for these relationships give language order and allow users to predict which units or symbols will be used. In addition, the rules permit language to be used creatively. A *finite* set of symbols and a *finite* set of rules governing symbol combinations can be employed to create an *infinite* number of utterances.

Language should not be seen, though, merely as a set of static rules. It is a process of use and modification within the context of communication. Language is a tool for social use.

Communication

Both speech and language are parts of the larger process of communication. **Communication** is the process participants use to exchange information and ideas, needs and desires. The process is an active one that involves encoding, transmitting, and decoding the intended message. Figure 1.2 illustrates this process. It requires a sender and a receiver, and each must be alert to the informational needs of the other to ensure that messages are conveyed effectively and that intended meanings are preserved. For example, a speaker must identify a specific female for the listener prior to using the pronoun *she*. The probability of message distortion is very high, given the number of ways a message can be formed and the past experiences and perceptions of each participant. The degree to which a speaker is

FIGURE 1.2 Process of Communication

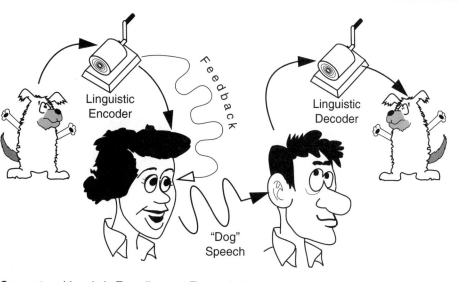

| Concept | Linguistic Encoding | Transmission | Linguistic Decoding | Concept |

successful in communicating, measured by the appropriateness and effectiveness of the message, is called **communicative competence** (Dore, 1986). The competent communicator is able to conceive, formulate, modulate, and issue messages and to perceive the degree to which intended meanings are successfully conveyed.

Speech and language are only a portion of communication. Figure 1.3 illustrates this relationship. Other aspects of communication that may enhance or change the linguistic code can be classified as paralinguistic, nonlinguistic, and metalinguistic. **Paralinguistic codes**, including intonation, stress or emphasis, speed or rate of delivery, and pause or hesitation, are superimposed on speech to signal attitude or emotion. All components of the signal are integrated to produce the meaning. *Intonation*, or the linguistic use of pitch, is the most complex of all paralinguistic codes and is used to signal the mood of an utterance. For

FIGURE 1.3 Relationships of Speech, Language, and Communication

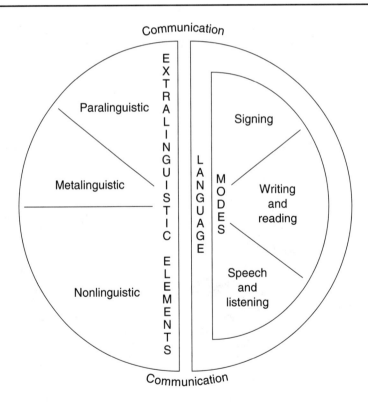

Communication is accomplished through a linguistic code and many means of transmission, such as speech, intonation, gestures, and body language.

example, falling or rising pitch alone can signal the purpose of an utterance, as in the following example:

You're coming, aren't you. ↓ (Telling)

You're coming, aren't you? ↑ (Asking)

A rising pitch can change a statement into a question. Pitch can signal emphasis, asides, emotions, importance of the information conveyed, and the role and status of the speaker.

Stress is also employed for emphasis. Each of us remembers hearing, "You *will* clean your room!", to which you may have responded, "I *did* clean my room!" The *will* and *did* are emphasized. Stress has been shown to speed memory retrieval and to aid comprehension, especially on the initial syllable where it confirms the listener's predictions of the word (Gow & Gordon, 1993).

Rate varies with the speaker's state of excitement, familiarity with the content, and perceived comprehension of the listener. In general, we tend to talk faster if we are more excited, more familiar with the information being conveyed, or more assured that our listener understands our message.

Pauses may be used to emphasize a portion of the message or to replace the message. Even young children recognize that a short maternal pause after a child's request usually signals a negative reply. Remember asking "Can Chris sleep over tonight?" A long silence meant that your plans were doomed.

Pitch, rhythm, and pauses may be used to mark syntactic divisions between phrases and clauses. Combined with loudness and duration, pitch is used to give prominence to certain syllables and to new information.

Paralinguistic mechanisms are called **suprasegmental devices** because they can change the form and meaning of a sentence by acting across elements, or segments, of a sentence. For example, a rising pitch can change a declarative sentence into an interrogative or question form without altering the arrangement of words. Similarly, "I did my homework" and "I *did* my homework" convey different emotions across words that signal the same information.

Nonlinguistic cues include gestures, body posture, facial expression, eye contact, head and body movement, and physical distance or proxemics. The effectiveness of these devices varies with users and between users. We all know someone who seems to gesture too much or to stand too close while communicating. Some nonlinguistic messages, such as a wink, a grimace, a pout, or folded arms, can convey the entire message with no need to rely on speech or language.

As with language, nonlinguistic cues vary with the culture. Perfectly acceptable gestures in one culture may be considered offensive in another (Axtell, 1991). Table 1.1 presents a list of common American gestures considered rude, offensive, or insulting in other cultures. Luckily, the smile is a universal signal for friendliness.

Metalinguistic skills are the abilities to talk about language, analyze it, think about it, judge it, and see it as an entity separate from its content. For example, learning to read and

TABLE 1.1   Nonlinguistic Cues

GESTURE	OTHER INTERPRETATIONS	COUNTRIES IN WHICH UNACCEPTABLE
Thumbs up		Australia, Nigeria, Islamic countries, such as Bangladesh
A-OK	Japan: *Money* France: Zero, worthless	Latin American countries
Victory or Peace sign		England (if palm toward body)
Hailing a waiter (One finger raised)	Germany: *Two*	Japan
Beckoning curled finger		Yugoslavia, Malaysia, Indonesia, Australia
Tap forehead to signify "Smart"	Netherlands: *Crazy*	
Stop		Greece, West Africa
Hands in the pockets		Belgium, Indonesia, France, Finland, Japan, Sweden
Strong handshake	Middle East: Aggression	
Good-bye	Europe & Latin America: *No*	
Crossing legs and exposing sole of the foot		Southeast Asia
Nod head for agreement	Greece, Yugoslavia, Turkey, Iran, Bengal: No	

Source: Adapted from Axtell, R.E. (1991). *Gestures: The do's and taboos of body language around the world*. Baltimore, MD: Wiley & Sons.

write depends on metalinguistic awareness of the component units of language—sounds, words, phrases, and sentences. In metalinguistics, language is abstract. Metalinguistic skills are used to judge the correctness or appropriateness of the language we produce and receive. Thus, **metalinguistic cues** signal the status of the transmission or the success of communication.

It is almost impossible not to communicate. If you tried not to communicate, your accompanying behavior alone would communicate.

PROPERTIES OF LANGUAGE

Several linguists have attempted to describe the general properties or characteristics of all languages. In general, language is a social interactive tool that is both rule-governed and generative, or creative.

Language as a Social Tool

It does little good to discuss language outside of the framework provided by communication. While language is not essential for communication, communication is certainly an essential and defining element of language. Even long-extinct languages such as Sanskrit are studied for what they can communicate to us about ancient peoples.

Language is a shared code that enables users to transmit ideas and desires to one another. It is shared by these language users because they wish to communicate. No one would devise or learn such a complex system without some purpose in mind. In short, language has but one purpose: to serve as the code for transmissions between people.

As such, language is influenced by its environment and, in turn, influences that environment. Overall, language reflects the collective thinking of its societal base, or culture, and influences that thinking. In the United States, for example, certain words, such as *democracy*, reflect meanings and emotions and influence our concepts of other forms of government. The ancient Greek notion of democracy was somewhat different and influenced the Greeks' thinking similarly.

Likewise, at any given moment, language in use is influenced by what precedes it and influences what follows. The utterance "And how's my little girl feeling this morning?" only fits certain situations that define the appropriate language use. It would not be wise to use this utterance when meeting the Queen of England for the first time. In turn, the sick child to whom this is addressed has only limited options that she can use to respond. Responses such as, "Go directly to jail; do not pass 'Go' " and "Mister Speaker, I yield the floor to the distinguished senator from West Virginia," while perfectly correct sentences, just don't fit. The reason is that they do not continue the communication but, rather, cause it to break down.

To consider language without communication is to assume that language occurs in a vacuum. It is to remove the very *raison d'être* for language in the first place.

A Rule-Governed System

The relationship between meaning and the symbols employed is an arbitrary one, but the arrangement of the symbols in relation to one another is nonarbitrary. This nonarbitrary organizational feature of language demonstrates the presence of underlying rules or patterns that occur repeatedly. These systems of rules are called **grammars**. Do not confuse the linguistic term *grammar* with the study of "parts of speech" that most of us endured in elementary school grammar lessons. Rather, a grammar is a finite set of underlying operational principles or rules that describe the relationships between symbols that form the structure of a language. As such, grammars describe the relationships between sounds, between words and smaller units such as plural *s*, between words and meaning, and between words and communicative intent or purpose. These shared rule systems allow users of a language to comprehend and to create messages. Language and grammar are not the same. Language includes not only the rules, but also the process of rule usage and the resulting product. For example, a sentence is made up of a noun plus a verb, but as noted previously, that rule tells us nothing about the process of noun and verb selection or the seemingly infinite number of possible combinations using these two categories.

A language user's underlying knowledge about the system of rules is called his or her **linguistic competence**. The specific rules a language user knows are called *intuitive grammar*. Even though the user can't state the rules, performance demonstrates adherence to them. The linguist observes human behavior in an attempt to determine these rules or operating principles. The results of such studies are called *formal grammars*, precise statements of the linguistic rules. To date, we still do not have a complete formal grammar for American English.

If you have ever listened to an excited speaker or a heated argument, you know that speakers do not always observe the linguistic rules. In fact, much of what we, as mature speakers, say is ungrammatical. Imagine that you have just returned from the New Year's celebration at Times Square. You might say the following:

> Oh, wow, you should have . . . you wouldn't be-believe all the . . . never seen so many people. We were almost . . . ah, trampled. And when the ball came down . . . fell, all the . . . Talk about yelling . . . so much noise. We made a, the mistake of . . . can you imagine anything as dumb as . . . well, it was crazy to drive.

Linguistic knowledge in actual usage is called **linguistic performance**. The linguist's formal grammar must be deduced from linguistic performance. Linguistic competence cannot be measured directly.

There are many reasons for the discrepancy between competence and performance in normal language users. Some constraints are long term, such as ethnic background, socioeconomic status, and region of the country. These account for dialects and regionalisms. We are all speakers of some dialectal or regional variation, but most of us are still competent in the standard or ideal dialect. Dialectal speakers, even those with relatively nonstandard dialects, do not have a language disorder. Other long-term constraints, such as mental retardation and language-learning disability, may result in a language disorder. Short-term constraints on nondisordered performance include physical state changes within the individual, such as intoxication, fatigue, distraction, and illness, and situational variations, such as the role, status, and personal relations of the speakers.

Even though much that is said is ungrammatical, native speakers have relatively little difficulty decoding messages. If a native speaker knows the words being used, he or she can apply the rules in order to understand almost any sentence encountered. In actual communication, comprehension is influenced by the intent of the speaker, the context, the available shared meanings, and the linguistic complexity of the utterance. Even kindergarteners know virtually all the rules of language. Children learn the rules by actually using the language to encode and decode. The rules learned in school are the "finishing touches." A child demonstrates by using words that he or she knows what a noun—or any class or category of words—is long before he or she can define the term.

On one family trip, we passed the time with a word game. My five-year-old daughter was asked to provide a noun. Immediately, she inquired, "What's that?" In my best teacher persona, I patiently explained that a noun was a person, place, or thing. She replied, "Oh." After some prodding, she stated, "Then my word is 'thing.'" Despite her inadequate understanding of the formal definition of a noun, my daughter had demonstrated for years in her everyday use that she knew how to use nouns.

Knowing the rules enables us to predict which symbols will come next. The following blank sentence will demonstrate this ability. Let's see how well you can identify the part of speech and the actual words in the following sentence.

_____ _____ _____ _____ _____ _____ _____

Above each blank, write the part of speech that will go into that blank; below the blank, write the actual word. Do one word at a time and then check your answer before going to the next.

- I'll help on the first word. It's an article. Can you guess which one? It's *the*. That's a clue to the second word. Try to predict the part of speech and the actual word.
- *Second word*: It could be a noun or an adjective; it's the latter. The word is *young*.
- *Third word*: You should get this one: a noun. What might the word be? It's *boy*. *Girl* or several others were equally likely.
- *Fourth word*: I hope you chose a verb. The word is *runs*. Boys can do lots of activities, such as eat, drink, jump, or walk. Thus, you may have missed the exact word.
- *Fifth word*: This one should be easy. It's a preposition, and the word is *to*.
- *Sixth word*: This word is also a noun. You may have missed the word, since boys usually run in the opposite direction of the one I've chosen. The word is *school*.
- *Seventh word*: One last chance. The part of speech is adverb. The word is *quickly*.

In this exercise, rarely does someone select all the correct parts of speech, and no one ever gets all the specific words. Almost everyone, however, does better than chance alone would predict. This sentence could have included any number of possibilities.

A sentence such as "Chairs sourly young up swam" is ungrammatical. It violates the rules for word order. Native speakers notice that the words do not fall into predictable patterns. When rearranged, the sentence reads "Young chairs swam sourly up." This is now grammatical in terms of word order but meaningless; it doesn't make sense. Other rules allow language users to separate sense from nonsense and to determine the underlying meaning. Although "Dog bites man" and "Man bites dog" are very similar, in that each uses the same words, the meanings of the two sentences are very different. Only one will make a newspaper headline. Likewise, a single sentence may have two meanings. For example, the sentence "The shooting of the hunters was terrible" can be taken two ways: either they shot poorly or someone shot them. Language users must know several sets of rules to make sense of what they hear or read.

A Generative System

Language is a generative system. The word *generative* has the same root as *generate*, which means to produce, create (as in *Genesis*), or bring into existence. Thus, language is a productive or creative tool. A knowledge of the rules permits speakers to generate, or form, meaningful utterances. From a finite number of words and word categories, such as nouns, and a finite set of rules, speakers can create an almost infinite number of sentences. This creativity occurs because words can refer to more than one thing or referent, because these referents can be called by more than one name, and because words can be combined in a variety of ways. Think of all the possible sentences you could create by combining all the nouns and verbs you know. When this task is completed, you could modify each sentence by adding adverbs and adjectives, articles and prepositions, and by combining sentences or creating questions.

The possibilities for creating new sentences are virtually endless. Consider the following novel sentence:

Large elephants danced gracefully beneath the street lights.

Even though you have probably never seen this utterance before, you understand its meaning because you know the linguistic rules. Try to create your own novel utterance. The process will seem difficult, and yet you form novel utterances every day and are not consciously aware of using any effort. In fact, ritualistic utterances such as "Hi, how are you?" aside, most of what you said today was novel or new. You didn't learn those specific utterances. As a young child, you deduced the rules for forming these types of sentences. Of course, I do not mean to imply that sentences are never repeated. Polite social or ritualistic communication is often repetitious. How frequently have you said the following sentences?

How are you?
Thank you very much.
I'm fine.
Can I, Mom, please?
See you soon.

You have probably repeated each one more often than you care to recall.

In summary, native speakers of a language do not learn all possible word combinations. Instead, they learn rules that govern these combinations. Knowing the linguistic rules allows each language user to understand and create an infinite variety of sentences.

COMPONENTS OF LANGUAGE

Language is a very complex system that can best be understood by breaking it down into its functional components (Figure 1.4). Language can be divided into three major, although not necessarily equal, components: form, content, and use (Bloom & Lahey, 1978). Form includes syntax, morphology, and phonology, the components that connect sounds or symbols in order. Content encompasses meaning or semantics, and use is termed pragmatics. These five components—syntax, morphology, phonology, semantics, and pragmatics—are the basic rule systems found in language.

FIGURE 1.4 Components of Language

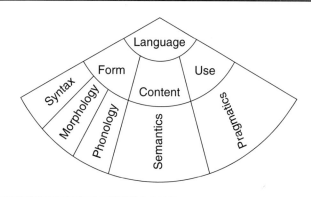

As each of us uses language, we code ideas (*semantics*); that is, we use a symbol—a sound, a word, and so forth—to stand for an event, object, or relationship. To communicate these ideas to others, we use certain forms, which include the appropriate sound units (*phonology*), the appropriate word order (*syntax*), and the appropriate words and word beginnings and endings (*morphology*) to clarify meaning more specifically. Speakers use these components to achieve certain communication ends or goals, such as gaining information, greeting, or responding (*pragmatics*). Let's examine the five components of language in more detail.

Syntax

The form or structure of a sentence is governed by the rules of **syntax**. These rules specify word, phrase, clause, and order, sentence organization, and the relationships between words, word classes, and other sentence elements. Sentences are organized according to their overall function; declaratives, for example, make statements, and interrogatives form questions. The main elements, or constituent parts, of a sentence are noun and verb phrases, each composed of various word classes or word types (such as nouns, verbs, adjectives, and the like).

Syntax specifies which word combinations are acceptable, or grammatical, and which are not. In addition to word-order rules, syntax specifies which word classes appear in noun and verb phrases and the relationship of these two types of phrases.

Each sentence must contain a *noun phrase* and a *verb phrase*. The mandatory features of noun and verb phrases are a noun and a verb, respectively. The short biblical verse "Jesus wept" is a perfectly acceptable English sentence: it contains both a noun phrase and a verb phrase. The following, however, is not a complete sentence, even though it is much longer:

The grandiose plan for the community's economic revival based upon
political cooperation of the inner city and the more affluent suburban areas

This example contains no verb and thus no verb phrase; therefore, it does not qualify as a sentence.

Within the noun and verb phrases, certain word classes combine in predictable patterns. For example, articles such as *a*, *an*, and *the* appear before nouns, and adverbs such as *slowly* modify verbs. Some words may function in more than one word class. For example, the word *dance* may be a noun or a verb. Yet there is no confusion between the following sentences:

The *dance* was attended by nearly all the students.
The children will *dance* to earn money for charity.

The linguistic context of the sentence specifies the word class of *dance* in each sentence—a noun in the first and a verb in the second—and clarifies any ambiguity.

Syntax can be conceptualized as a tree diagram or a hierarchy (Figure 1.5). Each noun phrase or verb phrase included in a sentence contains, in turn, constituent word classes. In

FIGURE 1.5   Hierarchical Sentence Structure

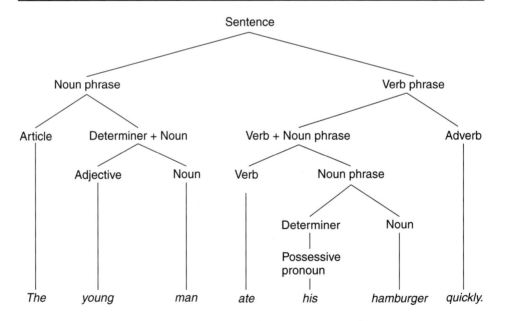

Within the noun and verb phrases, a number of different word classes can be arranged to form a variety of sentences. Many words could be used within each word class to form sentences such as "The young man ate his hamburger quickly" or "The mad racer drove his car recklessly."

a given phrase, word classes may be deleted or added. As long as the noun and verb remain, a sentence is produced. This hierarchical structure permits boundless elaboration within the confines of the syntactic rules. Words may be used within each word class to create an endless variety of sentences. Obviously, the tree diagram in Figure 1.5 has only limited use. Flexible use of language would require hundreds, if not thousands, of other possibilities. Children don't memorize diagrams; rather, they learn rules for ways of constructing such frames.

As language users, we sometimes get into difficulty when we must follow prescribed language rules. This usually occurs in writing. Spoken language is much more informal than writing and less constrained. In the nineteenth century, formal grammar guides were written, often prescribing rules used by the upper class. As a result, today we are saddled with the distinction between *who* and *whom*, the incorrectness of using *since* to mean *because*, the inadmissability of the split infinitive (*to finish quickly* is fine, but not *to quickly finish*), and the *not ending a sentence with a preposition* rule. Regarding the latter, Winston Churchill quipped, "That is the type of arrant pedantry up with which I shall not put." Grammatically, he's correct!

Languages can be divided into those with so-called free word order and those with word-order rules (Goodluck, 1986). The Australian aboriginal language, Warlpiri, has a relatively free word order. The same sentence may be expressed in several different word orders. Among word-order languages, rules fall into three classes based on the order of the subject, the verb, and the object. English is an example of the basic subject-verb-object (SVO) word order (*She eats cookies*). In contrast, Dutch, Korean, and Japanese have a basic verb-final form (SOV). The third type, represented by Irish, is verb-subject-object (VSO).

Morphology

Morphology is concerned with the internal organization of words. Words consist of one or more smaller units called *morphemes*. A **morpheme** is the smallest grammatical unit and is indivisible without violating the meaning or producing meaningless units. Therefore, *dog* is a single morpheme because *d* and *og* are meaningless alone. If we split the word into *do* and *g*, we have a similar situation, because there is nothing in *dog* that includes the meaning of *do*, and *g* is meaningless alone. Most words in English consist of one or two morphemes. In contrast, Mohawk, found in northern New York and southern Quebec, constructs words of several morphemes strung together.

Morphemes are of two varieties, free and bound (Figure 1.6). **Free morphemes** are independent and can stand alone. They form words or parts of words. Examples of free morphemes are *toy*, *big*, and *happy*. **Bound morphemes** are grammatical tags or markers that cannot function independently. They must be attached to free morphemes or to other bound morphemes. Examples include *-s*, *-est*, *un-*, and *-ly*, meaning plural, most, negative, and manner, respectively. By combining the free and bound morphemes, we can create *toys*, *biggest*, and *unhappily*. Bound morphemes are attached to words in the noun, verb, and adjective classes to accomplish changes in meaning. Furthermore, bound morphemes can be either *derivational* or *inflectional* in nature. Derivational morphemes include both prefixes and suffixes. Prefixes precede the free morpheme and suffixes follow. Derivational morphemes

FIGURE 1.6   Morpheme Classes and Examples

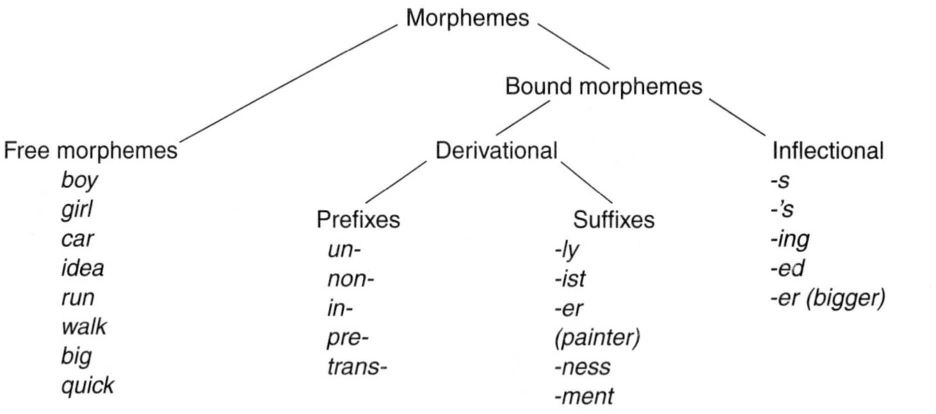

change whole classes of words. For example, *-ly* may be added to most adjectives to create an adverb, and *-ness* may be added to an adjective to create a noun: *mad, madly, madness.* Inflectional morphemes can be suffixes only. They change the state or increase the precision of the free morpheme. Inflectional morphemes include tense markers (such as *-ed*), plural markers, and the third-person singular present-tense verb ending *-s* as in "she walks." Because all of these modulations operate within the syntactic constraints of sentences, some linguists consider the morphological rules to be a subset of the syntactic rules.

Languages differ in their relative dependence on the syntactic and morphological components. In Latin, for example, meaning is changed through the use of many morphological endings. In contrast, in English word order is used more than morphological additions to convey much of the meaning of the utterance.

Phonology

Phonology is the aspect of language concerned with the rules governing the structure, distribution, and sequencing of speech sounds and the shape of syllables. Each language employs a variety of speech sounds or phonemes. A phoneme is the smallest linguistic unit of sound that can signal a difference in meaning. English has approximately forty-five phonemes, give or take a few for dialectal variations (see the appendix). Phonemes are actually families of very similar sounds. Allophones or individual members of these families of sounds differ slightly from one another, but not enough to sound like another phoneme and thus modify the meaning of a word. If you repeat the /p/[3] sound ten times, each production will vary slightly for a number of physiological reasons. In addition, the /p/ sound in *pea* differs from that in *poor* or *soup* because each is influenced by the surrounding sounds. Even so, each /p/ sound is similar enough so as not to be confused with another phoneme.

[3]Transcriptions of phonemes are placed within slashes, such as /p/. This book uses the notation of the International Phonetic Alphabet, as will be discussed in more detail in the appendix.

Thus /p/ is a distinct English phoneme. There is an obvious difference in the initial sounds in *pea* and *see* because each begins with a different phoneme. Likewise, the /d/ and /l/ sounds are different enough to be considered as different phonemes. Each can signal a different meaning if applied to other sounds. For example, the meanings of *dog* and *log* are very different, as are those of *dock* and *lock* and *pad* and *pal*. Phonemes are classified by their acoustic or sound properties, as well as by the way they are produced (how the air stream is modified) and their place of production (where along the vocal tract the modification occurs).

Phonological rules govern the distribution and sequencing of phonemes within a language. This organization is not the same as speech, which is the actual mechanical act of producing phonemes. Without the phonological rules, the distribution and sequencing of phonemes would be random. Distributional rules describe which sounds can be employed in various positions in words. For example, in English the *ng* sound, which is found in *ring* and is considered to be a single phoneme(/ŋ/), never appears at the beginning of an English word. In contrast, sequencing rules determine which sounds may appear in combination. The sequence /dn/, for example, may not appear back to back in the same syllable in English. Sequencing rules also address the sound modifications made when two phonemes appear next to each other. For example, the *-ed* in *jogged*, pronounced as /d/, is different from the *-ed* in *walked*, which is pronounced as /t/. On other occasions, the distributional and sequencing rules both apply. The combination /nd/, for example, may not begin a word but may appear elsewhere, as in *window*. The word *stew* is perfectly acceptable in English. *Snew* is not an English word but would be acceptable; *sdew*, however, could never be acceptable because in English words cannot begin with *sd*.

Semantics

This section might be subtitled, "What do you mean?" because the answer to that question forms the basis of semantics. **Semantics** is a system of rules governing the meaning or content of words and word combinations. Categories allow language users to group similar objects, actions, and relationships and to distinguish dissimilar ones. Some units are mutually exclusive, such as *man* and *woman*; a human being is not usually classified as both. Other units overlap somewhat, such as *female*, *woman*, and *lady*. Not all females are women and even fewer could be called ladies.

Semantics is concerned with the relationship of language form to our perceptions of objects, events, and relationships or to cognition and thought. The actual words or symbols used represent not reality itself but our ideas or concepts about reality.

It is useful at this point to make a distinction between *world knowledge* and *word knowledge*. **World knowledge** refers to an individual's autobiographical and experiential understanding and memory of particular events. This knowledge reflects not only the individual but the cultural interpretation placed on this knowledge. In contrast, **word knowledge** contains word and symbol definitions and is primarily verbal. If you will, word knowledge unites to form each person's mental dictionary or thesaurus.

The two types of knowledge are related because word knowledge is usually based on world knowledge. World knowledge is a generalized concept formed from several particular events. Thus, your concept of *dog* has been formed from several encounters with different types of dogs. These events become somewhat generalized, or separated from the original context, and are, therefore, more broadly useful. With more experience, knowledge becomes less dependent upon particular events. The resultant generalized episodes or scripts form the conceptual base for semantic or word knowledge. Language meaning is based on what we, as individuals, know.

According to this model, a concept is related to a whole class of experiences rather than to any single one. As an adult, you have experienced many very different creatures that can be classified as *dog*, yet your concept of *dog* is not limited to any one example. In general, all canines have enough in common to allow inclusion in the general concept of *dog*. Word meaning relates to this core concept. When the concept is paired with a linguistic unit or word, we can speak of semantic or word knowledge. Therefore, words do not refer directly to an object, event, or relationship but to a concept, which is the result of a cognitive categorization process, as in the previous example of the father (Figure 1.1).

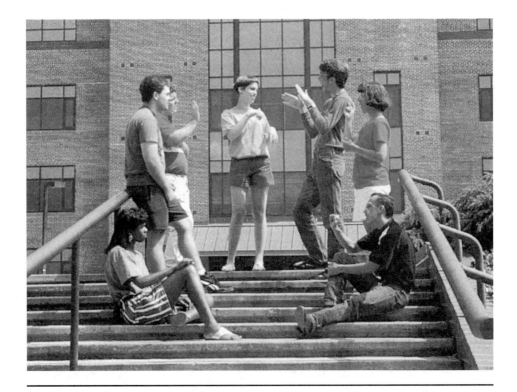

Deaf students at Gallaudet University are conversing with American Sign Language, a separate language from the dominant American English used in the United States.

As we converse with other users of the same language, we sharpen our concepts and bring them more to resemble similar concepts in others. In this way, we come to share definitions with others, thus making clear, concise, comprehensible communication possible.

Concept development results in increased validity, status, and accessibility. *Validity* is the amount of agreement between a language user's concept and the shared concept of the language community. *Status* refers to the addition of alternative referents: for example, *canine* can be substituted easily for the concept *dog*, and *dog* can be used to refer to the dry, hot, dog days of summer, to a dog-eared book, or to being dog-tired. *Accessibility* relates to the ease of retrieval from memory and use of the concept. In general, the more you know about the word and the more you use it, the easier it is to access.

Each word meaning contains two portions—semantic features and selection restrictions—drawn from the core concept. **Semantic features** are aspects of the meaning that characterize the word. For example, the semantic features of *mother* include parent and female. One of these features is shared with *father*, the other with *woman*, but neither word contains both features. **Selection restrictions** are based on these specific features and prohibit certain word combinations because they are meaningless or redundant. For example, *male mother* is meaningless because one word has the feature male and the other the feature female; *female mother* is redundant because biological mothers are female, at least for the foreseeable future.

In addition to an objective denotative meaning, there is a connotative meaning of subjective features or feelings. Thus, whereas the semantic knowledge of the features of *dog* may be similar, I may have encountered several large, vicious examples that you have not and may therefore be more fearful of dogs than you. Throughout life, language users acquire new features, delete old features, and reorganize the remainder to sharpen word meanings.

Word meanings are only a portion of semantics, however, and are not as important as the relationships between symbols. One important relationship is that of common or shared features. The more features two words share, the more alike they are. Words with almost identical features are **synonyms**. Some examples are *abuse* and *misuse*, *dark* and *dim*, *heat* and *warmth*, and *talk* and *speak*.

Antonyms are words that differ only in the opposite value of a single important feature. Examples include *up* and *down*, *big* and *little*, and *black* and *white*. (*Big* and *little*, for example, both describe size but are opposite extremes.)

Knowledge of semantic features provides a language user with a rich vocabulary of alternative words and meanings. To some extent, this knowledge is more important than the overall number of words in a language user's vocabulary. Because words may have alternative meanings, users must rely on additional cues for interpretation of messages.

Sentence meanings are more important than individual word meanings because sentences represent a meaning greater than the sum of the individual words. A sentence represents not only the words that form that sentence, but the relationships between those words. Mature language users generally recall the overall sentence meaning rather than the form.

Pragmatics

When we use language to affect others or to relay information, we make use of pragmatics. **Pragmatics** is a set of rules related to language use within the communicative context. That is, pragmatics is concerned with the way language is used to communicate rather than with the way language is structured.

Every speech utterance is called a **speech act**. In order to be valid, each speech act must meet certain conditions. It must involve the appropriate persons and circumstances, be complete and correctly executed by all participants, and contain the appropriate intentions of all participants. "May I have a donut, please" is valid only when speaking to a person who can actually get you one and in a place where donuts are found. If you just said "May I" without nonlinguistic communication, the speech act would be incomplete and incorrect. Finally, the utterance encodes my intention, which is to get a donut. Some acts, called *performatives*, are actually performed by the very act of saying them. Each of the following is a performative:

> I *apologize* for my behavior.
> I *christen* this ship the U.S.S. Schneider.
> I now *pronounce* you husband and wife.

Again, certain conditions must be met before each is valid. When someone apologizes but is overjoyed by another's discomfort or when a child or nondesignated adult pronounces a couple husband and wife, the act is invalidated.

Not all speech acts are performatives. For example, saying "John should apologize for his behavior" doesn't make the apology. In this case, the act is an expression of opinion.

Speech acts may be *direct* or *indirect*. Direct speech acts are reflected in their syntactic form. "Answer the phone" is a direct order or request to perform that act. On the other hand, the syntactic form of an indirect speech act does not reflect the intention. For example, "Could you answer the phone?" is an indirect way of requesting. You know that the expected outcome is for you to answer the phone, not to respond to the question with a "yes." If the question seems to merit action rather than a verbal response, then the speech act is probably indirect. Indirect forms are generally used for politeness.

Speech acts may also be *literal, nonliteral,* or both. In a literal speech act, the speaker means what he says. After a ten-mile hike, you might exclaim, "My feet really hurt," and no doubt they do. In contrast, the nonliteral speech act does not mean what the speaker has said. Upon discovering that transportation home has not arrived, the same tired hiker might state sarcastically, "Just what I need, more walking." Both literal and nonliteral meanings might be heard in the comment of a mother as she enters her child's messy room: "Mommy really likes it when kids pick up their room."

Three general categories of rules concern alternation, co-occurrent constraint, and sequence. The *alternation* rules relate to the selection of linguistic forms. Contextual variables and the speaker's intention influence the choice between "Gimme a cookie" and "May I have one, please," or between a direct and an indirect speech act. One choice may work with a school friend, whereas the other is best with the teacher. Listener characteristics that influence speaker behaviors are sex, age, race, style, dialect, social status, and role.

Rules for *co-occurrent constraint* limit the forms that may be used when speakers assume roles or use another dialect. For example, if you are in a less dominant conversational role, you are more likely to be polite. *Sequential* rules regulate the use of certain ritualized sequences in various social situations. We can all recall an occasion when we felt close to death and yet responded, "I'm fine! How are you?"—a response that has become ritualized in casual greetings.

Conversation is governed by the "cooperation principle" (Grice, 1975): Conversational participants cooperate with each other. The four maxims of the cooperation principle relate to quantity, quality, relation, and manner. Quantity is the informativeness of each participant's contribution: No participant should provide too little or too much information. In addition, the quality of each contribution should be governed by truthfulness and based on sufficient evidence. The maxim of relation states that a contribution should be relevant to the topic of conversation. Finally, each participant should be reasonably direct in manner and avoid vagueness, ambiguity, and wordiness.

Since language is transmitted primarily via the speech mode, pragmatic rules govern a number of conversational interactions: sequential organization and coherence of conversations, repair of errors, role, and speech acts (Rees & Wollner, 1981). Organization and coherence of conversations include taking turns; opening, maintaining, and closing a conversation; establishing and maintaining a topic; and making relevant contributions to the conversation. Repair includes giving and receiving feedback and correcting conversational errors. The listener attempts to keep the speaker informed of the status of the communication. If the listener doesn't understand or is confused, he might assume a quizzical expression or say, "Huh?" Role skills include establishing and maintaining a role and switching linguistic codes for each role. In some conversations you are dominant, as with a small child, and in others you are not, as with your parents, and you adjust your language accordingly. Finally, speech acts include coding of intentions relative to the communicative context.

Relationship of Language Components

Language is heavily influenced by context. Context, both situational and linguistic, determines the language user's communication options. In addition, a need to communicate exists prior to the selection of content and form. Thus, linguists generally agree that pragmatics is the overall organizing principle of language (Figure 1.7). It is only when the child desires a cookie and is in an appropriate context to receive one that he employs the rules of syntax, morphology, phonology, and semantics in order to form the request.

Obviously, the components of language are linked in some way. For example, the syntactic structure may require the morphological marker for past tense which, in turn, changes phonetically to accommodate the affected word. In development, components may also influence one another in that changes in one may modify development in another.

FIGURE 1.7   Model of Language

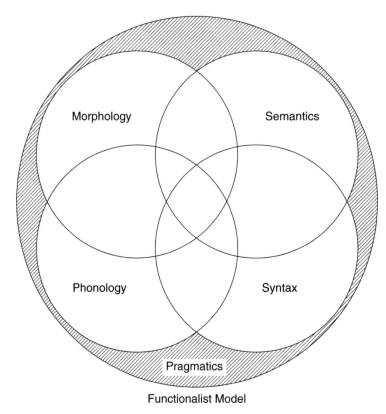

Functionalist Model

Pragmatics is the overall organizing
aspect of language.

CONCLUSION

Language is a social tool consisting of a very complex system of symbols and rules for using those symbols. Native speakers of a language must be knowledgeable about the symbols employed and the acceptable usage rules, including concept, word, morpheme, and phoneme combinations.

Humans may be the only animals with a productive communication system that gives them the ability to represent reality symbolically without dependence on immediate context support. Although animals clearly communicate at some level, this communication is limited in topic and scope and usually is dependent on the context. For example, bees have an elaborate system of movements for conveying information, but it is extremely iconic (it looks like what it conveys) and unitopical (the topic is always where to find nectar). Whether or not higher mammals, such as chimpanzees and other primates, are capable of complex symbolic communication will be discussed in the next chapter. In any case, it is only after intensive, long-term training that these animals learn what the human infant acquires in a few short months with little or no training.

DISCUSSION

Well, I did warn you! Yes, you're right; this is complicated and it can be confusing. It's good to reflect on what we've read at the end of each chapter and to ask ourselves "So what?"

The highlights in the chapter are the distinction between speech, language, and communication. Too many speech-language pathologists (SLPs) are still referred to as the "Speech Teacher" despite the fact that in school case loads, the largest percentage of cases are now language impairments. If you told someone that you worked with language impairments, not speech, and he or she replied "Aren't they the same thing?," how would you respond? Think about it. You have the ammunition from this chapter.

Other important aspects of this chapter include the characteristics of language. It's a social tool that's rule-based, and those rules enable it to be used in a generative fashion. Language can also be characterized by its five areas: syntax, morphology, phonology, semantics, and pragmatics. Of these, pragmatics seems to be the organizing area because context determines the other four. All areas are interdependent and changes in one area, either because of development or the dynamics of language use will result in changes in the others.

This last item—the interdependence of the five areas of language—has important implications for development and also for intervention. When an SLP intervenes with a child or an adult with a language impairment, there may be unforeseen consequences. For example, working on writing with an adult with aphasia or language loss often due to stroke may have a beneficial and unintended effect on spoken language. Likewise, adding too many new words to a child's language lesson may increase phonological precision but slow the child's delivery and decrease sentence length. The effect will vary with the amount of change, the individual child, and the type and severity of the impairment.

As we travel through this text, note the changes that occur and the overall effect on communication. Where appropriate I will characterize change based on the five areas of language.

REFLECTIONS

1. Speech, language, and communication are different aspects of the same process. Can you contrast all three?

2. Not all of the message is carried by the linguistic code. How do the other aspects of communication contribute?

3. Language is a social tool that is rule-governed and generative. Explain these three properties of language.

4. Language consists of five interrelated components. Describe these components, as well as the units of morpheme, phoneme, and speech act.

2

Language-Development Models

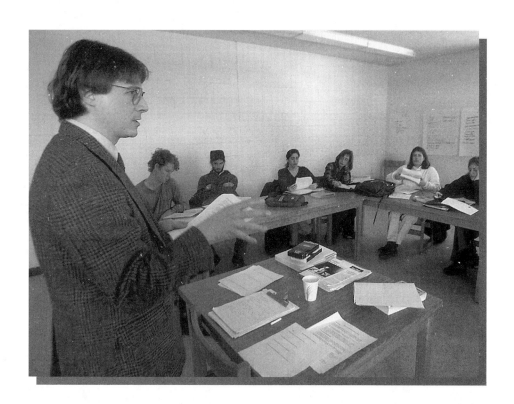

CHAPTER OBJECTIVES

Models of language development help us understand the developmental process by bringing order to our descriptions of this process and providing answers to the questions *how* and *why*. Of the many linguistic theories proposed, we will examine four that have had the greatest impact on language-development study. Each contains a core of relevant information, and the overall evolution reflects our changing view of language and child development. When you have completed this chapter, you should understand

- the language-development process described in the behavioral theory.
- the two rule systems employed in the psycholinguistic-syntactic model of linguistic processing and their sources.
- the advances of government-binding and biology-based theories.
- the contributions of the semantic revolution.
- the relationship between cognition and semantics.
- the context in which language is said to develop in the sociolinguistic model.
- the following terms:

case	propositional force
cognitive determinism	punisher
constituents	reinforcer
deep structure	rich interpretation
extinction	segmentation
government-binding theory	speech act
illocutionary forces	surface structure
joint (shared) reference	topic-comment
noun phrases	transactional model
operant conditioning	transformational rules
phrase-structure rules	verb phrases
primitive speech act (PSA)	

The study of language and language development has interested inquiring persons for thousands of years. Psammetichus I, an Egyptian pharoah of the seventh century B.C., supposedly conducted a child language study to determine the "natural" language of humans. Two children were raised with sheep and heard no human speech. Needless to say, they did not begin to speak Egyptian or anything else that approximated human language. Both St. Augustine and Charles Darwin published narratives on language development. Several modern researchers have devoted their professional careers to the study of child development.

People study language development for a variety of reasons. First, interest in language development represents part of a larger concern for child development. People who specialize in early childhood education are eager to learn about this developmental process in order to facilitate child behavior change. Special educators and speech-language pathologists study child language to increase their insight into normal and other-than-normal processes. A second reason for studying language development is that it is interesting and can help us understand our own behavior. There is a slightly mystical quality to language development. The developmental process has been called "mysterious" (Gleitman & Wanner, 1982) and "magic" (Bloom, 1983). As mature language users, we cannot state all the rules we use; yet, as children, we deciphered and learned these rules within a few years. Few of us can fully explain our own language development; it just seemed to happen. Finally, language-development studies can probe the relationship between language and thought. Language development is parallel to cognitive development. Hopefully, the study of language development may enable language users to understand the underlying cognitive processes to some degree.

Since language and language development are so complex, professionals are often at odds as to which approach provides the best description.

- The linguist is primarily concerned with describing language symbols and stating the rules these symbols follow to form language structures. The psycholinguist is interested in the psychological processes and constructs underlying language. The psychological mechanisms that let language users produce and comprehend language are of particular concern.
- The sociolinguist studies language rules and use as a function of role, socioeconomic level, and linguistic or cultural context. Dialectal differences and social-communicative interaction are important.
- The behavioral psychologist minimizes language form and emphasizes the behavioral context of language. The behaviorist is concerned with eliciting certain responses and determining how the number of these responses can be increased or decreased.
- The speech-language pathologist concentrates on disordered communication. Of greatest interest are the causes of disorder, the evaluation of the extent of the disorder, and the remediation process.

The study of how children learn language is like many other academic pursuits in that different theories that attempt to explain the phenomenon compete for acceptance. Occasionally one theory predominates, but generally portions of each are used to explain different aspects. Part of the problem in designing an overall theory is the complexity of both language and communication behavior. In recent years, four theoretical approaches to language development have evolved and become predominant: behavioral, syntactic, semantic/cognitive, and sociolinguistic. This chapter explores these four approaches, examining their overall theories, limitations, and contributions. Students might find it helpful to read each theory separately and allow time for processing before going on to the next.

BEHAVIORAL THEORY

At the turn of the twentieth century, the study of language development emphasized language form. Much of the information was anecdotal, data collection was inconsistent, and many important aspects of development were overlooked. In general, language forms were identified and classified into categories related to sentence types, parts of speech, and so on.

By the 1930s and 1940s, data collection had become more formalized. Researchers were interested in observable behaviors. Many of the child language studies of the period are called *count studies* because they cataloged and made distributional measurements of many language behaviors. Researchers observed regularities in language behavior that they accepted as evidence of underlying language knowledge (McCarthy, 1954; M. Smith, 1933; Templin, 1957).

During this period, the major influences on the psychological study of language were information theory and learning theory. Both approaches were concerned with the probability of production of a response or response unit, such as a word. According to information theory, the linguistic and nonlinguistic contexts determined the probability of a response being produced (Shannon & Weaver, 1949). Thus, some information theorists suggested that the occurrence of an individual word is determined by the immediately preceding word or phrase. Critics countered that there is no intrinsic order to words and that a given word can be followed by many different words (Lashley, 1951). The word order is governed by the speaker's intention to convey a certain message. Thus, the organization of the message involves larger units than words and follows a generalized pattern.

Learning theorists, such as Mowrer (1954), Skinner (1957), and Osgood (1963), considered language a subset of other learned behaviors. Language, as a set of associations between meaning and word, word and phoneme, and statement and response, is learned or conditioned through association between a stimulus and the following response. The strength of the stimulus-response bond determines the probability of occurrence of a certain response. Complex linguistic behaviors represent chains or combinations of various stimulus-response sequences.

Operant Conditioning

The most widely known proponent of language as a learned behavior was the psychologist B. F. Skinner. According to Skinner and his followers, all behavior is learned or *operant*. Behavior is modified or changed by the events that follow or are contingent upon that behavior. Any event that increases the probability of occurrence of a preceding behavior is said to be a **reinforcer** of that behavior. Any event that decreases the probability is said to be a **punisher**. The resultant behavior change is called *learning* or **operant conditioning**. Complex behaviors are learned by chaining or by shaping. In chaining, a sequence of behaviors is trained in such a way that each step serves as a stimulus for the next. In shaping, a single behavior is gradually modified by reinforcement of ever-closer (successive) approximations of the final behavior. Thus, language results from the active role of the environment. The learner is secondary to the process.

In 1957, Skinner published a classic language text, *Verbal Behavior*. He described language as a set of use or functional units. Traditional linguistic units, such as syntactic forms, are irrelevant. Instead, language is viewed as something we do (Lee, 1981). The "how" of language use takes precedence over the "what" of language form. Thus, language is defined as a verbal behavior, a learned behavior like any other, subject to all the rules of operant conditioning. As such, verbal behavior is modified by the environment.

A child acquires language or verbal behavior, stated Skinner, "when relatively unpatterned vocalizations, selectively reinforced, gradually assume forms which produce appropriate consequences" (p. 31). In other words, parents provide modeling and reinforcement and, as a result, establish the child's repertoire of sounds. For example, an infant produces many sounds that do not appear in the language she will use later. By nine months, the child vocalizes primarily the sounds she or he will later use in speech. In the interim, parents have reinforced only those sounds used in the native language. Reinforcement has included soothing the child, feeding and handling, and attending to the child when she or he produces sounds of the parent language.

Once acquired, a behavior requires only occasional reinforcement to be strengthened and maintained. Speech sounds that are ignored are produced less frequently and eventually disappear. This process of decreasing a behavior without punishment is called **extinction**.

Word learning is more complex. When the child says "mama" in her mother's presence, she or he is reinforced with attention or some other reinforcer. Should the child say "mama" when Mother is not present, she will not be reinforced. Thus, the presence of mother becomes a stimulus that evokes or elicits the verbal response "mama." Mother has become a *discriminative stimulus (SD)*, a stimulus in the presence of which "mama" will be reinforced. Therefore, a bond is built between the referent "mother" and the word *mama*. Meaning is attached to the speech sound. This process is illustrated in Figure 2.1. Obviously, other word-referent associations would be more elaborate because some other mature language user must be present in order for any word to be reinforced. According to Skinner, the child hears a word, such as *horsie*, in the presence of many examples of *horse*. Extracting similar attributes from each example of *horse*, the child associates these common attributes with the word *horsie*. The child's initial imitative attempts to say *horsie* will be reinforced by language users in the environment.

More complex responses are learned through successive approximation. Skinner (1957) summarized this process as follows: "Any response which vaguely resembles the standard behavior of the community is reinforced. When these begin to appear frequently, a closer approximation is insisted upon (pp. 29–30). Mature language users provide a model of the standard behaviors. For example, the child hears "I want a cookie, please" and produces the imitation "Want cookie." Initially, this response is acceptable, but the adults

FIGURE 2.1   Behavioral Model of Early Language Acquisition

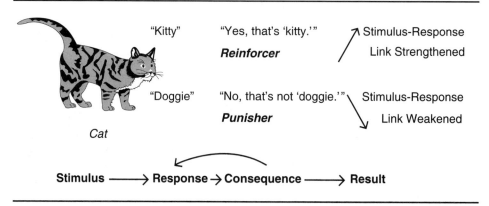

require gradual modifications that more closely approximate the adult model. Eventually the child will produce the full adult form. Thus, language learning is based on modeling, imitation, practice, and selective reinforcement.

Longer sentences are also learned through imitation and chaining. By hearing and imitating enough examples, the child learns word associations rather than grammatical rules.

Individual verbal behaviors fulfill one of several language functions, defined in terms of their effect. Skinner calls these functions mand, echoic, intraverbal, tact, and autoclitic. A *mand* is a verbal behavior that specifies its reinforcer, such as "Want cookie." In general, mands include behaviors known variously as commands, demands, and requests. The form of the utterance may vary, but the goal of "May I have a cookie, please" and "Gimme cookie" is similar. In contrast, *echoic* responses are imitative.

Intraverbal responses include social small talk and rituals, verbal responses with no one-to-one correspondence with the verbal stimuli that evoke them. For example, when I say that I went to New York for the weekend, you might reply, "Oh, I love the Metropolitan Museum." My initiating statement requires no reply, nor was the form of your utterance specified by my utterance. Conversations depend on intraverbal responses in which participants reply without a direct request to do so.

A *tact* is used in response to a nonverbal stimulus and to the things and events that speakers discuss. Tacts fill the function of naming, labeling, or commenting.

Finally, *autoclitic* responses are those that are influenced by, or influence, the behavior of the speaker. In addition, the autoclitic function includes sentence frames for the ordering of words, such as subject-verb-object. A child acquires grammar by learning these frames or chains, in which each word acts as a stimulus for the next. Thus, grammatical units are controlled by surrounding words.

Grammar develops through the learning of structured phrases and sentence frames. Syntactic and semantic "slots" within each frame are filled by substituting words or phrases that fulfill the same requirements. The child can comprehend or produce novel phrases and sentences by substituting units within these frames. Simply put, the child learns "I eat cookie" by chaining, with *I* acting as the stimulus for *eat*, which in turn is a stimulus for *cookie*. Gradually the child learns that *mommy, daddy*, and other words can be substituted for *I*; that *cut, drink*, and so on can replace *eat*; and that *meat, juice*, and others can replace *cookie* in the frame. Thus, word ordering is learned as adults reinforce chains of symbols that are increasingly more adultlike. Early language behavior is not rule-governed but rather shaped by the contingencies of the environment.

Limitations

There are several inadequacies in a strict behavioral theory of language acquisition. Perhaps these limitations were delineated best by psycholinguistic theorists. Noam Chomsky, a leading psycholinguist of the late 1950s and 1960s, summarized many of these inadequacies in his 1959 review of Skinner's *Verbal Behavior*. Specifically, Chomsky addressed the issues of reinforcement, imitation, and syntactic development.

"I have been able to find no support whatsoever," Chomsky (1959) stated, "for the doctrine . . . that slow and careful shaping of verbal behavior through differential reinforcement is an absolute necessity" (p. 42). In fact, parents of young language-learning children directly reinforce only a small percentage of their children's utterances. Parents of young children tend to ignore grammatical errors and to reinforce for truthfulness of utterances. Thus, the two-year-old girl who says "That bes a horsie" while pointing to a cow will be corrected. If she is pointing to a horse, however, her parent will probably respond with "Yes, that's a horsie." Chomsky also faulted Skinner for attempting to explain the process of acquisition while ignoring the content being learned.

Likewise, imitation may account for little syntactic learning. The value of imitation as a language-learning strategy has been questioned because of its infrequent use by children above age two. When young children do imitate, they correctly imitate structures they have produced without imitation on a previous occasion. In general, imitation is reserved for learning new words and stabilizing forms the child already produces. An overall imitative language-acquisition strategy would be of little value, according to Chomsky (1957) and McNeill (1970), because adult speech provides a very poor model. Adult-to-adult speech is characterized by false starts and revisions, dysfluencies or breaks in speech flow, and slips of the tongue. In addition, imitation cannot account for common child language structures, such as "I eated," that are presumably absent from adult speech.

Finally, the autoclitic function provides an insufficient explanation of complex syntactic development. The child could not possibly learn through imitation all the sentences she has the potential of producing later. Nor could the child experience all possible sentences in order to become aware of successive word associations, as Skinner suggested. In general, behavioral theory fails to explain the generative aspect of language, the ability to create novel utterances. The generative quality of language suggests underlying rules of language formation. Rather than learning specific sentences through imitation, the child learns rules that can be used for comprehension and production. Thus, children frequently produce the full form "Mommy is eating" before the contracted "Mommy's eating," although adults prefer to use the contracted form.

In conclusion, Chomsky criticized Skinner's explanation as superficial because it did not consider what the child brings to the learning task. By emphasizing production, Skinner minimized comprehension and underlying cognitive processes. Chomsky summarized this point as follows:

> The magnitude of the failure of this attempt to account for verbal behavior serves as a kind of measure of the importance of the factors omitted from consideration, and an indication of how little is really known about this remarkably complex phenomenon. . . . It is futile to inquire into the causation of verbal behavior until much more is known about the specific character of this behavior. (pp. 28, 55)

Contributions

The behavioral explanation of language development should not be dismissed entirely. Theorists such as Skinner have attempted to explain a complex process within the environmental context in which that process occurs. In that sense, behavioral notions have influenced later sociolinguistic theories. Chomsky may have been correct in stating that Skinner's efforts were premature. In subsequent years, we have learned much about language structure. This knowledge has provided new categories to use in analyzing development within the social environment of the child who is learning language. In addition, environmental input is now recognized as critical to language development.

Behaviors identified by Skinner and other operant psychologists have also proven very useful in language training. Today, structured behavioral techniques provide a basis for many remedial programs used with children who have delayed or disordered language.

PSYCHOLINGUISTIC THEORY: A SYNTACTIC MODEL

In contrast to the behavioral emphasis on language use, **psycholinguistic** theorists of the late 1950s and 1960s stressed language form and the underlying mental processes these forms represent. The linguistic structures, it was reasoned, are a key to the methods employed by language users to understand and generate language. The leading proponent of psycholinguistic theory was Noam Chomsky. Chomsky tried to describe language from a scientific perspective and thus to create a theoretical explanation for the manner in which humans create and make judgments about language. He attempted to provide simplified operating principles that explained both the similarities and the differences within human languages.

Biological Basis

Chomsky and his peers reasoned that there must be some universality or commonality to the rules followed in the diverse languages of humans. For example, all languages make temporal or time distinctions, have some means of negating a proposition, require both a subject and a predicate for correct sentence formation, and so on. Of central importance is the fact that some form of language is common to almost all human beings. Even humans with very limited mental abilities can communicate using simple conventional linguistic rules. The differences between humans are differences in degree of acquisition.

Are humans the only species to use linguistic systems? Lenneberg (1964), another psycholinguist, asserted that "there is no evidence that any nonhuman form has the capacity to acquire even the most primitive stages of language development" (p. 67).

If complex language and its use seems specific to the human species and nearly universal, the early psycholinguists reasoned that it must be biologically based. In other words, humans possess a specific, innate capacity for language. But even though language use is nearly universal, it doesn't follow that underlying language rules are also universal. Human languages seem to be very diverse. Chomsky found that human languages differ only superficially but that underlying principles are more uniform. These underlying principles are based on universal features. Chomsky proposed to describe these linguistic universals.

Primate Studies: Do Other Species Have Language?

Until the late 1960s, all previous primate language studies had failed because they attempted to train speech. The vocal mechanism of a chimpanzee is not capable of the great variety of human speech sounds. In contrast, Washoe, a chimpanzee, was trained to communicate using American Sign Language. Although she was able to learn approximately 130 signs and to create new words, such as *water-bird* for *duck*, Washoe seemed incapable of learning other than a very simple word order.

In a separate study, a chimpanzee named Sarah was trained to communicate using colored plastic shapes. Like Washoe, Sarah was capable of using very simple symbol-order rules expressively. For example, Sarah produced "Randy give banana Sarah" (although this example may be the result of word substitution, as she had previously learned "Randy give *apple* Sarah"). Success seemed to be based on matching the abilities of these chimpanzees with a mode of communication.

Critics were quick to note that this language use occurred only after an extraordinary training effort, which is not needed in human language acquisition. Much of the reported early success may have been due to trainer prompting and to imitation. Controversy often results from linguists' definition of language and from the results of specific methods of training, such as the use of imitation (Premack, 1986). Although primates appear to be capable of creating sentences, they have failed so far to master the more difficult task of conversation.

More recent studies with Koko (the mountain gorilla best known for her adoption of a kitten she named "All-ball") and with other primates have caused a reevaluation of earlier conclusions. Some promising studies have found that pygmy chimpanzees will repeat symbols when in agreement, requesting, promising, excited, or selecting alternatives (Greenfield & Savage-Rumbaugh, 1993). Thus, some distinct pragmatic functions are present. These same chimpanzees have demonstrated conversational turn-taking skills and cohesive conversations. Other aspects of human conversations have not been reported to date.

In very tightly controlled studies, Kanzi, a pygmy chimp, has demonstrated that he can respond symbolically to different human partners and without seeing them, thus putting to rest concerns about trainer prompting. In addition, Kanzi has learned language much as humans do with little direct instruction. Washoe taught her adopted son Loulis, who had never seen humans sign, to form signs. She gently molded his hands into the correct shape. Still, Kanzi and the others are capable of "proto-grammar," equivalent only to that of the human two-year-old.

Recent brain studies have revealed a larger panum temporale in the auditory-association cortex of the left hemisphere of chimpanzee brains similar to that found in humans (see chapter 4). Lateralization or development on one side of the brain suggests development of a specialized function. Given the location of this specific area, it seems to imply that chimpanzees may possess the neurological anatomy for development of language. Further research does not find this lateralization in the brains of lower primates. Obviously, we haven't heard the last word in this controversy. Further brain scans will help us understand whether these neural areas function during language processing.

Even the harshest critics of the chimpanzee studies admit that both in the wild and in signing studies, chimpanzees do demonstrate intentional communication and that their natural gestures do communicate meaning. Further questions arise: At what point does gesturing become symbolic communication? Where do syntax and generative language use begin?

Linguistic Processing

In *Syntactic Structures* (1957), Chomsky described language from the psychological perspective of the capacity of a language user to produce and comprehend language. Thus, he concentrated on the linguistic process instead of the grammatical products. He was interested in a theory of the universal grammatical rules of language, rules with biological bases.

Chomsky proposed two levels of linguistic processing. The initial level operates using phrase-structure rules; the second employs transformational rules. **Phrase-structure rules** delineate the basic relationships underlying all sentence organization, regardless of the language being used; they are universal. **Transformational rules**, on the other hand, govern the rearrangement of phrase-structure elements based on a specific language and are not universal.

The units within each sentence are known as **constituents**, and a description of sentence units is called a *constituent analysis*. Sentence constituents can be nominal, verbal, adverbial, or adjectival. Nominal constituents, or **noun phrases**, consist of a single word or phrase that can act as a noun, such as *he, the boy*, or *the nearly 1,000 college graduates*. Several different types of words can form a noun phrase, but the only obligatory word is the noun; without it there is no noun phrase. Verbal constituents, called **verb phrases**, must include the verb plus any additional words or phrases that might be needed to complete the verb. For example, some verbs, such as *walk*, may be used without a direct object, whereas others, such as *sell*, need a direct object to be complete. Thus, a verb phrase also might include a noun phrase, as in *sells used cars*. Adverbial constituents serve the function of an adverb, thus marking the manner, place, or time of an action. For example, a word such as *easily* or *late* or a phrase such as *in the gymnasium* may serve as an adverbial constituent, as in *danced in the gymnasium*. Finally, adjectival constituents serve as an adjective to modify a noun and may be a word, such as *big, handsome,* or *inarticulate*, or a phrase, such as *in sheep's clothing*, as in *wolf in sheep's clothing*. Each of these constituents may be combined with or embedded within the others.

Sentence constituents or elements are organized hierarchically, which means that each, in turn, may be broken into its constituent parts, as in Figure 2.2. Chomsky's phrase-structure rules begin with the sentence as the basic unit. A rule common to all languages is that each sentence must contain at least a noun and a verb. You will remember this rule from chapter 1. Thus, the Bible's shortest verse, "Jesus wept," is a perfectly acceptable sentence.

FIGURE 2.2 Phrase Structure Hierarchical Rules

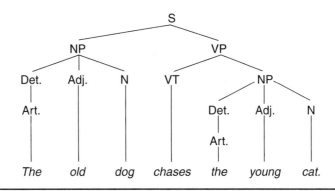

Most sentences, however, contain longer phrases and more modifiers. The basic relationship is written as follows:

$$S \rightarrow NP + VP$$

This formula is read as, "A sentence can be rewritten as a noun phrase and a verb phrase." (Remember, however, that only the noun and the verb are mandatory.)

Phrase-structure rules may be successively rewritten because each symbol to the left of the arrow can be replaced by the symbol(s) to the right. In the final step, actual words may be selected for each constituent, as in Figure 2.2. For example, a noun phrase may be rewritten as

$$NP \rightarrow Det + (Adj) + N$$

In this rule, the noun phrase is rewritten as a determiner, an optional adjective (as noted by the parentheses), and a noun. Determiners can be further rewritten as articles (*the, a, an*), demonstratives (*these, those*), or possessive pronouns (*his, her, their*). Constituents can be added or deleted to form a variety of noun phrase types. For example, under this phrase-structure rule, we can form *the big hat, those red apples, his car, the baby, my yellow shirt*, and so on.

Likewise, verb phrases can be subjected to the same element or constituent analysis. For example,

$$VP \rightarrow VI$$
$$VP \rightarrow VT + NP$$

These rules are interpreted to mean that a verb phrase may be rewritten as an intransitive verb (VI) or a transitive verb (VT) with a direct object, which is a noun phrase. Intransitive verbs, such as *walk* and *arrive*, do not act upon another noun. When I say "I walked quickly" or "I arrived on time," I am following the verb with an adverb of manner (*quickly*) or an adverbial phrase of manner (*on time*). In contrast, transitive verbs, such as *buy, give*, or *eat*, act upon a noun. Thus, we say "I should buy a new car" or "She is eating ice cream." *Car* and *ice cream* are nouns used as direct objects. They answer the questions "What did I buy?" and "What is she eating?" Transitive verbs occasionally have indirect objects, so another variation of the rule might read

$$VP \rightarrow VT + (NP) + NP$$

The noun phrase in parentheses is optional and represents an indirect object. An example might be *bought me a car*. The *me* is not necessary for a complete verb phrase, but it is needed to understand for whom the car was bought. These noun phrases might be analyzed further into their constituent parts. Thus, as before, each noun phrase might be rewritten as determiner, adjective, and noun. The verb phrase might now result in *bought his old uncle the antique automobile*.

In this manner, Chomsky attempted to provide a finite set of universal rules from which language users of all languages generate an almost infinite number of sentences. By rearranging the rules, we can construct a tree diagram, such as the one in Figure 2.2. Each rule previously formed can be seen by reading down the tree diagram from one level to the related constituents on the next lower level. Once a terminal category has been delineated, the variety of sentences that can be produced is limited only by the number of words available for each constituent. For example, for the rule given in Figure 2.2, let's assume that available nouns include *man, woman, dog,* and *cat* and that verbs include *chases* and *sees*. We can now construct numerous sentence variations; several examples are:

> The old dog chases the young cat.
> The old man chases the young dog.
> The old cat chases the young woman.
> The old woman chases the young woman.
> The old man sees the young cat.
> The old dog sees the young dog.
> The old woman sees the young man.

The particular constituent structure presented in Figure 2.2 will result in thirty-two different sentences if four nouns and two verbs are available. If the adjectives *young* and *old* are used interchangeably, 128 sentences can be produced. If we expand the article constituent to include both *a* and *the*, then 512 sentences are possible. It is easy to see how humans can theoretically create millions of sentences when over 500 are possible from one constituent structure using four noun choices, two verbs, two adjectives, and two articles. While our examples have been in English, keep in mind that Chomsky was interested in universal rules. Therefore, we would actually be operating at a conceptual level, not at a spoken, signed, or written level.

Although the phrase-structure rules can be used to construct many sentences, the rules do not apply to all sentence types. For example, phrase-structure rules are of only limited use for interpreting ambiguity or for explaining the similar meanings found in very different sentences. Ambiguous sentences have two different possible meanings. The sentence "They are arresting officers" can be interpreted in two ways. The ambiguity can be resolved by assigning different constituent structures to the sentence. The word *arresting* may be a verb or an adjective, thus modifying the sentence's interpretation. But not all ambiguity can be resolved this easily. In a second example, the sentences "The dog chased the cat" and "The cat was chased by the dog" are very different but have the same meaning. The phrase-structure rule for both is NP + VT + NP. In addition, the form "The cat was chased by the dog" is not universal but represents English syntax, so it is not found in the phrase-structure rules.

Theoretical inadequacies such as these are addressed in a second set of rules called *transformations*. These are language-specific syntactic rules that rearrange the structure of the basic phrase-structure sentence. By operating on the phrase-structure frame, transformational rules create general sentence types, such as questions, negatives, passives, and imperatives, and more complex sentences, such as those with embedded or subordinate clauses. These sentences cannot be formed by phrase-structure rules because of the interrelated operations needed and because the forms used to make questions, negatives, and the like are not universal, as are the phrase-structure rules. For example, selection of the correct verb form depends on the number and person of the noun and on the temporal or time aspect of the sentence. In the sentence "Mark was late last evening," the verb form *was* agrees with the singular noun and with the notion of time past. Transformational rules are an attempt to describe this contextual relatedness. Changing one element causes changes in the sentence, as in the following examples:

Mark and Ray *were* late last evening.
Mark *will be* late tomorrow.

In addition, the verb form used and the manner of use are English-based, not universal.

Using a combination of the universal phrase-structure rules and the transformational rules for English, Chomsky tried to explain the human ability to create all possible English sentences. Although transformational rules are specific to each language, the operations they describe are common to all languages, such as replacing one element with another or changing the location of one element. These operations are written as rules or formulas for changing the basic phrase structure of the sentence. For example, a transformational rule for passive sentences in English might be as follows:

$$PASS \rightarrow NP_2 + be + V + \text{-}ed + by + NP_1$$

This rule can be read as "noun phrase two followed by the verb *to be*, followed by the verb plus *-ed*, followed by *by*, followed by noun phrase one." This rule is a transformation of the phrase-structure rule NP + VT + NP. The two noun phrases have been redesignated as one and two, respectively. Applying the rule:

The boy likes the girl.

$(NP_1 + VT + NP_2)$

becomes

The girl is liked by the boy.

$(NP_2 + be + V + \text{-}ed + by + NP_1)$

The process seems quite simple; but if we modify the sentence slightly, the rule does not apply:

Cindy drives horses.

becomes

The horses are driv*ed* by Cindy.

A related but separate rule is needed in which *-en* is added to the verb instead of *-ed*.

These theoretical constructs need some psychological model within which to operate. Chomsky proposed a two-tier mental model that includes a deep structure and a surface structure (Figure 2.3). Each sentence has both structures. The **deep structure**, found in the brain, is generated by the phrase-structure rules and as such contains the basic meaning of the sentence. All the syntactic relationships needed to express the meaning correctly are present. The basic concept relationship "Mother eat something," for example, is universal.

An actual sentence that we produce is called the **surface structure**. The deep structures of a surface structure declarative sentence, such as "Mother is eating something," and an interrogative sentence, such as "What is she eating?" are the same. The meanings of the two sentences are similar, and the basic relationships are maintained in the surface structure.

The relationship between the deep and surface structures is expressed in the transformational rules. By changing, reordering, and modifying the deep-structure elements, transformational operations create the surface structure. For example, the deep-structure elements "Charlie open gift" must be modified for the present progressive verb tense by the transformational rule $NP_1 + be + V + -ing + NP_2$, resulting in "Charlie is opening the gift." As surface-structure complexity increases, more transformational operations must be performed and the relationship between the deep and surface structures becomes less obvious. In the example in Figure 2.3, the phrase-structure rule $NP_1 + V + NP_2$ is changed by the transformational rule NP_2 (*What*) $+ be + proN_1 + V + -ing$.

In *Aspects of the Theory of Syntax* (1965), Chomsky stated that a complete grammar must have three parts: syntax, phonology, and semantics. Syntax is the most important element, according to Chomsky, because it enables language users to generate sentences. Phonology and semantics are purely "interpretive." The syntactic element specifies a deep structure that determines the semantic interpretation and a surface structure that determines the phonetic interpretation. Thus, the transformational rules link semantics and phonology.

In addition, transformational rules specify an underlying relationship, not only between surface and deep structures but also between various surface structures. Thus, the transformational rules help language users recognize the close meanings of sentences with

FIGURE 2.3   Syntactic Psycholinguistic Language-Processing Model

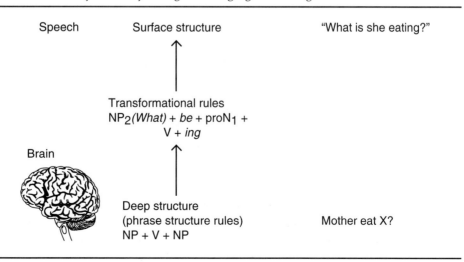

Speech   Surface structure   "What is she eating?"

Transformational rules
NP_2*(What)* $+ be + proN_1 +$
$V + ing$

Brain

Deep structure
(phrase structure rules)
$NP + V + NP$

Mother eat X?

shared constituents. For example, there is a meaningful relationship between all of the following sentences:

> The woman drove the car.
> Did the woman drive the car?
> Who drove the car?
> What did the woman drive?
> The car was driven by the woman.
> Was the car driven by the woman?

The interrelatedness can be explained in terms of the underlying phrase-structure rule system.

Language Acquisition

The child learning language is similar to a linguist in the field. Presented with a finite set of examples, the child must form hypotheses about the underlying rules and test these hypotheses in actual use. We would expect to see very individualistic patterns of language develop. Yet there appear to be developmental similarities within and across languages. Children progress from single to multiword utterances and then to modification of these structures. In addition, the developmental milestones are very similar across children. Most children say their first word at about one year of age. At around eighteen months, two-word utterances appear. These utterances are so predictable that children must be using some common method of analysis and generation, linguists concluded.

The early psycholinguists assumed that language universality and the developmental similarities across children pointed to an innate or inborn language-acquisition mechanism. Chomsky called this mechanism the *language acquisition device*, or LAD. The LAD contains universal underlying linguistic principles or phrase-structure rules. Thus, the infant is "prewired" for linguistic analysis. The LAD contains universals in the form of a catalog of semantic or meaning classes and the rules for generating sentences. These universals form a primitive theory for analyzing any potential natural language. The LAD enables each child to process incoming language and to form hypotheses based on the regularities found in that language. Through hypothesis testing, the child derives an accurate concept of the syntactic rules of his or her native language.

Although the LAD is innate, linguistic input is needed to activate the analysis mechanism. Hypotheses are formulated on the basis of the speech the child hears. Often ungrammatical, this linguistic input cannot serve as a complete model for language learning. However, it is regular enough to enable the child to extract linguistic rules based on his or her innate knowledge.

If the innateness theory is correct, we would expect the child first to use the phrase-structure rules and only later to use the transformational rules. Since the universal features of phrase structure rules exist in the infant, they should emerge in early child speech. Transformations appear later, it is reasoned, because they are peculiar to specific languages and must be deduced by the child using the phrase-structure rules. In fact, the early multiword utterances of children are not similar to the phrase-structure rules.

Child language is not a mirror of adult language. It has some unique qualities of its own. Chomsky's delineation of adult generative rules sparked an interest in describing the operating rules of child language. Initially, child language was described as "telegraphic speech" (R. Brown & Bellugi, 1964)—"Throw ball me" or "Airplane up," for example—reflecting a lack of sophisticated rehearsal and memory strategies, which prevent the child from exhibiting more mature memory performance. This model is inadequate because it offers only a superficial description of child language. It does not explore word relationships or provide an explanation of language acquisition. At this point, child development experts and linguists began to study the organization of child language in earnest.

Government-Binding Theory

It is only fair that we update Chomsky somewhat and not leave him in the late 1960s. In recent years, Chomsky (1981, 1986, 1992, 1995) attempted to formulate a theory of language to account for all and only all well-formed, acceptable sentences and the mental machinery necessary to form and comprehend these sentences and to make judgments of acceptability (Shapiro, 1997). The result, called **government-binding theory**, attempts to describe the way in which the human mind represents the autonomous system of language. His goal was to present a theory that can account for the great diversity in human languages and that can explain the development of grammars by children on the basis of limited input (Leonard & Loeb, 1988).

Obviously, not every verb, noun, or other grammatical unit could fill the spaces in the tree diagram in Figure 2.2. Each word in your lexicon or personal vocabulary must carry certain restrictions, he reasoned, that specify those sentence environments in which the word is allowed. For example, some verbs take a direct object, others do not; some require a prepositional phrase, others do not; and the number of nouns attached vary. The verbs *fix* and *make* require a direct object to complete the thought, as in *fix the leaky roof*. In contrast, the verb *sleep* does not require a following noun object. A prepositional phrase is required with a verb such as *send* as in *send in the mail* or *send to my sister*. In addition, *send* requires a direct object as in *sent **the letter** in the mail*.

The varying number of nouns or participants attached can be illustrated by the verbs *kiss* and *put*:

> The *puppy* kissed your *sister.*
> *Juan* put the *tickets* on the *table.*

In the first sentence, *kiss* requires only two nouns, while in the second, *put* requires three.

When we learn a new word, we also learn about these syntactic constraints or "privileges." Each noun (*Juan*) or noun phrase (*the tickets*) plays a role, such as location (*The table*), assigned by the verb. The meaning of a word may include the number of participants and the roles (Grimshaw, 1990; Jackendoff, 1990; Levin, 1993).

Universal grammar consists of four levels—D-structure, S-structure, phonetic form, and logical form—and several subtheories. D-structures consist of sentence-formation rules and the lexicon or personal dictionary. The lexicon specifies meaning but, more importantly, the manner in which each word is to be treated syntactically. For example, the word *see* should be followed by a noun phrase, as in *see the dog*. More complex terms such as *before* might be followed by a noun phrase (*before school*) or a clause (*before I had eaten*). D-structures are formed by placing the lexical items in the appropriate sentence forms.

Unlike phrase-structure rules, however, D-structures are expanded to explain other sentence forms, such as questions. Phrase-structure rules have been rewritten as follows:

$$S \rightarrow COMP + S$$

$$S \rightarrow NP + INFL + VP$$

A COMP or complementizer, such as *that* or *what*, is assumed to be contained in every sentence, whether stated or not. In addition, every verb is assumed to contain an INFL or inflection, such as a tense marker or auxiliary verb. The formation of questions would involve the use of the COMP and/or INFL, unavailable under the older phrase-structure rules of S → NP + VP.

The INFL marker is now theorized to be responsible for the shape of the verb phrase, tense, and person markers on the verb, and the semantic characteristics or case of the noun (Radford, 1988). If correct, lack of INFL might explain the simplified structure of children's early multiword utterances, such as "Mommy throw." (Loeb & Leonard, 1991).

S-structures are derived from D-structures by the *move alpha rule*, a single movement of sentence elements that replaces the separate transformational rules. Thus, the sentence "Joell can throw [what]" becomes "What can Joell throw?" The object noun phrase is moved to the initial position and replaced by the COMP, as in Figure 2.4.

Phonetic-form rules include phonological rules and the use of inflections (INFL). Logical-form rules govern the sense making of sentences. These two alone, however, can-

FIGURE 2.4   Sentence Formation Applying the Rules of Government-Binding Theory

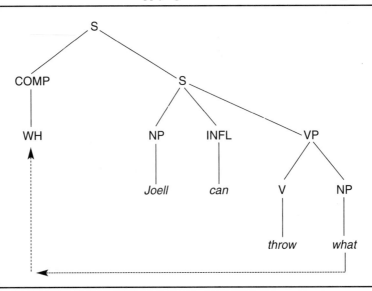

not handle potential confusions and ambiguities. For example, the sentence "Mary could not decide what she should do" is well-formed and makes sense, but the word *she* might refer to Mary or another female mentioned outside of this sentence.

Chomsky expands well beyond his previous theories, reasoning that the universal rules, by their very simplicity, can result in so many different sentences that children could never learn language in the short time in which they do. Therefore, he proposes several sub-theories: bounding theory, government theory, case theory, binding theory, θ-theory, and control theory governing the allowable amount of constituent movement, allowable constituent use, semantic case, reference, and roles (Leonard & Loeb, 1988).

Mature speakers use all of these processes to encode and decode the language around them, confounding the universal grammar with the peculiarities of their individual languages. Cross-language studies have demonstrated the application of government-binding theory to other languages (Frazier, 1993; Nagata, 1993).

Although government-binding theory tries to incorporate many aspects of language, primary interest is still language form. Too few child studies have been performed to make a definite statement about the contribution of government-binding theory to our understanding of language development.

Limitations

Transformational grammar emphasizes syntactic structures but virtually ignores the contributions of phonetics, semantics, and pragmatics. This approach fails to recognize the underlying semantic structures upon which language form is heavily dependent. A linguistic theory that ignores semantics cannot adequately explain why a syntactically correct sentence such as "Lively tables leap narrowly under the ceiling" does not make sense. Even government-binding theory focuses almost exclusively on syntax.

In addition, a syntax-based model seems inappropriate for describing single-word and two-word levels of development. The organization of these structures seems to be devoid of syntactic processes. Nor does later language learning follow transformational models. Children do not use one transformational rule, followed by two, and so on until multiple transformations are accomplished.

The inadequacies of transformational grammar and government-binding theory as an explanation for language development stem from the nature of that grammar. Chomsky's theoretical grammar is based on adult data. Difficulty arises when this preconceived adult model is imposed upon child language, which is different from adult language. There is a risk of losing information not included in the model. Looking for mature structures in child speech may result in missing important structures and underevaluating children's knowledge and capabilities.

The theory also negates children's uses of language. Children use language to describe and to accompany their experiences. Unfortunately, the theory deemphasizes the importance of the environment and of early social and cognitive growth. Chomsky did concede that children gain language through exposure to "scraps" of adult language, but he and his peers have described a process that occurs independently of cognitive development. While Chomsky and his followers concentrated on innate syntactic knowledge, they neglected innate cognitive abilities.

The issue of innateness is the weakest aspect of Chomsky's theory. The notion of a language-acquisition device is too simplified and provides an inadequate explanation. To assume that the ability to use language is innate does little to facilitate our understanding of the actual process of language development. Chomsky may have been describing the wrong innate qualities. It seems more appropriate to describe innate cognitive abilities such as problem solving and methods for processing information.

Contributions

It would be a great disservice to Chomsky to dismiss his contributions because of the inadequacies of his developmental explanations. In Chomsky's defense, we must note that he did not set out to describe language acquisition. Rather, his goal was to describe and explain linguistic processing.

Chomsky redefined linguistic behavior in psychological terms that were quite different from the older syntactic structural models. By emphasizing the generative feature of grammars, Chomsky formulated his own novel grammatical rules. His main concern was process or linguistic competence, not product or linguistic performance. Chomsky noted that operating rules exist and that some are universal. Cross-cultural studies continue to highlight underlying universal processes and the interaction of linguistic form and various linguistic systems. In the future, researchers will attempt to determine which part of language is innate and universal (Perara, 1994). Some linguists are even proposing a genetic link, a grammar gene.

Chomsky's and others' search for linguistic universals has led them to theorize about a Human Sentence Processing Mechanism (HSPM)(Altmann & Steedman, 1988; Frazier, 1987; Gibson, 1991; Hickok, 1993). Of interest is the relationship of the components of language and the steps in sentence processing which may be serial, parallel, or a combination of the two.

In redefining linguistic units, Chomsky also offered a different view of human beings than that presented by the behaviorists and learning theorists. Chomsky's human organism is psychologically active and linguistically creative. Language is not externally imposed but develops from internal processing mechanisms and is used in a generative fashion.

PSYCHOLINGUISTIC THEORY: A SEMANTIC/COGNITIVE MODEL

As early as 1963, the syntax-only theory of language processing was questioned. It was argued that a full account of language must include meanings, or semantics. These meanings should not be limited to individual words but should include the meanings expressed through syntactic relations as well. Although Chomsky discussed meaning at the deep-structure level, he minimized the contribution of semantics to syntactic processes. It is inadequate to say merely that a certain position in a sentence can be filled by any noun or by the subject of the sentence. Consider the vacancy in the subject position of the following sentence, for example:

The [noun] pushed the door angrily.

Only certain nouns can fill the vacancy. Inanimate nouns, such as *ball, door,* and *shoe*, though grammatically correct, do not make sense. Semantics helps us distinguish sense from non-sense. To have a generative language system, we must appreciate the semantic characteristics of each word. The word *mother* contains the semantic characteristics of being animate, human, female, parental, and so on. Such features govern the selection of appropriate verbs, pronouns, adjectives, and other words that are related in some way. Interpretation of any utterance must include the *referential context*, or its underlying semantic features and relationships.

Case Grammar: A Beginning

Case grammar is a generative system that attempts to explain the influence of semantics on the syntactic structure of language (Fillmore, 1968). It proposes that there is an underlying level of the deep structure. This level consists of a set of universal semantic concepts that specify the relationships of nouns to verbs. These semantic concepts are distinct from syntactic relations and from the form of the surface structure. They are not found in innate rules but represent the events and relationships found in all environments or in human genetic coding. With either source, the concepts are universal (Chafe, 1970).

A **case** is a distinct semantic role or function for a certain noun phrase. In the previous example, "The [noun] pushed the door angrily," only nouns of a certain case, those that cause action, can be employed. Thus, *ball*, which cannot cause action, does not make sense, while *girl*, which can, is perfectly acceptable.

Case function is marked by word order. Definitions and examples are listed in Table 2.1. The seven major universal cases are agentive, dative, experiencer, factitive, instrumental, locative, and objective. Each case has certain semantic features that mark it. For example, agentive and dative case nouns must be animate or alive. Instrumental case nouns must be inanimate. If the previous example had read "The boy pushed the [noun] angrily," the choice of noun would have been an objective case noun. With the objective case, almost any noun whose role fits the verb may be used. Therefore, the blank could be filled with *ball, door, bicycle,* or *chair*, but not with *skyscraper* or *airport*. The verb *push* implies movement or the possibility of movement, so skyscraper would not fit the role needed (unless we lived in a world inhabited by Saturday morning TV superheroes).

In general, cases are not exclusive, and a noun may be used in all cases in which it meets the criteria. The verb that is employed determines the case of the noun. Thus, case grammar accounts for structure through the semantic functions of nouns in relation to verbs (Chafe, 1970; Fillmore, 1968).

A general rule for surface structure is that "if there is an A [agent], it becomes the subject; otherwise, if there is an I [instrument], it becomes the subject; otherwise, the subject is O [objective]" (Fillmore, 1968, p. 33). This rule depends on the type of verb employed. In the following examples, the subject changes according to the case:

The *boy* used a *screwdriver* to open the *door*.
(agentive)　(instrumental)　　　(objective)

The *screwdriver* was used to open the *door*.
(instrumental)　　　　　(objective)

The *door* opened easily.
(objective)

The *door* was opened by the *boy* with his *screwdriver*.
(objective)   (agentive)   (instrumental)

Unlike other languages, English has few case markers other than position. Outside of the subject position, cases are marked by prepositions (see Table 2.1).

Much like Chomsky's transformational grammar, case grammar is an attempt to describe a generative system. These universal semantic cases form a structure that underlies, and provides a basis for, syntax.

TABLE 2.1   Case Relationships

CASE NAME	DEFINITION	EXAMPLE
Agentive (A)	The perceived instigator of action, typically animate with own motivation	*Mike* threw the ball. The ball was thrown by *Mike*. Mother gave *Joe* a big hug.
Dative (D)	The animate being affected by the state or action named by the verb	The clown gave a flower to *Grandma*.
Experiencer (E)	The animate being who experiences a given event, action, or mental disposition	*Mother* heard Stan. *Jeff* wanted a new car above all else.
Factitive (F)	The object or being resulting from the action or state of the verb	Father built a *treehouse*. Joyce wrote a *poem*.
Instrumental (I)	The inanimate object or force involved in a causal manner in the state or action named by the verb; the object brings about the process but is not the instigator	Lee battered the door with his *axe*. Martin ate peas with a *spoon*.
Locative (L)	The place, locus, or spatial orientation of the state, action, or process of the verb	The dog is in his *house*. *Seattle* is very humid. The game was played in the *stadium*.
Objective (O)	The animate or inanimate noun whose role in the state or action named by the verb depends on the meaning of the verb; the most semantically neutral case	Dad threw the *ball* to me. Mother heard *Tom* come in late.

Source: Based on C. Fillmore, "The Case for Case." In E. Bach & R. Harmas (Eds.), *Universals in Linguistic Theory.* New York: Holt, Rinehart & Winston, 1968; and on W. Chafe, *Meaning and the Structure of Language.* Chicago: University of Chicago Press, 1970.

The Semantic Revolution

Following the lead of other linguists, Lois Bloom attempted to apply a Chomsky-like syntactic analysis technique to child language in the late 1960s. She analyzed the language of three children at an early multiword stage. Bloom applied a reduction transformation process in which, presumably, the children know the underlying adult structure but delete certain elements. Thus, Bloom assumed that children have both a deep and a surface structure. Since children can process only a limited number of constituents at a given time, some must be omitted from the surface structure. Adult linguistic processing does not require this reduction because adults have greater memory and processing skills. Assuming that underlying meaning would help her analysis, Bloom recorded the verbal and nonverbal contexts of each child utterance. She was interested in the ongoing event and the communication partners.

Although Bloom was able to ascertain the children's meanings from the context, she found that syntactic rules were inadequate for describing these different meanings. In fact, without consideration of semantics, many of the syntactic relationships were missed. For example, on two occasions, Bloom's subject Kathryn said "Mommy sock." The contexts were very different. Once she said "Mommy sock" while picking up her mother's stocking; on the other occasion, she said those same words while her mother was putting the child's sock on Kathryn. The child's intended meaning was very different, but the surface structure was unchanged.

Bloom found that children's speech contains consistent relationships among entities in the children's world and that these relationships are expressed by simple word-order rules that underlie syntax. For example, one relationship is between the agent performing the action and the action itself. This is expressed as agent followed by action (agent + action), as in "Dad throw" or "Doggie run." The relationship of anything to its location is the entity followed by the location (X + location), as in "Go bed," "Throw me," or "Mommy car." Bloom assumed that word order marks semantic relationships that are expressed syntactically in later development.

With the publication of *Language Development: Form and Function of Emerging Grammars* in 1970, Bloom presented the conclusions of her study. Her results signaled the beginning of a new era in child language study. This move from a syntactic-transformational to a semantic analysis has been aptly dubbed the *semantic revolution*. Child language structure began to be examined in relation to the child's intended meaning interpreted from both non-linguistic and linguistic contexts. Such analysis is called a **rich interpretation** because it goes beyond the words of the speaker to attain the fuller meaning. "Baby bed," for example, may mean quite different things in different contexts. The child may be providing information while the baby sleeps or pointing to an empty crib. In the first instance, she may be telling her listener where the baby sleeps; in the second, she may be signaling ownership.

It was hypothesized that the underlying semantic basis of language develops prior to syntax. Researchers began to analyze child language for early examples of the case relationships.

Three other linguists, I. M. Schlesinger, Roger Brown, and Dan Slobin, reached the same general conclusions simultaneously with Bloom. Going beyond Bloom, Schlesinger (1971) proposed that child grammar is semantic, not syntactic. Schlesinger went on to identify the major semantic relationships of early child speech. Unlike case grammar in which semantic relationships are expressed in syntactic forms, in early child language semantic relationships are expressed very clearly in the word order. As the child develops, word-order rules give way to the syntactic devices adults use to signal case relationships. For example, possession is originally signaled by word order, then in English, by addition of the more mature possessive -'s. Thus, the word-order possessives "Mommy sock" and "Baby hat" become "Mommy's sock" and "Baby's hat." There is a continuity through child and adult language structure.

Greenfield and Smith (1976) found that semantic grammars could be used to describe children's initial, single-word utterances as well. Thus, the semantic approach assumes that content or meaning precedes language form. Later, acquired syntactic forms are used to express older semantic functions, as in the possession example. It is important to note that children have a range of semantic functions and can use a single-word utterance to express a number of meanings. For example, the questions to the child such as "What's that?" and "Where's cookie?" require a name and a location answer, respectively; yet both could receive the single-word reply "Table." Therefore, *table* can signify the inanimate thing (an objective case) or a place (a locative).

To you, the semantic-syntactic distinction may seem akin to the medieval argument over the number of angels who could sit on the head of a pin. Yet to describe a child utterance such as "Mommy sleep" as "noun plus verb," a syntactic distinction, is to do a disservice to children. Consider the following utterances:

A	B
Mommy eat	Eat cookie
Daddy throw	Throw ball
Baby drink	Drink milk

List A consists of "noun plus verb" sentences; list B, "verb plus noun" sentences. If children are just stringing two syntactically different types of words together, the order should be of no importance. Yet a reversal of the word order results in sentences that do not make sense or are awkward, such as "Throw Daddy" and "Cookie eat." There is a distinct difference between the nouns in lists A and B: those in the first list are agents—they cause action—and those in the second are objects—they receive action. It is important to note that young children have learned this distinction and can use it.

In addition to providing a new direction in child language study, the semantic revolution weakened the notion of the innateness of language rules. According to the semantic hypotheses, meaning, or semantics, is a method of representing mental experience. Support for the semantic structuring of early child language came from cross-cultural studies, suggesting that the early semantic rules, with some modifications, are universal. In fact, "a rather small set of operations and relations describe all the meanings expressed in the early multimorphemic utterances of . . . children, whatever the language they are learning" (R. Brown, 1973, p. 198).

Unlike Chomsky, the semanticists assumed that the common rules represent a general pattern of cognitive development, not innate structure. Children learn basic relationships between entities within the environment, and these relationships are reflected in the semantic structures produced by the child. These relationships form a general structure of language that children learn to express by actively attending to the linguistic environment, especially to the language addressed to them. Children begin to use language expressively to talk about the things they know. In other words, *thought precedes language*. Language is grafted onto existing knowledge about the world and serves as a means of representing the world.

The developmental order of language encoding of semantic relationships reflects the order of development of cognitive structures. This concept has been termed **cognitive determinism**. For example, children demonstrate a concept of object permanence, or of the existence of an object that cannot be seen, before they express relationships such as appearance, disappearance, and nonexistence in their speech. Thus, early utterances represent children's understanding and overall cognitive processing. Linguistic- and cognitive-processing patterns reflect an organization based on the relationships within children's environments. Children do not learn language and then use it to express relationships; rather, they learn entity relationships and express that knowledge in the language they learn subsequently.

Language Development

In some ways, the semantic/cognitive description of language development is a return to the earlier mentalistic approaches of the late 1800s, in which language was viewed as a key to the child's mind. By the very nature of the cognitive hypothesis, language development is rooted in early cognitive development, prior to the appearance of the first word. A particular level of cognitive achievement is necessary before language can be used expressively. There are several cognitive factors that must be present for a child to acquire language (Bowerman, 1974):

1. Ability to represent objects and events not perceptually present.
2. Development of basic cognitive structures and operations related to space and time, classification of types of action, embedding of action patterns within each other, establishment of object permanence and constancy, relationships between objects and action, and construction of a model of one's own perceptual space.
3. Ability to derive linguistic-processing strategies from general cognitive structures and processes.
4. Ability to formulate concepts and strategies to serve as structural components for the linguistic rules.

These cognitive abilities develop during the first year of life. The newborn is primarily a sensory detector. With maturity she begins to act upon the world, to explore, and to manipulate. The child's early sensorimotor interactions form a process that helps her organize the incoming stimuli from the real world.

The symbolic functioning may be rooted in imitation. The child learns to imitate or re-present her own motor behaviors and those of others. Later, the child imitates without an immediate model.

In a play mode, the child represents or re-presents reality symbolically. For example, a piece of paper can be used to represent a blanket. With language the child is able to represent the referent with an arbitrary symbol or word.

The child also uses sensorimotor behaviors to manipulate objects and explore their functions. The child groups these functional use features into classes—such as the category of things that cause action—to form the basis for early definitions.

Finally, with the development of the concept of object permanence, the child can represent entities that are not present in the immediate context. Presumably the child has stored the image of the object symbolically. If an object still exists, even though removed from the child's immediate perception, the child can cause it to recur by evoking the symbol for it.

Imitation, functional use, and object permanence can account for development of the young child's general ability to use symbols, but they are not directly translatable into semantic relationships (Rice, 1984). It is hypothesized that the child must have a concept of object permanence in order to develop semantic notions of appearance, disappearance, and recurrence. Other early cognitive relationships can also be seen in the presymbolic behavior of children.

Children are able to attend visually to location at five months of age. By nine months, children begin to discriminate between different agents that cause action and react to any changes in a situation. Children can discriminate between different actions by one year of age. This ability is an important prerequisite to classifying verbs for making case decisions.

Young children can distinguish between the agent and the object and will attend more to the agent in visual action sequences (Robertson & Suci, 1980). By age two, most children do not expect inanimate objects to move on their own. Agents in early multiword utterances are primarily animate, such as *mommy* and *daddy*.

The receptive abilities of young children also suggest underlying relationships. A number of studies have shown that children who produce predominantly one- and two-word utterances interpret longer unfamiliar sentences using certain familiar patterns later used by them in production (Golinkoff & Markessini, 1980). The inference is that children produce those linguistic forms of which they have prior knowledge.

Although single-word utterances are basically structure-free, they still demonstrate some of the underlying cognitive concepts. Nomination, or naming, is signaled by words such as *see, this*, and *that*. Recurrence is marked by *more* and *'nuther*. Nonexistence markers are phrases such as *all gone, no more*, and *no*. These words are later joined in longer utterances that signal semantic intent, or meaning.

Early two-word combinations are not just random sequences of words. Meaning is signaled by word order. Specific word orders fulfill specific functions. For example, children mark the possessive function in English with the possessor plus the possessed object, as in "Mommy car" and "Baby bed." Other relationships depend primarily on one or two words that signal the semantic function. The recurrence function, for example, is marked by a recurrent word followed by an object or action as in "more milk" or "'nuther jump." Approximately 70 percent of the two-word utterances of children who are learning language can be described by a few simple word-order rules. These rules are listed in Table 8.7 (p. 263) and will be discussed in detail in Chapter 8. Syntactic markers are later applied to the basic word-order rules to form more mature sentences and to mark semantic functions that do not comply with word order. Semantics, however, remains the key to sentence production and comprehension.

At higher language levels, cognitive development seems to precede linguistic development, although the relationship is not clearcut (Rice, 1984). For example, children are able to refer to time and space before they gain these concepts, although the concepts must be acquired before children gain adultlike use of prepositions that mark these concepts.

It has been recognized recently that conceptual knowledge is only a portion of what the child needs to know. The competent communicator has conceptual knowledge of persons, social categories, and events (Rice, 1984). Person knowledge involves knowing that certain features of persons and things are constant and that each individual has a unique perspective of the world. Constant features of persons include their identity, their perceptual fields and emotional states, their intention to communicate, and the like. Social category knowledge includes recognition of situational similarities and understanding of social relational terms, such as *mother* and *parent*. Event knowledge is an understanding of sequentially organized events and routines, such as a telephone conversation or a conversational opener, and of accompanying scripts, such as "Hi, how are you?" Thus, a cognitive basis for language presupposes more than mere knowledge of the concepts behind words.

The semantic/cognitive hypothesis of language acquisition can be summarized as follows (McLean & Snyder-McLean, 1978):

1. Children's early language utterances appear to be expressions of perceived *semantic* relationships as opposed to being expressions of innate preprogrammed syntactic relationships among language elements.
2. Semantic relationships necessarily reflect the perception and understanding of certain relationships between and among the entities and the actions which are present in a child's environment.
3. Such perception and the subsequent development of an understanding of these relationships [are] products of the cognitive domain of human functioning.
4. The products of the cognitive domain in the form of the perception and understanding of relationships among elements in the environment can be considered to be a child's *knowledge* of [the] world.
5. Therefore, a child's language utterances reflect . . . knowledge of the relationships among and between the entities and the actions which make up [the child's] world.
6. Thus, language "maps" onto or encodes a child's existing knowledge. (p. 22)

The semantic/cognitive hypothesis is characterized by an "information-processing approach" (Reber, 1973). The child must abstract basic relationships from the physical environment and rules from the linguistic environment. This information is internalized and categorized to appear later in the child's expressive language. Language input is interpreted using linguistic rules that reflect these cognitive relationships. Language development is a product of the strategies and processes of general cognitive development, although not a direct manifestation of it.

Limitations

The semantic/cognitive hypothesis has highlighted at least one correlate to language acquisition, although cognition alone is an inadequate explanation of the process. Some children with normal cognitive abilities do not acquire language. In addition, there is evidence that cognition does not always influence language. At around age three or four, there seems to be a crossover period in which language is equally likely to influence thought.

Some aspects of linguistic development cannot be explained without reference to earlier linguistic input. Presumably, young children are exposed to and process linguistic input in the same relational terms that are later evident in their linguistic production. These semantic relationships, which seem to explain the construction of early utterances, may be more "psychologically real" to the child than Chomsky's syntactic constituents. As with transformational grammar, however, the semantic relationships also represent an adult perspective. Although these semantic rules can be used to describe most child utterances, they do not necessarily explain linguistic processing or language acquisition.

The greatest limitation of the semantic/cognitive hypothesis is found in the how and why of language acquisition. The link between cognitive abilities and language acquisition is not adequately explained. The hypothesis does not explain why the child's cognitive concepts and relationships become linguistically coded because it ignores the contribution of early communication. An adequate description of language acquisition "must also include the basic nature and purpose of children's communicative transactions within the social context in which they reside or function" (McLean & Snyder-McLean, 1978, p. 41).

Contributions

The semantic/cognitive hypothesis has helped explain many of the phenomena of early language acquisition. The hypothesis offers a description of child language that seems to represent more closely the reality of the young child and to offer a clear relationship between child and adult language. Case grammar is particularly well adapted to the simple structure found in early multiword utterances.

In addition, the semantic/cognitive hypothesis presents a notion of language acquisition against the backdrop of general child development. Without certain cognitive attainments, the child could not ascertain the rules of her language or make the required behavioral associations found in the behavioral and earlier syntactic theories of language acquisition.

SOCIOLINGUISTIC THEORY

To view language from either a syntactic or a semantic perspective is to concentrate on the structural aspect of language. Although the structural units and rules differ, syntax and semantics are interdependent and tend to focus on discrete "bits" of language rather than larger, less finite units. **Sociolinguistic** analysis centers on the communication unit required to convey information. This unit could just as easily be an entire conversation as a word or sentence. The single word *yes*, for example, can convey much information. In contrast, the lengthy speech of a politician might convey only "vote for me," even though those actual words are not spoken.

A structure-only approach also removes language from its communicative context, thus ignoring language's primary function. According to sociolinguistic thought, language is used to communicate and does not occur in a vacuum. Only rarely is language the end in itself. Usually language serves as a means for accomplishing some end within the communicative context.

Theorists who adhere to a sociolinguistic model concentrate on the underlying reasons or social/communicative functions of language. According to the sociolinguistic model, language *use* in communication is central to the linguistic process and to development. An utterance is judged not in terms of its effectiveness in achieving the speaker's intention"

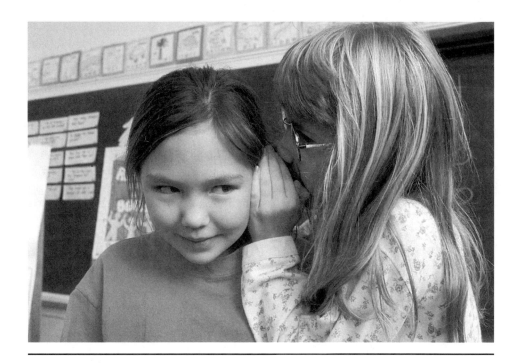

According to sociolinguistic theory, language use is crucial to the process of language development.

(Bruner, 1975, p. 3). Thus, the social/communicative context is essential to the process of conveying meaning.

The overriding motivation for language and language acquisition is effective communication. The speaker chooses the form and content that will best fulfill his or her intentions based on perception of the communication situation. Thus, the form of the speaker's utterance is controlled by (1) her or his knowledge of, and assumptions about, the listener's knowledge of the referent and (2) by the communicative context, which consists of the relative status, roles, and previous history of the participants, along with the social setting. Language rules do not operate independently of the context. Thus, the speaker decides what to say, how to say it, and when to say it. Meaning is inherent not in words but in the linguistic and referential contexts of those words. Conversational partners negotiate word meanings appropriate to the conversational context.

Speech-Act Theory

Two broad pragmatic functions of language are *intrapersonal* and *interpersonal* (Muma, 1978). The intrapersonal or *ideational* function (Halliday, 1975b) is found in the internal language used for memory, problem solving, and concept development. The interpersonal function of language is communication. One unit for analysis of this communicative function is called a speech act. A speech act is a unit of linguistic communication expressed according to linguistic rules that convey a speaker's conceptual representations and intentions. The speech act is a larger conceptual unit than the syntactic and semantic units discussed in previous theories and can thus be divided into other elements.

The **propositional force** of a speech act consists of the conceptual content of the utterance, or its meaning. The speaker's attitude toward the proposition, which is called *intention*, is found in the **illocutionary force**. For example, the one-word proposition *candy* can be altered in several ways with gestures and intonation. A rising intonation and a quizzical look might convey a question, whereas pointing might signify a labeling type of utterance. Reaching while whining the word *candy* might be considered a demand or request for the item. Thus, an utterance with fixed form and semantic content can fulfill several intentions. The reverse is also possible; several different forms or propositions can fulfill a single intention or function. For example, you can ask for the salt using many different forms, including:

> Please pass the salt.
>
> May I have the salt, please.
>
> Salt please.
>
> Does this dish taste like it needs more salt?
>
> Is that the salt over there?

The particular form of the speech act is somewhat dependent upon the communicative context.

The concept of *speech act* was first introduced by John Austin (1962). Searle (1965) theorized that "performance of the speech act . . . constitutes the basic unit of linguistic communication" (p. 222).

To further clarify the work begun by Austin, Searle (1965) proposed speech-act categories including the following:

- Representatives—Statements that convey a belief or disbelief in some proposition, such as an assertion.
- Directives—Attempts to influence the listener to do something, such as a demand or command.
- Commissives—Commitments of self to some future course of action, such as vowing, promising, or swearing.
- Expressives—Expressions of a psychological state, such as thanking, apologizing, or deploring.
- Declaratives—Statements of fact that presume to alter a state of affairs, such as "I confer upon you."

Several investigators have reported that initial child utterances can be categorized roughly into classes approximating Searle's representatives and directives. Others have found early prelinguistic cognitive precursors to speech acts and social-gestural precursors.

Two investigators, Michael Halliday and John Dore, developed separate child-based speech-act taxonomies. Halliday (1975a) concluded, after a longitudinal study of his son, Nigel, that a child emerges with limited adult functional abilities around age two, enabling the speaker to have multiple purposes within a single utterance.

Dore (1974) was primarily interested in preverbal and one-word communicative functions. The basic unit of Dore's taxonomy is the **primitive speech act** (PSA). A PSA is "an utterance, consisting formally of a single act or a single prosodic sound-intonation pattern which functions to convey the child's intention before he acquires sentences" (p. 345). Not merely truncated adult forms, PSAs are qualitatively different, composed of only some of the features of adult speech acts. Each PSA contains a lexical/semantic component and an illocutionary force or intention. The illocutionary component, the speaker's intention, is usually exhibited in intonational patterns. Thus, as described earlier, a word such as *candy* can be a request for action when the child wants candy, a request for an answer when the child is unsure of the name, or an answer to an adult question. Dore described nine categories of PSAs: labeling, repeating, answering, requesting action, requesting answer, calling, greeting, protesting, and practicing (see Table 8.1, p. 254). The components of these PSAs eventually develop into adultlike speech acts as the child's pragmatic intentions gradually become governed by syntactic and semantic structures. Language evolves from a nonverbal communication system.

Many sociolinguists have moved beyond the speech act. More recent research has examined the structure of conversational turns, topics, and whole conversations. Each of these units possesses its own internal organization influenced by the pragmatic rules of discourse.

In summary, the sociolinguistic model considers the communication effectiveness of language within linguistic and nonlinguistic contexts. Language use is central to linguistic coding, which is determined by speaker knowledge and perceived listener knowledge. From a developmental perspective, therefore, the role of the child's communication partners is crucial. The language-development process is "made possible by the presence of an interpreting adult who operates not so much as a corrector or reinforcer but rather as a provider, an expander and idealizer of utterances while interacting with the child" (Bruner, 1975, p. 17).

Language acquisition is a process of socialization. It follows a **transactional model** of child-caregiver give-and-take in which the child learns to understand the rules of dialog, not of syntax or semantics. A communication base is established first; language is then mapped on this base to express verbally those intentions or functions that the child previously expressed nonverbally. Social interactions and social relationships provide the needed framework that enables the child to decode and encode language form and content.

Language Acquisition

Within the sociolinguistic model of language acquisition, the primary communication context of interest is the child-mother or child-caregiver pair. As caregivers respond to their infants' early reflexive behaviors, the infants learn to communicate their intentions. Gradually, the infants refine these communication skills through repeated interactions.

The process is not one-sided, however; the direction of communication is more circular. The caregiver and child perform a communicative "dance" with each taking cues from the other. Within the first few months of life, infants are able to discriminate contrasting phonemes, different intonational patterns, and speech from nonspeech. Infants are also able to discriminate voices and to demonstrate a preference for the human face and human speech sounds. These discriminations and preferences provide the bases for early communication.

Parents or caregivers respond differentially to these infant behaviors and treat them as meaningful social communication. In other words, "the infant's mother . . . endows his behavior with meaning" (Dore, 1986, p. 17). Therefore, the infant receives input and confirmation of his or her own communication attempts. The degree of parental responsiveness appears to be positively correlated with later language abilities. In addition, parental responsiveness forges an attachment bond between the infant and the parent that fosters communication. By three to four months, interactions are regulated by eye gaze and form an early dialog that evolves into vocalization patterns and later into conversational exchanges. Infants engage in selective listening; by three months of age, they can distinguish and attend to utterances addressed to them.

These dialogs alone do not explain the language-acquisition process. Children receive highly selective language input within the routines of child-parent interactions, such as shared or joint action and joint reference. Within joint action routines or dialogs, such as "peekaboo" and "this little piggy," children learn turn-taking skills. Mothers provide a consistent set of behaviors that enable their children to predict the outcome and later to anticipate. Children learn to signal their intention to play. There are parallels between the attributes of play routines and early semantic relationships seen in child language. For example, the caregiver interacts with a ball in a certain ritualized way that helps the child learn that it can appear, disappear, reappear, and be acted upon.

Within joint action sequences, caregivers systematically train children through a process called *joint reference*. **Joint** (or **shared**) **reference** is the achievement of a common referent or the focusing of joint attention on an object or event. Mothers construct elaborate routines to establish joint reference, beginning with eye contact in the first few months and extending to calling the child, pointing, and naming an object. Children progress from following gestural to following verbal-only cues for the referent. Once the referent has been established, mothers provide linguistic input. A joint reference sequence might be as follows:

> *Mother*:   Gerry, see doggie. (Points.)
> *Child*:   (Looks at dog.)
> *Mother*:   Big doggie. Doggie bark.

The establishment of a joint or shared referent and the subsequent maternal verbalizations are important for early meaning development. Maternal speech is modified systematically so that it is comprehensible at the assumed level of the child.

The social interaction surrounding language input makes language acquisition possible (Ninio & Snow, 1988). One of the most important aspects of this input is the high degree of form-function relationship. Many maternal utterances are function-specific. In other words, they serve a single function and are used repeatedly for that function. Thus, it is possible that the child's own intentions arise from maternal input. The mother's pragmatically specific and predictable utterances may well provide a base from which the child can begin to decipher semantic and syntactic categories.

For their part, children evolve from using reflexive, nonintentional communication to expressing conventional verbal intentions in the second year of life. Three developmental stages of early communication functions have been identified: the perlocutionary, in which children's behaviors are undifferentiated; the illocutionary, in which children use conventional gestures and vocalization to express intent; and the locutionary, in which words convey children's intentions (Bates, 1976). Thus, communication functions or intentions are well established before the child acquires linguistic structures.

Before she or he expresses the first meaningful word or shortly thereafter, a child is able to express a range of early intentions. Language structure is acquired as a more efficient means of communicating these intentions. The structure of these early utterances seems to be governed by the nonlinguistic context and by the assumptions of both communication partners. Syntactic correctness appears to have very little influence on the form of the young child's productions.

Children's utterances are produced to accompany joint action or to establish joint reference, and the form reflects these purposes. Thus, the child produces utterances within the very sequences her caregiver has employed for selective language input. There are two possible toddler generative systems: segmentation of action sequences and topic-comment. In **segmentation**, children structure their utterances to encode the changing elements of a situation. While the father throws a ball, the child might say "Throw ball," "Daddy throw," "Daddy ball," "Ball go," or "Go up." By contrast, in **topic-comment** structure, children establish the topic and then provide information on some element of that topic (Gruber, 1967). Having established the topic *doggie*, the child might elaborate to form "Doggie big," "Doggie bite," "Doggie bed," and so on. Obviously, the processes of segmentation of action and topic-comment can occur together.

The earliest one-word utterances are purely functional. Many of children's first words perform some function, such as *bye-bye* and *hi*, or are names of persons from whom they seek attention or of objects they want retrieved. Even two-word combinations may be more pragmatically based than semantic. The semantic rules described in this chapter do not account for all two-word combinations. In addition, utterances categorized as *Recurrent + Head* ("More juice," "'Nuther cookie") fulfill a requesting function almost exclusively.

Borrowing somewhat from Chomsky, we can posit a similar model of communication (Ninio & Snow, 1988) (Figure 2.5). The deep structure would include the purpose or the intent of the speaker. There are limited ways in which to express this intention. For example, if a speaker desires something, there is a restricted set of language options that will satisfy this intention. Although "May I have X, please," "X, please" or "Give me X" fulfills this intention, many other forms do not. The speaker selects the appropriate symbols and form to express this intention. Context influences the choice of appropriate utterance.

Parents respond to a child's early utterances by expanding the form or extending the meaning of the utterance, by offering a reply or comment, by imitating, or by giving feedback. In addition, parents continue to provide a simplified model of adult speech. As children begin using new structures, parents systematically modify their language model. Children continue to learn those structures that most effectively encode their intentions. In short, the child's language acquisition is embedded in, and dependent upon, her social context. Development reflects the child's communication needs and her knowledge and expectations of that context (Snow, 1984). Thus, the language-development process is a reciprocal one involving the language-developing child and a "socializer-teacher-nurturer" who is a competent language user (Holzman, 1984). The caregiver's modeling and feedback differ with the language level of the child.

Limitations

Like the other theoretical approaches, the sociolinguistic position alone does not adequately explain language acquisition. Although the evidence of early communication is great, this

FIGURE 2.5   Sociolinguistic Language-Processing Model

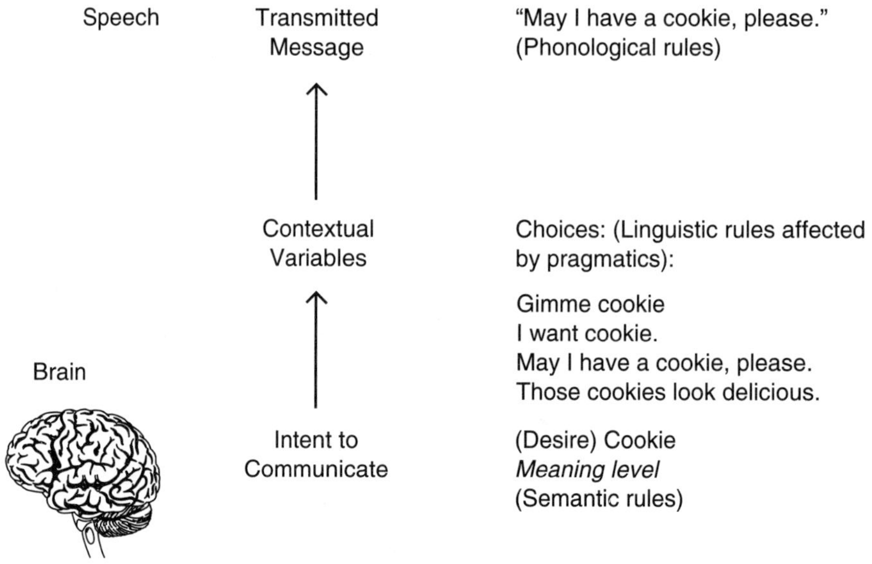

| Speech | Transmitted Message | "May I have a cookie, please." (Phonological rules) |

Speech — Transmitted Message — "May I have a cookie, please." (Phonological rules)

↑

Contextual Variables — Choices: (Linguistic rules affected by pragmatics):

Gimme cookie
I want cookie.
May I have a cookie, please.
Those cookies look delicious.

Brain

↑

Intent to Communicate — (Desire) Cookie
Meaning level
(Semantic rules)

evidence still does not explain how the child associates symbol and referent or how language structure is acquired. If, in fact, the child learns language to express intentions, there must be some underlying process by which intentions are linked to language form and content.

In addition, sociolinguistics as a field of study is so new that scholars have not had sufficient time to agree on classification systems. It is difficult to describe how a certain category of utterances developed when linguists cannot agree on the existence of that category of behavior.

Contributions

With the sociolinguistic approach, the study of child language has come almost full circle historically and theoretically. The sociolinguistic approach emphasizes language use or functions similar to Skinner's functional analysis. Language is employed to attain extralinguistic ends, and this attainment reinforces the linguistic behavior. The reinforcement in the sociolinguistic approach is qualitatively different, however, from that hypothesized by Skinner. Skinner envisaged a more direct type of reinforcement. In fact, the reinforcement process is more subtle and is grounded in the child-parent relationship. In most instances, the act of communication itself is reinforcing. The reinforcement may consist of closeness, caring, and needs fulfillment.

In addition to highlighting the social aspect of language learning, the sociolinguistic approach specifies the contribution of environmental linguistic input and the role of caregiver modeling and feedback. All of these contributions to children's learning are aspects of a general communication background established well before children begin to use language expressively.

The major conclusions of sociolinguistic thought are as follows (McLean & Snyder-McLean, 1978):

> Language is first acquired as a means of achieving already existing communicative functions . . . directly related to the . . . pragmatic aspect of later language.
>
> Linguistic structure is initially acquired through the process of decoding and comprehending incoming linguistic stimuli. . . .
>
> Language is learned in dynamic social interactions involving the child and the mature language users in his environment. The mature language users facilitate this process. . . .
>
> The child is an active participant in this transactional process and must contribute to it a set of behaviors which allow him to benefit from the adult's facilitating behaviors. (p. 78)

One outgrowth of this theory is the realization that many speech, language, and communication differences among children are just that, differences, and not disorders or improper usage. Communication effectiveness must be judged within the context in which it occurs. The question is, does the communication work? Child language behavior is now being examined using the same criteria, and there is a new appreciation for individual and cultural-ethnic-regional differences.

CONCLUSION

Within the past several decades, four major theories of language acquisition have been proposed: behavioral, psycholinguistic-syntactic, psycholinguistic-semantic/cognitive, and sociolinguistic. They are compared and contrasted in Table 2.2. Of course, there are hazards inherent in any summary table. These theoretical positions are much more complex than the table indicates. It reduces the linguistic theories to their most general common bases and ignores many minor differences. Such a summary can nevertheless be helpful.

Most linguists do not adhere strictly to one theoretical construct but prefer to position themselves somewhere between. This apparent fence-straddling reflects the complexity of language and language acquisition.

Initial language learning is "a process of cognitive socialization" (R. Brown, 1956, p. 247). The child's own meanings and uses become integrated with those of her or his environment through interaction. Language is interrelated with, but separate from, socioemotional and cognitive development. As the child matures, there is a gradual delineation of these separate aspects of development. To summarize:

> By nature of its content, language carries within it the products of the cognitive developmental domain; by nature of its function, language carries within it the products of human social development; by nature of its form, language carries within it the complex products of all of the inputs identified . . . plus the effect of the nature and functions of the human physiological and neurological systems. (McLean & Snyder-McLean, 1978, p. 43)

The relationship between language, cognition, and socioemotional development is not clearly understood (Howlin & Rutter, 1987). It is quite possible that for each child the

TABLE 2.2   Comparisons and Contrasts of Four Language Development Models

	BEHAVIORAL	PSYCHOLINGUISTIC-SYNTACTIC	PSYCHOLINGUISTIC-SEMANTIC/COGNITIVE	SOCIOLINGUISTIC
Language Form	Functional units (mands, tacts)	Syntactic units (nouns, verbs)	Semantic units (agents, objects)	Functional units: speech acts (requesting, commenting)
Method of Aquisition	Selective reinforcement of correct form	Language-acquisition device (LAD) contains universal phrase structure rules used to decipher the transformational rules of language	Universal cognitive structures help child establish nonlinguistic relationships later expressed as semantic relations	Early communication established through which child expresses intentions preverbally; language develops to express early intentions
Environmental Input	Reinforcement and extinction; parental modeling	Minimal	Cognitive relationships established through active involvement of child with environment	Communicative interaction established first; parental modeling and feedback

relative contribution of each of these aspects will differ greatly. Their contributions may also differ with the developmental level of the child. Indeed, there is evidence that, at certain stages of development, the relationships between the linguistic, social, and cognitive domains differ.

Finally, we must face the possibility that none of the descriptive units used within the four theoretical models has any reality for children. In each case, linguists have imposed adult classification models upon child language. Children may be organizing their worlds in very nonadult ways as they play and explore, as they fantasize and create, and as they think and speak.

DISCUSSION

You're probably wondering how you'll ever keep the theories separate in your mind. Well, you're not the first student to wrestle with this conundrum. It might help to see the contributions of each to our understanding of development.

Thanks to the work of Chomsky and other psycholinguists, we recognize that there is most likely a biological basis for language. It may not be as specific as the phrase–structure rules, but human brains are specialized for analyzing sequential information such as language.

The sociolinguists would also contend that the infant has certain innate social and communicative abilities that enable the child to establish early communication with care-givers. In turn, these caregivers interact in such a way as to insure the survival of the infant and, ultimately, the species. It is within these interactions that the child is exposed to language, the source of the child's own language use.

From a well-established communication system and armed with certain cognitive skills, as the psycholinguistic: cognitive/semantic theories suggest, the infant begins to use the language of those around him or her. As the sociolinguists remind us, this language has many uses, most already established through gestures. In other words, the language is not just an imitation of the language that surrounds the child.

The toddler uses language in many ways and treats different words in differing ways. One difference is the way in which words are combined and the specific placement of words. These reflect word order rules based on semantic categories of words. Language input is provided by caregivers who systematically modify their language to the child, as the sociolinguists suggest, and respond to the child in ways that keep the child communicating. In other words, replying to the child is reinforcing—something near and dear to behaviorists.

From this base, the child begins to explore language and to construct language rules, possibly following some of the constructs of the psycholinguists, such as the government-binding theory. In the process, the child takes his or her concepts and transforms them into language. Government-binding theories remind us of the interdependence of syntax, morphology, phonology, and semantics. Sociolinguists would insist that these four only make sense when we consider the effect of context on the production and comprehension of language.

Phew, we sure compressed that information. My take was necessarily a quick gloss over all of the information in this chapter, but it hopefully helped you see the big picture.

REFLECTIONS

1. Explain the several limitations of the behavioral model that are addressed within the psycholinguistic-syntactic model.

2. Describe how a sentence is produced using the two rule systems of the psycholinguistic-syntactic model.

3. The psycholinguistic-syntactic model demonstrates some limitations when applied to child language. Explain this inadequacy and the way it is addressed by the psycholinguistic-semantic model.

4. Describe the main features of the government-binding theory.

5. Part of the appeal of the psycholinguistic-semantic theory is the relationship between cognition and semantics. Explain this relationship.

6. In what way does the sociolinguistic model differ from the two psycholinguistic models?

7. Can you explain the relationship between deep structure and surface structure? The benefit of a rich interpretation and its relationship to child-based semantics?

3

Child Development

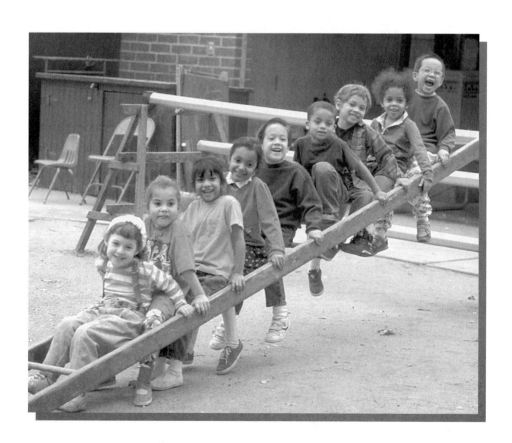

CHAPTER OBJECTIVES

Language is only one aspect, although a very important and complex one, of child development. To understand language development and keep it in perspective, we should have some knowledge of the overall development of the child. In this chapter we will explore this development, with special emphasis on the development of speech. When you have completed this chapter, you should understand

- the major patterns of development.
- the sources of speech production.
- the major reflexes of the newborn relative to oral movement.
- the characteristics of babbling and reduplicated and variegated babbling.
- the general behaviors of two-, three-, four-, and five-year-olds.
- the overall conclusions of several studies of speech sound development.
- the general changes that occur in the development of the school-aged child.
- the following terms:

articulation	neonate
babbling	oral cavity
cephalocaudal	pharynx
convergent semantic production	phonation
divergent semantic production	phonetically consistent forms (PCFs)
echolalia	quasi-resonant nuclei (QRN)
figurative language	reduplicated babbling
fully resonant nuclei (FRN)	reflexes
jargon	resonation
larynx	respiration
myelination	variegated babbling
nasal cavity	vocal folds

When studying language development, we can easily forget that children are also developing in many other ways. Far from being static and unchanging, children are growing and learning continually. We must understand children's growth and development to appreciate fully the behavioral changes associated with language.

In addition, students of language acquisition should remind themselves of the joy and wonder of childhood. Dry academic study can cause us to forget such youthful inquiries as the following from my daughter while riding in the car:

Daddy, do you think that maybe the trees are moving and that we're standing still? Maybe we just think that we're moving because the trees are.

Language is used by all of us to describe, explain, and inquire about the world around us. For children, this world is a fascinating wonder that often is controlled by unseen forces that we adults can only imagine.

DEVELOPMENTAL PATTERNS

Development is more than a cumulative list of changes and accomplishments. Each individual's growth reveals certain patterns. Several generalizations or principles are evident:

1. Development is predictable.
2. Developmental milestones are attained at about the same age in most children.
3. Developmental opportunity is needed.
4. Children go through developmental phases or periods.
5. Individuals differ greatly.

Developmental Predictability

The developmental pattern is predictable in character. There is an orderly sequence. For example, motor development proceeds from the head down. This is called **cephalocaudal** progression. Thus, a child is able to hold his head up before he can sit unsupported. In addition, he usually crawls prior to walking. Language development also follows a predictable pattern: initially, a child babbles, then says individual words, then sentences.

Developmental Milestones

In general, children attain certain skills or abilities at predictable ages. Although there is some individual variation, most children without disabilities reach such milestones as walking and talking at about the same age. For example, somewhere around the first birthday, a child will take the first unaided step and say his or her first meaningful word.

Developmental Opportunity

Although much development is the result of maturation, learning is also important. The opportunity for learning must be present in order for the child to develop. Walking will not occur on schedule without an opportunity to practice the needed prerequisite skills. A corollary to this principle is that opportunity is wasted if the child has not attained the required maturational level. A six-month-old child does not have the intellectual and physical abilities to read, and no amount of practice can compensate for these deficits.

In general, a child practices through play—an active, pleasurable, spontaneous, and voluntary involvement with the environment. Play is a nonserious, self-contained activity motivated by sheer enjoyment. Within play, a child imitates others or himself in endless repetition until a skill is perfected.

Developmental Phases or Periods

Development does not occur as a straight line. There are orderly, predictable phases in which certain areas of development are emphasized. For example, there are two phases of rapid physical growth: from prenatal development to about six months, and from age ten or twelve years to about fifteen or sixteen. As expected, nutritional needs are greatest dur-

TABLE 3.1   Height and Weight Ranges of Developing Children

AGE	HEIGHT	WEIGHT
Newborn	17–21 inches	6–8 pounds
4 months	23–24 inches	12–16 pounds
8 months	26–28 inches	
12 months	28–30 inches	26–30 pounds
2 years	32–34 inches	
5 years	40–42 inches	3–5 pounds/year
5 years–puberty	3 inches/year	

ing these periods. During other periods, the rate of growth is greatly decelerated. Within the first year of life, a child approximately triples in weight. If this rate of growth were to continue, he or she would weigh over 1,240,000 pounds by age eleven. In fact, the typical eleven-year-old weighs approximately seventy to eighty pounds. General height and weight data are presented in Table 3.1. Note the amount of change in the child's height and weight. Phases of physical growth do not necessarily coincide with other phases of development, such as cognition or socialization. Each area has its own developmental cycle.

Even within a given developmental area, the type of development changes as a child matures. For example, initial language development emphasizes vocabulary growth, which decelerates as syntactic growth is stressed. Physical growth of body parts also varies with the developmental level. Each part reaches maturity at its own rate, with its own growth phases; thus, the physical growth pattern is *asynchronous*. Some organs, such as the inner ear, the eyes, and the brain, reach mature size very early. Other parts of the body, such as the limbs, reach mature size only at the conclusion of puberty. This asynchronous growth is also reflected in the amount of development within different body parts. The head increases to twice its size from birth to maturity, whereas the torso increases to three times its birth size and the limbs to four to five times their size. As body proportions change, so does weight distribution. The brain, which accounts for one-eighth of total body weight at birth, equals only one-fortieth by maturity. The greatest gain in brain weight is within the first two years.

Individual Differences

Even though there are predictable stages and ages for development, the range of normality is broad. No individual child should be expected to conform to all of the averages or milestones presented. Mean ages, weights, or heights do not describe any given child but rather some fictitious "average" child, who is a combination of all children. A child who is outside the norms may be experiencing a momentary acceleration or delay or may be proceeding at his own individual pace. Even a child with severe retardation is a developing being; his personal schedule may be delayed beyond the normal period, but development proceeds nonetheless.

Normative data are meant as a guide. Beginning students of child development should avoid the pitfall of using this information in a diagnostic manner. Concerned parents must be cautious of normative data as well. Child–parent interactions do not need the added anxiety of slavish adherence to some normative timetable.

Individual development depends on many factors, including genetic inheritance, nutrition, gender, intelligence, overall emotional and physical health, socioeconomic level, ethnicity, and prenatal conditions. Other conditions being equal—which they never are—a child can be expected to develop more quickly if he or she has good nutrition, a high IQ, good overall health, a high socioeconomic status, and good prenatal conditions. The effects of these factors vary with age, and most of these factors are interrelated.

THE DEVELOPING CHILD

The remainder of this chapter presents a general child-development chronology, with emphasis on four related, but separate, developmental areas: physical, cognitive, socioemotional, and communicative growth.

Physical development refers to physical growth and motor control. Here several related hierarchies apply: cephalocaudal, proximodistal, and gross-to-fine development. Cephalocaudal, or head-to-foot, development was discussed earlier. Proximodistal development is from the center out and is related to the gross-to-fine hierarchy. We will be concerned with the proximodistal progression when we discuss the development of control of the speech mechanism. In addition, development proceeds from gross-motor to fine-motor control. Gross-motor, or large-muscle, movements are those of the head, torso, and limbs. These movements are used in walking, running, throwing, head turning, and so on.

Most children have attained gross-motor control by age four or five. Fine-motor, or small-muscle, control involves the eyes, hands, fingers, and so on. Much of this control is gained during the early school years. By age twelve, a child has adultlike control of the arms, wrists, and shoulders. Adultlike finger control is gained later, although a child can write, draw, and perform other fine-motor behaviors before adolescence. The muscular control needed for both types of motor control depends, in part, on nervous system maturation. At birth, the spinal cord is more mature than the higher centers of the brain. The senses send a signal to the spinal cord, brain stem, or midbrain, and an immediate, reflexive response is returned to the affected muscles. As a child matures, the higher portions of the brain develop and the child attains increased control over finer and finer muscle movement and there is less involuntary movement.

Cognitive development is intellectual growth. Beyond growth and internal development of the brain and spinal cord, cognitive development also involves the methods a child uses to organize, store, and retrieve information for problem solving and generalization. Each child perceives the world differently and must interpret incoming stimuli in light of his past experiences. Thus, even reception of new stimuli is not a passive process but involves interpretation and organization. As a child matures, he or she organizes incoming stimuli in different ways. Memory also increases. Part of this change is due to increased brain weight. Other changes can be attributed to learning. By age eight, the brain is nearly mature in size but not in structure. Further development concentrates on internal growth and maturation.

Socioemotional development is closely related to the other three areas. Physical size and prowess, intellectual growth, and communication abilities all contribute to a child's perceptions of self and of others. As a child matures, he or she becomes less egocentric and more social. By comparison, the seeming isolation of the child with autism stands out.

Although humans are social beings, each must learn social behaviors and the social rules and customs of his or her society.

Finally, communicative development is also related to the other developmental areas. The development and use of linguistic symbols depends on attaining certain cognitive, social, and motor skills. Speech requires the physical growth of certain neuromuscular structures and motor control of their functions.

The human body is, among other things, a sound–production source. As with any sound source, there must be power to drive the mechanism, and there must be a vibrating body. In speech, humans produce a great variety of sounds, so the human body must also be capable of modifying or resonating the vibrations produced.

The source of energy is compressed air in the lungs. Adults exchange this air with air in the environment approximately twelve times each minute. This process of inhaling and exhaling air, and the resultant gas exchange in the lungs, is called **respiration**. Air expelled from the lungs passes between the **vocal folds**, located in the **larynx** (Figure 3.1). In speech, the air may vibrate the vocal folds rapidly in a process called **phonation**, resulting in a series

FIGURE 3.1 The Speech Mechanism

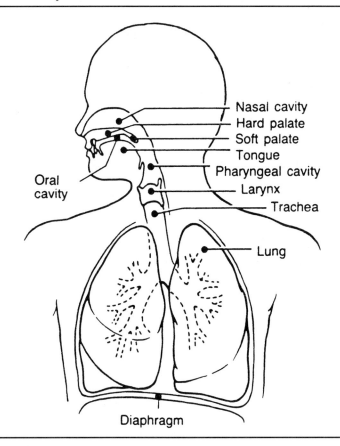

Nasal cavity
Hard palate
Soft palate
Tongue
Pharyngeal cavity
Oral cavity
Larynx
Trachea
Lung
Diaphragm

of short puffs of air that occur so rapidly that they are perceived as a sustained, low-pitched buzz or laryngeal tone. Above the level of the larynx, in the vocal tract, this tone is modified by the joint processes of **resonation** and **articulation**. The vocal tract consists of the throat, or **pharynx**; the mouth, or **oral cavity**; and the **nasal cavity**. By varying the shape of the vocal tract, the speaker changes the resonating characteristics of the laryngeal tone. Sounds are more precisely altered by articulation of specific speech sounds. This production is accomplished by restricting or momentarily blocking the exhaled air in the vocal tract using the tongue, palate, teeth, and lips. The resulting acoustic signals are perceived as speech sounds.

The following sections examine the different stages of a child's growth, with emphasis on the four types of development—physical, cognitive, socioemotional, and communicative—and the relationships among them.

The New Kid in Town: Age Birth to One Month

The newborn, or **neonate**, is hardly the "thing of beauty" that most people expect. Most neonates are very different from the plump, active, gregarious infants seen only a few months later. Usually, the skin is red and wrinkled and covered with a white, waxy material called *vernix*. This covering protects the newborn's skin and helps it slip through the birth canal. This passage may have left the newborn's face bluish and puffy, with his or her ears pressed against the sides of the head. Frequently, the top of the head is swollen and misshapen from the pressure of passage. The head is a third to a quarter of the total body length, as opposed to an eighth for adults, and makes the neonate appear top-heavy and awkward. In fact, the area above the eyes is much larger in relation to the total head size than the proportions found in adults. The head may be bald or covered by hair that may fall out later. The torso is small in comparison to the head, and the limbs are even more so. The newborn has narrow shoulders and a bulky middle, and a fine matte of hair called *lanugo* may cover his or her entire body.

Soon after birth, the newborn falls into a deep sleep of fourteen to eighteen hours to conserve energy for stabilizing such body functions as the rates of circulation and respiration and the process of digestion. At birth the newborn is generally unable to maintain homeostasis, a relatively stable condition of temperature, functioning, and chemical composition. In general, he or she breathes twice as fast as an adult, and his or her heart beats at 120 times per minute versus seventy for an adult. Frequently, the newborn is unable to digest milk for a few days, so fatty reserves must sustain him or her.

The newborn is unable to control motor behavior smoothly and voluntarily. Instead, behaviors consist of twitches, jerks, and random movements, most of which involve automatic, involuntary motor patterns called **reflexes**. There are two general types of reflexes: mass activity and specific activity. *Mass activity* occurs when the whole body responds to stimulation of one part, such as to temperature, light, and sound changes. *Specific activity* involves stimulation and response within a specific muscle group or portion of the body. The newborn's primary reflexes, listed in Table 3.2, allow him or her to react to things in the world while learning to control his or her body. In addition, reflexes help to ensure survival by protecting vital systems. For example, the gag reflex protects the lungs from inhalation of ingested fluids. Even smiling is reflexive in the newborn, occurring when the cheek or lips are touched.

Although some reflexes, such as gagging, coughing, yawning, and sneezing, remain for life, most disappear or are modified by six months of age. This disappearance is related

TABLE 3.2   Reflexes of the Newborn

REFLEX NAME	STIMULATION	RESPONSE
Babinski	Stroking side of foot from heel to toe	Big toe lifts and other toes spread out
Babkin	Applying pressure on both palms while child is lying on back	Eyes close, mouth opens, and head turns toward the midline
Biceps	Tapping tendon of bicep	Short contraction of the bicep
Blink	Flashing light	Both eyelids close
Doll's eye	Turning head slowly with hand	Eyes stay fixed instead of moving with head
Galant	Stroking back to one side of spine	Trunk arches toward side on which stroked
Knee jerk or patellar tendon	Tapping on tendon below patella or knee cap	Kick or quick extension of lower leg
Moro	Making a sudden loud noise or jarring; dropping head a few inches; or dropping baby a few inches	Arms extend and then come together as hands open and then clench; spine and legs extend
Palmar or automatic hand grasp	Pressing infant's palm	Fingers grasp object
Perez	Stroking baby's spine from tail toward head	Cry and head extension
Phasic bite	Touching or rubbing the gums	Bite-release mouth pattern
Plantor or toe grasp	Applying pressure to balls of feet	Toes flex
Rooting	Stroking cheek at corner of mouth	Head turns toward side being stroked; mouth begins sucking movements
Stepping	Holding infant supported with feet touching level surface; moving infant forward	Rhythmic stepping movements
Sucking	Inserting finger or nipple into mouth	Rhythmic sucking
Withdrawal	Pricking sole of foot with pin	Knee and foot flex

to the rapid rate of brain growth and to myelination. The rate of brain growth is greatest immediately following birth; in fact, no other body system develops as rapidly. Reflexes originate in the brain stem, the only part of the brain fully functional at birth. They are gradually replaced by more sophisticated motor skills as the brain learns to deliver increasingly more precise signals to the neurons. **Myelination** is the development of a protective myelin sheath around the cranial nerves. When myelination is complete, the organism has the capacity for full neural functioning.

The phasic bite and the rooting reflex are present at birth but disappear by three months of age. The phasic bite reflex is a bite-release action that occurs when the newborn's gums receive tactile stimulation. The rooting reflex results from tactile stimulation of the cheek near the mouth. In response, the newborn's lips, tongue, and jaw all move toward the area of stimulation. This reflex is often seen during nursing.

The reflex of most interest for speech development is the rhythmic suck-swallow pattern, which is first established at six months postconception, or three months before birth. Like other reflexes, sucking involves only the midbrain and brain stem. At birth, sucking is primarily accomplished by up-and-down jaw action. Within a few weeks, the newborn develops more lateral movement. Back-and-forth jaw movement appears at about one month. In order to suck, the neonate uncouples, or seals off, the nasal cavity by raising the velum, or soft palate; the newborn can then create a vacuum in the mouth, or oral cavity, by lowering the mandible or lower jaw, thus increasing the volume of the space. To swallow, the neonate opens his or her mouth slightly and protrudes and then retracts the tongue. Although this action is greatly reduced by three months of age, it is not until around three years of age that independent swallowing appears. To complete a swallow, the neonate must also close, or abduct, the vocal folds to protect the lungs.

The newborn is not totally helpless, however, but instead possesses many skills (Table 3.3). Shortly after birth the newborn is able to breathe on his or her own and ingest food,

TABLE 3.3 The Newborn's Behaviors

MOTOR	COGNITION	SOCIALIZATION	COMMUNICATION
Makes reflexive movements of head and limbs Makes nonspecific, random, nonreflexive movements Exhibits mass response to sudden changes Moves head side to side when on back Cannot raise head when on stomach Eyes frequently do not converge	Sees best at 7-1/2 inches; is sensitive to brightness and color; can follow a moving object; visually prefers movement, sharp contours, and contrasts Is sensitive to volume, pitch, and duration of sound (slight hearing loss until middle ear clear); discriminates sound sources; prefers hearing human voice Is sensitive to temperature changes Discriminates smells and tastes Screens out stimuli Is alert less than 5% of the day	Recognizes nipple Is comforted by sound of human voice Sleeps about 70% of the day Smiles reflexively	Cries Makes noncrying speechlike sounds, usually when feeding

coordinating the two to ensure that the food passes down the appropriate tube. In addition, the newborn is able to process ingested fluids, usually milk, and to eliminate waste. The newborn can turn its head from side to side and signal distress by crying.

Newborns produce predominantly reflexive sounds, such as fussing and crying, and vegetative sounds, such as burping and swallowing. Reflexive sounds are primarily produced on exhalation and consist of relatively lengthy voiced sounds of a vowel-like nature (Stark, 1986). In contrast, vegetative sounds, associated with activity and management of nutrients, are produced equally on inhalation and exhalation, voiced or voiceless, consonant- and vowel-like, and are of brief duration. Production of both decreases with maturation (Stark, Bernstein, & Demorest, 1993).

Some vegetative sounds, such as coughing, belching, and sneezing, which persist into adulthood, are defenses against penetration by substances that might choke the infant. Other sounds, such as gulping and clicking, result from unstable positioning of the vocal mechanism and from adaptations to oral reflexes and to swallowing.

Infant crying has been the subject of much study because of its early communication value. Initially, the newborn cries on both inhalation and exhalation, but there are many individual variations. The expiration phase of breathing gradually increases with crying. The relative amount of crying also varies with the time of day. Crying is most frequent before feeding and bed.

Although it has been claimed that a newborn's cries are undifferentiated, four basic cries have been identified within the first month. The first cry heard, of course, is the birth cry, consisting of two gasps followed by a wail that lasts for one second, with a flat, falling tone. Later, three cries can be differentiated: the basic cry, the pain cry, and the temper cry. The basic or hunger cry consists of a rhythmic pattern of loud crying, silence, whistling inhalation, and rest. During the rest, the infant may emit the sucking response. The pain cry, a loud, shrill cry, consists of one long cry followed by a long breath-holding silence and a series of short whimpers. Frequently, this cry is accompanied by tense facial muscles, frowns, and clenched fists. Finally, the anger cry is an exasperated sound because of the greater volume of air expended. By the end of the first month, the mother or the primary caregiver can usually ascertain the reason for the cry by its sound pattern.

Crying helps the child become accustomed to air flow across the vocal folds and to modified breathing patterns. Since speech sounds originate at the level of the larynx, this early stimulation is important. The modified breathing will progress to the lengthened exhalations of speech.

Usually, other noncrying sounds accompany feeding or are produced in response to smiling or talking by the mother. These noncrying vowel-like sounds with brief consonantal elements have been characterized as **quasi-resonant nuclei (QRN)**. QRN contain phonation, or vibration at the larynx, but the child does not have sufficient control of the vocal mechanism to resonate either consonants or full vowels. Resonation, you will recall, is a modification of the vibratory pattern of the laryngeal tone through changes in the size and configuration of the vocal tract, which consists of the nasal cavity; the oral cavity, or mouth; and the pharynx, or throat. QRN are probably the result of opening the mouth less than an adult would when resonating a sound. Considerable air is emitted via the nasal cavity, and the resultant sounds range from partial nasal consonants to a nasalized high-to-mid vowel. Initially, production of these sounds is caused accidentally by chance movements of the vocal folds. QRN tend to be individual sounds. Later, these sounds become sound sequences. The amounts of time spent in crying and cooing are inversely related: as vocal behaviors increase, crying decreases.

The vocal tract of the neonate resembles those of nonhuman primates more closely than that of an adult human (Figure 3.2). Thus, the noncrying sounds tend to be nasalized because of the relative height of the larynx and the close proximity of the larynx and the vocal tract. During crying, the lower jaw and tongue are dropped and the soft palate and pharyngeal wall move rearward, resulting in the vowel-like quality of distress sounds. At other times, the tongue is in close proximity to or touching the soft palate. Thus, many of the comfort sounds have a nasal consonantlike character.

The newborn also has perceptual skills of some magnitude, especially in sight and hearing. Nearsighted at birth, the newborn can see things best about eight inches away. Still, he or she is sensitive to both brightness and color and will close his or her eyes to a very intense light. Although the newborn can follow a moving object visually from side to side, its eyes don't always converge on the object. Generally, convergence is confined to non-moving objects.

FIGURE 3.2   Comparison of the Oral Structures of the Infant and Adult

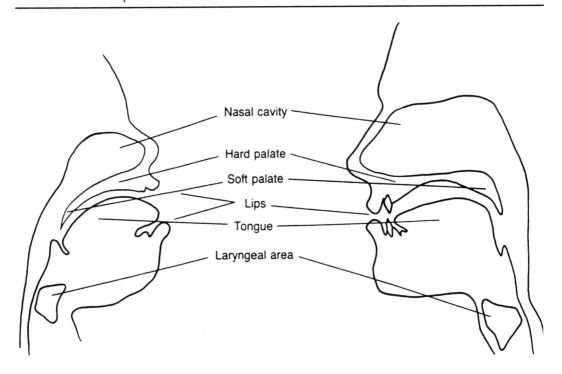

Nasal cavity

Hard palate

Soft palate

Lips

Tongue

Laryngeal area

In part, the differences in the sounds of infants and adults can be explained by the physical differences of the two. In this schematic, the infant has been enlarged to the approximate size of an adult.

Short-term visual memory is present in the newborn but is limited to recognition when the object reappears within two and one-half seconds. Within limits, the newborn learns to distinguish some people and objects. Newborns tend to rely on patterns for recognition, with special emphasis on high-contrast areas. For example, newborns concentrate on such features as the hairline and eyes when viewing the face. Concentration on high-contrast areas is an effective visual strategy when full-field focus is unavailable. It is not until about three months of age, when he or she gains full field vision and better eye control, that the infant prefers the complexity of a whole object. Prior to this age, the infant prefers to concentrate on particular attractive parts.

At birth, the newborn scans the environment visually during only about 5 percent of his or her waking hours. This amount increases to 35 percent by the tenth week. The newborn becomes "stuck" on any visually interesting object that comes into view. Not until about four or five months does the infant gain sufficient ocular control to move smoothly from object to object, thus gaining control over attending.

In general, newborns attend to objects of interest and have definite preferences. They prefer objects that move, have sharp contours, or have contrasts of light and dark. These preferences change with visual abilities. In general, the infant is attracted by visual stimuli that can activate his or her current level of neural activity (Haith, 1976). For example, the two-month-old infant has certain short-term mental images for common objects in the environment. He or she will attend to objects that differ slightly from the mental image already established.

In addition to visual skills, the newborn possesses auditory abilities. The middle and inner ears reach their adult size at twenty weeks of fetal development and, therefore, are ready to function at birth. The auditory cortex is not mature, however, and the middle ear is filled with fluid. The immaturity of the cortex and the lack of internal coordination of the brain's hemispheres make it difficult for the newborn to integrate sounds. In addition, the middle ear is not as sensitive to sound as it will be within two weeks after birth, when the fluid is absorbed. Despite these limitations, the newborn can distinguish loudness or intensity and duration of sound. The newborn blinks, jerks, draws in a breath, and increases his or her heart and respiration rates in response to sounds.

Within the first four days, the infant can discriminate between different sounds. In fact, infant and adult perceptual skills with phonetic contrasts are very similar. The only exception is the distinction between /f/ and the voiceless *th* (/θ/), which is difficult for children until about five years of age. Because infant perception studies use a constant phonetic context in which contrasted sounds always appear with the same adjacent sounds, as in *pet* and *bet*, it is not clear whether newborns are able to identify the same phoneme in different phonetic environments, as in *pet* and *poor*.

It must be stressed that discrimination of speech sounds is not the same as linguistic perception. Speech-sound discrimination does not involve sound–meaning relationships. The infant has only limited memory. In order to develop spoken language, the child must be able to store sounds, to use this information for later comparison and identification, and to relate these sounds to meaning.

The newborn has auditory as well as visual preferences. Above all, the infant seems to prefer the sound of the human voice which has a quieting effect.

Although vision and audition will be very important for later communication development, they are not the newborn's only sensory abilities. He or she can sense body temperature changes and respond accordingly. Within fifty-five hours of birth, newborns can differentiate smells. Finally, newborns can discriminate different tastes and prefer sweet tastes to sour ones.

At birth, the child is not the active, outgoing infant we will see later. He or she already has the abilities, however, to respond to the world. In the next few months, the infant will begin to explore the physical and social worlds around him or her.

The Examiner: Age One to Six Months

During the first six months of life (Table 3.4), the child gains voluntary muscle control rapidly and begins to examine objects, people, and events that occur close at hand. Increased motor abilities enable the infant to sit, thus freeing his or her hands for object appraisal. Vision and reach become coordinated, and the infant is able to reach and grasp. Social behaviors also increase as the child gains the ability to recognize and respond to familiar faces and situations.

The big events of the first six months are those that accompany the downward progression of large-muscle control and the further maturation of the brain. The infant goes from reflexive and random behaviors to rolling and creeping. Better control accompanies firmer muscles and bones and the building of new neural connectors.

Initially, the infant gains control of the head, lifting and then being able to hold it steady. This positioning provides a new perspective from which to examine the environment. At about the same time, approximately three months of age, the infant gains full focus, which enables him or her to appreciate all the new visual stimuli available. Head and neck control is followed by trunk control and sitting. In the upright position, the infant's hands are free to examine small objects. The infant is able to grasp voluntarily at two months of age but cannot control his or her reach. Increasing arm control enables the infant to hit, then reach for, and finally grasp objects. Toy or object play will begin shortly after some measure of hand control is achieved. Grasping is still somewhat primitive, however, with the fingers generally undifferentiated, as in a mitten. Most objects are brought to the mouth, a very sensitive and highly developed area, for tactile examination and identification.

As early as two months, the infant develops distinct nutritive and nonnutritive sucking behaviors. By four months of age, the infant engages in up to four hours per day of nonnutritive sucking of fingers and objects and of examining its face and mouth.

Neuromuscular control moves forward from the back of the oral cavity, reflecting the progression of myelination in the primary motor cortex and the proximodistal hierarchy. With greater control of the tongue, the infant exhibits tongue cupping and strong tongue projection. If you have ever attempted to spoon-feed a four- to six-month-old, you will recall the difficulty of inserting the spoon because the infant protrudes the tongue. Food constantly reappears on the infant's lips and chin. In sucking, the infant is also able to use the intrinsic muscles of the tongue rather than a whole-jaw movement as before.

The infant's bite is more volitional, and he or she no longer relies on tactile stimulation. The child can place its lips around a spoon and use them to ingest the contents.

Toward the end of the first half-year, large-muscle control has progressed so that the infant can crouch on his or her hands and knees and can roll over and creep, two early

TABLE 3.4   The Examiner: One to Six Months

AGE (MONTHS)	MOTOR	COGNITION	SOCIALIZATION	COMMUNICATION
1	Moves limbs reflexively Lifts head while on stomach but cannot support head while body held upright; head flops backward Has coordinated side-to-side eye movement; stares but does not reach	Cries from distress Prefers visual patterns Remembers an object that reappears within 2-1/2 seconds	Establishes eye contact with mother Quiets when held; adjusts body to person holding Follows own sleep schedule Smiles spontaneously	Responds to human voice, which usually has quieting effect Cries for assistance Makes pleasure sounds, quasi-resonant nuclei
2	Moves arms in circle smoothly; swipes at objects Holds head up briefly while on stomach; raises head while sitting supported but head bobs Opens and closes hand; holds for few seconds.	Visually prefers face to objects, regards own hands, and follows in a circle Repeats own actions Excites in anticipation of objects Increased awareness of environmental stimuli	Excites when sees people; has unselective social smile Quiets self with sucking Prefers touch and oral stimulation to social stimulation Sleeps on schedule closer to rest of household	Distinguishes different (speech) sounds Makes more gutteral or "throaty" gooing
3	Lifts head and chest while prone; holds head up with minimum bobbing while sitting supported Can swallow voluntarily Reaches and grasps; keeps hands open frequently Swipes at dangling objects Kicks more forceful with hip and knee flexibility.	Attains full focus; can glance smoothly between objects Visually searches for sounds Begins exploratory play; explores own body Stops sucking to attend to parents voice	Exhibits gregarious behavior Visually discriminates different people and things; recognizes mother Has selective social smile Sleeps most of the night	Coos single syllable (consonant-vowel) Turns head when hears a voice Responds vocally to speech of others Makes predominantly vowel sounds

(continued)

TABLE 3.4   Continued

AGE (MONTHS)	MOTOR	COGNITION	SOCIALIZATION	COMMUNICATION
4	Can turn head in all directions whether body is prone or seated; complete rollover. On stomach: Raises head and chest supported on arms. Occasionally opposes thumb and fingers, as a mitten; grasps small objects put in hand; brings objects to mouth	Localizes to sound Stares at place from which object is dropped Remembers visually for 5–7 seconds Recognizes mother in group; senses strange places and people	Pays selective attention to faces: Looks longer at joyful versus angry face; discriminates different faces Looks in direction of person leaving room Smiles at notice of another baby Anticipates being lifted; laughs when played with	Babbles strings of consonants Varies pitch Imitates tones Smiles at person speaking to him
5	Sits supported for up to half an hour Rolls from stomach to back Can be easily pulled to stand Has partial thumb opposition; swaps objects from hand to hand Grabs feet and brings to mouth	Begins to play Visually follows a vanishing object; recognizes familiar objects; anticipates whole object after seeing a part, is capable of 3-hour visual memory Explores objects by mouthing and touching Remembers own actions in immediate past	Reacts differently to smiling and scolding Discriminates parents and siblings from others Imitates some movements of others Frolics when played with Displays anger when objects taken away.	Vocalizes to toys Discriminates angry and friendly voices Experiments with sound Imitates some sounds Responds to name Smiles and vocalizes to image in mirror
6	Turns head freely Sits straight when slightly supported or in chair Balances well Reaches with one arm, grasps, and brings to mouth Holds bottle Turns and twists in all directions Creeps	Looks and reaches smoothly and quickly Inspects objects Reaches to grab dropped objects	Differentiates social responses Prefers people games, such as "peek-a-boo" Feeds self finger food Explores face of person holding him	Varies volume, pitch, and rate Vocalizes pleasure and displeasure: squeals with excitement, intones displeasure

forms of locomotion. When creeping, the infant keeps the stomach on the floor while pushing with his or her feet and steering with outstretched arms. Since the muscles for forward movement are not as strong as those for backward movement, the infant often goes in reverse. Small-muscle development enables the child to hold a bottle and to feed with its hands, although most of the food is smeared across the face.

Reaching and object examination become increasingly directed by vision, which now can focus on the hands at different distances. Even so, reaching seems to require the infant's total concentration.

The increased visual abilities used for directing reach also aid the infant's social development. As early as the first month, the infant becomes excited upon seeing objects and people, although he or she does not respond differentially. By the second month, periods of responsiveness expand to up to twenty minutes. They are accompanied by arching, turning, twisting, and kicking. Certain people become associated with particular behaviors. For example, the infant's mother becomes associated with feeding, and the infant will begin a sucking response upon seeing her. This recognition of familiar people, plus the infant's rapid habituation to, or boredom with, other visual stimuli, signify an increase in visual memory. By three months of age, the infant is able to discriminate different people visually and to respond accordingly.

This change is reflected in stages of smile development. At the end of the first month, the infant's smile becomes less automatic, but it is still unselective. The infant will respond to both people and objects with a whole-body movement that includes limb and trunk activation and vocalizations. During the third month, as the child becomes more responsive to people, he or she smiles less at objects. In turn, his or her smile becomes more social and physically broader, with a crinkling around the eyes. This responsiveness is reflected in the infant's selective attention at four months of age to specific individuals and to joyful expressions longer than to angry ones. Although the infant learns to suck and look simultaneously by four months of age, often he or she will ignore feeding in order to concentrate on "people watching." Such visual attending also reflects increased visual memory, which, by five months of age, has expanded to three hours, unless there are competing visual stimuli. By six months, the infant is very social. The infant smiles and vocalizes, examines faces visually and tactilely, and responds differentially. He or she cries or draws back from unfamiliar faces.

Visual responsiveness and memory are also reflected in increased communication skills. The two-month-old will search for its mother by visually tracking her voice but will avert his gaze from the direction of strange voices. Although the two-month-old infant can discriminate between /p/, which is made at the lips, and /g/, which is produced in the throat, he or she cannot discriminate between /p/ and /b/, both made at the lips.

By two months of age, the infant has developed oral muscle control to stop and start movement definitively, though tactile stimulation is still needed. This stage is characterized by laughter and nondistress "gooing." Gooing consists of "vocalizations in which QRN occur in the same breath group with a velar to uvular closure or near closure" (Oller, 1978, p. 534). Thus, the infant produces back consonant and middle and back vowel sounds with incomplete resonance. The consonant sounds consist of velar or soft-palate fricatives similar to /s/ and incomplete velar plosives similar to /k/ and /g/. See the appendix for a description of speech-sound production and terminology.

The infant does control the timing of vocalizations, and it is this timing that demonstrates his or her responsiveness. By three months of age, the infant vocalizes in response to the speech of others. An infant is most responsive if his or her caregivers respond. During vocal turn-taking with a caregiver, three-month-olds produce more speech-like syllabic vocalizations than isolated vowel sounds (Masataka, 1995). These are accompanied by index finger extensions, a possible early precursor to later developing gestures. These reactive vocalizations continue throughout the first year and into the second even though other vocal and verbal behaviors are added to the child's repertoire (Stark et al., 1993). As the infant's repertoire of responses expands, the amount of crying and vegetative sounds decreases markedly. By sixteen weeks, sustained laughter, characterized by a rapid alternation of voiced and voiceless sounds, emerges. A sample of the speech and language of a three-month-old child is presented on track two of the CD that accompanies this text. Note the random speech sounds in her babbling and the responsiveness to her mother.

At five months, an infant is able to imitate a few general sounds, usually vowels, immediately following a vocal model. He or she is even better at imitating tone and pitch signals. Most of the infant's imitative and nonimitative vocalizations are single-syllable units of consonant-vowel or vowel-consonant construction. These sound units and the early strings of sounds that begin at four months are called **babbling**. Vocalizing for attention, the infant will vary the volume, pitch, and rate of babbling. He or she will stop to listen to other sounds, especially to mother's voice.

With maturity, longer sequences and prolonged individual sounds evolve. Production is characterized by high and low pitches and glides between the two, growling and gutteral sounds, some friction sounds—produced by passing air through a narrow constriction—nasal /m/ and /n/, and a greater variety of vowels (Stark, 1986). The child produces increasingly more complex combinations of these features and conversational units in which the vowel duration may be highly variable and often very long.

The infant is capable of fully resonating the laryngeal tone to produce **fully resonant nuclei (FRN)**, vowel-like sounds similar to /a/. Constriction abilities become more mature in the forward portion of the mouth, and by six months labial, or lip, sounds predominate. The resultant sounds may be fricative, but more often they are vibratory, such as a "raspberry" or "Bronx cheer." Gutteral sounds, such as growling, tend to decrease. Increase in the size of the oral cavity and further development of discrimination to touch, pressure, and movement in the tongue tip and lips result in the increased variety of sounds heard.

Vowels such as /i/, /e/, and /ɛ/ require only jaw control. Later-developing vowels such as /u/ require coordination, jaw and longitudinal tongue movement, and lip rounding. Correct production of back vowels requires descent of the larynx and back tongue control (Buhr, 1980).

Babbling is random sound play of an almost infinite variety. Even infants with hearing impairments babble, which indicates the minimal effect of environmental auditory input on babbling. Hearing loss does, however, affect the number and variety of consonants in the prespeech vocalizations of infants (Stoel-Gammon, 1988). In general, infants with deafness have a smaller repertoire than hearing infants, and a greater proportion of labial sounds and prolongable consonants such as nasals (/m, n, ŋ/), approximants (/w, j/), and fricatives (i.e., /f, v, s, z/). A sample of the speech and language of a six-month-old child is presented on track three of the CD that accompanies this text. Reduplicated babbling, described on page 86, is more evident than noted at three months.

During the babbling period, the infant experiments with sound production. Often the sounds produced differ from those in his or her native language. Three explanations for this difference are possible (Ferguson, 1978). First, the infant's vocal tract differs in size and configuration from that of an adult. Therefore, laryngeal tones and subsequent resonated frequencies will differ. Second, the infant has not gained basic motor control for programming and sequencing the entire speech mechanism. Third, the infant has not acquired the phonological patterns of the surrounding language, such as sequencing and distribution of sounds. Despite these limitations, infants tend to produce sounds from the surrounding language more frequently than other speech sounds.

Linguists have argued for years about the relationship between babbling and later speech. The frequency of consonant appearance in babbling, not the order, seems to be reflected in the order of later speech-sound acquisition.

With age, the child's babbling increasingly reflects adult speech, especially in syllable structure and intonation. In addition, the reduplications of later babbling (*ma-ma-ma-ma*) often continue as the reduplications of early words (*mama*).

There is very little evidence that the infant's babbling is shaped gradually by selective reinforcement. Parents do not reinforce only those infant sounds used in their language. Even if parents did reinforce selectively, the results might be unforeseen. Social and vocal reinforcement used to modify the infant's range of sounds has little effect except to increase the overall amount of babbling. Furthermore, some qualities, such as the rate and pattern of development, depend on maturational factors. More research is needed before we can definitively state the relationship between babbling and speech production.

Within six months, the infant is able to examine with its hands and eyes and to remember familiar persons and objects. Very social, he or she will respond to smiles and vocalizations. Within limits, he or she can make wants known and influence environment.

The Experimenter: Age Seven to Twelve Months

The second six months of life are filled with new methods of locomotion and new abilities (Table 3.5). In addition, the infant experiments with speech and problem solving. Faced with a desired item, he or she will use a trial-and-error approach to achieve it. By twelve months of age, the infant begins to walk, to speak, and to use tools.

As the infant demonstrates increasing versatility in oral movements, speech progresses to repetitive syllable production and takes on more of the qualities of the surrounding language. By approximately six months of age, the infant is able to pout and draw its lips in without moving the jaw. Within two more months, the infant can keep his or her lips closed while chewing and swallowing semiliquids. At the same time, chewing changes from vertical to a more rotary pattern, reflecting changes in tongue-movement control. At eight months, the extension-retraction pattern of the tongue changes gradually to include more lateral, or sideways, movement. As a result, food is moved to the side for better chewing. In addition, the tongue can remain elevated, independent of jaw movement. By eleven months, the infant has the neuromuscular control to elevate the tongue tip and to bite soft

TABLE 3.5   The Experimenter: Seven to Twelve Months

AGE (MONTHS)	MOTOR	COGNITION	SOCIALIZATION	COMMUNICATION
7	Holds without palm; transfers object from hand to hand; bangs objects together Cuts first tooth; has better chewing and jaw control; can eat some strained solids Pushes up on hands and knees; rocks	Visually searches briefly for toy that disappears Imitates a physical act if in repertoire Sorts by size Remembers that jack pops up at the end of jack-in-the-box song	Resists Teases (beginning of humor); laughs at funny expressions Raises arms to be picked up	Plays vocally Produces several sounds in one breath Listens to vocalization of others Recognizes different tones and inflections
8	Holds own bottle Uses thumb-finger apposition Manipulates objects to explore Pulls up to stand but needs help to get down Crawls Drops and throws objects at will	Can store color and form separately; recognizes object dimensions Prefers novel and relatively complex toys Explores shape, weight, texture, function, and properties (example: in/out)	Acts positively toward peers Is clearly attached to mother Shouts for attention Reponds to self in mirror May reject being alone	Listens selectively Recognizes some words Repeats emphasized syllable Imitates gestures and tonal quality of adult speech; echolalia
9	Stands alone briefly; gets down alone; cruises Sits unsupported; gets into and out of sitting position alone Explores with index finger Removes and replaces bottle Puts objects in containers	Recognizes object dimensions Uncovers object if observes act of hiding first Anticipates outcome of events and return of persons	Explores other babies "Performs" for family ("so big") Imitates play Plays action games	Produces distinct intonational patterns Imitates coughs, hisses, tongue clicks, raspberries, etc. Uses social gestures Uses jargon May repond to name and "no" Attends to conversation
10	Crawls with bilateral leg-arm opposition Holds and drinks from cup Sits from a standing position Momentary unsupported stand	Points to body parts Attains a goal with trial-and-error approach Searches for hidden object but usually in a familiar place	Displays moods Helps dress and feed self Becomes aware of social approval and disapproval	Imitates adult speech if sounds in repertoire Obeys some commands

(continued)

TABLE 3.5 Continued

AGE (MONTHS)	MOTOR	COGNITION	SOCIALIZATION	COMMUNICATION
11	Stands alone; gets up from all-fours position by pushing up Climbs up stairs Feeds self with spoon	Imitates increasingly Associates properties with objects	Seeks approval Anticipates mother's goal and tries to change it by protest or "persuasion" May assert self	Imitates inflections, rhythms, facial expressions, etc.
12	Stands alone; pushes to stand from squat Climbs up and down stairs Has complete thumb apposition, uses spoon, cup, and crayon; releases objects willfully Takes first steps with support	Can reach while looking away Uses common objects appropriately Searches in location where an object was last seen Imitates an absent model	Expresses people preferences Expresses many different emotions	Recognizes own name Follows simple motor instructions, especially if accompanied by a visual cue ("bye-bye"); reacts to "no" intonation Speaks one or more words Practices words he knows and inflection; mixes word and jargon

solid foods with some control. He or she can draw lips and cheeks in during chewing and close the lips when swallowing liquids.

The downward bodily progression of motor skills continues during the second six months. The infant learns to sit unaided and to creep forward and back, then crawl, and finally walk. During the seventh month, the infant sits, creeps, and begins experimenting with standing. Within a month, standing has improved greatly but descent to the floor still needs practice. By ten months, the infant is able to push to a stand from a crawl and sit on the floor again. In the meantime, crawling speed and style improve. Two months later, the infant may walk unsupported for a few steps but still crawls when in a hurry. While walking, the infant extends the arms for balance. He or she stops by falling or grabbing nearby furniture or people. Both the unaided sitting and the crawling and walking expand the infant's range of exploration.

While sitting, the infant is free to examine and manipulate objects with the hands and to experiment with uses. The index finger probes incessantly. He or she experiments with sounds and reactions. For example, he or she may clear the highchair tray of all food and utensils while a horrified caregiver looks on. In addition, the infant is adept at emptying drawers and rearranging furniture. At eight months, the infant begins to experiment with perspective by shaking the head from side to side and looking upside down, thus noting the constancy of object shapes. The knowledge of object functions and characteristics gained from such experiments is important for early concept and definition development.

The infant also acquires the ability to search physically for a missing object. This skill depends on physical and cognitive development. In order to search, the infant must be able to remember the object while searching and be able to reach for it. During the second six months of life, searching progresses from a short glance for a missing object to a brief physical search. By the first birthday, the infant can reach while looking away. Physical searching leads to the early physical trial-and-error problem solving that begins to develop at ten months. For example, the infant must determine, through experimentation, the best method for attaining a toy that is on the floor on the other side of the coffee table. Only a physical attempt can result in success or nonsuccess. The infant is not capable of solving the problem through reasoning alone.

Toward the end of the second six months of life, the infant is also capable of solving problems by imitation, first direct and then indirect, or deferred. Imitation is an important learning strategy and requires a degree of representational thought. The infant develops the ability to remember a behavior in order to reproduce it. In addition, imitation is important for social interaction. At about nine months, the infant becomes an active game player and performer. He or she loves to play peekaboo and patty-cake, anticipating the end. Later the infant anticipates other routines and experiments with attempts to influence the outcome. He or she anticipates leaving and waves bye-bye, anticipates the mother's or father's arrival, and shows excitement. The infant also gains some measure of independence with self-help, such as feeding and dressing, but becomes very attached to mother, usually the primary caregiver.

The infant's increasing social and representational behavior is reflected most clearly in communication. At about six or seven months, babbling begins to change. Even though he or she still produces single-syllable sounds, the infant enters a brief stage of **reduplicated babbling** and begins to experiment with long strings of consonant-vowel syllable repetitions or self-imitations, such as "ma-ma-ma-ma-ma." Reduplicated babbling often occurs when holding an object or while exploring the environment and is similar to the rhythmic pattern of hand movement in this activity (Stark et al., 1993). Development of back sounds, followed by true vowel sounds and consonant-vowel babbling, has been found in infants from different language environments (Landberg & Lundberg, 1989).

Hearing ability appears to be very important in this imitative play, for at this point vocalizations of the child with deafness begin to decrease. In addition, the range of consonants within babbling decreases for the child with deafness, especially after eight months (Stoel-Gammon & Otomo, 1986). Whereas the hearing child increasingly produces true consonants, the child with deafness is limited increasingly to /h/, /l/ and /r/ sequences (Oller, Eilers, Bull, & Carney, 1985). Although the child with deafness may continue to babble until school age, without intervention the repertoire probably will not expand beyond that of the hearing infant (Locke, 1983).

Other differences in speech-sound production may appear earlier (Maskarinec, Cairns, Butterfield, & Weamer, 1981). Some hearing infants begin to produce more speech-like sounds as early as six weeks of age. Children with deafness, however, do not show the same trend. The hearing child practices speech sounds for long periods each day, seeming to enjoy this new ability. If mother responds to these sounds, the infant is likely to repeat them. He or she may repeat "ma-ma" at mother's urging but doesn't realize that this sound stands for or represents *mother*. The infant learns very quickly, however, that this behavior can be used to gain attention.

Initially, sound production passes through a period of marginal babbling consisting of "sequences of fully resonant vowels alternating with closures of the vocal tract" (Oller, 1978, p. 535). At first the child's repertoire of consonants is restricted to bilabial and alveolar plosives such as /p/, /b/, /t/, and /d/; nasals; and the approximant /j/ (Stark, 1979). (See the appendix for an explanation of speech sound symbols and their classification.) The phonemes are not fully formed or matured and are produced slowly. In contrast, the resonant quality and timing of reduplicated babbling more closely approximate mature speech. Reduplicated babbling is characterized by consonant-vowel syllable repetitions—CV-CV-CV—in which the vowel duration is very brief. Initially, reduplicated babbling is self-stimulatory in nature and is not used when communicating with adults. Gradually, the child uses reduplicated babbling in more contexts.

The six-month-old has some limited knowledge of speech (Griffiths, 1986). First, speech predicts the presence of humans. Second, the effects of speech on others vary along a predictable continuum. Finally, speech can fill a turn in conversational interactions. Beginning from this base, the child must discover what speech means.

Infants attend auditorily to sound patterns and search their own repertoires for the closest match (Locke, 1986). In fact, regardless of the language modeled for the infant, vocalizations and later first words have similar phonological patterns (Anderson & Smith, 1987; French, 1989; Locke, 1983; Stoel-Gammon & Dunn, 1985). For example, plosives or stops (/p, b, t, d, k, g/), nasals (/m, n, ŋ/), and approximants (/w, j/) constitute approximately 80 percent of the consonants in infant vocalizations and the first fifty words of English-speaking children (Leonard, Newhoff, & Mesalam, 1980). While the percentages may differ, these sounds often predominate in other non-English-speaking toddlers, such as Spanish-speaking Puerto Rican children, as well (Anderson & Smith, 1987). The ratio of single consonants to consonant clusters—roughly 9:1—is also similar in babbling and the first fifty words. Finally, the ratio of consonant-vowel to vowel-consonant syllables is also similar at roughly 3:1 in both English and Spanish (Anderson & Smith, 1987; Oller & Eilers, 1982).

Some characteristics of babbling may be affected by the "parent" language (Levitt & Aydelott Utman, 1992). There is evidence that vowels reflect the parents' language in type and distribution (deBoysson-Bardies, 1989; deBoysson-Bardies, Halle, Sagart, & Durand, 1989). Syllable structure and the consonant repertoire may also be affected by eleven months of age.

In the second half of the first year, the infant responds more consistently to speech. By approximately seven months, the infant will begin to look at objects that are named. Within another three months, he or she can recognize a familiar word within a phrase or a short sentence.

At around eight months, many changes occur in the infant's speech and interactional patterns. These include echolalia, gestures, variegated babbling, and jargon. First, the infant begins to react more to the environment by transferring the imitation stimulus to a second person. This period, ranging from eight to twelve months, has been called the *echolalic* stage. During this time the infant begins to imitate the communication of others, using echolalic speech. Echolalic speech, or **echolalia**, is speech that is an immediate imitation of some other speaker. Initially, the infant imitates gestures and intonation, but by eight months exhibits the identifiable pitch and contour patterns of his or her parent language (deBoysson-Bardies, Sagart, & Durand, 1984).

Soon the infant begins to imitate sounds, but at first only those he or she has produced spontaneously. Within a few months the infant will begin to use imitation to expand and modify his or her repertoire of speech sounds. Babbled speech sounds that are not in his or her native language decrease in number. The infant will also imitate stressed syllables in certain often-used words. For example, he or she may repeat "na-na" when mother says "banana," though he or she may not be associating the sound with the actual referent or object.

Second, the infant begins using gestures, with or without vocalizations, to communicate, although imitation is still very important. He or she begins to point, to show objects, to give objects, and to signal "no" or noncompliance, and seems to enjoy just plain showing off for attention. He or she waves bye-bye, gives kisses, and (perhaps to his parents' chagrin) shakes the head from side to side for "no."

Third, the speech during this period is characterized by **variegated babbling**, in which adjacent and successive syllables are not identical. Sound sequences may also include VCV and CVC structures, although vowel and consonant sounds do not differ within these syllables (Stark, 1986). In addition, reduplicated babbling changes in function, becoming less self-stimulatory. It is used more in imitation games with adults. The vocalizations of eight-month-olds also change with location and with significant changes in experiences (Hilke, 1988). It should be noted that not all child language researchers have found reduplicated babbling followed by variegated babbling (Mitchell & Kent, 1990). A sample of the speech and language of a nine-month-old child is presented on track four of the CD that accompanies this text. Babbling is more variegated than at six months and the babbling has more of the intonation of speech. Reduplicated babbling is also present.

Between babbling and the appearance of words, there is a reduction in the number of long babbled strings and an increase in the number of more wordlike utterances (Menyuk, Menn, & Silber, 1986). In the second half of the first year, children begin to notice contrasts in pitch contours, in vowels, and in initial consonants in consonant-vowel syllables. Children selectively listen more frequently to word-length utterances than to connected speech. They begin to recognize recurring patterns of sounds within specific situations.

Fourth, the infant begins to experiment with **jargon**, long strings of unintelligible sounds with adultlike prosodic and intonational patterns. Infants seven to ten months of age are sensitive to prosodic cues that help them segment speech into perceptual units corresponding to clauses (Hirsh-Pasek, Kemler Nelson, Jusczyk, Cassidy, Druss, & Kennedy, 1987). Mothers' speech to infants includes pauses at sentence boundaries, while mothers' speech to other adults does not. Thus, the child is given cues to a grammatical unit of language (Nelson, Hirsh-Pasek, Jusczyk, & Cassidy, 1989).

The child's babbling gradually comes to resemble the prosodic pattern of the language to which he or she is exposed. Babbling patterns become shorter and phonetically more stable. These prosodic features will continue into speech. Words and utterances are acquired as a "whole tonal pattern" (Lenneberg, 1967, p. 279). The resultant jargon may sound like questions, commands, and statements. Many parents will swear at this point that their child is communicating in sentences, although the parents aren't exactly clear on what the child is saying. Parental estimates of the infant's expressive abilities are frequently inflated. Apparently, the paralinguistic aspects of language are easier for the child to reproduce than the linguistic aspects. The amount of jargon produced and the number of months spent in this activity differ greatly across children (Stark, 1986).

Many speech sounds will develop sound–meaning relationships. Called **phonetically consistent forms (PCFs)** (Dore, Franklin, Miller, & Ramer, 1976), these sounds function as words for the infant, even though they are not based on adult words. The child may develop a dozen PCFs before he or she speaks first words. PCFs tend to be of four varieties: (a) single or repeated vowels, (b) syllabic nasals, (c) syllabic fricatives, and (d) single or repeated consonant-vowel syllables (syllables consisting of one consonant and one vowel) in which the consonant is a nasal or stop. Although PCFs have relatively stable sound and syllable forms, the prosodic pattern is even more consistent. PCFs are found across children regardless of the language they will later speak (Blake & deBoysson-Bardies, 1992).

PCFs may be a link between babbling and adultlike speech in that they are more limited than babbling but not as structured as adult speech. In short, they are "babbling-like sounds used meaningfully" (Ferguson, 1978, p. 281). PCFs display the creative role of the child as a language learner. The child does not use PCFs just because the adult models are too difficult or unavailable. Rather, he or she gets the idea that there can be sound–meaning relationships. Thus, the child demonstrates a recognition of linguistic regularities, though most PCFs are not found in adult speech.

By nine to thirteen months, children "understand" some words based on a combination of sound, nonlinguistic and paralinguistic cues, and context. In other words, in certain specific contexts children have limited comprehension of some phonemic sequences. The words are probably not comprehended alone. The exceptions are the child's name and *no*, which children seem to recognize out of context. As a result of continued exposure to recurring sound patterns in context, the child learns to reproduce aspects of these patterns in these situations. These sound patterns are most likely learned as a whole rather than as specific individual sounds.

Acquisition of single phonemes alone cannot explain word production. Some aspects of vocal development are progressively coordinated and recombined into meaningful speech, while others are dropped. Sound production depends on sound grouping and sound variation within individual words. Thus, the child adopts a problem-solving or trial-and-error approach to word production, gradually developing expressive strategies. Over time, these strategies become more general, less word specific, and more automatic.

Finally, at around the first birthday, the child produces the first meaningful word. Although he or she has previously responded to and produced words, the infant now produces them in the presence of the referent. The child associates the word with its meaning in some limited manner. Generally, first words name favorite toys or foods, family members, or pets. My own children began speaking with words such as *mama, dada, pepa* (the dog), *all gone,* and *bye*-bye. Single words are used for more than naming; the infant uses them to make requests, comments, and inquiries.

PCFs and first words are often used for a specific function, such as *mama* to gain attention or *more* to request. Gradually, the child expands this system so that a single word can signal a variety of functions by altering its pitch contour.

With the acquisition of words, the child's sound production becomes more constrained by the linguistic context. Children's speech is a complex interaction of the ease of production and the ease of perception of the target syllable. The success of both processes is a function of the phonemes involved and of syllable stress and position within the target word.

Infants can be trained to identify speech sounds and to organize speech sounds perceptually on the basis of auditory features (Hillenbrand, 1983). The order of appearance of the first sounds that children acquire—/m/, /w/, /b/, /p/—cannot be explained by the frequency of their appearance in English. Although not the most frequently appearing English sounds, /m/, /w/, and /p/ are the simplest consonants to produce. The /b/ is relatively more complex, although relatively easy to perceive.

After he or she acquires one word, the child will usually learn a few more within a short time and then plateau. More energy now goes into perfecting walking ability and exploring.

The Explorer: Age Twelve to Twenty-Four Months

With a beginning realization of self and a new (albeit shaky) method of locomotion, the infant begins the second year of life. During that year he or she will change from a dependent infant to a more independent toddler. Newly acquired walking skills and increased linguistic abilities give him or her mobility and tools to explore (Table 3.6).

Much of the second year is spent perfecting and varying walking skills. There is a deceleration in bodily growth rate in both height and in weight. Brain growth also decelerates, and head size increases only slightly. By age two, the brain is about 80 percent of its mature adult size. By fifteen months, the toddler is experimenting with different forms of walking, such as running and dawdling. Favorite games are hiding or being chased. The toddler learns to walk while carrying objects and to stoop and recover. My son Jason would stoop to pick up an object while forgetting the glass of juice clutched to his chest. After spilling the juice, he would turn to see what his parents would say, forget the puddle of juice, and inevitably sit in it.

By eighteen months, the toddler is able to walk backward and to stop smoothly but is not able to turn corners very well without assistance. He or she tries to climb out of the crib and to rearrange furniture. Walking is still not perfected, although he or she falls less often. The infant walks with toes pointed out, feet widely separated, and his or her body leaning forward. There is a rolling, "drunken sailor" quality to these movements. Within six months, he or she progresses to a stable walking rhythm. The two-year-old is able to walk on tiptoes, stand on one foot with assistance, jump with both feet, and bend at the waist to retrieve an object on the floor.

Unlike the somewhat sedentary world of the one-year-old, the toddler's environment becomes one of motion. New mobility, plus increasing control over his or her fine-motor abilities, gives the toddler new freedom to explore. If allowed by his parents, the toddler will get into everything and initiate an active and systematic exploration. The toddler turns over wastebaskets and sorts through the uncovered "treasures," empties cabinets and drawers, and hides objects. As a toddler, my brother went through the house dumping a liberal mound of baby powder into each opened drawer just after my mother had completed spring housecleaning.

Most of the toddler's play and exploration is solitary and nonsocial. As the pincer grasp becomes more coordinated, he or she demonstrates an interest in small objects, such as insects. By fifteen months he or she explores by fingering everything. A favorite game is carrying objects and handing them to others. He or she can release objects at will and has a primitive whole-arm throw. With this grasp, sticks become tools for retrieving and exploring.

TABLE 3.6   The Explorer: Twelve to Twenty-Four Months

AGE (MONTHS)	MOTOR	COGNITION	SOCIALIZATION	COMMUNICATION
15	Enjoys unceasing activity; walks with rapid runlike gait Walks a few steps backwards and sideways Carries objects in both hands or waves while walking Throws ball with elbow extension; dumps toys in container Takes off shoes and socks Points with index finger; picks up small objects with index finger and thumb	Imitates small motor acts Use toy phone like real one	Looks for adults when left alone Likes music and dancing Pushes toys Imitates housework Plays in solitary manner; but likes to act for an audience Begins make-believe play Laughs when chased	Points to clothes, persons, toys, and animals named Uses jargon and words in conversation Has four- to-six-word vocabulary
18	Walks up stairs with help; walks smoothly, runs stiffly Drinks unassisted Throws ball with whole arm Throws and catches without falling Jumps with both feet off floor Turns pages Has muscle control for potty training Sorts shapes	Recognizes pictures Recognizes self in mirror Remembers places where objects are usually located Uses a stick as a tool Imitates adult object use	Explores reactions of others; tests others Enjoys solitary play, engages in increased cooperative play from here on Pretends to feed doll Responds to scolding and praise Little or no sense of sharing	Begins to use two-word utterances Has approximately 20-word vocabulary Identifies some body parts Refers to self by name "Sings" and hums spontaneously Plays question-answer with adults

(continued)

TABLE 3.6   Continued

AGE (MONTHS)	MOTOR	COGNITION	SOCIALIZATION	COMMUNICATION
21	Walks up and down stairs with help of railing or hand Jumps, runs, throws, climbs; kicks large ball; squats to play; running is stiff Puts shoes on part way Begins to show hand preference Fits things together, such as easy puzzle Responds rhythmically to music with whole body	Knows shapes Sits alone for short periods with book Notices little objects and small sounds Matching objects with owners Recalls absent objects of persons	Hugs spontaneously Plays near but not with other kids Likes toy telephone, doll, and truck for play Enjoys outings Becomes clinging around strangers	Likes rhyming games Pulls person to show something Tries to "tell" experiences Understands some personal pronouns Uses I and mine
24	Walks smoothly, watching feet Runs rhythmically but unable to start or stop smoothly Walks up and down stairs alone without alternating feet Tiptoes for a few steps Pushes tricycle Eats with fork Transitions smoothly from walk to run	Matches familiar objects Comprehends one and many Recognized when picture in book is upside down	Can role play in limited manner Imagines toys have life qualities; engages in pretend play that is constrained by the objects Enjoys parallel play predominately Prefers action toys Cooperates with adults in simple household tasks Orders others around Communicates feelings, desires, and interests	Has 200–300-word expressive vocabulary; names most common everyday objects Uses short, incomplete sentences Uses some prepositions (in, on) and pronouns (I, me, you) but not always correctly Uses some regular verb endings (-s, -ed, -ing) and plural s

During the entire second year, the toddler tests objects' qualities by touching, pushing, pulling, and lifting. Mouthing decreases. Sensory exploration is still very important, however, and the toddler enjoys exploring new sights, sounds, and textures, later demonstrating definite likes and dislikes. As he or she nears eighteen months, the toddler begins combining skills. He or she can carry one or several small objects in one hand and throw objects with the other and begins to concentrate on fitting things together, rather than separating them, and on filling containers, rather than emptying them. Increased fine-motor skills and a longer attention span enable him or her to look at books. By eighteen months, the infant recognizes pictures of common objects. Six months later, he or she pretends to read books and has the fine-motor skills to turn pages one at a time. He or she is also capable of holding a crayon and scribbling circles and vertical and horizontal lines.

The toddler's exploration changes concepts of objects and people in the environment and, in turn, his or her concept of self. Increased memory aids this realization process. By fifteen months, the toddler demonstrates increased mental abilities at physical problem solving. He or she begins to plan new trial-and-error behaviors, without going through the actual physical events, by combining ideas from previous encounters. In addition, when moving objects disappear, he or she is able to anticipate their movement. By eighteen months, objects are used increasingly for their intended function; he or she "combs" hair with a comb, for example. In addition, toys are used increasingly in play. By eighteen months, the toddler plays appropriately with toy phones, dishes, and tools. He or she likes dress-up play. Dolls and stuffed animals become more important. My own children loved to pound pegs through a wooden toy workbench and to stack objects. The toddler often repeats daily routines with toys and demonstrates short sequences of role playing at age two. My son Jason loved to imitate his mother's morning ritual in the bathtub. All of this learning depends on better memory.

The toddler also enjoys routines and anticipates actions. From routines such as feeding, changing, and eating, the toddler develops a primitive sense of order and time. By two years of age, the toddler has gained a good grasp of the environment. He or she is able to predict routine behaviors and the location of familiar objects. With some confidence in the world and a better sense of self, the toddler tries to influence the outcome of many routines and interactions.

Much of the social interaction of the second year involves the toddler's attempts to be in the spotlight. Having learned in the first year to influence others, the toddler will do almost anything for attention. He or she becomes an active imitator of adults and siblings. The fifteen-month-old gains attention by "dancing" to music. He or she becomes more adept at imitating hand movements, such as clapping and waving. At around eighteen months, the toddler begins to imitate the family's housework, perhaps attempting to vacuum or sweep. One of our nieces, Angela, became quite domestic at this age.

Increasing self-awareness and the ability to influence others are reflected in the toddler's growing noncompliance with the wishes of the family. At sixteen months, the toddler begins to assert some independence by ignoring or dawdling in response to parental commands or requests. By twenty-one months, this behavior has evolved into a very defiant "no." The child frequently says "no" even when he or she really wants the help or advice being offered. One little friend, Dean, shouted "no" for *no* and "no" with up and down head nodding for *yes*.

Since the two-year-old has many self-help skills, he or she expresses the desire not to be helped. For example, the two-year-old can usually place food on a spoon and feed himself or herself, undress except for shoelaces, wash, turn on simple appliances, open easy doors, and straighten a bed. When the child needs help, he or she knows how to request it.

The toddler's growing sense of self is also reflected in the notion of possession. He becomes increasingly aware that objects have owners. At around eighteen months, the toddler becomes very possessive of toys, using words such as *mine*. By twenty-two months, the toddler may become more verbal in defense of possessions, although others may disagree as to just which objects are the child's. My son Jason insisted on sleeping with all of his toy cars in the bed. It was easy to tell how restless he was by the amount of clanking. The toddler's verbal defense of possessions reflects an awareness that adults attend to him or her when words are used.

Not all interactions are negative, however, and toddlers will play near other children. This play is usually parallel or side by side, with each child engaged in his or her own activity.

Language development also goes beyond the use of such single words as *no, mine,* and a few others. The second year is one of vocabulary growth and word combinations. Vocabulary growth is slow during the first few months, when the toddler is concentrating on gross-motor refinement. Much of the toddler's speech consists of single words or jargon. These words are used to name objects or people, to gain attention, or to attain some object or information. Phrases frequently used by adults in the child's environment may be repeated as single words. For example, many children say "Wassat?" and "Go-bye." A favorite of the eighteen-month-old is the *name game* in which the toddler touches an object, queries "Wassat?" and awaits a reply. Some words, such as *no, more,* and *gimme,* can be combined easily with others to form longer sentences. Other words represent common objects, foods, pets, or household members. Each toddler has his or her own **lexicon**, or personal dictionary, with words that reflect, in part, the child's environment. In general, the toddler's definitions are not the same as those of the adults in the same environment. For example, the word *horse* might apply to all four-legged animals. The toddler must therefore rely on extralinguistic cues to interpret adult speech accurately. This outcome is to be expected, since the child's experiences with the environment and with words are much more limited. A sample of the speech and language of a twelve-month-old child is presented on track five of the CD that accompanies this text. The child at this age will use all types of babbling, plus jargon, phonetically consistent forms (PCFs), and words.

During the second half of the second year, the toddler begins to combine words and to increase the rate of vocabulary growth. The early word combinations appear to follow predictable patterns, and the toddler is likely to produce phrases such as "More cookie," "Daddy eat," "No night-night," and so on. Within a few months, short-term memory has increased so that the child can attempt a few longer constructions, such as "Daddy eat cookie." At this time, the toddler seems to be absorbed in speech and language play. He or she likes rhymes, songs, and stories, and activities, such as playing and eating, often are accompanied by speech. Vocabulary increases rapidly. At age two the toddler has an expressive vocabulary of about 150 to 300 words. A sample of the speech and language of an eighteen-month-old child is presented on track six of the CD that accompanies this text. The child's vocabulary has increased and some word combinations and repetitions are evident. Compare this sample to that of a two-year-old child presented on track seven. The two-year-old is beginning to use longer, more sentence-like utterances.

Accompanying the increases in utterance length and vocabulary is a decrease in the use of jargon and babbling, although the child continues to use both. In general, the relationship of babbling to speech is very complex, although expansion of a child's expressive lexicon is positively correlated to continued babbling, especially consonantal babbling (Whitehurst, Smith, Fischel, Arnold, & Lonigan, 1991).

In summary, the two-year-old is a relatively independent sort, although still very dependent upon adults for protection and well-being. He or she has a good concept of the immediate environment and an expectation of daily routines. The child has the social skills to attain and hold the attention of others and to express some emotions. Increased mobility enables him or her to explore the environment and to modify it. In addition, he or she has the linguistic skills to influence the behavior of others.

The Exhibitor: Age Three to Five Years

As the preschool child develops, he or she exhibits new independence (Table 3.7). He or she is very mobile and very curious about the world. During the preschool years, the child acquires many self-help skills, including dressing and feeding. Increased memory enables him or her to solve problems with less dependence on physical input, to understand temporal concepts, and to recall the past. Language skills develop rapidly during the preschool years. By age five the child has acquired about 80 percent of the syntactic structures that he or she will use as an adult. Recall and increased language skills combine in the five-year-old to produce a delightful storyteller and recounter. The five-year-old, with a better-defined personality, is a more openly social being than he or she was at age two.

TABLE 3.7   The Exhibitor

AGE (MONTHS)	MOTOR	COGNITION	SOCIALIZATION	COMMUNICATION
3	Walks up and down stairs without assistance; uses nonalternating step Walks without watching feet, heel-to-toe gait; marches to music; tiptoes 3 yards Balances momentarily on one foot Rides tricycle Can spread with knife Explores, dismantles, dismembers Plays simple musical instrument	Creates representational art: one shape represents several things Matches primary colors and shapes Can show two objects: understands concept of *two* Enjoys make-believe play; is less constrained by objects Knows sage but no concept of length of a year	Labels some coins Plays in groups, talks while playing, selects with whom he'll play Shares toys for short periods Takes turns Insists on being in the limelight	Has 900–1,000-word expressive vocabulary, creates 3–4 word sentences Uses "sentences" with subject and verb, but simple sentence construction Plays with words and sounds Follows two-step commands Talks about the present "Swears"

(continued)

TABLE 3.7   Continued

AGE (MONTHS)	MOTOR	COGNITION	SOCIALIZATION	COMMUNICATION
4	Walks up and down stair with alternating steps Jumps over objects Hops on one foot Can copy block letters	Categorizes Counts rotely to five; can show three objects; understands concept of *three* Knows primary colors	Plays and cooperates with others Role plays	Has 1,500–1,600-word expressive vocabulary Asks many, many questions Uses increasingly more complex sentence forms Recounts stories and the recent past Understands most questions about the immediate environment Has some difficulty answering *how* and *why* Relies on word order for interpretation
5	Has gross motor control, good body awareness; plays complex games Cuts own meat with a knife Draws well, colors in lines; creates more recognizable drawings Prints simple words Dresses without assistance Still lacks eye coordination for sustained reading Has established hand preference	Carries a rule through a series of activities Knows own right and left, but not those of others Counts to 13; can show four or five objects; understands concept of *greater than three* Accepts magic as an explanation Develops time concepts of *today/tomorrow/yesterday, morning/afternoon/night, day/night* Recognizes relationship of parts to whole	Plays simple games Selects some playmates based on sex Enjoys dramatic play Shows interest in group activities Plays purposefully and constructively	Has expressive vocabulary of 2,100–2,200 words Discusses feelings Understands *before* and *after,* regardless of word order Follows three-step commands Has 90% grammar acquisition

FIGURE 3.3   Average Age of Acquisition of English Consonants

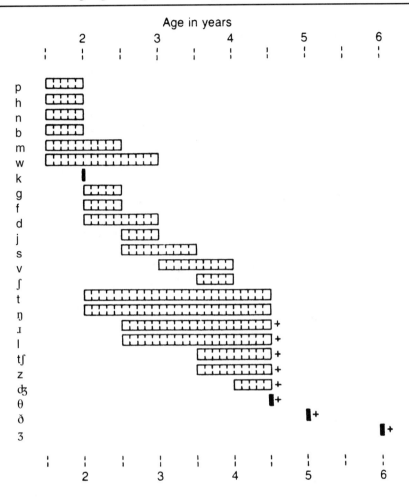

Compiled from Olmstead (1971) and Sander (1972), representing the ages at which 50 percent of English-speaking children can produce a sound correctly in all positions in conversation and formal testing.

Several studies have attempted to establish an order of phoneme acquisition by young children. Comparing the results of these studies (Figure 3.3), we can make the following statements:

1. As a group, vowels are acquired before consonants. English vowels are acquired by age three.
2. As a group, the nasals are acquired first, followed by the plosives, approximants, lateral approximants, fricatives, and affricatives.

3. As a group, the glottals are acquired first, followed by the bilabials, velars, alveolars and post-alveolars, dentals and labiodentals, and palatals.
4. Sounds are first acquired in the initial position in words.
5. Consonant clusters and blends are not acquired until age seven or eight, although some clusters appear as early as age four. These early clusters include /s/ + nasal, /s/ + approximant, /s/ + stop, and stop + approximant in the initial position and nasal + stop in the final position.
6. There are great individual differences, and the age of acquisition for some sounds may vary by as much as three years.

Samples of the speech and language of three-, four-, and five-year-old children are presented on tracks eight, nine, and ten, respectively, of the CD that accompanies this text. Note the speech sounds and the sentence construction.

Although the sequence of sound acquisition presented in Figure 3.3 is not universal and differs according to the sounds used in individual languages, surprising similarity exists (Amayreh & Dyson, 1998; Paulson, 1991; So & Dodd, 1995). Although motor control is a big determiner of sound development, the specific use patterns of different languages influence both the order and speed of acquisition. The acquisitional order of phonemes common to several languages is presented in Table 3.8.

The Three-Year-Old

By age three, the child has perfected walking on flat surfaces. He or she can run well, climb stairs without assistance, and balance on one foot. The newfound skill of tricycling expands horizons beyond the immediate household. He or she is still very home-oriented, however, and will remain so throughout the preschool period.

Fine-motor abilities continue to develop slowly. The three-year-old can dress except for shoe-tying and can use a knife for spreading but not cutting. He or she continues to be interested in fine-motor manipulation and explores by dismantling or dismembering house-

TABLE 3.8   Acquisitional Order of Consonant Sounds Across Languages

AGE	ENGLISH	SPANISH	CANTONESE	ARABIC
By 3	t, d, k, f, m, n, w	k, m, n, j	t, n, p, j, m, w	t, k, f, m, n, w
3–4	j, s	d, f, t	k	d
4–5		w	f, s	
5–6		s		s
6+				j

This data is the compilation of a liberal interpretation of several studies, often with differing criteria. Differences reflect the slight variation in phoneme production in different languages and the use patterns within each language. Only phonemes used in all four languages are presented. Despite some glaring differences, there is considerable similarity across languages.

Sources: Amayreh & Dyson, 1998; Paulson, 1991; Smit, Hand, Freilinger, Bernthal, & Bird, 1990; So & Dodd, 1995

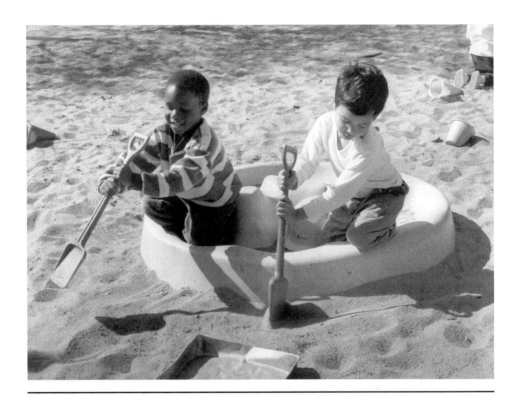

By age four children can engage in cooperative play, such as paddling a boat across the ocean.

hold objects or favorite toys. Scribbling has developed into more representational drawing. Often a single "drawing" will represent many very different things. The representation is not constrained by the object or person portrayed. Most adults have experienced the rough-drawn circle with two lines below it that the child calls "Mommy." Upon a second inquiry, the child announces that the same picture is now a doggie, next it's a tree, and so on.

The play of a three-year-old is also less constrained by actual objects. He or she uses toys in imaginative ways and exhibits much make-believe play. Thus, one object may symbolize another. Such an event is called *symbolic play*. Unlike two-year-olds, a child of three is likely to play in groups and to share toys and take turns. Play is often accompanied by sounds and words as he explains his actions, makes environmental noises, or takes various roles. Parents and teachers often hear themselves portrayed in the child's play—not always in flattering terms!

Speech and language are used in many other ways, and there is a tremendous relative growth in vocabulary. The three-year-old uses an expressive vocabulary of 900 to 1,000 words and employs about 12,000 individual words per day. Most three-year-olds have mastered the vowel sounds and the consonants /p/, /m/, /h/, /n/, /w/, /b/, /k/, /g/, and /d/.[1] There

---

[1]The appendix lists the phonetic symbols and words illustrating each one.

is much individual variation in speech-sound development, however, and at least 50 percent of the three-year-olds are also proficient in their use of /t/, /ŋ/, /f/, /j/, /r/, /l/, and /s/ (Figure 3.3).

The language of the three-year-old consists of simple sentences that frequently omit small, unstressed words. Most sentences follow a subject-verb-object format, although the child has begun to employ variations of adult negative, interrogative, and imperative forms. Negative words used are *no, not, can't, don't,* and *won't,* often employed interchangeably. The most frequent interrogatives are *what* and *where; why* and *how* are used infrequently, and the three-year-old cannot respond successfully to these types of questions. The three-year-old uses some noun modifiers and articles, the plurals of often used nouns, and possessive *-'s.* He or she also uses some pronouns and the prepositions *in, on,* and *under.* In addition, the child has learned to use the *-ing* and *-ed* endings. Unfortunately, most three-year-olds overgeneralize the *-ed* ending to irregular past-tense verbs, such as *goed* and *eated.* The three-year-old still has some difficulty with auxiliary verbs and the verb *to be.*

In short, the child's language is increasingly beginning to reflect the environment. This is not a passive imitative process, however. The child demonstrates processing of language rules by using such constructions as *eated* and *goed,* although he or she does not hear those constructions used by adults. The child is formulating language rules.

Two aspects of the linguistic environment more readily reflected in child speech of this age group are adult intonation and swearing. I recall eavesdropping on my three-year-old daughter Jessica as she warned one of her dolls, "Now listen here, young lady!" Her intonation was flawless. I cringed to think from whom that had come. Swearing also causes parents to cower, and every family has at least one embarrassing story about the incident at Grandma's house or in a crowded shopping mall. Our most embarrassing tale involved an alphabet game in which children were saying words that began with certain sounds. One of our cherubs strayed from the traditional *apple, boy, cat* format. The preschool teacher ended the activity abruptly.

The three-year-old exhibits good motor and language skills for his or her short period of experience. Much of the environment is reflected in play and in conversation.

The Four-Year-Old

The motor skills of the four-year-old reflect the increased control of independent movements of the right and left sides. The child of four can hop on one foot for a short period and can ascend and descend steps with alternating foot movements. Hand preference is also more pronounced, and the child is able to copy simple block letters with the dominant hand.

Increased memory helps the child recount the past and remember short stories. This memory and recall are aided by the child's increased language skills. The child also demonstrates categorization skills that seem to indicate more advanced procedures for storage of learned information. The four-year-old can name the primary colors and label some coins. Although the child can count to five by rote, he or she has a notion of quantity only through three. Socially, most four-year-olds play well in groups and cooperate well with others. Although there is still a lot of object play, role play becomes increasingly frequent.

The ability to carry a role through story play is reflected in the four-year-old's language. The child can tell simple stories of his or her own or others' authorship. Increased language skills enable the child to form more complex sentences. Vocabulary has increased to 1,500 to 1,600 words, with approximately 15,000 used each day. Most four-year-olds can correctly articulate the consonant sounds /p/, /m/, /h/, /n/, /w/, /b/, /k/, /g/, /d/, /t/, /ŋ/, /f/, and /j/. At least 50 percent of all four-year-olds can produce /r/, /l/, /s/, /tʃ/, /ʃ/, and /z/ (Figure 3.3). Most sentences average four or five words, and the four-year-old demonstrates good usage of declarative, negative, interrogative, and imperative forms. Although demonstrated infrequently, the four-year-old child also can join sentences together to form longer units, using conjunctions such as *and, but,* and *if* and relative pronouns such as *who.* Frequently, the child will begin sentences with *and* or use *and* to produce long run-on sentences that tell a story, as in ". . . and then . . . and then . . . and then. . . ." Events are relayed in the order in which they occurred.

Four-year-olds also rely on word order for interpretation of temporal information. For example, the four-year-old interprets the following sentences to mean the same thing:

After you eat, go right home.
Before you eat, go right home.

The child will ignore the words *before* and *after*. The order-of-mention strategy results in the interpretation, "Eat, then go home."

Language becomes a real tool for exploration, and the four-year-old is full of questions. He or she may ask several hundred in a single day, causing parents to wonder why they ever longed to hear their child speak. The child learns very quickly that he can exasperate Dad by continually asking "why?"

A subject is now used in all sentence forms except the imperative ("Throw the ball.") in which it is not required. Usually one modifier or an article is used with the noun. Many regular and irregular past-tense verbs are used correctly, as is the third-person singular, present-tense *-s,* as in "Mommy *eats* at work." Thus, four-year-olds can be expected to say "ate," not "eat*ed*," and "Mommy eats," not "Mommy eat." The specific verbs acquired and the speed of acquisition depend on many factors, including environmental input. Auxiliary or helping verbs are also used in the interrogative and negative sentence forms that require their use.

In general, four-year-olds are very social beings who have the linguistic skills and the short-term memory to be good, if somewhat limited, conversationalists. My daughter Jessica, now an adult, teasingly asked a four-year-old for a date. He responded, "No, I'm not grown up yet, but we could go to dinner as a family." Four-year-olds are very curious and very anxious to exhibit their knowledge and abilities.

The Five-Year-Old

By the fifth birthday, the child has a good sense of the person he or she has become. The child possesses a good awareness of the body and how to use it to accomplish complex tasks and games. The five-year-old knows left and right but can't transfer them to others. Each hand can be employed independently for tasks such as dressing and cutting meat with a knife. Small-muscle control enables the child to draw recognizable pictures, to color within the lines, and to copy short words.

The child uses its body in play and enjoys group games. With increased memory skills, the child of five is able to play organized games with simple rules. He or she can concentrate on playing and still carry through certain rules of play.

The five-year-old has a good temporal sense and understands words such as *yesterday, today,* and *tomorrow.* Temporal notions aid the child's understanding of explanations of cause and effect and comprehension of temporal terms such as *before* and *after.*

Although the five-year-old has good physical reasoning abilities, he or she still believes in magic and sorcery as explanations for much that happens. When my son Todd turned five, he asked for a magic kit. Mom and Dad complied. After opening it, he turned to us for a demonstration. We dutifully explained each trick and showed him how it was done. When we finished, he cried in a very disillusioned voice, "No, no, I wanted *real* magic."

Five-year-olds use very adultlike language, although many of the more subtle syntactic structures are missing. In addition, the child has not acquired some of the pragmatic skills needed to be a truly effective communicator. Expressive vocabulary has grown to about 2,200 words. Word definitions still lack the fullness of adult meanings, however, and this aspect continues to be refined throughout life. Most five-year-olds can correctly articulate the /p/, /m/, /h/, /n/, /w/, /b/, /k/, /g/, /d/, /t/, /ŋ/, /f/, /j/, /ɪ/, /l/, /s/, /tʃ/, /ʃ/, /z/, /dʒ/, and /v/ consonant sounds. At least 50 percent can produce the /ð/ or "th" in "*there*" sound correctly (Figure 3.2). Five-year-olds still have difficulty with a few consonant sounds and with consonant blends, as in "*street*" or "*clean.*"

The child of five uses regular and irregular past tenses of common verbs correctly but still has difficulty with the past tense of the verb *to be* (*was* and *were*). The future-tense *will* is also used correctly where required in context. Some of the other auxiliary verbs, such as *would, should, must,* and *might,* are used less frequently and often correctly. The five-year-old child also has limited use of the comparative (*more . . . than* or *-er*); the possessive *-'s* and possessive pronouns (*his, her, your*); the conjunctions *and, but, if, because, when,* and *so;* relative pronouns for embedded clauses ("I know *who* lives next door"); gerunds ("We go *fishing*"); and infinitives ("I want *to eat* now"). These syntactic structures do not appear rapidly, and many children struggle with acquisition well into the school years. It frequently takes the child several years of practice to gain complete control of many linguistic structures. The malnourished child or the child from a stimulation-poor environment may take longer to acquire the structures mentioned. Many other, less obvious linguistic changes are also occurring.[2]

Although there are still many aspects of speech, language, and communication to be mastered, the five-year-old has made spectacular progress in only a few years. The child of five is able to use language to converse and to entertain. He or she can tell stories, has a budding sense of humor, and can tease and discuss emotions. Over the next few years, language development will slow and begin to stabilize but will be nonetheless significant.

The Expert: School-Age Years

In the first six years of school, the child develops cognitive and communicative skills that by age twelve almost equal those of the adult. Physical growth follows shortly as the twelve-year-old begins adolescence. Increasingly the child becomes less home centered, as school and age peers become more important (Table 3.9).

---

[2]These changes will be discussed in greater detail in Chapters 8, 9, and 10.

TABLE 3.9 The Expert: The School-Age Child

AGE (MONTHS)	MOTOR	COGNITION	SOCIALIZATION	COMMUNICATION
6	Has better gross motor coordination; rides bicycle Throws ball well Begins to get permanent teeth	Has longer attention span Is less distracted by additional information when problem solving Remembers and repeats three digits	Enjoys active games Is competitive Identifies with sex peers in groups Transforms egocentric reality to more complex and relative reality view	Has expressive vocabulary of 2,600 words, receptive of 20,000–24,000 words; defines by function Has many well-formed sentences of a complex nature; uses all parts of speech to some degree
8	Has longer arms, larger hands Has better manipulative skills Has nearly mature-size brain Has more permanent teeth	Knows left and right of others Understands conservation Knows differences and similarities Reads spontaneously	Enjoys an audience Learns that others have different perspectives of a third person Has allegiance to gang, but also strong need for adult support	Talks a lot Boasts, brags Verbalizes ideas and problems readily Communicates thought Demonstrates little difficulty with comparative relationship
10	Has eyes of almost mature size Has almost mature lungs and digestive and circulatory systems	Plans future actions Solves problems with only minimal physical input	Enjoys games, sports, hobbies Discovers that he may be the object of someone else's perspective	Spends lots of time talking Has good comprehension
12	Experiences "rest" before adolescent growth (girls usually taller and heavier, may have entered puberty) Begins rapid muscle growth with puberty Can be on wide range of maturational levels	Engages in abstract thought	Has different interests than those of the opposite sex	Has 50,000-word receptive vocabulary Constructs adultlike definitions

Physically, the school-age child gains greater coordination of gross- and fine-motor movements. As the six-year-old attains better coordination and balance, he or she learns to ride a bicycle and to throw and catch a ball well. It takes six months to a year of practice to become a proficient bicyclist. In ball handling, throwing skills precede catching skills by several months. Throughout the period, physical coordination enables the child to perform more motor acts at one time and therefore to enjoy sports and coordinated games. In addition, better fine-motor abilities and eye–hand coordination enable the child to engage in hobbies and crafts. With more mature motor skills, he or she gains more self-help skills and increased independence.

Cognitive skills change markedly during the first six years of school. The brain is nearly adult in size by age eight, but development is not complete. Intracerebral association tracts must be better developed before the brain becomes mature. This internal growth is reflected in the relative weight of the brain to the whole body weight: By age ten the child's brain is one-fifteenth of the total body weight, compared to one-fortieth for the adult. Brain weight changes little; growth is internal. During the first six years of school, the child's mental abilities mature from concrete problem solving, requiring sensory input, to abstract thought. Four major cognitive developments in the period from age seven to eleven are inferred reality, decentration, transformational thought, and reversible mental operations (Flavell, 1977). *Inferred reality* is an inference about a physical problem based not only on perceived appearances but also on internal information. For example, a preschooler bases his judgment of a container's volume on its height alone. The school-age child bases conclusions on all physical characteristics and on his or her knowledge of the volume of liquid poured into the container. The ability to maintain a notion of size or quantity regardless of the shape of the object or container is called *conservation*. *Decentration* is the ability to consider several aspects of a physical problem at once, rather than focusing on only a few. *Transformational thought* refers to the ability to view a physical problem as existing in time and to anticipate future consequences effectively. Finally, *reversible mental operations* enable the child to recognize that change can be undone or reversed.

In addition, the child's selective attention, both visual and auditory, improves, and he or she is able to filter out unnecessary information more effectively. Increased memory enables him or her to process and organize the remaining information for more efficient problem solving. Along with these increased abilities, the child gains a better understanding of his or her own mental processes.

The school-age child is also a very social being, and peers, especially same-sex peers, become very important. Thus, this period of social development is called the "gang age." The child may begin to use slang or peer-group talk for added acceptance. This can be a trying period for parents, as children begin to establish an identity separate from their family. One afternoon my son Todd stormed into the house from his friend's house and demanded to know "the truth." "There's one thing you'll never tell me," he challenged. Fearing the worst, I suggested that he ask anyway. What a relief when he shot back, "Is there a real Easter Bunny?" With this peer socialization comes a less egocentric perspective. The child begins to realize that his or her own reality is not the only one.

The child also realizes how to manipulate and influence others, especially through the use of language. During the early school-age years, the child refines the conversational skills needed to be a truly effective communicator. He or she learns to introduce new topics and, once begun, to continue and to end conversation. While in a conversation, the child makes relevant comments and adapts roles and moods to fit the situation. In addition, the school-age child learns to make certain assumptions about the listener's level of knowledge and to adjust his or her conversation accordingly. This communication development reflects the child's growing appreciation for the perspective of others. A sample of the speech and language of a seven-year-old child is presented on track eleven of the CD that accompanies this text. Compare this sample to the mature sample of a twelve-year-old child presented on track twelve.

Toward more effective speech, the six-year-old acquires most English speech sounds, adding the /θ/ and /ʒ/ sounds, as in *th*in and treasure. By age eight, he or she also acquires consonant clusters, such as *str, sl,* and *dr.*

In addition, the child's vocabulary continues to grow. The first-grader has an expressive vocabulary of approximately 2,600 words but may understand as many as 8,000–10,000 root English words and 14,000 when various derivations are included (Anglin, 1993; Carey, 1981). Aided by school, this receptive vocabulary expands to approximately 50,000 words by sixth grade and to 80,000 words by high school. Multiple word meanings are also acquired. In general, the child learns verbs that describe a simple action first, then verbs for complex actions or specific situations. The age ranges for the following four verbs illustrate this trend:

Verb	Age Range of Understanding in Years-Months
hitting	4–3 to 5–5
balancing	7–6 to 9–5
directing	11–6 to 13–5
hoisting	13–6 to 15–5

Two aspects of school-age language development relative to vocabulary growth are divergent and convergent language abilities. **Divergent semantic production** is the process of producing a great variety of words, word associations, phrases, and sentences from a given topic. As such, divergent abilities add originality, flexibility, and creativity to language. **Convergent semantic production** is the process of selecting a unique semantic unit given specific linguistic restrictions. For example, there are only a few words that can complete the sentence, "The opposite of *up* is ___." Development of both abilities helps the school-age child become a more effective communicator.

In part, the school-age child's vocabulary growth reflects the systematic development of word-formation rules. First grade is a period of stabilization of rules previously learned and addition of new rules. The major learning period for the rules of pluralization of nouns may be kindergarten through first grade. By second grade, the child uses regular plurals correctly. Irregular plurals and plurals of nouns ending in *s* blends, such as *-sk* and *-st,* are accurately produced by third grade. In second and third grades, the child also attains accurate use of the rules for noun and adverb derivation. For example, a verb can be changed to a noun by adding *-er* to the verb, producing *teacher* from *teach*. Some nouns require *-man, -person,* or *-ist,* as in *fisherman, chairperson,* or *cyclist.* Adverbs are derived by adding *-ly* to adjectives, producing *quickly* from *quick.*

The sentence structure of the school-age child slowly becomes more elaborate as the child matures. Older children's sentences include increased embedding of subordinate clauses ("The man *who drives our bus* is crabby."). In addition, there are significant increases in the child's ability to comprehend comparative (*as big as . . .* ; *bigger*), passive ("The girl is chased by the boy"), temporal or time (*before; after*), and spatial and familial relationships (Wiig & Semel, 1984). The school-age child begins to comprehend the sentence and its relationships as a whole and does not depend on word order for interpretation. Conjunctions are added slowly with some, such as *although* and *however,* not acquired until early adolescence.

The school-age child also increases understanding and use of figurative language. **Figurative language** consists of idioms, metaphors, similes, and proverbs that represent abstract concepts not always stated in a literal interpretation. **Idioms** are expressions that often cannot be justified literally, such as "hit the roof" or "tied up." **Metaphors** and **similes** offer implied comparisons, such as "black as night" and "eats like a bird." **Proverbs** offer advice that differs from the concrete example used. For example, "look before you leap" concerns caution in decision making, not advice for long-distance jumpers. Figurative relationships add richness to language but require higher language functions to interpret the deeper meaning. General usage of figurative language does not begin until the child attends school.

One of the greatest changes in language comes with the learning of reading and writing. Because these skills are formally taught, the acquisition pattern is quite different from that for language learning via the speech and auditory modes. Reading and writing training removes language from the conversational context and thus requires the child to consider language in the abstract. It is not surprising, therefore, that reading, writing, and metalinguistic skills seem to be related (Kemper, 1985).

In conclusion, by age twelve the child has many of the cognitive and linguistic skills of an adult. The rate of development in these areas decreases as the child prepares for the physical changes that will accompany adolescence. Language development does not stop, however, and many complex forms and subtle linguistic uses are learned in the adolescent period.

CONCLUSION

Within twelve years, the child develops from a dependent newborn to an adolescent approaching adulthood. Although physical growth is slightly behind cognitive and linguistic maturity, the overall rate of development is amazing. Language development is all the more remarkable in the first five years, when there is rapid development of most English syntactic structures—without formal instruction. In the succeeding chapters, we will examine the language development process in detail. I hope you will return frequently to the tables in this chapter to remind yourself of the ongoing, multifaceted development of the child.

DISCUSSION

Did you memorize all that? If so, you're much smarter than I am. Focus on the broad aspects of development. The tables are meant by me as a reference. The text is the important part.

Most of the first two years are spent trying to gain some control over the body, including the oral musculature. Slowly, the child gains the ability to say adultlike sounds, to repeat them when desired, and finally, to put them together into words that others understand. Early developmental emphasis is on speech sounds and establishing communication between the caregivers and the child.

Try to visualize language development as three phases: toddler, preschool, and school-age and adult. In toddler development, emphasis is on pragmatics—broadening of the child's intentions—and semantics, especially the semantic rules. In preschool, development of these continues, but emphasis shifts to language form—syntax, morphology, and phonology—so that by age five, 90 percent of form has been learned. Most speech sounds are acquired and, with the added development of language form, the five-year-old sounds like a little adult. What's missing are the adult's topics and content and the flexibility provided by expanded language uses and increased vocabulary breadth and depth. As development of language form slows during school-age, pragmatics and semantics become more important again. The subtleties of meaning and language use are perfected in order to develop into the great communicator that you are today and the even better one you will be tomorrow.

REFLECTIONS

1. The diverse development of children exhibits several patterns. What are these patterns, and what do they mean?

2. Explain briefly the four processes in speech production.

3. Some of the reflexive behaviors the newborn exhibits are related to oral movement. Describe these oral reflexes and when they disappear.

4. Babbling and reduplicated babbling differ considerably. Can you describe each form of behavior?

5. What are the major differences between two-, three-, four-, and five-year-olds?

6. What generalizations can we make about preschoolers' development of speech sounds?

7. Describe the overall changes that occur in the behavior of school-age children.

8. Explain these semantic skills: divergent and convergent production; figurative language.

4

Neurolinguistics

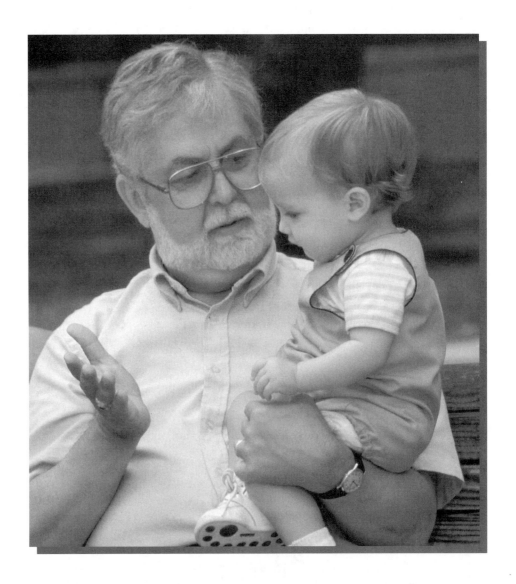

CHAPTER OBJECTIVES

The brain is the only primary organ in the body concerned with processing linguistic information. The study of the manner and location of this processing is called *neurolinguistics*. In this chapter, you will learn about the structures and functions of the brain relative to language. When you have completed this chapter, you should understand

- three basic brain functions.
- the major brain areas responsible for linguistic processing.
- the major theories of brain lateralization.
- the processes of language comprehension and production.
- the models that help explain linguistic processing.
- the following terms:

angular gyrus	information processing
arcuate fasciculus	neurolinguistics
Broca's area	neuron
central nervous system (CNS)	peripheral nervous system
cerebrum	reticular formation
corpus callosum	sulci
cortex	supramarginal gyrus
fissures	synapse
gyri	thalamus
Heschl's gyrus	Wernicke's area

Recently I met a preschool child with whom I'd been acquainted previously. After we exchanged greetings, he eyed me suspiciously for several seconds. When I inquired if anything was wrong, he asked, "Do I remember you?" In our study of language, we might ask our brains the same question regarding incoming and outgoing messages because memory is a large portion of linguistic processing. The study of the anatomy, physiology, and biochemistry responsible for language processing and formulation is called neurolinguistics.

In this chapter, we will examine the main structures of the central nervous system, specifically those involved in processing language. We will also discuss the functioning of these structures and construct a model for language processing.

CENTRAL NERVOUS SYSTEM

The human nervous system consists of the brain, spinal cord, and all associated nerves and sense organs. The brain and spinal cord make up the *central nervous system (CNS)*. Any neural tissue that exists outside the CNS is part of the *peripheral nervous system,* which conducts impulses either toward or away from the CNS. These two systems are responsible for monitoring the body's state by conducting messages from the senses and organs and responding to this information by conducting messages to the organs and muscles. These messages are transmitted through nerves.

The *neuron* is the basic unit of the nervous system. There are approximately 100 billion neurons in the human nervous system. Each neuron consists of three parts: the cell body, a single long *axon* that transmits impulses away from the cell body, and several branchy *dendrites* that receive impulses from other cells and transmit them to the cell body. A nerve is a collection of neurons. Neurons do not actually touch each other but are close enough to enable chemical-electrical impulses to "jump" the minuscule space, or *synapse,* between the axon of one neuron and the dendrites of the next. In short, the electrical charge of one neuron is changed by the release of neurotransmitters at its axon, which in turn affects the release of other neurotransmitters at the dendrite end of the second neuron.

Most of the nervous system's neurons (approximately 85 percent) are concentrated in the CNS. At its lower end, the CNS contains the spinal cord, which transmits impulses between the brain and the peripheral nervous system. At the top of the spinal cord is the brain stem, consisting of the medulla oblongata, the pons, the thalamus, and the midbrain. These structures regulate involuntary functions, such as breathing and heart rate. Within the brain stem is a compact unit of neurons called the *reticular formation.* This body acts as an integrator of incoming auditory, visual, tactile, and other sensory inputs and as a filter to inhibit or facilitate sensory transmission. The *thalamus* acts as a switching station that relays incoming sensory information (with the exception of smell) to the appropriate portion of the brain for analysis. Thus, the thalamus prepares the brain to receive certain select inputs (Lemme & Daves, 1982). To the rear of the brain stem is the cerebellum, which controls equilibrium (Figure 4.1).

Atop the brain stem and the cerebellum is the *cerebrum.* The cerebrum is divided into two halves, designated the left and right hemispheres. In general, sensory and motor functions of the cerebrum are *contralateral,* which means that each hemisphere is concerned with the opposite side of the body. With a few exceptions, the nerves from each side of the body cross to the opposite hemisphere somewhere along their course. Two exceptions to this crossover are vision and hearing. In vision, nerves from the left visual field of each eye, rather than from the left eye, pass to the right hemisphere, and those from the right visual field pass to the left hemisphere. Hearing is predominantly contralateral but not exclusively. Thus, in the sensory and motor functions, the cerebral hemispheres are roughly symmetrical. For specialized functions such as language, however, the hemispheres are asymmetrical, and processing is the primary responsibility of one or the other hemisphere.

Each hemisphere consists of white fibrous connective tracts covered by a gray *cortex* of cell bodies approximately one-fourth of an inch thick. The fiber tracts are of three types: association, projection, and transverse. Association fibers run between different areas within each hemisphere; projection fibers connect the cortex to the brain stem and below; and transverse fibers, as the name implies, connect the two hemispheres. The largest transverse tract, containing approximately 200 million neurons, is the *corpus callosum.* The cortex has a wrinkled appearance caused by little hills called *gyri* and valleys called *fissures,* or *sulci.* Each hemisphere is divided into four lobes labeled frontal, parietal, occipital, and temporal (Figure 4.1).

FIGURE 4.1 Schematic Lateral Surface of Cerebral Hemisphere

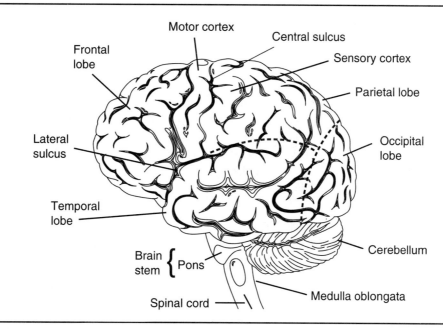

The *fissure of Rolando,* or central sulcus, separates the frontal lobe from the parietal lobe. As in other mammals, large portions of the human cortex are designated for sensory and motor functions. Immediately in front of the central sulcus is the *primary motor cortex,* a two-centimeter-wide strip that controls motor movements. Discrete sets of muscles are controlled from discrete areas of the motor cortex. In general, the finer the movement, the larger the cortical area designated for it. In other words, the fingers have a proportionally greater cortical area devoted to motor control than does the trunk (Figure 4.2). Behind and parallel to the motor cortex is the somatic sensory strip, which receives sensory input from the muscles, joints, bones, and skin. Other motor and sensory functions are found in specialized regions of the cortex. For example, the occipital lobe is primarily concerned with vision, and the temporal lobe processes auditory information. It is simplistic, however, to conceive of the brain as merely consisting of localized sensory and motor mechanisms because of the integration of sensory and motor information required for the body to respond. Rather, we must consider integrated processes.

Three basic brain functions are regulation, processing, and formulation (Luria, 1970). The regulation function is responsible for the energy level and for the overall tone of the cortex. By maintaining the brain at a basic level of awareness and responsivity, this process, located in the reticular formation of the brain stem, aids the performance of the other two functions.

FIGURE 4.2   Schematic of Motor Cortex

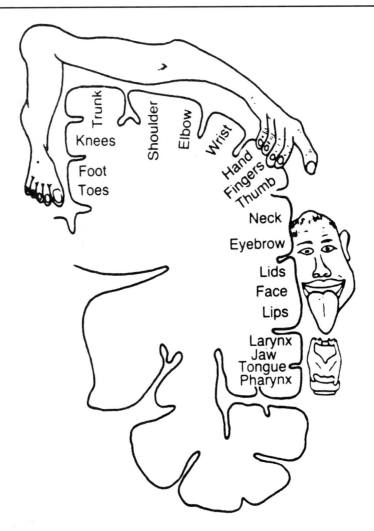

Parts of the body drawn to represent the portion of the motor cortex devoted to each.

The processing function, located in the rear of the cortex, controls information analysis, coding, and storage. Highly specialized regions are responsible for the processing of sensory stimuli, such as optic, acoustic, and olfactory stimuli. Data from each source are combined with those from other sensory sources for analysis and synthesis.

Finally, the formulation process, located in the frontal lobe, is responsible for the formation of intentions and programs for behavior. This function serves primarily to activate the brain for regulation of attention and concentration. Motor behaviors may also be planned and coordinated, but not activated, within this function. Motor movements are sequentially organized based on the integrated information supplied by the tertiary zone from incoming sensory information. Movement is accomplished through a complex process of outgoing (efferent) signals to muscles and incoming (afferent) signals from muscles, joints, and bones.

Of course, these functions are not accomplished in an unconscious brain. The individual thinker is aware of many functions and directs their outcomes by both executive and self-regulating processes (Singer & Bashir, 1999). The executive function is a decision-making and planning control process through which the individual attends selectively, sets goals, plans, and organizes. The overlapping self-regulating process enables the individual to monitor, evaluate, and flexibly adjust behavior for successful performance.

Hemispheric Asymmetry

Although there is symmetry between the left and right hemispheres for many motor and sensory processes, there is a marked asymmetry for certain specific functions such as language. In other words, the distribution of specialized functions is different, usually lateralized to one hemisphere or the other. Although they may possess these separate functions, the two hemispheres are complementary, and information passes readily between them via the corpus callosum and other subcortical bodies. Overall, neither hemisphere is dominant, since each possesses specialized talents and brings different skills to a given task. Neither hemisphere is competent to analyze data and program a response alone. In fact, the brain functions as an interconnected whole with activity throughout and differing levels of response with various activities.

Specialization, or lateralization, of the brain is not unique to humans, although the human brain may be the most asymmetrical. It may be advantageous for an organism to be able to receive and process a greater variety of information through specialization than to duplicate such processing in both hemispheres (Geschwind & Galaburda, 1985). In short, right hemispheric processing is nonsegmental, holistic, and successive, while left processing is segmental, analytic, and sequential (Witelson, 1987).

The right hemisphere in humans is specialized for holistic processing through the simultaneous integration of information. When a specific ability is housed primarily in one hemisphere, we generally say that the hemisphere is *dominant* for that ability. In other words, the primary processing centers are located in that hemisphere. The right hemisphere, for example, is dominant in visuospatial processing such as depth and orientation in space and perception and recognition of faces, pictures, and photographs. In addition, the right hemisphere is capable of holistic or simultaneous recognition of printed words but has difficulty decoding information using grapheme-phoneme (letter-sound) correspondence rules. (See the discussion of reading in Chapter 12.) Other language-related skills include comprehension and production of speech prosody and affect; metaphorical language and semantics; and comprehension of complex linguistic and ideational material and of environmental sounds, such as nonspeech sounds, music, melodies, tones, laughter, clicks, and buzzes (Gainotti, Caltagirone, Miceli, & Masullo, 1981; Millar & Whitaker, 1983; Ross, 1981; Shapiro &

Danley, 1985). In general, these abilities seem limited to the receptive aspects of language. Interestingly, individuals who sign, whether deaf or hearing, have better memory for faces and objects than individuals who do not sign, suggesting that at least the visuospatial aspects of sign may be associated with the right hemisphere (Arnold & Murray, 1998)

In almost all humans, the left hemisphere is specialized for language in all modalities (oral, visual, and written), temporal or linear order perception, arithmetic calculations, and logical reasoning. Whereas the right hemisphere engages in holistic interpretation, the left is best at step-by-step processing. As such, the left hemisphere is adept at perceiving rapidly changing sequential information, such as the acoustic characteristics of phonemes in speech (Mateer, 1983; J. Schwartz & Tallal, 1980; Yeni-Komshian & Rao, 1980). Processing these phonemes for meaning, however, involves representation in both hemispheres (Molfese, Molfese, & Parsons, 1983). The left hemisphere is also dominant for control of speech- and non-speech-related oral movements (Tognola & Vignolo, 1980).

Not all human brains are organized as described. In general, all right-handers are left-hemisphere dominant for language. This condition might be expected, given the crossover of nerve fibers from one side of the body to the opposite hemisphere. But approximately 60 percent of left-handers are also left-hemisphere dominant for language. The remainder of left-handers, approximately 2 percent of the human population, are right-hemisphere dominant for language. A minuscule percentage of humans display bilateral linguistic performance, with no apparent dominant hemisphere. Thus, approximately 98 percent of humans are left dominant for language. In actuality, lateralization may be a matter of degree, rather than the all-or-nothing patterns suggested.

Brain Maturation

Language development is highly correlated with brain maturation and specialization. Whether this relationship is based on maturation of specific structures or on the development of particular cognitive abilities is unknown. (See Chapter 5 for a discussion of cognitive growth in the infant.)

One overall index of neural development is gross brain weight, which changes most rapidly during the first two years of life, when the original weight of the brain at birth triples. Average brain weights are presented in Table 4.1. In addition, chemical changes occur and internal pathways become organized, connecting various portions of the brain. By age twelve, the brain has usually reached its fully mature weight. The number of neurons does not change appreciably, but they increase in size as dendrites and axons grow to form a dense interconnected web. Malnutrition or sensory deprivation may result in less density (Maxwell, 1984).

Most of this increase, however, is the result of myelination, or the sheathing of the nervous system, discussed in Chapter 3. In general, the myelined areas are most fully developed and rapidly transmit neural information. Myelination is controlled, in part, by sex-related hormones, especially estrogen, which enhances the process (Geschwind & Galaburda, 1985). This fact may account for the more rapid development of girls. In general, sensory and motor tracts undergo myelination before higher functioning areas.

TABLE 4.1   Gross Brain Weight of Child

AGE	WEIGHT (GRAMS)	PERCENTAGE OF ADULT BRAIN WEIGHT
Birth	335	25%
6 months	660	50
12 months	925	70
24 months	1065	80
5 years	1180	90
12 years	1320	100

Adapted from *Neurology for the Speech-Language Pathologist* by R. Love and W. Webb, 1986, Boston: Butterworths.

The brain is not simply growing. Microscopic "connections" are being made as neural pathways are identified. Genes determine the basic wiring, and approximately half of the 80,000 genes in our bodies are involved in the formation and operation of the CNS. It is experience, however, that determines the pathways. In the first month of life, synaptic firings may increase fifty-fold to over one thousand trillion. Use of these neural pathways stimulates and strengthens them.

Cell differentiation within the brain of the fetus begins during the sixteenth week of gestation. Subsequent brain maturation is differential and is reflected in the behavior of the infant at birth. During prenatal existence, growth occurs rapidly in the brain stem and in the primary motor and somatic sensory cortices. After birth there is rapid growth in the cerebellum and in the cerebral hemispheres, especially in the visual receptor areas of the occipital lobe. The auditory receptor areas of the temporal lobes mature somewhat later than the visual receptor areas, possibly explaining the relatively early visual maturity of the infant compared to later-developing auditory maturity. The association tracts devoted to speech and language are not fully mature until the late preschool period or later (and some not until adulthood).

In the neonate, vocalization is controlled by the brain stem and pons. The emergence of reduplicated babbling may coincide with maturation of portions of the facial and laryngeal areas of the motor cortex of the brain. Maturation of the auditory association pathways, such as the arcuate fasciculus, that link auditory and cortical motor areas is not achieved until early in the second year and may be essential for imitation of sounds and speech intonation (Stark, 1986).

The primary anatomical asymmetry in the brain is found in the left temporal lobe. This area, enlarged even in the fetal brain, may account for the dominance of the left hemisphere in speech and language reception and production, although it is difficult to pinpoint functions. In addition, this area continues to grow even larger in the mature brain and to myelinize at a slower rate than corresponding areas of the right hemisphere (Geschwind &

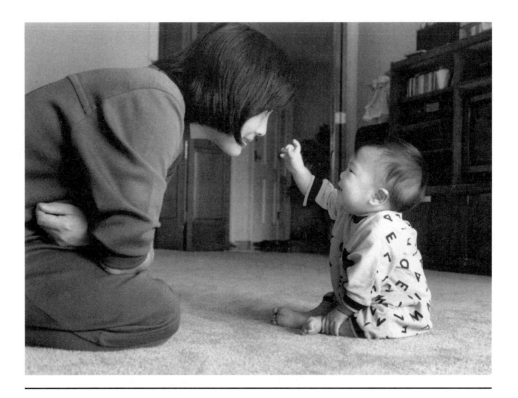

The young child's brain develops rapidly with different sections receiving varying amounts of energy as the child matures.

Galaburda, 1985). The white fiber tract beneath the temporal lobe, called the *planum temporal,* is larger in the left hemisphere of about two-thirds of the adult population.

Brain measurement and the reported *plasticity* of the CNS in young brain-injured children suggest that lateralization of language in the left hemisphere may be progressive. In the infant brain, clear regions for specific abilities have not been delineated, so the brain is plastic, or capable of change. Early brain damage can result in shifts in cortical functional responsibilities to other areas of the cortex. Adjacent or surrounding areas may function in place of the damaged area. Possibly, these areas share functional specialization with the damaged area. This specialization does not occur as long as the primary area is functioning normally. While the language of adults is severely affected by a left hemispherectomy (removal of the left hemisphere), children who undergo the same procedure may have near normal language (Springer & Deutsch, 1985).

We should be careful, however, in drawing conclusions about healthy brain maturation from the study of injured brains (Kinsbourne, 1981). We cannot assume that behavior and specialization represent a one-to-one relationship. A second and differing view holds that language may be fully lateralized from the start. Electrophysiological studies of infants have supported the idea that lateralization occurs long before the development of specific abilities.

A third view assumes that much lateralization occurs during fetal development and that the environment contributes less to lateralization with age. Thus, important factors may be "variations in the chemical environment in fetal life and to a lesser extent in infancy and early childhood" (Geschwind & Galaburda, 1985, p. 431).

Whichever thesis we accept, there can be little disagreement on left-hemisphere dominance for most oral language processing in almost all adults. Let's explore the neural pathways and the processes involved.

LANGUAGE PROCESSING

Linking language processes with specific cortical locations is difficult because these processes are often not localized in particular areas. The processes often overlap, and a particular region may be responsible for both incoming and outgoing information. In addition, language processing is extremely complex, requiring a broad range of functions. The brain functions holistically, not as separate, individualistic, isolated units, and few operations are accomplished by one portion acting alone (Goldman-Rakic, 1987).

Recent advances in brain imaging, such as position emission tomography (PET), single photon emission tomography (SPECT), and functional magnetic resonance imaging (fMRI) have enable researchers to monitor cerebral blood flow while a subject is conducting specific linguistic tasks (Raichle, 1994). Such on-line or "real-time" studies have helped researchers to realize that linguistic processing, such as word retrieval and word and sentence comprehension, often relies on contributions from differing areas of the brain. These results, in turn, have fostered a theoretical move away from processing models based on sensory input and motor output channels of language processing. Syntactic knowledge and word retrieval, for example, transcend the mode of reception or production (Goodglass & Wingfield, 1998).

With all of these advances in mind and forwarned that anatomical localization is not an explanation of function, we will venture into the brain. As a new introductee to this field, you may still find it useful to be able to locate the main area of comprehension and production of language.

Comprehension consists of linguistic auditory processing and language symbol decoding. Auditory processing is concerned with the nature of the incoming auditory signal, whereas symbol decoding considers representational meaning and underlying ideational concepts. Linguistic auditory processing begins with attending to incoming auditory stimuli. The reticular formation of the brain stem sets the tone for the brain and determines to which modality and stimuli the brain will attend. Undoubtedly, this focusing is directed by "orders from higher up." Since it has a limited capacity to process incoming data, the brain must allocate this capacity by focusing its attention on certain stimuli while ignoring or inhibiting others.

Auditory signals received in the brain stem by the thalamus are relayed to an area of each auditory cortex called *Heschl's gyrus* (Figure 4.3). Most of the nerve signal is received at Heschl's gyrus from the ear on the opposite side of the body. Heschl's gyrus and the surrounding auditory association areas separate the incoming information, differentiating significant linguistic information from nonsignificant background noise. This decision is made on the basis of stored knowledge. Linguistic information receives further processing. Coded linguistic input is sent to the left temporal lobe for processing, while paralinguistic input (intonation, stress, rhythm, rate) is directed to the right temporal lobe. Separate processing of linguistic and paralinguistic information may lead to separate but related storage (Gow & Gordon, 1993).

Linguistic analysis is accomplished in *Wernicke's area,* located in the left temporal lobe (Figure 4.3). The *angular gyrus* and the *supramarginal gyrus* assist in this process, integrating visual, auditory, and tactile information and linguistic representation. Damage to these areas disrupts the connection between oral and visual language and may necessitate the use of oral reading for comprehension. The importance of these gyri and of multi-modality input may be signaled by the relatively late myelination of the association areas, occurring in adulthood, often after age thirty. Although their functioning is not totally understood, the angular gyrus aids in word recall and the supramarginal gyrus is involved in processing longer syntactic units, such as sentences. Wernicke's area and the two gyri function "by deriving representational meanings based on established linguistic rules" (Lemme & Daves, 1982, p. 355). Written input is received in the visual cortex and transferred to the angular gyrus, where it may be integrated with auditory input. This informa-

FIGURE 4.3   Receptive Linguistic Processing

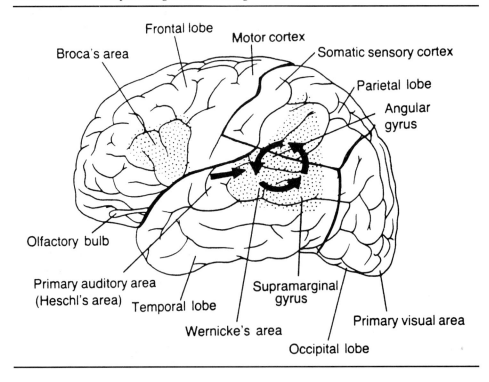

tion is then transmitted to Wernicke's area for analysis. Figure 4.4 presents a quick review of receptive linguistic processing.

Obviously, analysis for comprehension depends on memory storage of both words and concepts. The lexical store of word meanings required for semantic interpretation is diffusely located, centered primarily in the temporal lobe, although the exact location is unknown. Incoming information is transmitted to the *hippocampus* and related structures for consolidation prior to storage. Conceptual, experiential memory is stored throughout the cortex.

The exact method of linguistic analysis is unknown. Sentence processing may consist of a number of autonomous processes that don't interact until each is finished. In contrast, the process may be a highly interactive one in which all components interact from the onset. In either scenario, the processing system is so robust that you can even comprehend sentences in which the word order has been digitally recorded and reversed.

Production processes are located in the same general area of the brain as comprehension functions, many sharing the same structures. One difficulty in describing the

FIGURE 4.4   Following the Path of Receptive Processing

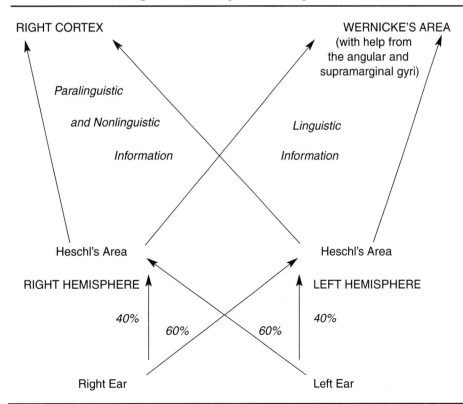

process is that "oral language is highly redundant, only a portion of the signal being necessary for transmission of meaning" (Mateer, 1983, p. 146). The conceptual basis of a message to be produced forms in one of the many memory areas of the cortex. The underlying structure of the message is organized in Wernicke's area; the message is then transmitted through the *arcuate fasciculus*, a white fibrous tract underlying the angular gyrus, to *Broca's area*, in the frontal lobe (Figure 4.5). Broca's area is responsible for detailing and coordinating the programming for verbalizing the message. Signals are then passed to the regions of the motor cortex that activate the muscles responsible for respiration, phonation, resonation, and articulation. This is an active process of symbol selection and message formulation.

Damage to any of these areas results in disruption of linguistic production, but with different effects. Injury to Wernicke's area causes disruptions in both expressive and receptive language abilities. If damage occurs to the arcuate fasciculus, speech is unaffected

FIGURE 4.5   Productive Linguistic Processing

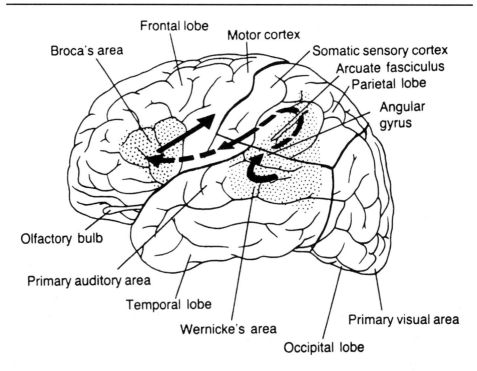

Messages are transmitted from Wernicke's area to Broca's area via the white fibrous tract of the arcuate fasciculus.

except for repetitive movements but the resultant speech may not make sense. Finally, damage to Broca's area results in speech difficulties, but writing and language comprehension may be relatively unaffected.

The message is conceived abstractly and given specific form as it passes from the posterior ideational areas to anterior motor execution areas. Writing follows a similar pathway, passing from Wernicke's area to the angular and supramarginal gyri. From here the message passes to an area similar to Broca's called *Exner's area* for activation of the muscles used for writing.

The actual processes are much more complex than our quick description suggests. Many areas have multiple or as yet unknown functions. Also, describing the location of a function does not explain how that function is performed. Several models of brain functioning have attempted to fill this need.

Models of Linguistic Processing

Several models help explain how language processing occurs. The model that actually applies varies, depending on the task and the individual language user. First, we must distinguish between structures and control processes. Structures are the fixed anatomical and physiological features of the CNS. Structures and their functions are similar across the healthy brains of most individuals. How these structures respond to organize, analyze, and synthesize incoming linguistic information varies with the individual and with the task involved. The way information is processed represents the voluntary problem-solving strategies of each person, called *information processing*.

Information Processing

While the structures of the CNS probably vary little from person to person, processes or the manners of dealing with incoming stimuli or sensory information and formulating outgoing information or responses are more individualized. Although the exact nature of these cognitive processes is unknown, there is a relationship between measured intelligence and the speed of information processing.

Information processing can be divided into the processes of *attention* and *discrimination, organization, memory,* and *transfer* (Figure 4.6). Qualitative differences may reflect operational or processing differences. For example, there may be differences between the automatic and effortful processing abilities. Automatic processes are those that are unintentional or that have become routinized and thus require very little of the available cognitive capacity. Automatic processing neither interferes with other tasks nor becomes more efficient with practice. Effortful processing, on the other hand, requires concentration and attention by the brain. For some, effortful processing is slower to develop and requires greater effort.

Attention and Discrimination. Attention includes both awareness of a learning situation and active cognitive processing. The individual does not attend to all stimuli. Attending can be divided into orientation, reaction, and discrimination. *Orientation* is the ability to sustain attention over time. Humans attend best when motivated and are especially attracted

FIGURE 4.6 Information-Processing Model

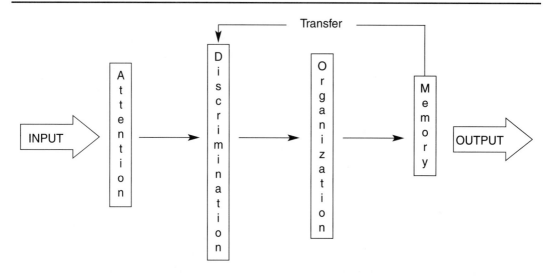

Incoming information to which the brain attends is first subjected to discrimination to determine its relative novelty or familiarity. On the basis of this discrimination, information is organized for storage. The organization aids retrieval by making information readily available. This information can then be transferred to novel problems to aid in their solution.

by high-intensity stimuli that are moving or undergoing change. In part, orientation is related to the individual's ability to determine the uniqueness of the stimulus. *Reaction* refers to the amount of time required for an individual to respond to a stimulus. In part, reaction time is a function of the individual's ability to select the relevant dimensions of a task to which to respond. *Discrimination* is the ability to identify stimuli differing along some dimension. If an individual cannot identify the relevant characteristics, she or he will have difficulty comparing the new input with stored information.

In general, less developmentally mature populations are less efficient at attention allocation and have a more limited attentional capacity (Nugent & Mosley, 1987). These processes are relatively automatic for more mature individuals and require only minimal allocation of the available resources of the brain. Thus, children must allocate more of the limited resources of the brain at this level, leaving fewer resources available for higher level processes.

Organization. The organization of incoming sensory information is important for later retrieval. Information is organized or "chunked" by category. Poor organization will quickly overload the storage capacity of the brain and hinder memory. It is theorized that memory capacity is fixed and, thus, that better memory results from better organization. In other words, better organization results in more efficient use of the limited capacity. The lack of chunking hinders later recall, because it is more difficult to recall unrelated bits of information. Two organizational strategies seem to predominate, mediational and associative. In mediational strategies, a symbol forms a link to some information. For example, an image might facilitate recall of an event. In associative strategies, one symbol is linked to another, as in such common linkages as "men andwomen" or "pins andneedles."

Memory. Recall or memory is the ability to recall information that has been learned previously. It may be helpful to think of three types of memory: sensory information storage, working memory, and long-term memory. Sensory information storage is the most peripheral and separates incoming and stored information by sensory modality.

Working or short-term memory is very limited, and most adults can hold fewer than ten items simultaneously (Baddeley, 1986; Klatsky, 1980). An item may include information that has been "chunked" or organized for easier recall. Incoming information is discarded or held in working memory while encoded and rehearsed for more durable long-term memory. In addition, working memory tracks tasks at hand, such as conversations, and holds messages to be communicated.

Information is retained in long-term memory by rehearsal or repetition and organization. Encoding of information affects ease of retrieval. Memory is best when information is deep processed, which includes semantic interpretation and elaboration and relating to prior experience and existing knowledge. In addition, learning is also facilitated by relating it to experience and knowledge (Chi, 1985; Rabinowitz & Glaser, 1985). Words may be stored in various locations based on meaning, word class, sound pattern, and various associational categories.

Every stimulus event has both a sensory impression or signal, which is inherent in the event, and an abstract or symbolic representation for that event. The signal is meaningful but nonlinguistic. For example, the sound of an engine may signal an automobile. In contrast, the abstract representation or word is linguistic in nature. In early presymbolic development, children seem to use sensory images in their cognitive processing. After the acquisition of language, children have two available memory codes. In other words, the early meaning of *doggie* is based on the perceptual attributes of the examples of *dog* that are encountered. The symbol or word *doggie* is superimposed later.

Echoic memory is "the ability to hear a sound for some time after physical stimulation has ceased" (Watkins & Watkins, 1980, p. 252). In other words, echoic memory is the ability to remember what is heard when it is no longer present. It is a passive retention strategy related to immediate recall of linguistic stimuli, especially during the relatively rapid rates of presentation found in conversation. This echo decays rapidly, requiring the signal to be processed quickly.

Transfer. Transfer or generalization is the ability to apply previously learned material in solving similar but novel problems. The greater the similarity between the two, the greater the transfer. When the two are very similar, generalization is called *near transfer*. When very dissimilar, it is called *far transfer*.

Other Processing

The general nature of information-processing theory makes it an inadequate explanation of purely linguistic processing. Several other types of processing have been proposed for linguistic information. These are *top-down/bottom-up, passive/active,* and *serial/parallel* processes.

Top-Down/Bottom-Up Processing. Top-down and bottom-up processing differ with the level of informational input. (See the discussion of reading in Chapter 12.) Top-down processing is *conceptually driven,* or affected by the expectations of the individual concerning incoming information. In a sense, the cortex prepares other areas of the brain to receive certain kinds of information. The linguistic and nonlinguistic contexts enable individuals to predict the form and content of incoming linguistic information. Hypotheses are formed regarding incoming data. Knowledge, both cognitive and semantic, is used to cue lower order functions to search for particular information. For example, when we hear "The cat caught a . . . ," we predict the next word. Syllable stress in that word, especially on the initial syllable, may be important for confirmation (Gow & Gordon, 1993).

In contrast, bottom-up processing is *data driven.* Analysis occurs at the levels of sound and syllable discrimination and proceeds upward to recognition and comprehension. For example, analysis of the word *mouse* would begin at the phoneme level with /m aʊ s/. The two processes may occur simultaneously or may be used for particular processing tasks.

Passive/Active Processing. Passive and active processing are based on recognizing patterns of incoming information. In passive processing, incoming data are analyzed in fragments until enough information can be combined for the individual to recognize a pattern. This method is similar to bottom-up processing. The contrasting active process involves the use of a comparator strategy that matches input with either a previously stored or a generated pattern or mental model. World knowledge forms a basis. This model forms gradually from active engagement with the environment and helps each of us make sense of the world, anticipate or predict, and plan. In actual practice, both processes probably occur simultaneously.

Serial/Parallel Processing. Finally, serial and parallel, or successive and simultaneous, processing vary with the speed and volume of information flow. Serial, or successive, processes are one-at-a-time in nature. Located in the left frontal and temporal lobes, successive processes analyze information at one level and then pass it on to the next level. For example, the incoming frequency, intensity, and duration of a signal are synthesized to determine the phonemic features. These features are bundled into phonemic characteristics, then syllables, words, and so on until the message is understood.

Parallel, or simultaneous, processing accesses multiple levels of analysis at the same time. Located in the occipital and parietal association areas and possibly in the right hemisphere, simultaneous processing deals with underlying meaning and relationships all at once.

In practice, the two processes occur together, with overall comprehension dependent on the one that most efficiently processes incoming information or outgoing signals. Although successive processing is more precise, it necessarily takes more of the brain's processing potential and is relatively slow. It is therefore quickly overwhelmed, so simultaneous processing must carry the bulk of the responsibility for comprehension. When the incoming rate slows, successive processing takes over again.

Imagine that your brain is writing out each message that enters, in the way you do when taking notes. If the lecturer goes slowly over important points, you can write every word or process successively. Since this situation is rare, however, you usually scramble to summarize what the lecturer has said, recording the overall meaning of the information. This situation is similar to the two functions of successive and simultaneous processing.

Signing, unlike speech, has a greater capacity to express information simultaneously (Emmorey, 1993). Although signs take longer to produce than words, only a minimal portion is needed to identify a sign. The visual nature of signs provides greater initial information and few signs have similar initial shapes. Thus, confirmation is more rapid for signs than words (Grosjean, 1980). The effect on overall linguistic processing is unclear.

Metacognition. Overriding the entire process is metacognition or our knowledge about our processes and our use of that knowledge. Knowledge of our own cognitive and memory processes can facilitate encoding and retrieval and the use of problem-solving strategies. Decisions to execute these processes help manage their use and guide attending; make decisions to attempt, continue or abandon; and monitor progress.

CONCLUSION

Language processing, both expressive and receptive, is located primarily in the left hemisphere of the brain in most adults. Anatomical differences between the hemispheres have been noted in the fetus, but specialization for language develops later in the maturing child. Although most major language-processing functions are generally situated anatomically within the brain, their exact location and function are not totally understood. The effects on these processes of past learning, problem-solving ability, memory, and language itself are also unclear. It is known, however, that cognition, or the ability to use the resources of the brain, is closely related to the overall language level of each individual.

When I was a child we used to play "Button, button, who has the button," in which the child in the middle tried to guess which of the children in the circle around him or her held a button. Neurolinguistics can seem like this when we try to discern where language functions reside in the brain. Don't be troubled by the fact that functions may not be located exactly where we've said they are. The human brain is very flexible, and information is often storied in very diffuse areas.

Let's do a quick retracing. Comprehension goes from the ear to Heschl's area with 60 percent of the information crossing to the opposite hemisphere and 40 percent staying on the same side; then the two Heschl's areas divide linguistic from paralinguistic data, sending the linguistic to Wernicke's area in the left temporal lobe. Wernicke's area processes the linguistic information with aid from the angular and supramarginal gyri. What do they do? Easy to remember. Supramarginal starts with an "s," and so do sequential and syntax. The supramarginal gyrus processes units larger than words and the way they're joined together —syntax. The angular gyrus is left with word recall. Good!

Production is easier to remember. Wernicke's area formulates the message and sends it via the arcuate fasciculus to Broca's area in the frontal lobe. Broca's area is a computer that programs the motor strip, which in turn sends nerve impulses to the muscles of speech. Broca's area does not send nerve impulses to the muscles.

Just as the infant must learn to control its muscles, it must also learn to operate its brain. Different parts of the brain become more active during the first year and mature with myelination. As the child adds more and more information, he or she must learn to organize that information for access. Information processing helps us describe the process. For example, the child's lexicon will eventually be organized by categories based on word meanings, rhymes, alliteration, opposites, and the like. With improved organization and repeated use, the brain's ability to remember increases, making greater language use possible.

DISCUSSION

No discussion of neurolinguistics would be complete without the story of Alex, a young man born with a rare brain disorder known as Sturge-Weber syndrome, which resulted in seizure activity and severely limited blood supply to the left hemisphere of his brain (Trudeau & Chadwick, 1997). As a result, the left hemisphere atrophied, while the right seemed normal. At age eight, when Alex's left hemisphere was removed as a last resort effort to stop his violent seizures, he was nonspeaking and seemingly unable to comprehend language.

Unexpectedly, at age nine, after recovery from surgery, Alex began to speak. Although at first beginning with single words and immature speech, his language began to grow rapidly. In a few months, Alex developed the language of a late preschooler. By age sixteen and still improving, his language was equivalent to that of a ten- to eleven-year-old.

The experience of Alex calls into question much that we have discussed in this chapter, in addition to the notion of a critical period or age—considered to be the preschool years—for language learning, after which such learning was believed to be extremely difficult. The brain of children is extremely "plastic" or malleable. In other words, functions such as language may be be assumed by other areas of the brain whether in the course of normal development or as a result of injury.

As a practicing speech-language pathologist, educator, or psychologist, you will see many children with either brain injury or pathology. While it is important to know the area of injury, we cannot make assumptions about a client's language based on this information. Nor is the size of the damaged area directly related to the resultant deficits, if any. Nothing substitutes for a thorough assessment of speech, language, and communication. It is more important to thoroughly describe what a client can do than to be able to name the site of injury or to name the neurological condition.

REFLECTIONS

1. Describe three basic brain functions: regulation, processing, and formulation. Explain how these functions, especially processing, relate to linguistic material.

2. In most humans the left hemisphere is dominant for linguistic processing. Can you name the major areas responsible for this processing?

3. Few theorists would argue with the notion of brain lateralization for language. Can you explain the major theories on how this lateralization occurs?

4. Explain briefly how language is processed relative to specific areas of the brain.

5. Describe information processing theory and the several models of language comprehension and production processes associated with it.

5

Cognitive and Perceptual Bases of Early Language

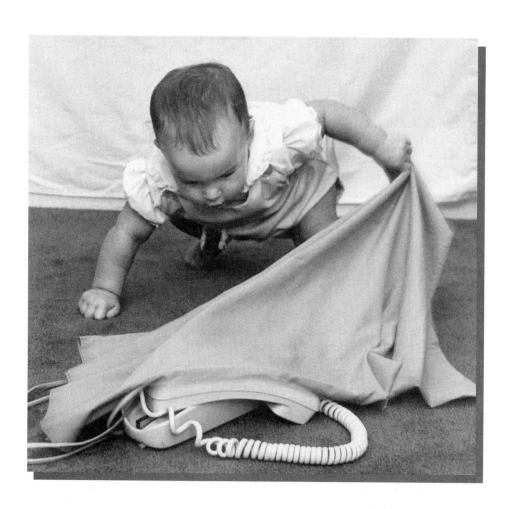

CHAPTER OBJECTIVES

Congratulations, you've made it through the necessary background chapters. Now we're all using the same terms and are ready to begin discussing language development.

The use of symbols requires a certain level of cognitive or mental skill, as well as certain perceptual abilities and social and communication skills. In this chapter, we shall explore both cognition and perception and relate them to the early development of symbols. When you have completed this chapter, you should understand

- the relationship of cognition to language.
- the main aspects of information processing theory.
- the developmental characteristics of the sensorimotor stage of development.
- the aspects of the sensorimotor stage that contribute to the ability to symbolize.
- the basic principles of Piaget's theory of development.
- the contribution of perception to early learning.
- the following terms:

accommodation	linguistic determinism
adaptation	linguistic relativism
assimilation	organization
cognitive stimulation	perceptual stimulation
distancing	rehearsal
equilibrium	schemes
habituation	sign
index	signal
information processing	symbol
integrative rehearsal	

In the first four chapters, we looked at some cognitive developmental milestones and at the relationship of cognition to language. Many (though not all) theorists would agree that "the pacesetter in linguistic growth is the child's cognitive growth" (Slobin, 1973, p. 184).

The purpose of this chapter is not to reopen this "cognition-first" argument. Rather, it is to examine early cognitive development for clues to the child's ability to use symbols. In addition, this chapter will add substance and order to the cognitive development information provided in Chapter 3 and place these milestones in perspective. In this chapter I am assuming that a certain level of cognitive functioning is required before a child uses expressive language. Further, I am assuming that certain perceptual abilities are also required for the child to learn language by hearing it, as most children do.

The infant is not a passive creature but is actively engaged in his or her environment, organizing his experiences into general classes and larger concepts. Of particular importance for students of language development is the means by which the child learns to represent, or symbolize, these ideas and concepts. The importance of this representational ability cannot be overemphasized. The ability to represent one thing with another is one of the most fundamental cognitive prerequisites bases for language acquisition. For example, a child can use a piece of wood to represent a doll's chair. In a similar fashion, the word *chair* can also symbolize a chair.

In this chapter we will first explore the general question of the relationship of cognition and language. Next, we will examine and try to explain early cognitive development. Finally, we will discuss early perceptual growth and its importance for language development.

WHICH CAME FIRST, COGNITION OR LANGUAGE?

In general, we can divide theories on the relationship of thought and language into four types (Figure 5.1). Piaget and others hypothesize a strong cognitive model, represented in Figure 5.1 by model A. According to this theory, cognition is responsible for language

FIGURE 5.1   Models of the Cognition–Language Relationship

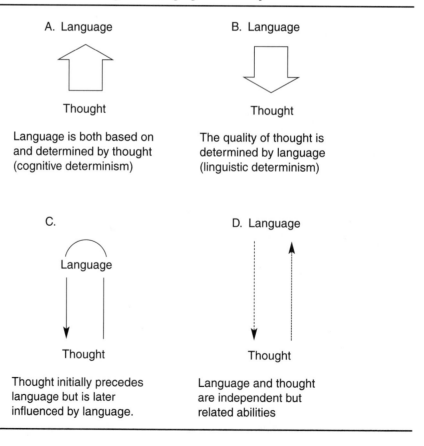

A. Language

Thought

Language is both based on and determined by thought (cognitive determinism)

B. Language

Thought

The quality of thought is determined by language (linguistic determinism)

C.

Language

Thought

Thought initially precedes language but is later influenced by language.

D. Language

Thought

Language and thought are independent but related abilities

acquisition and cognitive knowledge is the basis for word meanings. (See the discussion of *cognitive determinism* in Chapter 2.) In contrast, others, such as Whorf, favor a model of language influencing thought called *linguistic determinism,* represented by model B. Whorf proposed that language strongly influences the very quality of thought. A more moderate position is that of Vygotsky, represented by model C, in which cognition precedes language but, in turn, is influenced by linguistic structures. Finally, in Chomsky's independent theory, represented by model D, the two are considered to be relatively separate but related abilities, each having some limited influence upon the other.

Piaget proposed a model of cognitive functioning that clearly places language on a cognitive base. According to Piaget, cognitive growth is responsible for language. In Piaget's words, "Language is not enough to explain thought, because the structures that characterize thought have their roots in action and in sensorimotor mechanisms that are deeper than linguistics" (Piaget, 1954, p. 98). While cognition and language are interrelated, cognition is clearly the dominant member. Not all theoreticians and child-development specialists agree.

Lev S. Vygotsky, a Russian psychologist and linguist, formulated a theory of specific cognitive development that is somewhat different from Piaget's theory. In *Thought and Language* (1962), Vygotsky theorized that thought and language have different genetic origins and separate curves of development. At about two years of age, these curves join to initiate a new behavior. According to Vygotsky (1962), "[i]nitially thought is nonverbal and speech nonintellectual" (p. 49), but at the point at which they come together, "thought becomes verbal and speech rational" (p. 44). He called this overlap of thought and language *verbal thought.*

In early development, Piaget's and Vygotsky's accounts are similar, with the exception that Vygotsky postulates that human mental activity is the result of social learning. Rather than the self-initiated, solitary child-as-learner proposed by Piaget, Vygotsky describes a collaboration between the child and social environment in the form of parents who mold the child's thinking in culturally adaptive ways.

In later development, Piaget continues to concentrate on cognition with language as a peripheral concern. Language is one of many symbolic processes used to represent reality and is relatively unimportant for cognitive development.

In other words, language is a symptom of the child's underlying cognitive development. In contrast, Vygotsky viewed language as the force that drives later cognitive development because language mediates the child's participation in intellectual and social environments.

Vygotsky did not stress the symbolic development of early thought, as Piaget did. Rather, he claimed that first words are not symbols for objects but actual properties of those objects. Vygotsky (1962) stated, "The word, to the child, is an integral part of the object it denotes" (p. 128).

According to Piaget, the child develops egocentric speech or self-talk to label his environment and then later participates in social interaction. While Piaget considered language to be relatively independent of its social-interactive context, Vygotsky considered the two to be intrinsically linked (Hickman, 1986). Vygotsky claimed that, initially, language merely accompanied ongoing actions in the context and served as a means of social contact. Gradually, language becomes differentiated and serves both a social and an internal function.

Thought can be represented by language, but language also enables humans to develop cognitively. According to Vygotsky, language leads to new forms of cognitive organization. The child develops cognitive skills through social interaction and then uses these skills in intrapersonal behavior. Thus, reversing Piaget, Vygotsky hypothesized that language is learned in interpersonal interaction and then used by the child in self-thought.

Counter to Piaget's cognition-first position, Vygotsky (1962) theorized that "the speech structures mastered by the child become the basic structures of his thinking. . . . The child's intellectual growth is contingent on his mastering the social means of thought, that is, language" (p. 51). As a result, language is multifunctional, serving as a social-interactive tool and also as an abstract representation for internal logical reasoning. As such, language is the most significant achievement of childhood (Blanck, 1990). Language learned within a social interactive context likewise influences thought. As a result, the child exhibits a socially formed mind (Rogoff & Chavajay, 1995; Wertsch & Tulviste, 1992).

Gradually, according to Vygotsky, the regulative behavior of adults in interactions with the child is internalized by the child. Adults use language to guide the child's behavior in problem-solving tasks that the child cannot perform alone. The adults' communication patterns vary with the age and competence of the child and the nature of the problem-solving task. Thus, the language of the adult and, later, of the child is context-related. Vygotsky was interested in these functions of language much more than in the structure of language; he was more interested in the process than in the product (Girbau, 1996).

Benjamin Whorf (1956) also proposed an interdependent theory of thought and language (often referred to as the *Whorf hypothesis*) but emphasized the dependence of thought on language. This position, called **linguistic determinism**, states that all higher thinking is dependent on language; language determines thought. The more lexical richness or breadth in a language, the more superior the resultant cognitive development. In addition, Whorf proposed a **linguistic relativism**: If language determines thought, Whorf reasoned, then the world must be experienced differently by speakers of different languages. In other words, experiences are interpreted relative to the linguistic base. One way in which language influences the interpretation of reality is by classifying it. For example, the Inuit of northern Canada have several different words to describe the quality of snow. We could hypothesize that these arctic dwellers have a different perception of reality than English speakers, who use only the word *snow*. This is a lexical classification. There are also grammatical classifications such as the particular manner used to describe an event. Some languages require gender markers; all nouns are either male or female. Others do not require articles or verb endings. Both of these classification systems influence thought.

Furth (1966, 1971) found that children with deafness performed as well as hearing children, who had much better oral and written language skills. Therefore, Furth concluded that language was not required for some forms of thought. Jerome Bruner viewed language as one instrument of thought. In his view, possession of language is not enough, for the child must learn to organize thinking and experience within the linguistic framework. Thus, lexical hierarchy, or organization, is more important than lexical richness, or breadth.

Finally, Noam Chomsky, with his psycholinguistic emphasis on innate structures, took issue with the experiential nature of Piaget's cognition-first notions. He had dismissed the cognition-first notion of language acquisition. "The child acquires language . . . at a time when he is not capable of complex intellectual achievement in many other domains. This achievement is relatively independent of intelligence or the particular course of experience" (Chomsky, 1957, p. 66). Language and thought are related but independent, he concluded.

Despite all the theories, the exact relationship of thought and language is unknown. For every example of thought influencing language, there is another of the opposite relationship. I. Schlesinger (1977) has proposed four hypotheses, any one of which may explain the relationship. First, cognitive attainment may explain some linguistic achievements, and linguistic attainment may explain others. Second, some children may use a sensorimotor approach to language acquisition, while others may use a linguistic approach. Third, both cognitive and linguistic factors may operate within the same child, but at different points in language acquisition. In other words, cognitive and linguistic factors do not operate simultaneously. Fourth, cognitive and linguistic factors may operate simultaneously and be mutually supportive. It may be that thought and language are so closely aligned that it is difficult to separate them. Possibly the relationship changes at various stages of development or with the task involved. Jenkins (1969) posed the question as follows:

What is the relationship between thought and language?

1. Thought is dependent on language.
2. Thought is language.
3. Language is dependent on thought. . . .
4. None of the above. Or perhaps, all of the above. (p. 212)

The correct answer, according to Jenkins, is "all of the above." Stated another way, as the child's "capacity to communicate symbolically develops, language and thought become so inextricably intermixed [that] it becomes almost impossible to separate [them]" (Lindsay & Norman, 1977, p. 437).

NEUROLOGICAL DEVELOPMENT

The human brain seems wired for development of language, and most linguists agree that there is a biological basis for human language (Pinker, 1994). But biology alone is insufficient to explain the process of language development.

Still, there is compelling evidence within brain maturation that suggests the importance of physiological changes within the infant for the development of language. Thanks to the new imaging techniques mentioned in Chapter 4, researchers are now able to map brain activity on-line and also to follow infant development as different portions of the brain "turn on" or become more active with maturation. A correlation exists between neurological areas becoming active and cognitive functions known to reside in those areas.

At around two month of age, the motor cortex in the frontal lobe becomes more active. During this time, the child is gaining more control of volitional motor behaviors, and many reflexive patterns are disappearing. Likewise, the visual cortex becomes more active at three months when the child gains a full-range focus, enabling her or him to focus on things close in or far distant.

During the second half of the first year, both the frontal cortex and the hippocampus become more active. This is not suprising given the child's increasing ability to remember stimuli and the initial associations between words and the entities to which they refer. In similar fashion, development of gestures, which require the child to plan for the desired response, appear at about eight months when the prefrontal cortex, responsible for fore-thought, becomes more active. The experiences and interactions of the infant are helping him or her to organize the framework of the brain. Organization reflects experience.

The neurons of the newborn are relatively unorganized and unspecified. Over time, the child begins to construct auditory maps from the phonemes heard in the environment. Sounds must be heard thousands of times before neurons are assigned. Eventually, differ-ent clusters of neurons will respond to each phoneme, firing when that phoneme is heard.

The effect of language spoken to the child cannot be overemphasized. There is a direct correlation between the number of words heard by a child during early development and the cognitive abilities of the child even into the late preschool years (Hart & Risley, 1995).

EARLY COGNITIVE DEVELOPMENT

Theories of early cognitive development fall in and out of fashion. Piaget may be popular for a while, then Vygotsky, followed by neo-Piagetians and information processing theory. None fully explains the process. At the risk of doing the same thing, I shall try to weave my way through these theories, finding common ground and using logic to try to explain what I believe is happening cognitively in the first and, to some extent, second years of life. From the preceding section, we recognize that various portions of the brain are becoming more active. I shall attempt to sketch the experiential aspects of cognitive development that pro-vide the overall organization.

Information Processing Change During Infancy

Information processing, presented in Chapter 4, is concerned with cognitive functioning and with the steps involved in handling incoming and outgoing information. These include, but are not limited to, attention and discrimination, organization, memory or recall, and transfer. Of particular importance for learning are sensory information storage, short-term memory, and long-term memory, explained in Chapter 4.

It has been posited that, the structural components of memory do not change with age. Rather, substantial changes reflect changes in the control processes or strategies chil-dren use to encode information. Changes in memory performance are related to changes in long-term memory strategies. Children of different ages vary in the techniques they use to control information flow between parts of the system. Infants require more repeated rehearsals in order for information to be coded in long-term memory. As memory strategies change to accommodate increasing amounts of information, the child's ability to hold infor-mation increases. Cognitive development represents an increase in information processing capacity as a result of use of more efficient processing strategies (Case, 1985, 1992).

The newborn's very limited attending abilities hamper discrimination abilities (which are quite impressive), including auditory discrimination of phonemic differences and of changes in loudness, duration, and frequency. "A stimulus is first feature-analyzed, percep-tually, then matched against stored abstractions, or pattern-recognized, or meaning-associated; and then it may undergo further processing by enrichment or elaboration through association with past experiences" (N. Myers & Perlmutter, 1978, p. 192). Increasing or decreasing attention to an item during encoding produces a corresponding increase or decrease in memorability (Adler, Gerhardstein, & Rovee-Collier, 1998).

Discrimination abilities, already formidable within a few weeks of birth, continue to develop. Perception of speech and speech sounds is described at the end of this chapter. With increasing memory, the child moves from recognition to evocation. After repeated exposures, entities and faces will elicit signs of recognition from the young child. The sight of the bottle will elicit sucking. With increasing memory, the child is able to recall a storied image with minimal stimulation. For example, mother's footsteps may elicit her memory. Within the child's memory, differing aspects of a concept become linked, such as the sight, sound, smell, feel, and name of the family pet. The word *dog* may elicit a searching behavior from the seven-month-old. At some time around the child's first birthday, any stimulus may be enough to elicit the name from the child. For example, seeing the dog or hearing it bark may elicit "Doggie." By about eighteen months, the child is able to evoke the word with no external stimulus.

If memory capacity is fixed, increased organization must account for more efficient processing. In early development, action patterns are probably poorly organized and, therefore, less efficient than they will be later in development. As a result, more memory capacity is used. Through experience, the patterns become better organized and leave more capacity for other schemes. Information is "chunked" to aid storage and also retrieval.

The limited time constraints of sensory memory and the limited capacity constraints of short-term memory enhance the importance of long-term memory for learning. Information is maintained by repetition, a process called **rehearsal**. Transferral to long-term memory requires a special type of rehearsal, **integrative rehearsal** in which new material is integrated into the structure of information already stored in long-term memory. Memory is the transfer of information within the system. It includes acquisition, storage, and retrieval.

Initially, the child has few memories beyond his or her own physical movements or sensorimotor schemes. A stimulus is retained only briefly and may elicit a recognition response if repeated immediately. Gradually, the child develops a "representation" of the stimulus and may display recognition upon encountering the stimulus repeatedly. Thus, Mother's face may aid the child in retrieving the representation for this pattern. When the two—the actual face and the representation—are matched, the child demonstrates recognition by getting excited or by smiling.

In general, infants learn best from repeated presentation of the stimulus. Only later are fewer physical stimuli needed for learning. As cognitive capacity to generate memory cues develops, there is less dependence on external stimuli. Deliberate strategic memory behaviors develop and increase with age as the child's cognitive demands become more extensive.

Over time, with repeated exposure, the child becomes better able to retrieve the representation without the stimulus input. In addition, associations are made between the physical characteristics and the name of the stimulus. Mother's voice or the word "Mommy" may elicit the representation.

Finally, the child is able to retrieve the representation him- or herself. The child can use the word "Mommy" with no input stimulus, such as the presence of mother. As memory becomes less context-bound, the child is free to experiment and to use objects and symbols in novel ways. With increased memory, the child is able to understand and produce more than one symbol at a time.

With maturation and repeated exposure to the environment, working memory or short-term memory, the memory needed to solve immediate problems, expands and less attentional space is needed for the operational processes of the brain, which become more automatic. The child forms broad central concept structures consisting of networks and relations that enable the child to think about a wide range of topics and to bring these interconnected networks to bear on problem-solving tasks (Case, 1985, 1992).

At the same time, the child is learning individual skills to apply to particular tasks, such as attracting attention. The breadth of application of the skill, such as attracting attention to a broad range of gestures, is also dependent on brain maturation and repeated exposure to the environment (Fischer & Bidell, 1991; Fischer & Farrar, 1987). During the extended skill learning, the child learns new competencies, integrates them with other skills, then gradually transforms these skill networks into more general, higher level skills. In the process, he or she becomes more automatized and more efficient. Developmental changes represent increased memory and increased speed in the use of problem-solving strategies.

Stages of Development

Some developmentalists, such as Swiss psychologist Jean Piaget, have proposed a stage theory of cognitive development in which each stage represents qualitatively different cognitive structure evident in the cognitive abilities of the child. Not everyone agrees. There is some danger in viewing development in stages. Beginning students often treat stages as real divisions when they are merely attempts to describe the changes that characterize development. Stages also give the impression that development is sudden when, in fact, it is a slow, gradual evolution.

Nonetheless, Piaget's stages do offer some explanation of these changes and some examples of the infant's evolving ability to represent reality in other cognitive areas in addition to the area of language. For example, cause and effect may be demonstrated in the operation of certain toys at the same time it is noted in the development of gestures. While development in one cognitive area does not necessarily cause development in another, its description does help us to witness the evolution of the infant's thought.

I will not be presenting pure Piagetian theory. For Piaget cognitive advances result from the infant acting directly on the physical world, but infants are rarely left on their own to explore. Rather, the child experiences the world as it is filtered by the adults and older, more mature children. This interactionist or sociocultural view is that of Vygotsky. I will attempt to blend these two philosophical positions, which are often placed at odds.

During interactions with the world, the child is engaged in cooperative dialogues with others who assist him or her. During these interactions, cognitive processes adapted for a particular culture are transferred to the child. Language used by these "teachers" is crucial to cognitive change. Through these interactions with more mature members of the culture, the child develops skills and learns to think in a manner consistent with that culture. As such, the child serves a sort of apprenticeship, as his or her participation is guided through culturally relevant activities by a skilled partner.

As an organism develops, its conceptual system changes. For Piaget, the conceptual system consists of organized patterns of reaction to stimuli he called *schemata*, or schemes. **Schemes** are an individual's cognitive structures that are used for processing incoming sensory information. As new stimuli are received, the organism (the person) tries to fit this information into existing schemes. An event is perceived in a certain way and organized or categorized according to common characteristics. This is an active process involving interpretation and classification. In addition, new information may require the reorganization of the cognitive structures.

An individual's response to a given stimulus is based on his or her cognitive structures and his ability to respond. For example, successive viewings of different dogs may confirm the concept of *dog* as four-legged, fur-covered, and with a tail; dogs can therefore be organized within that general concept. *Cat* fits into this concept, so the scheme for *dog* must be disregarded, redefined, or reorganized, or a new concept formed.

With experience, schemes change and become more refined. Thus, there is no one intelligence for a given person; rather, there is a succession of "intelligences" as schemes evolve. An individual's response to stimuli at a given time reflects his or her concepts or schemes.

The infant experiences tremendous cognitive growth during the two years following birth. It is within this period that the basic structures of intelligence begin to evolve. Whereas the newborn possesses only a few reflexive schemes, the two-year-old child is capable of symbolic thought. By the end of the **sensorimotor** period, the child can solve

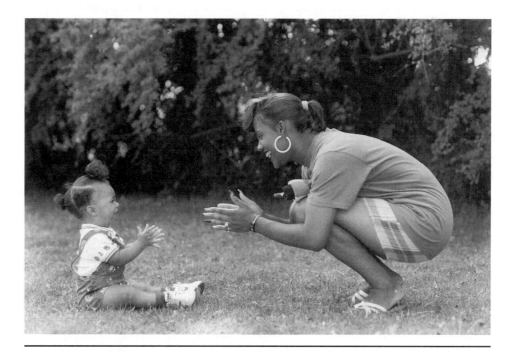

Infants and toddlers gradually learn to symbolize and represent the elements of their environment.

many physical problems through thought and can communicate through the use of language.

As noted in Chapter 3, the infant is capable of many complex cognitive behaviors. This functioning is demonstrated in organized patterns of actions that can be characterized as *pre-representational.* Sensorimotor intelligence is similar to the level of cognition used by adults for routine motor tasks, such as putting on socks.

The sensorimotor child "thinks" to the extent that he or she interacts with familiar people and objects in predictable ways that demonstrate recognition. Thus, the child's cognitive structures, or schemes, represent action-oriented functioning. For example, rather than labeling or classifying an object, the sensorimotor child will behave toward that object in a way that indicates that he knows its function. His schemes are organized according to sensory input and motor responses. Schemes may be coordinated or combined for more complex interactions.

Piaget has divided the sensorimotor period into six stages of progressively more complex cognitive structures. The major accomplishments of each stage are listed in Table 5.1. Let's discuss the major observable changes in imitation, object concept, causality, and means-ends, looking for examples of cognitive growth and an increasing ability to use symbols.

Stage 1: Birth to One Month

According to Piaget's theories, the behavior of the stage 1 child is almost totally reflexive. The child makes no differentiation between stimuli and understands no causality beyond his or her own egocentric view of the environment; the child is a part of all objects and causes all events. Some reflexes, such as the sucking and rooting reflexes, undergo significant changes as a result of interaction with the environment. The child demonstrates *adaptive intelligence,* continually adjusting his behavior to unfamiliar environmental conditions. By the end of stage 1, the child has already begun to differentiate the sucking response to accommodate the environment. These small, yet significant, experience-based changes indicate cognitive growth.

Stage 2: One to Four Months

In stage 2, reflexive behavior is further modified. As the infant reacts reflexively, he or she assimilates and accommodates to sensory information, producing the initial changes in his or her schemes. Continual practice of schemes, such as sucking, looking, and reaching, results in elaboration and refinements of these behaviors. Toward the end of stage 2, the sucking response begins to occur in anticipation of eating: The nipple becomes a sign for the event that will follow, and the child responds with sucking.

In addition to the continued change in sensorimotor schemes, there is a gradual coordination and integration as evidenced in eye–hand coordination, visual following of a moving object, localization to sound, and purposeful thumb sucking. Eventually, the child will be able to reach without watching his or her hand and the object simultaneously. In other words, the child will hold a representation of the location of each in space.

Localization of sound results from coordination of vision and audition. It represents an early object concept because of the association of the object with a specific sound. In

TABLE 5.1 Piaget's Sensorimotor Stages

STAGE AND AGE (MONTHS)	GENERAL	IMITATION	OBJECT CONCEPT	CAUSALITY	MEANS–ENDS
Stage 1 Birth–1	Reflexive	Notion not present	No differentiation of self from objects	Egocentric	Notion not present
Stage 2 1–4	Coordination of sensory schema	Self-imitation of actions with unexpected results "Preimitation"	Object followed with eyes until out of view Change in perspective interpreted as change in object	No differentiation of self and moving objects	Notion not present Intentionality lacking
Stage 3 4–8	Repetition of actions of others	Imitation of others' actions already in repertoire	Anticipation of position of moving objects; no manual search	Self as cause of all events	Repetition of events with unexpected outcomes; heightened interest in event outcome Intentionality follows initiation of behavior
Stage 4 8–12	Known means applied to new problems	**Imitation of* behaviors different from those in repertoire** Facial imitation	**Manual search for object where last seen** **Object constancy**	**Some externalization or causality** Realization that objects can cause action	Coordination and integration of schemata **Establishment of goal prior to initiation of activity** Anticipation of outcomes
Stage 5 12–18	Experimentation	Imitation of behaviors markedly different from repertoire	Sequential displacements considered Awareness of object spatial relations	Realization that he is one of many objects in environment	New means through experimentation Tools used

(continued)

TABLE 5.1   Continued

Stage and Age (Months)	General	Imitation	Object Concept	Causality	Means–Ends
Stage 6 18–24	Representational thought	**Deferred imitation**	Representation of displacements Awareness of unseen movements	Representation of causality Able to predict cause–effect relationship	Language used to influence others Representation of outcome or end

*Words in bold indicate sensorimotor schemes considered to be especially important for the development of symbol use.

addition to making object–sound associations, the child begins to associate people with their voices in stage 2.

In general, the child does not initiate behaviors with a desired end in mind. His or her behavior is reflexive for the most part, and goals are not identified until after the child begins an action sequence. For example, the child will reach for an object in front of him or her but is incapable of uncovering or searching for an object that is not in view.

Imitation in stage 2 is primarily self-imitation. The child produces an action pattern, and the resultant feedback further elicits the behavior. For example, sucking produces the tactile pressure in the mouth to elicit more sucking. The child exhibits *preimitation:* and will repeat a habitual behavior if someone imitates the behavior immediately after the child has performed it.

Stage 3: Four to Eight Months

The third stage of cognitive development is characterized by imitation in which feedback is not solely proprioceptive, or from within the organism, but also from external stimuli. The child will repeat his or her own actions in an attempt to sustain an event. In this early goal-directed, or intentional, behavior, the child continues to repeat a behavior for which he or she has a scheme. As before, however, the goal of the behavior is established only after the activity begins.

Even though the child attempts to sustain an activity, it cannot be said that he or she has a concept of causality, or cause and effect, beyond himself. The stage 3 child remains egocentric, believing that he or she causes events to happen. The child makes little attempt to explore the effect of its behavior. Yet in stage 3 there is an increased interest in environmental effects. The child's increased interest in events beyond the body is also reflected in an increased orientation toward objects. The child reaches for familiar objects even if they are partially hidden from view and grasps the object and manipulates it for inspection, thus exhibiting greater coordination between vision and prehension. Although the child is able to anticipate the future position through which a moving object will pass, he or she does not search for a hidden object.

The stage 3 child applies its limited behavior repertoire rather indiscriminately to objects. His primary behaviors include mouthing, banging, looking, and shaking. There appears to be little knowledge of, or concern for, the objects' properties. Near the end of stage 3, the child goes through a transition and begins to combine or sequence schemes into an "examining" scheme. In addition, the child begins to coordinate actions on different objects.

During stage 3 the child begins to imitate others when two conditions are met. First, the child will only imitate behaviors that he or she produced spontaneously on another occasion. Second, the child must see and hear himself or herself while producing the imitations. For example, the child can see his or her own hands and hear the sound when banging an object on the table. If the child has performed this motor act before on his or her own, then during stage 3 he or she is likely to imitate this action when it is performed by others.

Stage 4: Eight to Twelve Months

According to Piaget, the stage 4 child exhibits the first clear evidence of thought. The stage 4 child is able to establish a goal and select a means to that end before taking action. Often the means are coordinated for an end that is not immediately directly attainable. For example, the child may realize that it must put down one object in order to pick up another or that he or she can pull a string to obtain an object at the other end.

In part, this means-ends behavior reflects the child's developing ability to anticipate events independent of those currently in progress. The child is able to associate certain indices with actions that will follow, even though these signs may not be directly related. For example, the child may cry when mother turns away but before she actually departs.

Stage 4 imitation is more flexible than that exhibited in stage 3. Physical imitation has now become a learning tool because the child can imitate behaviors that differ to some degree from those already in the repertoire. In addition, he or she can imitate motor behaviors that he or she cannot actually see on him- or herself, such as facial expressions. That imitation requires a limited degree of short-term memory of motor behaviors.

The stage 4 child can also remember objects and realizes that they exist even when they are not seen. If an object is hidden, the child will manually search for it, usually in the location in which the object disappeared.

In addition to this early form of object permanence, the child shows evidence of concepts such as object constancy and causality. By stage 4 the child demonstrates that he or she is aware that an object has not changed when it appears to be smaller or when it is viewed from a different perspective. The child has learned that qualities such as shape and size do not change and that objects can cause action.

The child recognizes that some objects have more interesting or important features than others. Thus, the child plays longer and manipulates more complex toys more often. Object manipulation is characterized by differentiated actions as the child's action repertoire is applied more discriminately.

In stage 4, the child begins to externalize causality. He or she realizes that other people and objects may be the source of activity.

In summary, stage 4 is a very important stage in cognitive development. Several behaviors indicate an externalization of cognitive functioning. Through interaction with the environment, the child has become less egocentric in thought and action. In addition, the stage 4 child is able to interpret indices and thus anticipate actions. The use of indices is a step toward truly symbolic representation. Finally, the child demonstrates limited short-term motor memory. All of these behaviors will be significant for later symbol use.

Stage 5: Twelve to Eighteen Months

Stage 5 is the last totally sensorimotor stage. It is filled with experimentation with objects and with exploration. This stage is characterized by the coordination of new schemes to solve problems. New means are established through trial-and-error experimentation. Thus, the stage 5 child is very adaptable to new situations. The child explores real properties of objects and experiments with object potentials. There appears to be an ongoing search for new methods of interaction. In addition, the child exhibits true experimentation and waits to see the outcome of his or her behavior.

The stage 5 child is a skilled imitator. Within its motor limitations, the child is capable of imitating behaviors that are markedly different from those in his or her repertoire.

Finally, the concept of object permanence has developed to the point that the child will manually search for an object through sequential or multiple displacements. This searching will be situationally oriented and not dependent on previous patterns of success.

Stage 6: Eighteen to Twenty-Four Months

In sensorimotor stage 6, the child progresses to *representational* intelligence. In this stage the child is able to represent objects internally and to solve problems through thought, demonstrating real symbolic functioning. Object representation is exhibited in the child's ability to search for an object even though he or she did not see it hidden. Thus, the child is freed from a reliance on immediate observational and perceptual information. This change is also noted in the child's problem-solving abilities. Experimentation is accomplished in thought, through symbolization of actions rather than through actions themselves. The child is able to solve problems in part because he or she can predict the cause-effect relationship.

The ability to use symbols is also exhibited in the child's ability to produce and comprehend words when the referents are not physically present. Most children produce their first words well before this stage, but only in the presence of the referent, or entity.

Deferred imitation, which appears in stage 6, is another example of representation. The stage 6 child can observe a behavior, store it, and retrieve it later for production. It is not unusual for the child to reproduce other children's behaviors, such as tantrums, at a later time.

Summary

The infant is born with certain reflexive schemes. These reflexes are gradually modified through interaction with the environment. During the sensorimotor period, several developmental trends are evident. The child becomes less reflexive and less egocentric as he or she begins to act on the environment. In addition, the child develops increased memory skills and increased ability to represent reality symbolically.

It is difficult to believe that the newborn is the same individual two years later. The overall cognitive changes are monumental. The child has moved from sensorimotor intelligence to truly symbolic thought. With this development, the child is freed from the slower process associated with motor actions and is less bound by actions or concrete objects. In addition, symbolic intelligence is a shared system that encourages communication with others. Symbols can be transmitted via speech to those who share the coding system.

Relation of Sensorimotor Development to Language

Although there is no one-to-one relationship between cognition and language, the principles of cognitive organization apply to language. Children learn object functions, such as rolling a ball, through manipulation and then use these functional characteristics to relate classes of objects, such as things that roll. These common features may form the semantic basis for early words.

The sensorimotor development of language is a progression from signal to sign (Morehead & Morehead, 1974). Toward the end of sensorimotor stage 3, the child learns to respond to signals. A **signal** is "any indicator which elicits an action scheme and in which there is no differentiation between the form of the action (signifier) and its content (significant)" (Morehead & Morehead, 1974, p. 161). For example, the bottle becomes a signal for *eat*. As you can see, many movements or vocalizations of the child and parent have the potential of becoming signals. Games such as peekaboo, for example, evoke a predictable child response; the actions of the game signaling a response.

In stage 4 an index becomes an early form of prerepresentation. An **index** is a shared property of some motor act of the child and others. The child uses similar or shared properties as a means of interpreting the actions of others. The action need not be part of its immediate context, as before. For example, when mother puts on her coat, the child infers that the mother is leaving, although she is not actually in the process of going out the door. Each occasion of putting on her coat is similar enough to allow the child to generalize the meaning of this behavior. Before reaching stage 4, the child would respond to mother's physical leave-taking as a signal but might not infer leave-taking from the isolated action of simply putting on a coat. In part, this change reflects the child's increased ability to anticipate behavior based on environmental cues.

The shared features of actions also aid the child's learning and are reflected in more mature motor imitation behaviors. In turn, the motor imitation is reflected in the child's beginning use of gestures and vocalizations. Children begin to imitate adult vocalizations at about nine months of age. At about the same age, the child begins to shift from signals that represent response to an internal stimulus, such as crying, to signals, such as gestures that represent an intention to communicate.

Symbols begin to appear as first words in stage 5. A **symbol** is an entity used to represent another entity that has similar features; thus symbols incorporate more than just words. Just as a word can stand for *doggie* in the presence of a dog, a shoe may be used to represent a telephone receiver. This kind of representation presupposes an understanding of object use and properties.

Finally, in stage 6, the child begins to use signs. True **signs** denote thought about an entity or event. The sign, or word, represents cognitive structures, not the real entity or event. For example, when the stage 6 child discusses *doggie,* he or she is using a concept, not just the name of an entity in the context. Thus, the stage 6 child can talk about objects or events that are not present or are present in a novel context.

Piaget theorized that stage 6 functioning is required for word use. Yet, stage 6 behaviors are not required for single-word production. Single-word language begins late in stage 4 or early in stage 5 (Kelly & Dale, 1989). On the other hand, if we accept the premise that true symbol-word use does not occur until the child is capable of representing absent referents, then the theory is more acceptable. In addition, stage 6 seems to be correlated closely with early multiword communication.

To understand the importance of cognitive development to language development, we will examine five specific aspects separately: imitation, object permanence, causality, means-ends, and play. The available research data are mostly correlational and the exact nature of the relationship is unknown. Correlational results do not imply cause and effect.

Imitation

A number of studies have called early physical imitation a prerequisite to speech, to language, and to communication. In general, imitation is important because of the developing ability to construct internal representations of the behavior of others and to duplicate them. To imitate physically, the child must be able to perform at least three tasks: turn-taking, attending to the action, and replicating the action's salient features.

Vocal imitation and gestures are significantly correlated at about nine months of age: an increase in one thus results in an increase in the other. Gestures are learned through imitation. Early gestures are *recognitory,* or functional, representing the use of objects. Children "label a known object by carrying out an action typically associated with it" (Bates & Snyder, 1987). For example, using a spoon for its intended purpose signifies a knowledge of object function. In addition, the appearance of multiaction imitation schemes coincides with initial two-word utterances.

It is generally accepted that imitation is important for speech production. Physical imitation is not, however, a necessary prerequisite for facial and vocal imitation, although there is a strong correlation. The speech sounds made during vocal play generally reflect environmental input. The tonal qualities of adult speech are also imitated very early.

The link of imitation to language is less certain. Children begin to use words before stage 6 deferred imitation occurs. Although imitation is significantly correlated with gestural development, this correlation occurs at nine to ten months of age, well before stage 6. In short, there is a strong correlation between naming and the emergence of recognitory gestures and deferred imitation (Bates & Snyder, 1987).

In summary, imitation may aid early speech development and is correlated with symbolic representation. True symbol functioning is assumed to occur when deferred imitation is acquired because the referent need not be present. This occurs after the first birthday when children are already using single words. The importance of imitation may be as a social behavior seen in child–parent interactions. Such early turn-taking will be discussed in Chapter 6.

Object Permanence

Object permanence is "the cognitive basis for 'knowing' that an object which has been removed from . . . immediate perception still exists and thus can be made to recur" (McLean & Snyder-McLean, 1978, p. 23). One method of recurrence is through speech. By naming an entity, the speaker can cause the object to exist symbolically for the listener. Object permanence may be related to such early semantic functions as nonexistence, disappearance, and recurrence.

Although there is some correlation between object permanence and language, other aspects of early cognitive development correlate more strongly with language acquisition. At nine to ten months of age, the infant's development of imitation, play with toys, and means–ends seems to be most highly correlated with language development in the form of gestures. Object permanence is not related.

Stage 6 object permanence does seem to be related to the large growth in vocabulary at the end of the second year. Some stage 6 behaviors are found among children at the single-word level, but vocabulary increase seems to occur when children exhibit all stage 6 object permanence schemes.

Although stage 6 memory for absent objects is not a prerequisite for first words, such memory may be related to developmental changes noted late in the second year of life (Bates & Snyder, 1987). Stage 6 memory may indicate a stabilization of the ability to represent reality. Perhaps stage 4 object permanence is sufficient for development of single words. In stage 4 the child recognizes objects when they reappear. This may be sufficient to enable the child to refer to present objects. Stage 6 object permanence requires memory of absent objects. This skill is unnecessary for initial word use. Object use, or manipulation, may be more closely related to language than is object permanence.

Causality

Several authors have concluded that a sensorimotor notion of causality is a prerequisite for communication and for language. Once the child realizes that he or she and others can be a source of action, then the means are available for language to become a vehicle of change. With the development of causality, the child can solve problems by representing them internally. This ability is a portion of the symbolic function of language. It should be obvious that recognition of self and others as sources of action is closely related to recognition of the means for solving problems. The latter is demonstrated in means–ends development.

Causal development in interactions with people and with objects seems to mature differently. Causality in social behavior may develop well before the first birthday, whereas causality applied to objects may not occur until late in stage 4 (Sexton, 1980). Stage 5 causal understanding may be a necessary but not sufficient condition for communication development, as measured by expression of intentions. There appears to be a strong relationship between causality and understanding of verbs and semantic relations (J. Miller, Chapman, Branston, & Reichle, 1980).

Means–Ends

Sensorimotor means–ends schemes appear to be a critical feature in language development. Examples of means–ends behaviors are pulling a cord to get an attached toy or pulling the tablecloth to get an item on the table. Means–ends skills are significantly correlated with language development at nine months of age, early in stage 4. At nine months the child begins to use gestures to communicate. Thus, the development of stage 4 means–ends appears to be related to development of intentionality.

Initially, the child approaches the task with an anticipation of the outcome. He or she selects from among the appropriate means to attain the desired end. Once a means is selected, the child maintains that behavior. The action is terminated when the end is attained. Finally, if the end is not totally appropriate, the action taken to attain it is slightly modified.

Gestures have received considerable attention, because they are an early communication form used to attain a desired end. Gestures and early words refer to the same content. Each begins in rigid, context-bound routines and gradually becomes more flexible. Sequences of gestures appear at about the same time as multiword utterances.

Object retrieval and early tool use have generated particular attention. Attempts to retrieve an object help the child learn that one object can be used to attain another. Words can serve a similar function. Tool use may be related to symbolization in three ways (Bates, Benigni, Bretherton, Camaioni, & Volterra, 1979). First, each requires analysis of the problem into part–whole relations. Second, the child must locate the missing part in order to solve the problem. Finally, a substitution must be found for the missing part. This process is analogous to using a word to represent, or substitute for, a referent.

Although means–ends abilities seem to be significantly correlated with communication and language development, there is little support for the notion that stage 6 is required for symbol use. Children use very low-level gestures at stage 4 means–ends. At stage 5, children use words to communicate. Stage 6 means–ends appears to be related to higher language functioning, such as the emergence of syntax. The appearance of two-word utterances also correlates significantly with stage 6 means–ends.

Play

Several studies have demonstrated the importance of play for language development. There is a significant correlation between object play and language at ten to thirteen months.

While play is an important learning strategy, symbolic play is of particular importance for development of language. Symbolic play occurs when the child uses one object to represent another, such as a spoon for a telephone receiver. Words are used similarly to represent referents. This level of play does not occur until the middle of the second year of life. Children able and willing to drink from toy cars or to use a block as a spoon make significantly more progress in language than children who are symbolically less flexible (Bates, Bretherton, Snyder, Shore, & Volterra, 1980). The number of schemes that children demonstrate during symbolic play and the number of symbolic schemes used in language have been found to be similar.

The level of play required for symbol use has been questioned. Early schemes with objects are a good indicator of later language growth, but children use single words before they fully develop symbolic play.

Conclusion

It would seem that a notion of object permanence develops early, as does causality relative to interactions with people. Other cognitive skills, such as means–ends, take longer to develop but are nonetheless significant, especially for the development of gestures. Finally, skills such as deferred imitation, invisible displacement, and symbolic play may be critical for vocabulary growth and early multiword combinations but unnecessary for single-word speech.

Certain semantic functions correlate well with cognitive development of specific skills rather than with stages of development (Gopnik & Meltzoff, 1984, 1986). For example, the ability to solve complex object permanence problems correlates well with the appearance of disappearance words and phrases, such as *all gone*. The ability to sort objects correlates with the appearance of naming or labeling.

Some representational abilities may even be present at birth. For example, two- or three-week-old infants are capable of limited facial self-imitation. At this age, the child reproduces actions that he or she "feels" himself or herself producing. This proprioceptive imitation is quite different from later imitations, which serve a representative function. In those situations, which occur at around nine to ten months of age, the child imitates others with the realization that he or she now mimics the model. If the neonate is capable of facial imitation, the ability to represent the external world may not be the culmination of infant cognitive development but the beginning.

Throughout this period, the child learns to cope with changes in surface appearance by discovering underlying stability. This cognitive process relates to language acquisition in two ways. First, cognitive abilities allow infants to understand the consistencies in the non-linguistic context so that their communication partners share mutual meanings. Second, cognitive abilities help the infant learn how the speaker's words relate to these shared meanings. Most early shared meanings include object identity. It is this identity that enables the child to detect the relationship between adult speech and the nonlinguistic context of objects. Thus, the rules for object identity, not Piaget's action schemes, may be the organizing principles of cognitive development. At about five months of age, the child uses the object identity rules to construct a notion of object invariance across transformations, or changes. Later, the child learns words that name transformations or that do not vary across transformations or objects. This feature is reflected in children's first words. First words name actions, the sources or recipients of actions, and attributes. In language development, adult linguistic input also serves a greater function than Piaget theorized.

Studies have shown that sensorimotor stage 6 is not a necessary prerequisite for language. It appears that only a subset of sensorimotor abilities correlates closely with language development.

Infant Learning

Cognitive development is not a quantitative accumulation of ideas and facts. It is a qualitative change in the process of thought. An organism organizes and stores material in qualitatively different ways as a result of this maturation. These changes occur through a child's active involvement with the environment as mediated by a mature language user who interprets and facilitates interaction for the child. The motivation for cognitive change or learning is internal as the child attempts to reach a balance between new and previously held concepts or schemes.

All organisms adapt to changes in the environment. Such adaptations are cognitive as well as physical. According to Piaget, cognitive evolution or development is the result of organization and adaptation, two complementary processes.

Organization and adaptation are two basic functions found in all organisms (Figure 5.2). **Organization** is the tendency to systematize or organize processes (either physical or cognitive) into systems. The human body has several physical systems, including circulation and respiration. According to Piaget, behavioral and cognitive structures are also organized coherently into systems. The organized cognitive structures are the schemes. **Adaptation** is the function or tendency of all organisms to change in response to the environment. Adaptation occurs as a result of two related processes: assimilation and accommodation.

Assimilation is the use of existing schemes or cognitive structures to incorporate external stimuli (Figure 5.2). In other words, assimilation is an attempt to deal with stimuli in terms of present cognitive structures. In this way, an organism continually integrates new perceptual matter into existing patterns. For example, an Irish setter is similar enough to be incorporated into the dog category along with collies and German shepherds. Obviously, these types of dogs are not identical, but the similarities are great enough to allow their assimilation into the same category. Without such categorization, we could make little sense of the environment. Not all stimuli fit into available schemes, however, and mental structures must be adapted to these stimuli.

Accommodation is a transformation of cognitive structures in response to external stimuli that do not fit into any available scheme and, therefore, cannot be assimilated (Figure 5.2). As such, an individual has the option of modifying an existing scheme or developing a new scheme. The Irish setter could be included in the dog concept. An elephant, however, is sufficiently different to require a new category. Once the organism has accommodated its schemes to the external stimulus, the new information is assimilated, or incorporated, into the new or modified scheme. The new scheme does not replace the old one. They are both retained. Thus, the processes of assimilation and accommodation are complementary and mutually dependent. New or modified structures are created continually and then used to aid the organism's comprehension of the environment.

Each organism is more effective in interacting with the environment if that organism is in equilibrium with the environment. **Equilibrium** is a state of cognitive balance, or harmony, between incoming stimuli and the organism's cognitive structures. Obviously, equilibrium is only momentary for any given stimulus, but nonetheless it is the state toward which all organisms strive. Equilibrium is the "driving force" of cognitive and other biological changes. Intelligence, or cognitive functioning, changes with each adaptation, or attempt to achieve equilibrium. The results of these changes are different cognitive structures that occur in fairly predictable patterns.

Role of the Caregiver

The child's interaction with the environment is moderated by an adult or a more mature child who uses language to help explain and describe the child's experiences. While not directly teaching the child, this caregiver provides the opportunity for learning.

FIGURE 5.2 Piaget's Cognitive Learning Process

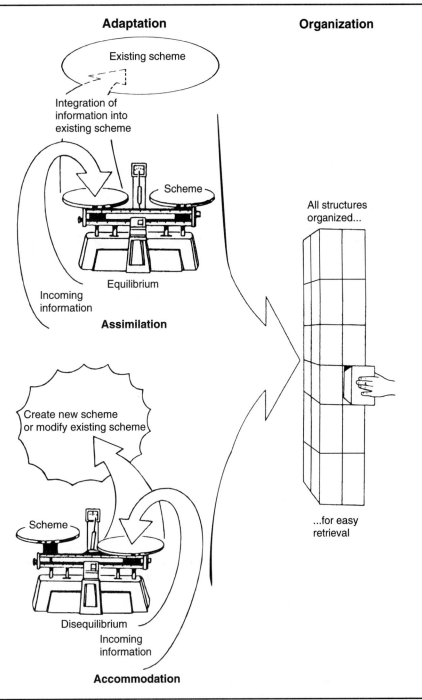

The caregiver regulates not only the amount of stimulation but also the timing. Caregiver behavior is not random but fits into the child's behavior. By modifying his or her behavior, the caregiver maintains an interactional dialog with the infant. There are six techniques that mothers use to create opportunities for their children to participate (R. Schaffer, 1977). These techniques—phasing, adaptive, facilitative, elaborative, initiating, and control—are listed in Table 5.2. The mother monitors the child's behavior continually and

TABLE 5.2   Maternal Techniques for Infant Participation

TECHNIQUES	BEHAVIORS	EXAMPLES
Phasing	Monitors infant behavior to determine when to slot her behavior for most impact; must know when to intervene to attain predictable outcome	Mother attains infant's attention to an object before using it in some way. Mother monitors infant's gaze and follows it for clues to infant interest.
Adaptive	Exhibits behaviors that enable infant to assimilate information more rapidly; maintains infant's attention and provides highly ordered, predictable input	Mother uses slower arm movements than with adults. Mother has more emphatic gestures and more exaggerated facial expressions than with adults. Mother's speech is simpler and more repetitive than with adults.
Facilitative	Structures routine and environment to ensure infant success	Mother holds toy so child can explore. Mother assists infant physically. Mother supplied needed materials for task completion.
Elaborative	Allows child to indicate an interest, then elaborates upon it; talks following the infant's activities and interests closely	Mother demonstrates play with object of infant's interest. Mother talk about infant's behavior as she performs (parallel talking).
Initiating	Directs infant's attention to objects, events, and persons; follows sequence of gaining infant's attention, directing it, and looking back to ensure that the infant is attending	Mother points to direct attention. Mother brings object into child's view.
Control	Tells infant what she is to do; pauses after key words that are emphasized and makes extensive use of gestures	Mother insists that infant eat. Mother stresses what she wants the infant to do.

Source: Adapted from R. Schaffer, *Mothering.* Cambridge: Harvard University Press, 1977.

adapts her behavior accordingly. Her modifications enable the infant to enter the dialog as a partner. These mutual dialogs seem to reach their greatest frequency at around an infant age of three or four months (S. Cohen & Beckwith, 1975).

EARLY PERCEPTUAL DEVELOPMENT

In addition to cognitive abilities, such as representation or symbol use, the infant must be able to discriminate between different sights and sounds within his environment. The ability to discriminate differences in incoming information is a portion of perception, a process of gaining awareness of what is happening around us. Of most interest for a study of linguistic development are the auditory perceptual skills related to voice and speech, but other perceptual skills are also important for the formation of early meanings based on the characteristics of various entities, such as the way they look or feel. Some of these perceptual abilities were mentioned in Chapter 3, so I will review them only briefly.

Perceptual development appears to have at least four aspects: growth, stimulation, habituation, and organization (T. Bower, 1977). Growth includes not only internal development of individual nerve cells but also development of the entire system, with an increased number of cells. Each cell becomes thicker, to carry more signals, and better insulated, to decrease close channel interference. Stimulation is environmental input. Several studies have demonstrated the importance of early stimulation for later development. Habituation is the result of schemes formed for frequently occurring stimuli. The child comes to expect certain stimuli that occur frequently. If that expectation or scheme is fulfilled, then the stimulus does not elicit a significant response. Thus, habituation enables the infant to attend to new stimuli without competition from competing, but less novel, stimuli. Finally, organization enables the child to store information for later retrieval.

The newborn is capable of many auditory discriminations. For example, the newborn can discriminate between different sound durations, different loudness levels, and different consonants in CVC syllables (Bertoncini, Bijeljac-Babic, Blumstein, & Mehler, 1987; Davis & DeCasper, 1989; Moon, Bever, & Fifer, 1992; Prescott, 1985). Newborns are also capable of discriminating different pitches or frequencies, especially in the human speech range. In addition, the neonate responds to the human voice more often and with more vigor than to other environmental sounds.

From birth, the infant is an active stimulus seeker who will even work to attain certain types of stimulation. In general, there are two types of stimulation, perceptual and cognitive (D. Stern, 1977). **Perceptual stimulation** (sometimes called *sensory stimulation*) refers to the recognition of the existence of a stimulus and of its parameters, such as loudness, pitch, or complexity. **Cognitive stimulation** involves the relationship between the incoming stimulus and a stored referent and includes evaluation and comparison of a new stimulus with previously received information. In the neonate, most stimulation is solely perceptual. Cognitive stimulation develops later but still depends on perceptual modalities or channels and thus has a perceptual component.

The neonate is somewhat at the mercy of perceptions, although he or she can shut out visual images by closing the eyes or averting the gaze. If the level of stimulation is too low, the infant loses interest quickly. Attention is captured more easily by moderate stimulation. At a moderate level of stimulus strength, the infant's attention is maintained longer and more frequently. As the stimulus strength increases, so does attention, until a point is attained at which stimulus strength reaches the infant's tolerance threshold. The child will then avert his or her face, become restless, or cry for assistance.

Many of the infant's behavior-state changes reflect internal changes or intrinsic brain activities. During the first month of life, the infant is frequently asleep or drowsy. Even so, external stimuli can influence the duration of these states. The infant is most receptive to external stimuli when alert but not moving excessively. As can be seen, the ability to attend is influenced by the infant's internal state. Within a few months, the level of external stimulation is a greater determinant of attending than the infant's internal state. By this time the infant is capable of maintaining a rather stable internal condition.

By two months of age the infant exhibits selective attending skills. He is not stimulus bound and can remain unresponsive to background stimulus events. When presented with a stimulus repeatedly, the infant will react less strongly to each successive presentation. This habituation is exhibited in both vision and audition, or hearing.

At one month or less, the infant is able to discriminate different phonemes (Aslin & Pisoni, 1980). Initially, these phonemes must be very different in order for the infant to discriminate between them. This ability is gradually refined. By two months, the infant is also able to distinguish his mother's voice from those of others The infant is also able to discriminate frequency changes by this age, or by four to six months at the latest. As intonational patterns are closely related to frequency shifts, we can expect to see discrimination of intonational patterns shortly after frequency shift discriminations; this occurs by seven months.

These abilities demonstrate that at a very early age the infant engages in cognitive stimulation, evaluating and comparing stimuli. A face is not sufficient to hold the infant's attention for long periods. Rather, the infant focuses on the contrast between the face and the infant's scheme or internal representation of a face. Thus, stimulation is coming from both the stimulus and its relationship to the internal scheme. These schemes provide the infant with an expectation of the properties of objects, events, and people in the environment.

At about seven to nine months, the infant begins to understand words. Not only does he or she perceive sequences of arbitrary phonemes, but the infant begins to associate these sound sequences with entities in the perceptual world. Each incoming acoustic stimulus is compared with stored sound traces and associated meaning and is thus analyzed.

Naturally, this analysis requires increased memory capacity. The first step in the memory process is organization and storage of perceptual information. Structuring or organizing incoming information is essential because the child is exchanging information with the physical environment continually. This underlying organization can be inferred from the similar way in which infants interact with objects of similar perceptual attitudes. Although objects may have an infinite variety of characteristics, the infant has only a limited or finite quantity of motor responses. Therefore, the infant generalizes and classifies objects into general response classes.

Stored sensory information "maintains a rather accurate and complete picture of the world as it is received by the sensory system" (Lindsay & Norman, 1977, p. 304), albeit for only a few tenths of a second. Memory may be short or long term. Short-term capacity is very limited and is not a complete image of events that have taken place. Only about five to eight items can be retained at one time, although this is increased with chunking. In contrast, long-term storage has unlimited capacity, although retrieval may be problematic. The amount of information contained is so large that it would be difficult to find individual bits. Thus, the information must be highly organized. The key is not physical capacity but the ability to retrieve selected pieces of data on request. Retrieval is the process of following organized pathways through the stored structure in order to find a particular bit of information.

Memory and retrieval can be seen in the infant's gradual differentiation of the sucking response. The early recognition of his mother's face and voice is also a good indicator. By five months, the infant can remember geometric patterns for approximately three hours, but human faces for much longer.

Distancing

Perceptual behavior may contain some clue to the development of representational skills in the process of distancing (Moerk, 1977). **Distancing** is a gradual increase in the perceptual distance of infants and the accompanying shift from the senses of touch, taste, and smell to vision and hearing. As the distance increases, the infant has less contact with the actual object and must rely on a longer range visual or auditory image. For example, when the infant notices people at a distance, he or she recognizes them even though he or she cannot see all of their attributes. These long-range images may be symbols for the original perceptual attributes.

A gradual process of distancing seems to be part of the play activities of the child. Toys are one step removed from the real object, pictures even more so.

Finally, real or even imaginary objects are manipulated solely through language in stories. Symbolization is a more efficient way of manipulating objects because mental representation can be accomplished more quickly and with less effort than physical movement.

Summary

Perception of speech sounds is critical for later speech and language development in normal children. If some disability precludes normal use of these abilities, then extraordinary measures must be taken to ensure speech and language acquisition. Frequently, an augmentative mode of communication, such as signing, must be employed.

For normal speech and language development, the child should be able to do the following:

1. Attend selectively to speech.
2. Discriminate "mother tongue" phonemes.
3. Hold a speech sound sequence in the correct order for processing.
4. Discriminate speech-sound sequences.
5. Compare a sound sequence to a stored model.
6. Discriminate intonational patterns.

The loss of these abilities, even in a mature user of a language, usually results in speech and language deterioration unless some clinical intervention occurs.

At one year of age, the infant becomes master of the perceptual system, using it rather than only responding to it. According to Piaget, shortly after this age the infant begins to represent reality internally through the use of symbols.

CONCLUSION

The strongest form of the cognitive hypothesis states that cognition precedes language development, that is, that the child expresses in his or her language only those relationships that are understood intellectually. Scholars continue to argue about this relationship. Without entering this battleground too far, it seems safe to assert that there are certain levels of cognitive functioning that must precede expressive language. It is also plausible that this relationship changes with maturation.

The child needs perceptual skills to discriminate the smallest units of speech and to process speech-sound sequences. Both skills require good auditory memory. At a linguistic-processing level, these sound sequences are matched with the referents they represent. These representational abilities develop in the infant during the first two years of life through adaptation to, and organization of, incoming sensory stimuli. Sensorimotor stage 5 representational abilities are adequate for expressive single-word utterances; stage 6 for early multiword utterances. Those aspects of early cognitive development that are most highly correlated with language development are means–ends, causality, and symbolic play.

Unfortunately, there are still many unanswered questions about this early relationship of cognition, or thought, and language. The mental processes involved in word–referent association and in the use of true signs have not been adequately explained.

The cognitive basis of language is best illustrated in early semantic development. Much early expressive language development involves the child's learning how to express what he or she already knows. Stated somewhat differently, the child must develop a certain number of meanings before he or she can begin to confer information intentionally on the environment. By interacting with objects and persons in the environment, the infant forms primitive definitions that are later paired with the word and the referent. This relationship will be discussed in more detail in Chapters 7 and 8.

In the final analysis, the cognitive and perceptual prerequisites for early language appear to be necessary for early language development but are not adequate for a full explanation of the process. This does not detract from the importance of early perceptual and cognitive development, but it begs for consideration of other factors. Language does not develop in a vacuum but, rather, within an environment of well-developed communication.

Sociolinguistic studies emphasize environmental influences, especially the social interactions between the child and the primary caregiver. It is possible that *event knowledge* or the child's understanding of daily routines and events, rather than knowledge of objects, forms the conceptual foundation for language (Farrar, Friend, & Forbes, 1993). This possibility will be explored in Chapter 6.

DISCUSSION

Language doesn't just happen. A child needs certain cognitive perceptual, social, and communicative skills. In the future, you may work with children who lack the cognitive skills to use language. As a group, we might label these children as having mental retardation. A child might also lack perceptual skills. We might say these children have a severe learning disability. Other children may lack the motor skills for speech, such as those with cerebral palsy, or may have a sensory deficit, such as those who are deaf, but may be able to develop language through some augmentative or alternative method of communication, such as pictures, sign, or the use of computers. As an SLP you will need to decide whether to train cognitive skills with a child, or social or perceptual skills, or whether to go directly to communication and possible use of symbols.

Cognitive development may be thought of in terms of information processing. Recall how the four steps—attention, discrimination, organization, and memory—change during the first year. In addition, remember how we believe infants learn through trial-and-error involvement with the environment. Piaget gave us some ideas. Finally, recall what children learn. They need to develop the skill to represent reality in their minds. More importantly, they must be able to recall the symbols that are used to represent that reality so that they can transmit these concepts to others. It is the development of that skill that we addressed.

REFLECTIONS

1. Explain briefly the several models of the cognition–language relationship that have been advanced.

2. Describe information-processing changes that occur in infancy?

3. Describe the major developmental changes that occur in the sensorimotor stage.

4. Describe the sensorimotor aspects of imitation, object permanence, causality, means–ends, and play and the relative contribution of each to language.

5. According to Piaget, organisms learn and evolve through the processes of organization and adaptation. Explain how learning occurs and describe the effect of the environment on the child's schemes.

6. Perceptual development can be divided into four aspects: growth, stimulation, habituation, and organization. How does each one relate to early perceptual development?

6

The Social and Communicative Bases of Early Language

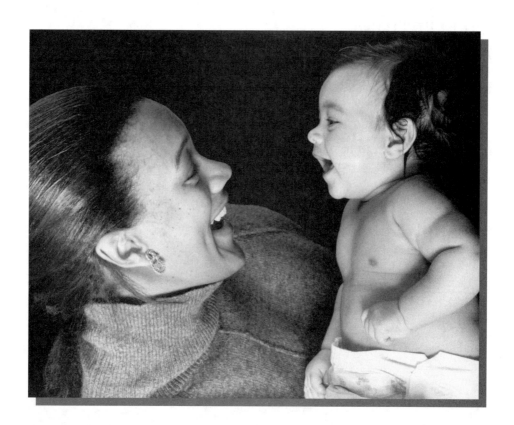

CHAPTER OBJECTIVES

Language is acquired within the context of early conversations between the caregiver and the child. In this chapter we will describe the early interactions of these individuals and the contributions of each to the conversational context. In addition, we will explore the child's development of both communication skills and the intention to communicate. When you have completed this chapter, you should understand

- the communication behaviors of the newborn.
- the importance of gaze coupling, ritualized behavior, and game playing.
- the development of gestures.
- the effects of baby talk, gaze, facial expression, facial presentation and head movement, and proxemics on the child's development.
- the importance of joint reference, joint action, and turn-taking on the development of communication.
- the following terms:

bracketing	mutual gaze
clustering	protoconversation
communication functions	referencing
deictic gaze	script
joint action	social smile
joint reference	

The word *infant* is derived from the Latin *infans*, which means "not speaking." In fact, terms such as *prelinguistic* and *nonverbal* are frequently used to describe infants. All these terms indicate a subtle prejudice which is reflected in the common assumption that it is the development of language and speech that lets children become communicating beings. This supposition does not reflect the actual behavior of infants, who communicate before they have language. Actually, language is a communication tool whose development depends on the prior development of communication.

In Chapter 5 we discussed the cognitive and perceptual bases of language. Words and symbols have meaning only as they relate to these underlying cognitive representations. This process of association, however, does not occur in isolation. Although the child can, to some degree, understand the entities and relationships in the world by exploring with his or her own body, this knowledge can be expanded only by interacting within the social environment.

Language is a social tool and we must look to the child's interactive environment to understand development. Simply put, children learn language to communicate better or to maintain better social contact. Use is the motivating factor.

The social context in which language occurs helps the infant understand that language. Both the nature of communication situations and the process of communication exchanges aid linguistic development. In fact, the situational appropriateness of language is a necessary part of understanding and learning language. As we shall see, context is employed heavily by the mother, or other caregivers, to augment verbal communication. Caregivers talk about objects that are immediately present in the environment. In addition, infant–caregiver communication exchanges have a predictable quality that also facilitates comprehension and learning. The child's knowledge of give-and-take exchanges and non-linguistic signaling equip him or her to interpret or "crack the code" used in such exchanges. The routines of the caregiver enable the child to predict events. The caregiver's speech in these situations also becomes predictable and, therefore, more understandable.

Language represents only a portion of a larger interactional pattern that reflects the way we socialize our children. In short, human babies become human beings because that's the way they are treated. In the communication context, the caregiver assumes that the child is attempting to communicate meaningfully. Thus, in their early dialogs, the caregiver imparts the child's behaviors with social significance, thereby providing an opportunity for the child to take a conversational or pseudoconversational turn. Initially, any child response is treated as a meaningful turn. If the child gives no response, the caregiver proceeds with the next conversational turn. As the caregiver communicates with the child, the child learns that people can reciprocate feelings and meanings.

In this chapter we will discuss infant–caregiver interactions almost exclusively. In middle-class American culture, the mother tends to be the infant's primary caregiver and, therefore, the primary socializing agent. Certainly, in some homes the father or a sibling ful-fills the "mothering" function, but nearly all infant interactive studies have focused on the female parent. You should keep in mind that we will be discussing a "generic" mother–child duo.

In lower socioeconomic groups, the mother's need to work, the family structure, and the neighborhood environment may result in older children becoming the primary care-givers. Studies indicate that these children behave in much the same way as middle-class mothers in their communication adaptations. Even so, these older children or mothers from either lower socioeconomic groups or ethnic cultures may interact differently with their children than middle-class mothers do.

There are many different ways to learn language. In some African cultures, the mother and child have little face-to-face interaction. Instead, the mother spends the day reciting rit-ualized rhymes or songs. Through this process, the child learns that language is predictable. These interactions provide the vocal and nonvocal components of a culturally appropriate language-learning environment.

Within the middle-class American infant–caregiver exchange, the infant develops the essential skills for learning language. The dialog is one of mutual participation. The infant's contribution is as important as that of the caregiver. The caregiver integrates her behavior into the infant's behavior system, and both seem to adjust their behaviors to maintain an optimal level of interaction.

Although the content and intonation of these dialogs can be characterized as "baby talk," the dialog pattern is adult. Each partner takes a turn within the dialog and signals shifts in topic, either nonverbally or verbally. From these dialogs the infant learns initiation and ter-mination of conversation, turn-taking patterns, pacing, and verbal and nonverbal elements.

Naturally, the roles taken by the infant and mother are different. There are five basic differences in the infant–mother exchange (Kaye, 1979):

1. The mother has superior flexibility of timing and anticipates the infant's rather rigid behavior schedule.
2. The mother has an intuitive curriculum. She has an agenda for the infant's development and leads the infant slightly.
3. The mother is able to monitor and code her changes of expression rapidly. The infant has less mature monitoring abilities and responds less rapidly.
4. The mother can alternate among different means to attain her desired ends. The infant does not have the cognitive ability to assess situations and determine alternative strategies to attain goals.
5. The mother is more creative in introducing variations of her repetitions. Thus, she is able to hold the infant's attention by varying her vocalizations only slightly each time.

Communication is maintained because the mother is socially sensitive to the effect of her behavior on the infant. The mother displays this sensitivity and tailors her speech to the task and to the child's abilities. Mothers learn this skill in order to sustain the exchange and to hold attention. In addition, the mother assumes that the child is fully responsive and infers meaning from the child's behavior. For example, if the infant smiles, the mother assumes that he or she is happy. For the child, however, the smile may have a different meaning. The mother's attribution of meaning to the infant's behavior enables a dialog to begin. The mother acts as if she has a competent communication partner.

Much of this early prelinguistic dialog occurs in specific situations, or is situation-dependent. Within these situations, the mother attempts to divide the incoming stimuli into more readily comprehensible segments to which the child can attach meaning. Daily routines also provide predictable patterns of behavior, which aid interpretation. As a result of its mother's behavior, the infant learns the conventions of conversation and a method for interpretation. It would be incorrect, however, to assume that the child does not influence the infant–caregiver interaction. Communication is not implanted in the child. Rather, mother and child engage as partners in a dialog.

In summary, the child is capable of expressive communication long before he or she develops formal verbal language. The infant communicates prelinguistically for at least four purposes: relief from discomfort; attainment of desired ends; reestablishment of proximity; and initiation, maintenance, and termination of an interaction (McLean & Snyder-McLean, 1978). Gradually, these early intentions attain a linguistic form.

In this chapter we will examine the behavior of both the caregiver and the infant in their early interactions. Of importance are the communication strategies that facilitate later speech and language development. The discussion will be developmental in nature and will concern, specifically, interaction and communication development in newborns and during the first year. Later in the chapter, we will explore adult communication strategies and interactional behaviors such as joint reference and joint action, game playing, and turn-taking.

DEVELOPMENT OF COMMUNICATION: A CHRONOLOGY

The infant's world is a world of people—people who do things for, to, and with the infant. Uniquely prepared for interacting with these individuals, the infant learns the conventions of communication into which he or she will eventually place linguistic elements. Every mother will verify the fact that her child began to communicate long before developing language. By the time the child begins to use words, he or she is already able to indicate intentions, to orient himself or herself, to interpret others' responses, and to elicit repetitions and variations.

The Newborn

Chapter 5 highlighted the newborn's perceptual and cognitive abilities. Taken together, these abilities might suggest that the neonate is "prewired" for communication. For example, vision attains best focus at seven and one-half inches, where most infant–caregiver interactions occur. Within a few hours of birth, the infant can follow visually at this close range. During feeding, the mother's eyes are at a distance of almost seven and one-half inches exactly, and she gazes at the infant 70 percent of the time. The child is most likely, therefore, to look at and focus on mother's face, especially mother's eyes.

Visual preference is for the human face or a face pattern. Several studies have found no particular face configuration to be preferential. Rather, newborns prefer visual stimuli with angularity, light and shade, complexity, and curvature. The infant is exposed frequently to the human face which contains all these preferred parameters. "From the very beginning, then, the infant is 'designed' to find the human face fascinating; and the mother is led to attract as much interest as possible to her already 'interesting' face" (D. Stern, 1977, p. 37).

One example of the neonate's predisposition to speech is movements in relation to speech patterns. Undoubtedly, the newborn has been exposed in utero to sounds, such as the mother's heartbeat and digestive sounds. He or she has also been hearing mother's voice and experiencing the rhythmic movements that accompany mother's speech. In response to speech, adults make discrete and continuous synchronous movements at the phoneme, syllable, phrase, and sentence levels. This interactional synchronization, called *entrainment,* is also exhibited by the neonate within twenty minutes of birth. The neonate will not produce synchronous movements to disconnected vowel sounds or to tapping. Body motion changes when the sound pattern changes. If the mother, while pregnant, recited to her fetus, her newborn will prefer these acoustic patterns (DeCasper & Spence, 1986).

The neonate's optimal hearing is within the frequency range of the human voice. As noted in Chapter 5, he or she is able to discriminate some parameters of voice and speech. The neonate has definite auditory preferences. Using the sucking response to maintain or change an auditory stimulus, newborns have registered a preference for the human voice over nonspeech sounds in several studies. Newborns also have a preference for their own mother's voice (DeCasper & Fifer, 1980).

Typically, the newborn will search for the human voice and demonstrate pleasure or mild surprise when finding the face that is the sound source. Upon sighting the face, the newborn's eyes widen, face broadens, and he or she may tilt the head and lift the chin toward the source. Body tension increases, but the infant remains quietly inactive. Upon finding a nonhuman sound source, however, the infant does not demonstrate these recognition behaviors. When the infant demonstrates this preference for human stimuli, it is almost impossible for a caregiver not to become "hooked" on the infant.

The importance of eye contact cannot be overstated. Parents of children with congenital blindness or children who avoid eye contact, such as those with autism, may have difficulty relating to their children.

The newborn will stop crying to attend to its mother's voice. In turn, the mother will stop doing almost anything to attend to her infant's voice. The selective attention of each partner and the ease of interacting predict later communication between the infant and caregiver.

Newborns have individual personalities that affect the patterns of interaction. Differences may include the infant's general mood, intensity of activity and response, sensitivity to stimuli and adaptability to change, persistence, distractability, and approach–withdraw. The best interaction is one in which there is a "good fit" between contextual demands and the child's temperament.

The neonate also has a limited set of behaviors that will help him or her begin to communicate. In fact, the newborn was communicating prior to birth, generally with kicks to express discomfort resulting from the mother's position.

The newborn's facial expressions demonstrate the high degree of maturity of the facial neuromuscular system, resulting in neonatal expressions resembling displeasure, fear, sorrow, anger, joy, and disgust. No experts attribute these actual emotional states to the infant, but caregivers act as if these emotions are present. Infant expressions have definite recognizable patterns.

Eye gaze is another behavior in the neonate's repertoire. Almost from birth, the infant selectively attends to visual stimuli. Visual preferences, mentioned previously, suggest that the angles at the corners of the eyes and the dark-light contrast of the eye itself and the eyebrow might be particularly attractive. The caregiver interprets eye contact as a sign of interest or attention.

Infant head movements also have high signal value for the caregiver. The face and head become important for communication very early because of the relatively advanced maturational level of these structures compared to the rest of the infant's body. The newborn will turn its head to view a human face. Initially, the head and eyes move together, but not to the same degree. Three head positions, illustrated in Figure 6.1, are important because the caregiver interprets them as communication signals.

The infant's state of wakefulness also influences adults' behaviors, such as adjustment of timing of behaviors. The caregiver learns the appropriate times to play with the neonate and to leave him or her alone. The caregiver learns the signals for engagement. The refinement of the baby's state signals and responsiveness to the caregiver reinforce further communication (Brazelton, 1979).

Initially, there is little synchrony between the newborn's sleep-awake cycle, or state of wakefulness, and caregiver behavior; but the synchrony increases as the newborn becomes a few days older. The newborn establishes rhythmic patterns in utero, but these change rapidly at birth. States become regulated by bodily processes such as ingestion, elimination,

FIGURE 6.1   Head Positions of Newborn

TYPE	DESCRIPTION	RESULT FOR INFANT AND MATERNAL INTERPRETATION
Central 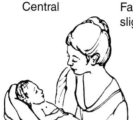	Faces mother or turns away slightly to either side.	Infant: Can discern form Mother: Interprets as an approach or attending signal
Peripheral 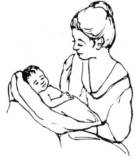	Turns head 15 to 90 degrees	Infant: Cannot discern mother's facial features so form perception lost; motion, speed, and direction perception maintained, so can monitor mother's head Mother: Signal of infant aversion or flight
Loss of visual contact 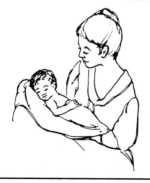	Turns head more than 90 degrees or lowers head	Infant: Loss of motion, speed, and direction perception Mother: Termination of interaction; head lowering interpreted as more termporary

Source: Drawn from D. Stern, *The First Relationship.* Cambridge: Harvard University Press, 1977.

respiration, and hunger. The sleep–awake patterns of the caregiver and child provide shared periods of wakefulness as a context for specific interactions. Under the caregiver's direction, the awake periods become specific action sequences. With each successive awakening, the child's interactions become increasingly predictable. This common context aids infant interpretation and becomes the forum for later introduction of new content.

The mother appears to maintain an optimal state of infant wakefulness by holding the child in close proximity and by speaking. Both of these behaviors become more frequent in the first two weeks of the infant's life. Manipulation by the mother is maximally effective at points of shift or change in the infant's state and can bring the infant back to alertness or facilitate the shift to sleep. Thus, the infant's state influences the mother's behavior, which in turn influences the infant's state.

Finally, the newborn has in its behavioral repertoire the ability to express needs, albeit primitively. The expressive function of communication can be found, from birth, in reflexive crying, which expresses a general form of excitement.

Socialization and Early Communication: Age Birth to Six Months

Shortly after birth, the infant becomes actively involved in the interactive process with the mother. By one month of age, the infant engages in participant exchanges, interactional sequences that began shortly after birth. When awake and in the appropriate position with the adult, the infant will gaze at the adult's face and vocalize. In turn, the infant responds to the mother's vocalizations and movements.

As was noted, the infant is especially responsive to the caregiver's voice and face. In fact, the young infant will attend to the human face to the exclusion of just about everything else. Within the first week of life, the infant begins to "imitate" gross hand gestures, tongue protrusions, and mouth opening. This "imitation" is reflexive in nature, similar to a yawn. The caregiver treats the behavior, however, as if it is social in nature. She embellishes the infant behaviors with communicational intent in the context of these early dialogs. By one month of age, the infant may approximate imitations of the caregiver's pitch and duration of speech sounds.

In addition, the infant responds differentially to mother's face and voice. By as early as two weeks, the infant is able to distinguish its mother from a stranger. The infant will turn toward the adult and fix its gaze upon the adult's mouth or eyes. The infant's facial expression will be one of interest or mild surprise, followed by a smile. At about three weeks of age, this smile of recognition is one of the first examples of a **social smile**, one not contingent upon the infant's internal physical state. At around three to six weeks of age, the infant begins to smile in response to external stimuli, such as the human face and eye gaze; to the human voice (especially if high-pitched); and to tickling. The caregiver, of course, responds in kind.

The young infant is so tuned to the human face that he or she will even smile at a very simplified outline with two large dots for eyes but will not respond to the outline or to the eyes separately. Infants find eyes to be the most attractive part of the human. This preference for the human face, especially the eyes, increases even more during the second month of life. Infant cooing also increases and is easily stimulated by attention and speech, and by toys moved before the baby. The infant coos when not distressed, and this behavior develops parallel to social smiling. By two months of age, the infant is stronger and mouth movements are more distinct. Cooing often occurs in bursts or episodes accompanying other expressions.

By fourteen weeks, the infant has a visual preference for complexity. The three-month-old infant's cognitive abilities are such that the expressionless human face alone does not have the stimulus power to hold her attention. He or she may have internal schemes of certain familiar objects, events, and persons. The stimulus power of any one face resides in that face's similarity to, or difference from, the infant's internal scheme. The degree of stimulation for the infant relates to the degree of stimulus–scheme mismatch. If the mismatch is too great, however, the infant loses interest or gets upset.

To maintain attention, the caregiver must modify her behavior to provide the appropriate level of stimulation. She therefore exaggerates her facial expressions and voice and vocalizes more often. In turn, the infant responds to this new level of stimulation. "There is a progressive mutual modification in the child's and mother's behavior in that changes in the baby's development alter the mother's behavior and this, in turn, affects the baby" (R. Schaffer, 1977, p. 53). In this developmental dance, first one partner leads and then the other. An example of this meshing of infant behavior and caregiver expectations is the infant's sleep-awake cycle. Initially, the infant's sleep pattern is random: sleeping about two-thirds of the time, both day and night. By week sixteen he or she sleeps about ten hours at night, with time out for a feeding or two, and about five hours during the day. The infant moves from an individual synchrony to an interpersonal one. As can be seen, both partners affect their mutual interaction. Infants do affect caregivers and vice versa (Worobey, 1989). Development is not cause and effect; instead, developmental changes affect the dynamic relationship between child and caregiver behaviors and the context (Sameroff & Fiese, 1990).

At any given moment, the caregiver must determine the appropriate amount of stimulation based on the infant's level of attention. By three months, the infant can maintain a fairly constant internal state, so he or she can be attentive for longer periods. The infant's level of excitation is positively related to the level of incoming stimulation. If the caregiver provides too much stimulation, the infant overloads and turns away or becomes overexcited.

Dialogs also become more important as handling decreases. By the third month, handling has decreased by 30 percent from that at birth, but dialog has increased. The infant is a full partner in this dialog, and its behavior is influenced by the communication behavior of the caregiver. The twelve-week-old infant is twice as likely to revocalize if the caregiver responds verbally to the child's initial vocalization rather than responding with a touch, look, or smile. Similar revocalization patterns are also reported for six-month-olds. There is a greater tendency for the infant's vocalizations to be followed by caregiver vocalizations, and those of the caregiver by the child's, than would be expected by chance. The caregiver may perceive her role as that of "replier" to the infant's vocalizations. Caregivers seem to prefer babbling that sounds like speech (Bloom & Lo, 1990).

This "conversational" turn-taking by adults with three-month-olds benefits the infants' babbling and turn-taking (Bloom, 1988). Random responding by adults does not. In addition, this babbling may become more speechlike and mature, containing syllables rather than individual sounds. A sample of the speech and langue of a three-month-old child is presented on track two of the CD that accompanies this text. Note that even at this age the child is very responsive to her mother. Listen to the exchange.

There appears to be a shift in the infant–caregiver vocalization pattern beginning at about twelve weeks (Ginsberg & Kilbourne, 1988). Prior to this, the infant produces predominantly concurrent vocalizations that overlap with those of the mother. Mothers are more likely to initiate and less likely to terminate their vocalizations if their infants are vocalizing. For their part, infants are more likely to initiate vocalizations when their mothers are vocalizing. Although vocal exchanges between mothers and infants are rather simple and contain little useful information, later, more complex messages will necessitate a turn-taking pattern rather than a concurrent one. In addition, both interactive partners make extensive use of smiles, head movements, and gestures. At twelve to eighteen weeks, there is a sharp increase in the alternating vocalization pattern, although concurrent vocalizations still occur more frequently. During alternating vocalization, both American and Japanese infants will pause as if awaiting a response (Masataka, 1993). If none is forthcoming, the child may revocalize.

Mothers begin to imitate their infants' coughing at two months of age. Initially, this behavior is performed to attract attention, but eventually an exchange emerges. By four months, the infant will initiate the exchange with a smile or a cough.

Eye gaze is also very important in these early dialogs. By six weeks of age, the infant is able to fix visually on its mother's eyes and hold the fixation, with eye widening and brightening. The infant is more likely to begin and to continue looking if the caregiver is looking. In return, the caregiver's behavior becomes more social, and play interactions begin. At three months of age, the infant has a focal range that almost equals the mother's, and he or she becomes a true interactional partner in this modality.

Two types of gaze patterns have been identified. **Deictic gaze** is directed at objects. Mothers monitor their infants' gaze and follow its orientation. **Mutual gaze** or looking at each other may signal intensified attention. At about three months, mutual gaze may be modified occasionally into gaze coupling, a turn-taking interaction resembling later gaze patterns observed in mature conversation. Mutual eye gaze may be important for the formation of attachment or bonding.

Infant–caregiver bonding is determined by the quality of their interactions. Several factors influence bonding and the infant's subsequent feelings of security. The levels of maternal playfulness, sensitivity, encouragement, and pacing at three months have been found to be positively related to the security of attachment at nine months.

During the first three months, the caregiver's responding teaches the child the signal value of specific behaviors. The infant learns the stimulus–response sequence. If he or she signals, the caregiver will respond. When the infant cries, the caregiver answers. Thus, the infant develops an expectation that he or she can change or control the environment. In addition, the child learns that a relatively constant stimulus, or signal, results in a predictable response: the world has predictable outcomes. Possibly as high as 77 percent of infant crying episodes are followed by maternal responses, while only 6 percent are preceded by maternal contact. As a result of maternal responses, the cry becomes an infant's means of gaining contact with mother.

Immediate positive parental responsiveness increases the child's motivation to communicate. If motivation is high, the infant will attempt more frequent and varied interactions. Motivation to communicate at nine months is best indicated by earlier exploration behavior and displays of curiosity (Brockman, Morgan, & Harmon, 1988).

The degree of parental responsiveness varies with the culture, as does the amount of infant crying. In general, more mobile societies, such as hunter-gatherer cultures, exhibit little child crying. Carried by the mother in a sling, the child is often attended to before crying begins.

Mothers not only respond to their infants' cries but can identify the type of cry produced. Mothers can reliably rate their three- to four-month-olds' cries along a continuum immediately following the infant's vocalization and even three weeks later on audiotape (Petrovich-Bartell, Cowan, & Morse, 1982). This is of interest when we consider that fewer nonacoustic and contextual cues are available in the latter condition.

By three to four months, two additional response patterns have emerged: rituals and game-playing. These will be discussed in some detail later in this chapter. Rituals, such as feeding, provide the child with predictable patterns of behavior and speech. The child becomes upset if these rituals are changed or disrupted in any way. Games, such as "peekaboo," "this little piggy," and "I'm gonna get you," have all the aspects of communication. There is an exchange of turns, rules for each turn, and particular slots for words and actions. Although the interaction reflects adult communication, it is constrained by the abilities of each partner.

There are identifiable interactional phases in rituals and game-playing. Mothers and their three-month-old infants exhibit initiation, mutual orientation, greeting, a play dialog, and disengagement. However, any given exchange may not contain every phase. To initiate the exchange, the mother smiles and talks to her infant. For its part, the infant vocalizes and smiles at her mother when her mother has paused too long. When the partner responds with a neutral or bright face, the mutual orientation phase begins, and one partner speaks or vocalizes. The greeting consists of mutual smiles and eye gazes, with little body or hand movement. Turn-taking is seen in the play-dialog phase. The mother talks in a pattern of bursts interspersed with pauses, and the infant vocalizes during the pauses. Finally, disengagement occurs when one partner looks away. Within any phase, the behaviors of either partner may differ. These interactional exchanges called **protoconversations**, contain the initial elements of emerging conversation.

Both partners are active participants in these exchanges. The infant moves face, lips, tongue, arms, hands, and body toward the mother, whose behavior reflects that of her infant. In turn, the infant imitates the mother's movements. Frequently, the behaviors of the mother and infant appear to be so simultaneous as to constitute a single act. The infant frequently leads by initiating the behavior. Mother does not simply follow, however, but maintains a mutual exchange.

By five months the infant shows more deliberate imitation of movements and vocalizations. Facial imitation is most frequent at four to six months of age. By six to eight months, however, hand and nonspeech imitation become most frequent. The behaviors imitated are not new to the child but are a remodeling and integration of behaviors previously exhibited in the child's spontaneous behavior.

Between three and six months of age, the period of peak face-to-face play, the infant may be exposed to over 30,000 examples of facial emotions (Trotter, 1983). In interactions with mother, the child mirrors mother's expression and she, in turn, imitates the infant. The infant's repertoire of facial emotions is listed in Table 6.1.

The five-month-old also vocalizes to accompany different attitudes, such as pleasure and displeasure, satisfaction and anger, and eagerness. He or she will vocalize to other people and to a mirror image, as well as to toys and objects.

TABLE 6.1   Infant Emotions

EMOTION	DESCRIPTION	EMERGENCE
Interest	Brows knit or raised, mouth rounded, lips pursed	Present at birth
Distress	Eyes closed tightly, mouth square and angular (as in anger)	Present at birth
Disgust	Nose wrinkled, upper lip elevated, tongue protruded	Present at birth
Social smile	Corners of mouth raised, cheeks lifted, eyes twinkle; neonatal "half smile" and early startle may be precursors	4–6 weeks
Anger	Brows together and drawn downward, eyes set, mouth square	3–4 months
Sadness	Inner corners of brows raised, mouth turns down in corners, pout	3–4 months
Surprise	Brows raised, eyes widened, oval-shaped mouth	3–4 months
Fear	Brows level but drawn in and up, eyes widened, mouth retracted	5–7 weeks

Source: Drawn from work of Carroll Izard as reported by R. Trotter in "Baby Fact," *Psychology Today*, August 1983, *17*(8), pp. 14–20.

As the infant approaches six months of age, this interest in toys and objects increases. Prior to this period, the infant is not greatly attracted to objects unless they are noise-producing or made mobile and lively by an adult. By six months, however, there is a small shift in interest away from people and toward objects. This change reflects, in part, the development of eye–hand coordination, which is exhibited in reaching, grasping, and manipulation. From this point on, interactions become more triadic; they include the infant, the caregiver, and some object.

Development of Intentionality: Age Seven to Twelve Months

During the second six months of life, the infant begins to assert more control within the infant–caregiver interaction. He or she learns to communicate intentions more clearly and effectively. Each success motivates the infant to communicate more and to learn to communicate better. The primary modes for this expression are gestural and vocal.

By seven months, the infant begins to respond differentially to his or her interactional partner, staying close to the caregiver, following her movements, and becoming distressed if she leaves. Even infant play with objects is influenced by maternal attending. Infants play with toys as long as their mothers look on, but when their mothers turn away, infants leave their toys 50 percent of the time and attempt to retrieve the lost attention. This maternal attachment is related to the predictability of the mother's behavior.

In recognition of the infant's interest in objects and increasing ability to follow conversational cues, the caregiver makes increasing reference to objects, events, and people outside of the infant–caregiver dyad. Increasingly, the infant demonstrates selective listening to familiar words and compliance with simple requests.

The infant imitates simple motor behaviors, by nine to ten months responding to requests to wave bye-bye. Infant response rates to maternal verbal and nonverbal requests increase with age (Liebergott, Ferrier, Chesnick, & Menyuk, 1981). At nine months, infants respond to 39.5 percent of the maternal requests, compared to 52.0 percent at eleven months. Requests for action are answered one and a half times as frequently at both ages as requests for vocalization. By modifying forms and frequencies of reply, the infant gains considerable control over the communicative exchange.

Nine-month-olds can also follow maternal pointing and glancing or regard. The infant cues on a combination of maternal head and eye orientation and on eye movement.

Visual orientation of both the infant and mother is usually accompanied by maternal naming to establish the topic of a protoconversation. The mother watches her infant's face more than the infant observes hers. She monitors the infant's glance and signs of interest. Mothers of eight- to fourteen-month-olds look at their infants so frequently that the responsibility for maintaining eye contact really rests with the child. This monitoring by the mother decreases as the infant gets older.

Caregivers also monitor infant vocalizations. Parents of eight- to twelve-month-olds can consistently recognize infant intonational messages that convey request, frustration, greeting, and pleasant surprise.

Gaze and vocalization seem to be related. The infant's gaze is more likely to be initiated and maintained when the mother is vocalizing and/or gazing back and, in turn, the mother is more likely to initiate and maintain vocalization when the infant is looking at her. In addition, mothers and one-year-olds exhibit very little vocal overlap. Mothers and one-year-olds depart from their turn-taking behaviors when they laugh or join in chorus or when the mother attempts to fill nonexistent pauses. The exchange is one of reciprocal actions, intonations, and gestures.

A temporal relationship exists between the infant's gaze and vocal behavior addressed to interactive partners (D'Odorico, Cassibba, & Salerni, 1997). At around one year of age, children who have learned to coordinate gaze and vocalization look at their partners at the beginning of a vocal turn, possibly for reassurance. Six months later, they tend to use a more adult pattern and to look at their partners at the end of a turn to signal a turn shift.

The communication between infant and caregiver is closely related to the infant's resultant behavior state, and the child will show signs of distress when communication sequences end. The infant will vocalize and gesture for attention, then exhibit sadness or grimace.

Communication Functions

At about eight to nine months, the infant begins to develop *intentionality* or goal directedness and the ability to share goals with others. Up to this point, the child has focused primarily on either objects or people. Even complex action sequences are really a series of discrete behaviors directed toward one or the other. For example, the child might look at a person, smile, and touch. Outcomes are not predicted by the child.

Intentionality is exhibited when the child begins to encode a message for someone else. For the first time, he or she considers the audience. The child may touch mother, gain eye contact, then gesture toward an object. An explicit bid for attention is coupled with a signal behavior, although the order may vary. The child's uses of these signals are called **communication** functions, and they are expressed primarily through gestures. In other words, functions, such as requesting, interacting, and attracting attention, are first fulfilled by prelinguistic communicative means and only later by language. A sample of the speech and langauge of a nine-month-old child is presented on track four of the CD that accompanies this text. Accompanied by gestures, these speech sounds will be used to accomplish several intentions.

A three-stage sequence in the development of early communication functions includes perlocutionary, illocutionary, and locutionary levels (Bates, Camaioni, & Volterra, 1975). In Table 6.2, these stages are related to the infant's cognitive developments.

TABLE 6.2 Development of Intentionality

STAGE	AGE (MONTHS)	CHARACTERISTICS
Perlocutionary	0–8 (approx.)	Intention inferred by adults *Attentional interactions* • No goal awareness • Attends to and responds to stimuli *Contingency interactions* • Awareness of goal • Undifferentiated behavior to initiate or continue a stimulus, anticipates events, vocalizes for attention
Substage 1		Shows self *Differentiated interactions* • Design, plan, and adjust behavior to achieve goal • Raise arms to be picked up, pull string to get object, look at adult and desired object
Illocutionary	8–12	Emergence of intentional communication *Encoded interactions* • Coordinated plan to achieve goals • Gestures, brings objects to caregiver for help, climbs for desired objects
Substage 2		Shows objects
Substage 3		Displays a full range of gestures • Conventional gestures: requesting, pointing or signaling notice, showing, giving, and protesting • Unconventional gestures: tantruming and showing off • Functional gestures
Locutionary	12+	Words accompany or replace gestures to express communication functions previously expressed in gestures alone or gestures plus vocalization *Symbolic interactions*

Adapted from Wetherby & Prizant (1989) and Bates et al. (1975).

Perlocutionary Stage. The perlocutionary stage begins at birth and continues into the second half-year of life. Throughout this stage, the infant fails to signal specific intentions beyond those behaviors that will sustain an interaction, such as cries, coos, and use of the face and body nonspecifically.

Initially, the infant's behavior is characterized by *attentional interactions* in which he or she attends to and discriminates stimuli (Wetherby & Prizant, 1989). The child responds to stimuli with diffuse undifferentiated behaviors, such as crying.

Crying indicates general pain, discomfort, or need but does not identify the cause of the problem. The mother interprets her infant's behavior and responds differentially. The infant's cry has a directive function for the mother, alerting her to some disorder, the cause of which she will investigate. Crying thus aids the development of intentionality by teaching the child the signal value of behavior.

The communication system becomes more effective as the caregiver learns to interpret the child's increasingly more interpretable behavior. Interactions become more predictable. Only later does the infant recognize the means–ends potential of his or her communication. Gradually, the infant's greater cognitive ability will enable him to her to understand the outcome of behavior (see Chapter 5). Soon the infant will begin making deliberate attempts to share specific experiences with caregivers, fully expecting them to respond. Characterized by *contingency interactions,* behavior is directed toward initiating and sustaining interactions (Wetherby & Prizant, 1989). Affective signals, such as crying, will become more conventional and more directed toward and responsive to the communication context (Adamson & Bakeman, 1985).

The referential function, in which an infant calls attention to the environment, is exemplified by infant scanning and searching. The mother follows her infant's visual line of regard and provides a label or comment.

When aware of the child's desire to continue an interaction, the caregiver can respond to the child and help sustain their "dialog." When more mature, the child will initiate a behavior and repeat it in order to sustain these interactions.

Toward the end of the perlocutionary period, the infant becomes more interested in manipulating objects and begins to use recognitory gestures (Bates, Bretherton, Shore, & McNew, 1983). These gestures demonstrate an understanding of object purpose, or functional use, and include such behaviors as bringing a cup to the lips or a telephone receiver to the ear. As such, these gestures constitute a primitive form of naming and a categorization of an object, or referent, as belonging to a particular conceptual class. Thus, the infant demonstrates recognition that objects have stable characteristics and functions that necessitate specific behaviors. Occasionally, the recognitory gestures are applied to objects that are related or look similar. These early gestures are usually brief and incomplete, often with some element missing. For example, the child may drink from an empty cup (the liquid being the missing element). In the early stages, sequences of events are also rare.

At this stage, the infant begins reaching for desired objects. For objects that are beyond its grasp, the infant's reach will become a pointing gesture.

Illocutionary Stage. The second, or illocutionary, stage of functional communication development begins at eight to nine months of age. Within this stage the infant uses conventional gestures or vocalizations to communicate intentions. The child's behavior becomes differentiated to signal different intentions. Several behaviors mark the emergence of intentional communication (Scoville, 1983):

- Gestures are accompanied by eye contact with the child's communication partner.
- The child uses consistent sound and intonation patterns of his or her own invention as signals for specific intentions. For example, the child might say "eh-eh" to express a want.
- The child persists in attempting to communicate. If not understood, he or she may repeat the behavior or modify it for the communication partner.

In each behavior the child considers both the message and the partner's reception of it, thus exhibiting an intention to communicate.

Three sequential substages in the development of gestures have been noted (Bates et al., 1975). In the first substage, which begins prior to the illocutionary period, the infant exhibits or shows self. The infant hides its face, acts coy, raises the arms to be picked up, or plays peekaboo. Characterized by *differentiated interactions,* behavior becomes coordinated and regulated to achieve goals (Wetherby & Prizant, 1989).

In the second substage, the infant shows objects by extending them toward the caregiver but does not release them. The child draws attention to these objects as a way of sharing attention.

Finally, in the last substage, fully within the illocutionary stage, the infant displays a full range of gestures, including conventional means of showing, giving, pointing, and requesting (Figure 6.2). Other nonconventional gestures, such as having tantrums and showing off, are also present. In general, each infant develops its own style with nonconventional gestures. Finally, each infant develops one or more functional gestures or gestures that are shaped for specific meaning, such as touching the mouth repeatedly to signal *eat* or running to the door to signal *out.* My daughter would weave her legs around each other to signal *potty.*

Giving, unlike showing, includes a release of the object. Frequently, giving follows a maternal request for the object. A favorite game becomes "the trade," in which the partners take turns passing an object between them.

Pointing may include the whole hand or only a finger with the arm extended. The infant makes only the minimal effort needed to convey the intention. Unlike requesting, pointing is not accompanied by movement of the upper trunk in the direction of the object.

Requesting is a whole-hand grasping reach toward a desired object or a giving gesture accompanied by a call for assistance. In its most mature form, each gesture contains a visual check to ensure that the communication partner is attending.

These initial gestures are used to signal two general communication functions (Bates et al., 1975). *Protoimperatives,* such as requests, signal an adult to attain an object. In contrast, giving, showing, and pointing, called *protodeclaratives,* use an object to attain adult attention. Protoimperatives or requests generally request objects, participation, or actions (Bruner, 1983). The infant begins to realize with requests that she cannot be unreasonable or ask for something that she can do herself.

FIGURE 6.2   Infant Standardized Gestures

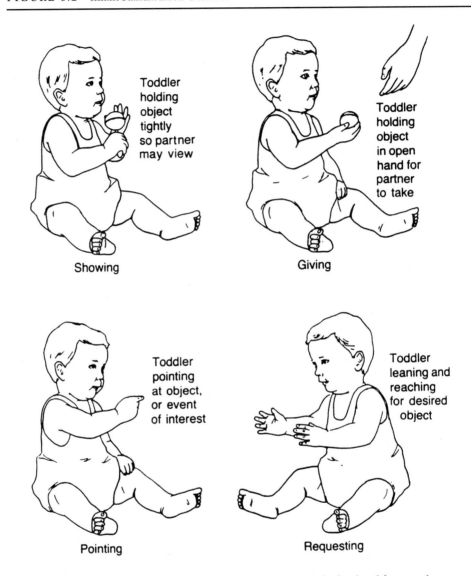

Infants develop a set of standardized gestures in addition to nonstandardized and functional gestures.

Protodeclaratives, such as pointing or showing, have the goal of maintaining joint or shared attending. Thus, children communicate to share information as well as to request (Golinkoff, 1993). Nearly 30 percent of the communication episodes between presymbolic children and their caregivers have nonmaterial goals. The infant will point in the presence of a communication partner but not when alone.

The appearance of gestures or *encoded interactions* signals a cognitive ability to coordinate a plan to achieve a desired goal. Gestures demonstrate preplanning rather than the trial-and-error behavior noted previously.

Initially, gestures appear without vocalizations, but the two are gradually paired. Consistent vocal patterns, dubbed *phonetically consistent forms (PCFs)*, accompany many gestures. PCFs occur with pauses that clearly mark boundaries and function as words for the child. Often imitations of environmental sounds, such as a dog's bark or a car's engine, or of the child's own or others' sounds, PCFs usually accompany events or actions in the environment (Reich, 1986). My granddaughter Cassidy started barking at about seven months. Once the infant begins to use PCFs, mother will no longer accept other, less consistent vocalizations. PCFs are a transition to words in a highly creative developmental period when the child is also adept at employing gestures and intonation.

The appearance of intentional communication in the form of gestures requires a certain level of cognitive, as well as social, functioning. Children use very low-level gestures at stage 4 means–ends. The infant must attain stage 5 means–ends behaviors, or at least object-to-object use, by the time she begins to use intentional speech. Person–object sequences, such as requests, begin at eight to ten months, along with a shift to complex social interactions.

Locutionary Stage. The final stage of functional communication development is the locutionary stage, which begins with the first meaningful word. In these symbolic interactions, the child's intent becomes encoded in a language symbol. Conventional verbalizations are used with or without gestures to accomplish the functions previously filled by gestures. For example, pointing develops within a shared attention context, then vocalization within pointing, and naming within vocalization. Words and gestures are used to refer to the same content. The gesture, which initially stands for the entire message, gradually becomes the context for more symbolic ways of communicating the message.

Comprehension

During the second six months, the child also begins to attach meaning to symbols. Infants use both bracketing and clustering strategies to segregate speech directed at them (Goodsitt, Morgan, & Kuhl, 1993). **Bracketing** is the use of prosodic cues to detect divisions between clauses and phrases (Gleitman & Wanner, 1982; Morgan, 1986; Peters, 1985). Divisions are marked by maternal pauses, pitch changes, vowel lengthening, changes in vowel rhyming or alliterative patterns, or by use of specific words (Morgan, Meier, & Newport, 1987). These cues are especially helpful for identifying clauses and phrases but of little aid for deciphering words. Words possess inconsistent forms and are more easily identified using a clustering strategy.

Clustering is the use of predictable units within the word to synthesize words. In order to accept this explanation, we must assume that the child has some basic unit of perception such as the syllable or phoneme. Each language permits only certain syllable and phoneme structures, so predictability is high within words. Between words, predictability is low, highlighting word-to-word transitions.

Using a combination of these strategies, the infant is able to divide caregiver speech into manageable units. Predictable, familiar words and phrases become associated with familiar contexts and early meanings begin to form.

Summary

During the first eight months of life, the infant learns the rituals and processes of communication through interaction with her caregiver (Table 6.3). The caregiver treats the infant as a full conversational partner and acts as if the infant communicates meaningfully. The infant also learns that behavior can have an effect upon the environment. At first, the infant's communication is general and unspecified. During the second six months, he or she develops functional communication, first gesturally, then vocally. When the infant begins to use meaningful speech, it is within this functional context of gestures and vocalizations.

TABLE 6.3   Infant Social and Communicative Development

AGE	BEHAVIORS
Newborn	Vision best at 8 inches; prefers light–dark contrasts, angularity, complexity, curvature Hearing best in frequency range of human voice; prefers human voice; exhibits entrainment Facial expressions
1 week	"Self-imitation"; reflexive actions but treated as meaningful by caregiver
2 weeks	Distinguishing of caregiver's voice and face
3 weeks	Social smile
1 month	Short visual exchanges with caregiver; prefers human face to all else
2 months	Cooing
3 months	Face alone not enough to hold infant's attention: in response, mother exaggerates her facial movements More frequent dialogs; decrease of handling by 30% Revocalization likely if caregiver's verbal response immediately follows child's first vocalization Vocal turn-taking and concurrent vocalization Gaze coupling Rituals and games Face play
5 months	Purposeful facial imitation Vocalization to accompany attitude
6 months	Hand and nonspeech imitation
8 months	Gestures
9 months	Imitation of more complicated motor behaviors Following of maternal pointing
11 months	Response to about half of maternal verbal and nonverbal requests
12 months	Use of words to fill communicative functions established by gestures

MATERNAL COMMUNICATION BEHAVIORS

As we have noted, the infant and caregiver engage in mutual dialog soon after birth. It is a complex interaction between infant character/temperament and maternal speech (Smolak, 1987). To some degree, both partners control this exchange. The infant sets the level of exchange because of limited abilities. The initial infant responses are rather rigid and fixed. Only gradually does the infant expand this behavioral repertoire.

The mother provides the framework and adjusts her behaviors to the information processing limitations of the infant. As a result, many important experiences occur "because of the mother's willingness to learn from the infant and respond to his patterns" (Bateson, 1979, p. 70). The mother's observation of the child's regular hunger rhythms, reflected in the child's readiness to nurse, instructs the infant on the nature of order.

Within a given exchange, both partners adjust their behavior continually to maintain an optimum level of stimulation. The mother maintains the infant's attention at a high level by her behavior. In response, the infant coos, smiles, and gazes alertly. Reinforced for her efforts, the mother tries even harder to maintain the infant's level of stimulation. Each party is responsive to the other. In addition, the mother helps expand the infant's abilities by deliberately "messing up" more consistently than expected. By exceeding the limits of the infant's behavior, the mother forces the infant to adjust to new stimuli.

Four caregiver behaviors form the background or foundation of infant–caregiver face-to-face exchanges: preparatory activities, state-setting activities, communication framework maintenance, and infantlike action modifications (Tronick, Als, & Adamson, 1979). Table 6.4 describes and gives examples of each behavior category. Among mothers' infantlike modifications are exaggerated facial expressions, body movements, positioning, timing, touching, prolonged gaze, and baby talk. These modifications also occur in the behavior of other adults and children as they interact with infants. Prior experience with infants does not affect the behavior of either adults or preschoolers, and prior learning seems to be unimportant. Three factors appear important in influencing the initial interactions of the newborn and its mother: the medication used in delivery, the number of pregnancies, and the mother's socioeconomic and cultural background.

Most adults respond to the "babyness" of the infant, particularly the face, which they find irresistible. The infant's head is large in proportion to the body, with large eyes and round cheeks. In brief, the child looks cute. To this physical image the infant adds smiles, gazes, mouth opening, and tongue thrust. Infants with a deviant look may elicit very different or negative responses.

In the following sections, we shall explore the modifications made by caregivers in response to their infants. This behavior varies with culture, class, and gender of the infant.

Infant-Elicited Social Behavior

Caregiver responses can be characterized as "infant-elicited social behaviors." They appear in response to infants but occur infrequently in adult-to-adult exchanges. Infant-elicited social behaviors have three characteristics. First, they are exaggerated in space, and the exaggeration may be maximal. Second, they are exaggerated in time, usually being slow or

TABLE 6.4   Caregiver Foundations for Face-to-Face Communication

BEHAVIOR	DESCRIPTION	EXAMPLES
Preparatory activities	Free infant from physiological state dominance	Reduce interference of hunger or fatigue Sooth or calm infant when upset
State-setting activities	Manipulate physical environment to optimize interaction	Move into infant's visual field Attain attention by modifying vocalizations
Maintenance of communication framework	Use of continuates by caregiver	Modulate speech, rhythmic tapping and patting, rhythmic body movements; provide infant with a focus of attention and action, a set of timing markers
Infantlike modifications of adult actions	Variation of caregiver activities in rate, intensity modulation, amplitude, and quality from those of adult-adult	Use baby talk—slowed and exaggerated Imitate baby movements—close, oriented straight ahead, parallel, and perpendicular to plane of infant

Source: Drawn from E. Tronick, H. Als, and L. Adamson. "Structure of early face-to-face communicative interactions." In M. Bullowa (Ed.), *Before Speech*. New York: Cambridge University Press, 1979.

elongated. Finally, they form a select, limited repertoire that is performed frequently. The purpose of these modifications is to enhance recognition and discrimination of the behaviors by the child. The behaviors of one mother differ from those of another. Each caregiver develops her own style. Infant-elicited social behavior consists of maternal adaptations in speech and language (sometimes called *baby talk*), gaze, facial expression, facial presentation and head movement, and proxemics.

Baby Talk

The speech and language of adults and children to infants is systematically modified from that used in regular conversation. This adapted speech and language has been called *baby talk* or *motherese*. For our purposes, we shall use *baby talk* to signify the speech and language addressed to infants (Table 6.5). We will use the term *motherese* or *parentese* later to denote speech and language used with toddlers. Use of the term baby talk does not imply that mothers use forms, such as *horsie* or *ni-night*. Parents do not use such babyish forms until the child is old enough to understand them (Kaye, 1980).

Maternal input is very important for the infant's own communication development. Children who are deaf achieve all developmental milestones at or before the expected age

TABLE 6.5 Characteristics of Baby Talk

Short utterance length (mean utterance length as few as 2.6 morphemes) and simple syntax
Small core vocabulary, usually object centered
Topics limited to here and now
Heightened use of facial expressions and gestures
Frequent questioning and greeting
Treating of infant behaviors as meaningful: mother awaits infant's turn and responds even to nonturns
Episodes of maternal utterances
Paralinguistic modifications of pitch and loudness
Frequent verbal rituals

for hearing children when exposed to sign from birth (Petitto, 1984, 1985a, 1985b, 1986, 1987, 1988; Petitto & Marentette, 1990, 1991).

Baby talk is characterized by short utterance length and simple syntax. These qualities reflect, in part, the small core vocabulary used. Possibly to facilitate understanding or word–referent association by the infant, mothers paraphrase and repeat themselves. Topics are limited to the here and now. The mother's choice of content, type of information conveyed, and syntax appear to be heavily influenced by the context (D'Odorico & Franco, 1985). In addition, mothers use paralinguistic variations, such as intonation and pause, beyond those found in adult-to-adult speech. Employing more frequent facial expressions and gestures and an overall higher pitch, any one of us might engage in the following monologue:

> See the dog. (turn, look, pause)
> Big dog. (gesture, pause)
> Nice dog. (pause)
> Pet dog. (pet, pause)
> Can you pet dog? (pause)
> Nice dog. Do you like dog? (pause)
> Un-huh. Nice dog.

This little monolog contains most aspects of baby talk.

Maternal speech measured at six, thirteen, and twenty-three weeks of infant age averages only 2.8 morphemes per utterance (Kaye, 1980). This average may increase to about 3.5 morphemes at six months. In part, this rise may reflect the increasingly complex communication of the mother and her infant, since there is a shift at five to seven months to a more conversational mode with greater turn-switching and more incorporation of objects. After one year, average maternal utterance length is reported to be between 2.8 and 3.5 morphemes. These low values may represent maternal modeling in anticipation of the infant's first words. An adult-to-infant average of 2.8 to 3.5 morphemes per utterance is well below the adult-to-adult average, which is around 8 morphemes. Although researchers disagree on the degree of syntactic simplicity they concede that adult-to-infant speech is less complex structurally than adult-to-adult speech. In general, mothers who use more short sentences when their children are nine months of age have toddlers with better receptive language abilities at eighteen months (Murray, Johnson, & Peters, 1990). Such short, simple utterances can be found in the baby talk of different languages.

Mothers use a considerable number of questions and greetings with their infants. These conversational devices may enable the mother to treat any infant response as a conversational turn, since both questions and greetings require a response. In turn, the mother responds to her infant's behavior as a meaningful response to her own initial cue. Even the infant's burps, yawns, sneezes, coughs, coo-vocalizations, smiles, and laughs may receive a response from the mother. Approximately 21 percent of maternal utterances are greetings such as *hi* and *bye-bye* or acknowledgments such as *sure, uh-huh,* and *yeah,* given in response to infant behaviors (Kaye, 1980). This maternal response pattern does not occur with nonsignaling infant behaviors, such as arm waving or bouncing.

Responsivity or the adult's consistent tendency to recognize the infant's signal and provide an appropriate and consistent response is very important in the emergence of early communication (Hanzlik & Stevenson, 1986; Siegel-Causey & Ernst, 1989). Communication results when the caregiver attributes meaning to these behaviors. Gradually, the child learns that behavior results in consistent, predictable effects and thus gains an appreciation of the signal value of that behavior (Snow, 1981). Responsivity is highly partner–child specific (Wilcox, Kouri, & Caswell, 1990).

For its part, the infant responds selectively. As mentioned previously, the twelve-week-old infant is most likely to vocalize if the mother has just vocalized. Situational variations are also important: The infant is least likely to vocalize when engaged in activities such as being changed, fed, or rocked, or when its mother watches television or talks to another person. In contrast, some maternal nonvocal behaviors, such as touching, holding close, looking at, or smiling at the infant, increase the likelihood of infant vocalizations.

Maternal utterances often occur in strings of successive utterances referring to the same object, action, or event. Verbal episodes may facilitate understanding because speech is less difficult to understand if recognizable strings of utterances are produced referring to the same object. Information gained from preceding utterances assists comprehension of following ones. Most episodes with infants begin with object manipulation and naming by the mother. At the beginning of the episode, pauses between utterances are twice as long as pauses within the episode itself. Young children receive help with object reference and *episodic* boundaries. Within each episode there is also a high proportion of naming. A typical episode might proceed as follows:

> (shake doll) Here's baby! (pause)
> Mommy has baby. (gesture, pause)
> Uh-huh, Betsy want baby? (gesture, pause)
> Here's baby! (pause)
> Oh, baby scare Betsy? (facial expression, pause)

High rates of redundancy also occur in mothers' speech to their infants (Kaye, 1980). Maternal repetitions exceed the number expected by chance, and there is a great degree of semantic similarity between successive utterances. The high rate of syntactic and semantic redundancy increases the predictability and continuity of each episode. Mothers repeat one out of every six utterances immediately and exactly. These self-repetitions decrease as the child assumes increasing responsibility in the conversation. The probability of a content word's appearing again within the next three utterances is high.

Early content tends to be object-centered and concerned with the here and now. For the mother, topics are generally limited to what her infant can see and hear. As the child's age approaches six months, mother tends to use a more informational style. The mother's affective and contentless speech decreases, and she talks more about the environment and the infant's behavior (Penman, Cross, Milgrom-Friedman, & Meares, 1983).

Within an episode, the infant and mother engage in a dialog in which the infant's new communication functions can emerge. Certain elements appear over and over in the mother's speech. The mother presents "standard interactional routines" (Bruner, 1975) to give her infant the opportunity to predict and engage in the dialog. These predictable maternal behaviors may aid the infant's comprehension, allow the infant to concentrate her attention, and provide models of the expected dialog.

One of the most common sequences is that of joint, or shared, reference. **Referencing** is the noting of a single object, action, or event and is signaled by either indicating or marking. In **indicating**, the mother follows her infant's line of regard or visual attending and comments on the object of their joint attention. With *marking,* the mother shakes an object or exaggerates an action to attract her infant's attention.

In addition to linguistic modifications, mothers use paralinguistic variations. The manner of presentation may be more important than the form or content. Infants will respond to intonation patterns before they comprehend language. The mother uses a broad range of pitch and loudness, although overall, her pitch is higher than in adult-to-adult conversations (Sachs, 1985). This pitch contour has been found in a number of languages, although there is some variation (Bernstein, Ratner & Pye, 1984). In general, four-month-old infants seem to prefer a high, variable pitch (Fernald, 1981; Fernald & Kuhl, 1987). Conversational sequences may include instances of falsetto or bass voice and of whispers or yells. Content words and syllables receive additional emphasis.

The mother also modifies her rhythm and timing. Vowel duration is longer than in adult-to-adult discourse. The mother uses longer pauses between utterances, although this delay may be a function of her infant's nonvocalization. Signing mothers of children who are deaf maintain similar rhythms with their hands (Fernald, 1994).

After speaking, the mother waits approximately 0.6 second, the average adult turn-switching pause. Next, she waits for the duration of an imaginary infant response and another turn switch. Since many maternal utterances are questions, the duration of an infant response is relatively easy for the mother to estimate. Thus, the infant is exposed to a mature time frame in which later discourse skills will develop.

There are many similarities in intonation across parents from languages as different as Comanche, English, French, Italian, German, Japanese, Latvian, Mandarin Chinese, Sinhala, and Xhosa, a South African language (Fernald & Simon, 1984; Fernald, Taeschner, Dunn,

Papousek, deBoysson-Bardies & Fukui, 1989; Grieser & Kuhl, 1988; Masataka, 1992; Mee-gaskumbura, 1980; Papousek, 1987; Papousek, Papousek, & Haekel, 1987). Parents use a higher pitch, greater variability in pitch, shorter utterances, and longer pauses when talking to their preverbal infants than when talking to other adults. For example, Japanese mothers use responding to alter the duration of their infant's vocalizations. The length of maternal pauses is reflected in the child's subsequent response (Masataka, 1993). In general, regardless of the language, mothers use a wider pitch range than fathers.

Parents who speak American English seem to have more extreme modifications in their speech than do parents in other languages, especially Asian languages (Fernald et al., 1989; Shute & Wheldall, 1989). These differences may reflect the more open American style of communicating and the more reticent and respectful Asian style. In any case, infants seem to prefer the intonational patterns of "baby talk" from a very young age (Cooper & Aslin, 1990; Fernald, 1985; Fernald & Kuhl, 1987; Sullivan & Horowitz, 1983; Werker & McLeod, 1989).

In elicitation sequences with their infants, mothers use all of the baby talk behaviors just mentioned. Unlike games, elicitation sequences continue even when the infant does not respond. In such situations, the mother redoubles her efforts with increasing use of baby talk. There is no fixed repertoire of behaviors and mothers are very adaptable.

Two events lead mothers to talk to their infants. First, selected infant behaviors are treated as meaningful communication turns and the mother responds. For the three-month-old infant, these behaviors include smiling, burping, sneezing, coughing, vocalizing, looking intently, and gaze shifting. The second occasion occurs when the mother talks about what she is doing. She employs baby talk, asks her infant's permission, and gives reasons for her own actions.

On other occasions, mothers talk to their infants for the fun of it. Three specific occurrences of "fun talking" are game playing, attempting to elicit infant vocalizations, and offering objects for play.

Language development experts differ as to the purpose of baby talk (Fernald et al., 1989). Why do mothers and other adults and children use this style of talking with prelinguistic infants? Some experts suggest that these behaviors maintain the infant's attention; others believe that the goal is language teaching. Another group attributes the maternal linguistic adaptations to conversational constraints. A fourth rationale is based on evaluation.

First, a mother probably uses both repetition and variation to capture and maintain her infant's attention (Fernald et al., 1989). Maternal patterns of repetition are found in nonverbal as well as verbal behaviors (D. Messer, 1980). There are also prosodic and intonational variations, which reach a peak at four to six months, corresponding to a period of extensive face-to-face interaction (D. Stern, Spieker, Barnett, & MacKain, 1982). This variety helps keep the infant alert and interested. As the infant gets older, mother introduces more variety and rhythm declines.

The second rationale is that simplified speech aids children in learning language. The maternal modifications differ only slightly from what the infant already knows. Such stimuli provide an optimal level of training.

It seems improbable that maternal speech adaptations serve a specific language-learning function for very young infants. Although mothers' responses to two-month-old infants are stimulating and inject meaning into infants' expressions, it seems doubtful at this stage that verbal meaning has any influence on the infant.

A third reason for the maternal modifications may be to maintain the child's responsiveness at an optimal level (Fernald et al., 1989). However, explanations of the mother's speech modifications based purely on responsiveness to attention and comprehension from the child may be simplistic. The mother assumes that her infant is a communication partner. Thus, maternal speech modifications are an attempt to maintain the conversation despite the conversational limitations of the infant. With a three-month-old infant, the mother structures the sequence so that any infant response can be treated as a reply.

A fourth, compromise rationale for maternal modifications is that mothers use baby talk "to communicate, to understand, to be understood, to keep two minds focused on the same topic" (R. Brown, 1977, p. 12). The mother's modifications are highly correlated with the level of her infant's performance. The main goal is to maintain a conversation in order to provide a context for teaching language use rather than form or content.

Finally, it is suggested that maternal adaptations may reflect evolutionary developments in the human species (Fernald, 1994). The long period of offspring dependency found in humans may necessitate the use of such adaptations as an important part of nurturing and survival of the infant.

Specific goals aside, maternal speech adaptations fulfill three functions. First, the mother's speech modifications gain and hold the infant's attention. Second, the modifications aid in the establishment of emotional bonds. Third, maternal speech characteristics enable communication to occur at the earliest opportunity.

Gaze

The mother modifies her typical gaze pattern, as well as her speech, when she interacts with her infant. Mature adult gaze patterns, which rarely last more than a few seconds, can evoke strong feelings if extended. In a conversational exchange, the mature speaker looks away as he or she begins to speak and checks back only occasionally. When the mother gazes at her infant, however, she may remain in eye contact for more than thirty seconds. During play, gazing may occur up to 70 percent of the time. In addition, play is an activity in which gaze and vocalization can occur simultaneously.

The mother also monitors her infant's gaze. Infant gaze is a good predictor of the mother's conversational topic. In fact, the very young infant doesn't look where mother points, even though he or she behaves as such. Actually, mothers point quickly following the infant's gaze so that the infant's behavior only seems to follow. Gradually, the infant's gaze behavior comes to follow her mother's pointing or naming, although the infant is still free to gaze where it chooses.

Maternal gaze modifications help maintain the infant's interest and focus attention on mother's face. The mother's monitoring of the infant's gaze enables them to establish joint reference before they can establish a shared topic. Caregivers also learn that the infant will look into their faces for interpretation of novel events.

Facial Expression

The mother uses facial expression skillfully to complement her verbalizations. Facial expressions can fulfill a number of conversational functions, including initiation, maintenance and modulation of the exchange, termination, and avoidance of interaction. Mock surprise is frequently used to initiate, invite, or signal readiness. In this expression, the mother's eyes open wide and her eyebrows rise, her mouth opens, her head tilts, and she intones an "o-o-o" or "ah-h-h." Owing to the brevity of most episodes, the mother may express mock surprise every ten to fifteen seconds.

An episode can be maintained or modulated by a smile or an expression of concern. Similar to adult exchanges, a smile signals that communication is proceeding without difficulty. An expression of concern, characterized by open eyes but knitted brows and a partially opened mouth, signals communication distress and a willingness to refocus the exchange.

Termination is signaled by a frown, accompanying head aversion, and gaze breaking. A frown is characterized by low, knitted eyebrows, narrowed eyes, a downwardly curved or pursed mouth, and tense nostrils. Occasionally, the frown is accompanied by a vocalization with decreased volume and dropping pitch.

Finally, avoidance of a social interaction can also be signaled by head aversion, but with a neutral or expressionless face. There is little in the mother's face, therefore, to hold her infant's attention.

Naturally, the mother's repertoire includes a full range of affective facial expressions. Mothers use these expressions to maintain their infants' attention and to aid comprehension.

Facial Presentation and Head Movement

The mother uses a large repertoire of head movements to help transmit her messages, including nodding and wagging, averting, and cocking to one side. The sudden appearance of the face, as in "peekaboo," is used to capture and hold the child's attention. In a variation of this procedure, the mother lowers her face and then returns to a full-face gaze accompanied by a vocalization. Many games, such as "I'm gonna get you" and "raspberries for your tummy," are accomplished by a full-face presentation. Frequently, the mother also exhibits mock surprise.

Proxemics

Proxemics, or the communicative use of interpersonal space, is a powerful interactional tool. Each person has a psychological envelope of personal space that can be violated only in the most intimate situations. When communicating with her infant, however, the mother acts as if this space does not exist and communicates from a very close distance.

Cultural, Socioeconomic, and Sexual Differences

The interactional patterns just described reflect the infant–caregiver behaviors found in the mainstream American culture. In other cultures, the caregiver provides different types of linguistic input. Extended families, common in many cultures, offer multiple caregivers unlike the American middle-class model (Werner, 1984).

Although mothers in other cultures may speak to their children less often in one way, they engage in other communication activities found less frequently in the American culture. Differences in the interactions of mothers and infants may reflect cultural differences, especially as regards the assumed intentionality of infants to communicate (Toda, Fogel, & Kawai, 1990). Mothers in the United States are more information-oriented than mothers in Japan. U.S. mothers are more chatty and use more questions, especially of the yes/no type, as well as more grammatically correct utterances with their three-month-olds. In contrast, Japanese mothers are more affect-oriented and use more nonsense, onomatopoetic, and environmental sounds, more baby talk, and more babies' names. These differences may reflect each society's assumptions about infants and adult-to-adult cultural styles of talking that are direct and emphasize individual expression in the United States and are more intuitive and indirect and emphasize empathy and conformity in Japan.

Japanese mothers also vocalize less with their three-month-old infants but offer, in turn, more physical contact than do mothers in the United States (Otaki, Durrett, Richards, Nyquist, & Pennebaker, 1986; Sengoku, 1983; Shand & Kosawa, 1985). This difference is also reflected in more frequent nonverbal responding by Japanese mothers and more frequent verbal responding by U.S. mothers (Fogel, Toda, & Kawai, 1988). The types of utterances to which mothers are most likely to respond also differ. U.S. mothers are more likely to respond to their three-month-old's positive cooing and comfort sounds, while Japanese mothers are more likely to respond to discomfort or fussing sounds (Morikawa, Shand, & Kosawa, 1988). Japanese mothers try to soothe their infants with speech. These purposes may also differ across cultures, with U.S. mothers more likely to talk to maintain attention and Japanese mothers talking within vocal activities to elicit more vocalizations.

Mothers make use of pitch very early. In English, a rising contour is used to gain the infant's attention (Stern, Spieker, & MacKain, 1982). This pattern is not universal. For example, mothers speaking Thai to their infants use a falling pitch pattern (Tuaycharoen, 1978), and those speaking Quiche Mayan use a flat or falling contour (Pye & Ratner, 1984). Differences in maternal speech modifications to infants reflect cultural differences (Ingram, 1995). Speech patterns are acquired behaviors within the culture in which the mother was raised.

Within the American culture, race, education, and socioeconomic class each influence maternal behaviors toward the child. For example, although inner-city, working-class African American mothers reportedly engage in vocal behavior at about the same rate as middle-class African American mothers, data reveal other more subtle differences (Hammer & Weiss, 1999). Middle-class mothers incorporate language goals more frequently in their play with their infants. In response, middle-class African American infants initiate verbal play more frequently and produce twice as many vocalizations as working class infants.

Children may be expected to learn language through observation, not interaction (Ochs, 1982; Westby, 1986). In one Piedmont, South Carolina, African American community, infants are not viewed as capable of intentional behavior, so their cries and vocalizations often go unattended (Heath, 1983). Middle-class American mothers ask more questions, while those from the lower socioeconomic classes use more imperatives or directives. Similarly, better educated mothers are more verbal. Siblings and peers are more important in the infant socialization process within the homes of minority and lower socioeconomic class families.

Cultural and socioeconomic differences are not maladaptive. Quite the contrary, they reflect the values and beliefs of a society or class. It is not known which aspects of maternal adaptation are most important for a child's communication development. It would be inappropriate, therefore, to suggest that one culture's infant linguistic environment is more productive than another.

As an infant gets older, the American mother communicates more and more from a distance. The resultant decrease in touching is accompanied by increased eye contact. In general, mothers tend to maintain closer proximity to their daughters than to their sons, at least until the age of four years. This sexual difference is reflected in other ways. At two years of age, female infants receive more questions, male infants more directives. With female infants, mothers are more repetitive, acknowledge more child answers, and take more turns. In short, more maternal utterances of a longer length are addressed to daughters than to sons. This difference is not related to the child's linguistic behavior, there being very few if any gender differences in children's language performance at this age.

INTERACTIONS BETWEEN INFANT AND CAREGIVER

Some interactional behaviors are of particular interest for language development. These behaviors, which we will examine in detail, are joint reference, joint action, turn-taking, and situational behaviors. Language may develop as a means of regulating both joint reference and joint action.

Joint Reference

As mentioned previously, *reference* is the ability to differentiate one entity from many and to note its presence. The term **joint** reference presupposes that two or more individuals share a common focus on one entity. "The deep question about reference is how one individual manages to get another to share, attend to, zero in upon a topic that is occupying him" (Bruner, 1978, p. 69).

Joint reference is particularly important for language development, because it is within this context that infants develop gestural, vocal, and verbal signals of notice. Many initial words serve a notice function. The child calls attention to an object, event, or action in the environment, thus conveying the focus of attention to his or her mother.

One of the first uses of language is naming. Approximately 65 percent of the first fifty words the child uses may be nouns, although these nouns may be used for intentions other than naming.

There appear to be three aspects of early referencing: indicating, deixis, and naming (Bruner, 1977). *Indicating* can take a gestural, postural, or vocal form. At an early age, the infant and mother engage in a system to ensure joint selective attention. For example, the mother will shake an object before her infant to attract the infant's attention to it. These routines are used to attain eye contact, the first step in establishing joint reference. As the infant matures, indicating behaviors change. First, indicating behaviors become less dependent on specific situations for interpretation. Next, indicating becomes more economical, thus requiring less effort. As other forms develop, a gesture may carry less of the message content. In its turn, the gesture becomes the context for other content. A reaching gesture changes from an actual reach to a mere indication of a reach. Finally, indicating is gradually conventionalized. Indicating methods become more standardized, more recognizable by others.

Deixis, the second aspect of referencing, is the use of spatial, temporal, and interpersonal features of the content to aid joint reference. Spatial cues relate the object to other aspects of the context, such as *next to* or *in front of.* Temporal cues fix the object in time, as in *after* or *before.* Interpersonal cues relate to role from the speaker's perspective, such as *you* or *me.* The listener must convert deictic aspects to her or his own perspective.

The third aspect of referencing is *naming.* Infants are able to associate names with their referents prior to developing the ability to produce names.

Development of Joint Reference

Four phases in the development of reference have been identified (Table 6.6). Phase I, lasting for the first six months of life, is characterized by mastery of joint attention. The goal is for the infant to look at objects and events in the environment in tandem with mother. The infant must be able to maintain eye contact. The early presence of this behavior is well-documented (Bruner, 1975; Stone, Smith, & Murphy, 1973; Wolff, 1963).

Initially, the mother interests her infant by using direct face-to-face techniques. She does not use objects until the infant is four to six weeks old. At this point, the mother elects to bring the object into the infant's field of vision or to follow the child's line of regard. Both strategies are accompanied by shaking or moving of the object and talking, frequently using the infant's name or phrases such as "Oh, look." The mother's comments on the object of their joint attention become routine. As a result, interactional expectations are established for the infant. Initially, these routines mean little to the infant.

The infant's understanding develops slowly. By eight weeks the infant is able to follow her mother's movements visually. At three months infants can distinguish and attend to utterances addressed to them. The four-month-old infant is able to follow mother's line of regard or pointing. Within a short time, the infant's response quickens with mother's directives, such as "Look!" Later the mother uses the object or event name to establish joint reference. By six months the mother's intonational pattern signals the infant to shift attention. By six months the mother and infant use a number of cues to regulate reference.

Phase II is characterized by the beginning of intentional communication. The infant's heightened interest in objects is accompanied by reaching. With the onset of reaching, face-to-face contact decreases from 80 percent to 15 percent of infant–mother contact time.

Initially, the infant's reach is solely a reach and is not intended to communicate any other meaning. The infant does not look toward mother to see if she has received the message. Instead, the infant orients toward either the object or mother. By eight months the reach is less exigent, and the infant begins to look at mother while reaching. At this point, the infant has two reaches, a "reach-for-real" and a "reach-for-signal," indicating that he or

TABLE 6.6 Development of Joint Reference

PHASE	AGE	DEVELOPMENT
Phase I:	4–6 wks.	Caregiver places object in child's field of vision, shakes object, says "Look"
Mastering	8 wks.	Infant visually follows caregiver's movements
Joint	12 wks.	Infant attends to utterances addressed to her
Attention	4 mos.	Infant follows caregiver's line of regard and response quickens with caregiver's "Look"
	6 mos.	Infant may respond to object or event name and/or intonational pattern to establish joint reference
Phase II: *Intention to Communicate*	7 mos.	Infant establishes joint reference by pointing to or showing objects or events but without looking at adult for confirmation
	8 mos.	"Reach-for-real" and "reach-for-signal" with gaze shift between object and caregiver
Phase III: *Gestures and Vocalization*	8–12 mos.	Reaching or requesting, pointing and showing • Protoimperatives and protodeclaratives • Gesture only becomes gesture plus vocalization
Phase IV: *Naming and Topicalization*	12 mos.	Joint reference established more within the structure of dialogues. • Child assumes more control and parental questioning decreases

Based on Bruner (1975, 1977), Lewis & Freedle (1973), Ryan (1974), Scaife & Bruner (1975)

she expects maternal assistance. The infant's reach-for-signal becomes a stylized indicating behavior. He or she shifts gaze from the object to mother and back again. Mother responds with the object or with encouragement of an even greater effort.

There are thematic changes in mothers' speech to their infants at five to seven months. Mothers move from a social mode, in which they discuss feelings and states, to an activity mode, in which they discuss children's activities and events outside the immediate context. The concentration is on objects as children's focus of interest.

In phase III the infant begins to point and to vocalize. Gradually, the full-hand reaching grasp becomes a finger point. The pointing behavior becomes separated from the intention to obtain an object. In response, the mother asks questions and incorporates the child's pointing and interests into the dialog.

Finally, in phase IV the child masters naming and topicalizing. With this change in the child's behavior there is a corresponding increase in the mother's use of nouns. Increasingly, exchanges involve objects. Initially, the mother provides object and event labels. This strategy is modified when the child begins to talk. The mother attempts to get the child to look, to point, and to verbalize within the ongoing dialog. She uses object-related questions to elicit these verbalizations. As the child assumes more control of the dialog, the mother's questioning decreases.

Summary

The reference function, established months before meaningful language appears, is the vehicle for the development of naming and establishing a topic. More important, joint reference provides one of the earliest opportunities for the infant to engage in a truly communicative act of sharing information. Specific speech and language skills develop as more precise means to transmit the signal to a communication partner.

Joint Action

Throughout the first year of life, the caregiver and infant develop joint behaviors in contexts that support each participant. These routinized actions, called **joint action** provide a structure within which language can be analyzed. Routinized activities, such as game playing and daily routines, have an aspect of convention that lets the child encounter rules within a pleasurable experience. From game playing and routines, the child learns turn-taking and conversational skills. Thus the infant learns to "slot" his or her behavior in the ongoing dialog.

These social interactions are among the most crucial infant learning and participating experiences. Within these joint action sequences, the infant begins to learn the conventions of human communication.

The infant's cry is gradually differentiated into recognizable signals by mother's repeated response. Crying shifts from a demand mode to an anticipatory request mode. As the mother responds to the infant's demand cry, she establishes an expectation within her infant. The resultant request cry is less insistent. The infant pauses in anticipation of her mother's response. This shift is a forerunner of early dialogs in which a behavior or a vocalization is followed by a response.

Early examples of dialogs can be found in the anticipatory body games of infant and mother, such as "peekaboo" and "I'm gonna get you." Gradually, the infant's and mother's contingent play evolves into an exchange mode in which the partners shift roles. For example, when passing an object back and forth, each partner plays the passer and the recipient in turn. Exchange, rather than possession, becomes the goal. Within these exchange games, the infant learns to shift roles, take turns, and coordinate signaling and acting. Role-shifting and turn-taking become so important that the infant will react with frustration, often accompanied by gestures and vocalizations, if the turn is delayed. The infant may even reach for an object being passed before mother offers it. In coordinating his or her signals and actions, the infant learns to look at mother's face in anticipation of the signals.

Finally, a reciprocal mode of interaction replaces the exchange mode. With the reciprocal mode, activities revolve around a joint task format, such as play with an object.

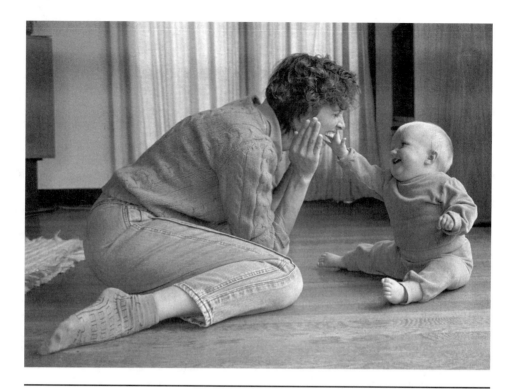

The first year of life is filled with communication and protoconversations between the infant and its caregivers.

Game Playing

The infant and caregiver(s) engage in play almost from birth. Each mother and infant develop a unique set of games of their own. As each mother becomes familiar with her infant's abilities and interests, she creates interpersonal games. These games, in turn, become ritual exchanges that comment upon or emotionally mark familiar patterns of interaction.

The most striking feature is the consistency of each mother's behavior both within and between these play sequences, especially the repetitiveness of the mother's vocal and non-vocal behaviors. Approximately one-third to two-thirds of maternal behavior directed toward the infant occurs in *runs,* or strings of behavior related to a single topic. This form of stimulation may be optimal for holding the infant's attention.

Early face-to-face play occurs in alternating cycles of arousal. The infant is aroused by maternal stimulation. A strong positive correlation exists between the sensory modality of the mother's stimulation and her infant's responses. For example, if the mother stimulates vocally, the child is likely to respond vocally.

An infant as young as six weeks old can initiate games by modifying its internal state of alertness. By thirteen weeks the infant has adopted a true role in social games and thus signals readiness to begin play. When the mother approaches with a still face, her infant initiates the interaction by performing its repertoire of facial expressions and body movements. If the infant fails to get a response, it turns away. This behavior is modified, in turn, to independent exploration play by twenty-three weeks.

Over time, the infant's vocalizations accompanying game playing change and reflect the changes seen in overall language development (Rome-Flanders & Cronk, 1995). The percentage of vocalizations and single syllables gives way to jargon and phonically consistent forms (PCFs), which in turn are pushed aside for single words and multiword expressions. Although vocalizations decrease as a percentage of overall communication, the overall amount of vocalizing remains constant. It is possible that these sounds signal an availabilty to play and a willingness to participate. PCFs and accompanying gestures—in which one establishes a topic and the other a comment, such as making a sound associated with cookie and making an eating gesture—are found in games long before multiword utterances appear.

The mother adjusts gradually to these developmental changes and to changes in her infant's internal state with changes in timing, infant arousal, and agenda. First, the mother adjusts her timing to the infant's arousal to find the appropriate slot for her behavior. She is most likely to respond when the infant looks at her. By modifying her timing, the mother attempts to alter the interactional pattern, to prolong the interactions, or to elicit a response from the infant. Second, the mother buffers her infant's arousal state to maintain a moderate level of arousal. Thus, the infant maintains an optimal state for learning. In turn, the mother is reinforced by her infant's responsiveness. Finally, the mother maintains a balance between her agenda and her infant's behavior. For example, when the infant does not interact for a period of five to ten seconds, the mother responds with her bag of tricks. She makes faces, smiles, protrudes her tongue, moves her limbs, or vocalizes. In so doing, she is careful to leave an opportunity or slot for the infant to respond.

One very popular infant–mother game is "copycat" in which the mother's imitative behavior is dependent on the infant's behavior. Much of this imitation appears to be an unconscious following of the infant's most demonstrative behaviors. The importance of this particular game for later imitation by the infant cannot be overemphasized.

Maternal imitation is not an exact imitation, however, and the mother pulls her child in the direction of the mother's goals or agenda. First, the mother may maximize the imitation by exaggerating her infant's behavior and thus calling attention to it. Second, she may minimize the imitation to a short, quick flash, used to draw the infant back to the mother's ongoing behavior. Third, the mother may perform a modulating imitation such as responding with a mellowed version of the infant's behavior. For example, the mother may perform mellow crying in imitation of the child's wail.

In contrast, infant behaviors that can be interpreted as having communicative intent receive a conversational response. Mothers do not usually imitate prespeech or small hand movements such as pointing. Instead, they reply to these with baby talk.

Early play consists primarily of social behaviors. During the first six months, the focus of play is social; there are no specific game rules. Interpersonal rules are employed. Social play is usually spontaneous and occurs frequently during routines. Once play begins, all other external tasks end.

In a typical social play period, play begins with a greeting when the partners catch each other's glance. This initiation is followed by a moment of mutual gaze. If either partner breaks the gaze pattern, play ceases momentarily. Maintenance of the gaze signals readiness and is usually followed by a maternal mock surprise, in which she raises her eyebrows, widens her eyes, opens her mouth, and repositions her head. Her infant responds with wide eyes, an open mouth, a smile, and head reorientation. The infant may wag its head or approach mother's face, but the result is a full-face positioning. Play begins.

The initial exchange in actual play is a greeting. This exchange, which may last for only a second, accomplishes two things. First, all other activities stop; second, there is a reorientation to a face-to-face position, in which signals will be most visible. Often the infant is not prepared, and there are false starts.

Two subunits, or episodes, of the play sequence that may occur several times per minute are engagement and time out. Episodes of engagement are variable-length sequences of social behaviors separated by clearly marked pauses. Each sequence begins with a greeting that is less full than the initial greeting. Within each episode, the rate of caregiver verbal and nonverbal behaviors is relatively constant. These behaviors occur in discrete bursts within each episode. The mother keeps most of her behaviors under half a second in duration. Tempo can be used to soothe or arouse the infant. For example, the mother increases her rate to exceed that of a fussy child, then gradually slows in order to soothe the infant. Although the rate of maternal behaviors within an episode is constant, the tempo between episodes may vary considerably. For example, the excitement caused by "I'm gonna get you" is due to changes in tempo. Generally, each episode has one major purpose: to establish attention, to maintain attention, or to enter into play. Within each episode, therefore, the mother's behavior is fairly predictable for her infant. These maternal consistencies, accompanied by slight variations, are ideal for gaining and maintaining the infant's attention.

Episodes of time out consist of rests used to readjust the interaction. Time out, usually lasting for three seconds or longer, occurs when the infant signals, often by fussing or averting the gaze, that he or she is no longer excited. Time out provides an opportunity to retune the interaction. The mother changes the focus of the interaction by glancing away or at some other infant body part or by sitting quietly.

Maternal behaviors often occur in repetitive runs within each episode. The average run is three or more units in length. For example, the mother may introduce a topic and then vary it systematically, as in the following sequences:

> You're so big, aren't you?
> So big.
> Oh, so big.
>
> No, we can't do that.
> No, not that.
> Oh, no.

These repetitive maternal speech patterns have already been discussed (see p. 179). Between these repetitive runs, the mother may vary the tempo. Although these repetitions have enormous instructional potential, they also reflect the mother's limited repertoire. In short, she runs out of things to do. Nonetheless, these behaviors expand the infant's range of experience and maintain her attention.

During the second six months of life, object play increases. Object play is almost nonexistent at three months of age. By six months, play often begins with the body but is repeated with a toy. Infant and mother participate in a ritualized give-and-take of objects that occurs frequently after seven months of age. Infant possession time decreases steadily from thirty to ten seconds during the period from seven to ten months. By eleven months the child does not need coaxing before releasing an object. Another popular infant game is "retrieve" in which the child drops an object in anticipation that mother will return it. Infants in all cultures seem to enjoy the shared anticipation and the predictable sequence under their own control. Games allow for lots of shared meaningful communication at a nonverbal level. Throughout the first year, play demonstrates many of the characteristics of later conversation.

Routines

The context for communication can be dynamic, complex, and difficult to predict. This is not the best learning environment. In contrast, routines, such as bathing or dressing, offer conventionalized, predictable contexts in which caregivers provide order. The infant can rely on the order and on caregiver cues. The frequency of routines increases throughout the infant's first year.

Routines provide **scripts,** or scaffolds, that have "slots" for the infant's behavior and aid meaningful interpretation of the event. Just as a fast-food restaurant has a script that constrains adult behavior, dressing and feeding also have similar scripts. By providing a framework, scripts reduce the cognitive energy needed to participate and to make sense.

Infants' event knowledge, which is one of the conceptual foundations of later language development, is gained within familiar daily routines and events (Mandler, 1984; Nelson, 1986). Event knowledge includes information on the actors, actions, props, causality, and temporal aspects of an event.

The content of the child's language may come from these daily interactions. Specific words and phrases, plus presentation formats, vary with each event context (French & Nelson, 1985; Lucariello & Nelson, 1986; Snow & Goldfield, 1983). When children begin to talk, they display greater semantic complexity and range, longer utterances, and more unique words in familiar situations (Farrar et al, 1993; Lucariello & Nelson, 1986).

Summary

Although each infant–caregiver pair evolves different patterns of interaction, there are similarities that are important for later communication development. These include the "process" of conventionalization, the mutual topic-comment, routines, and learning to anticipate partner behavior change. Play is particularly relevant to language acquisition. First, play usually occurs in a highly restricted and well-understood *semantic domain*. Games such as "peekaboo" and "I'm gonna get you" have a restricted format, limited semantic elements, and a highly constrained set of semantic relations. The mother is frequently the agent of some action upon an object. Second, play has a well-defined task structure. The order of events enables the child to predict. The rules of language provide similar boundaries. Third, play has a role structure similar to that of conversation. The infant learns to recognize and to play various roles. In addition, she learns that roles have a property of reversibility.

Turn-Taking

Most of the interactional behaviors discussed so far have contained an element of turn-taking. The infant's development of this skill is essential for development of later conversational skills.

In very early feeding sessions, "turn-taking . . . is a matter of the mother's fitting her behavior into the infant's natural rhythms" (Kaye, 1979, p. 196). Initially, mothers jiggle the nipple to increase or to elicit feeding. Infants respond by decreasing their sucking behavior. Within two weeks mothers learn to cease their jiggling to elicit sucking. The resultant cycle becomes one in which an infant pause is followed by a jiggle. The jiggling stops. After a short delay, the infant begins to suck. Thus, early feeding behaviors represent a pattern of turn-taking.

Most infant and mother turns last for less than one second. The pattern is more like a waltz in which "both partners know the steps and music by heart and can accordingly move precisely together" (D. Stern, 1977, p. 85). As a result, sequences of infant–mother behavior emerge.

Even body games, such as tickling, lifting, and bouncing, contain pauses for infant responses. The pauses are initially short, but they lengthen as the infant gains the ability to respond more fully. This gradual pause lengthening is also found in the maternal responses of Japanese mothers (Masakata, 1993). A lack of pauses can result in overstimulation and a less responsive infant. At three to six months of age, the infant responds or attends quietly. Gaze, facial expression, body movement, or vocalization can all fill a turn.

A set of conversational behaviors evolves from these infant turn-filling behaviors. Several child development specialists have noted the development of reciprocal and alternating patterns of vocalizations called *protoconversations*. Gestures and, later, words will develop to fill the infant's turn in the conversation.

Situational Variations

Mothers use a variety of naturally occurring situations to facilitate language and communication development. Prelinguistic behaviors may be situationally bound, even at an early age. Certain infant–mother situations occur frequently. Eight interactional situations accounted for almost all locational activities of the three-month-old infant. From most to least frequent, these situations are mother's lap, crib/bed, infant seat, table/tub, couch/sofa, playpen, floor, and jumper/swing. The frequency of occurrence is less significant, however, than the frequency of vocalization within each situation. In other words, it is not the location itself that is significant but the function associated with that location.

Within each situation, certain infant–mother behaviors occur regularly. This regularity is the basis for the development of meaning, which emerges from nonrandom action sequences, especially vocalization sequences associated with different "situational" locations. For example, the infant is usually placed in the crib to sleep. Therefore, the mother neither responds nor initiates vocalizations. On the other hand, at the table or in the tub, the infant is subjected to many vocalizations and nonrandom maternal behaviors. Situations provide a context within which the child can process the nonrandom content. Nonrandom behaviors form an early meaning base.

CONCLUSION

Symbolic communication in the form of spoken language develops within the context of a very early communication system that is integrated and nonspeech in nature. Presymbolic communication enables the child to learn language. Over the first year, the infant's early behaviors acquire intentionality and serve several communication functions.

The child's initial behavior communicates little, if anything, beyond the immediate behavior itself. Infant behaviors are not as significant overall as the mother's response to these behaviors. Mothers perceive their infants as persons and interpret their baby's behavior as communicative, verbal, and meaningful.

Humans are social animals who live generally within a social network. The infant is dependent on others, especially mother. The mother is controlled to a great extent by the infant's biological needs. In addition, the infant is adaptable to the social world. The mother is very responsive to the infant's behavior and mindful of the infant's current abilities. She accommodates quickly to infant behavior changes, but her own behavior always has a direction. In general, the mother modifies her behavior by simplifying her speech, by increasing the amount and quality of her nonverbal communication, and by relying heavily on the context. She gives linguistic input while providing an opportunity or turn in which the infant can respond.

Both semantic structure and pragmatic functions are derived from social interaction. The child infers meaning from mother's vocalizations and nonrandom behaviors in interactional situations. Case relationships are learned through joint action routines, such as games, in which the child takes a particular semantic role within the interaction.

The reference function derives from joint attention. The mother and child attend jointly to a rather limited array of objects they share in common. These form the initial concepts that are later named by the child. In addition to reference, other communication functions, such as requesting and giving, are also expressed preverbally.

Functions develop as a result of the mother's responsiveness to her child's earliest interactional behaviors. As the infant learns to control the behavior of others, he or she begins to modify and conventionalize signals in order to communicate more specifically. The particular words that the infant later uses expressively will be determined by pragmatic factors, such as functions, or the intentions these words express. The infant will use those words that are most accurate for expressing its intentions.

Social communication is found in mother–infant discourse over the first year of life. In turn, communication skills developed within the infant–mother dyad provide a basis for the infant's learning of the linguistic code.

It may not be glaringly obvious, but in both chapters 5 and 6, we have addressed the *how* of language development but not the *why*. There is a simple explanation for this omission: We don't know why children develop language.

Although behaviors that the child learns may lead to language, we cannot conclude that the child learned them for that reason (Locke, 1996). The infant does not understand the long-term consequences of its learning, nor is it storing away knowledge for an unknown future. Even if the young infant did sense a need for attaining linguistic competence, he or she is incapable of planning for this eventuality.

The social and communicative bases for language development can be used to explain, in part, the motivation for learning language. The child and caregivers establish strong communicative bonds. Because of the enjoyment or reinforcement each partner receives from these communicative interactions, he or she is desirous of even more communication. The frustration of being misinterpreted and the joy of being understood are strong motivators for both the child and caregivers to modify their language. The infant attempts the code used by the caregiver, who, in turn, simplifies that code to enhance the infant's comprehension. The outcome for the infant is that he or she understands and uses more language within communicative interactions as an attempt to participate even more.

DISCUSSION

Within a discussion of the social and communicative bases of language, we get to the motivation for learning language in the first place. Language is learned within well-established communication. Learning language makes the learner a better communicator.

Most importantly, children become communicators because we treat them that way. We expect them to communicate. If an SLP or teacher doesn't expect his or her clients to communicate, they won't. Not to expect better performance is to give up.

The child seems prewired for communication, but it is what the caregiver—primarily the mother—does with this "predisposition" that is important. Recall how the child progresses to gestures, the first signs of intention to communicate, and how words fulfill the intentions expressed through these gestures. Remember the early learning within joint action routines and game playing that teaches the child about predictability in interactions and about turn-taking. Think of all the things an infant can do socially. The first word is merely the icing on the cake.

REFLECTIONS

1. Discuss the abilities and behaviors of the newborn that suggest prewiring for communication.

2. Describe the aspects of conversation found in gaze coupling, ritualized behaviors, and game playing.

3. Why are gestures particularly important? Describe the sequence of gestural development.

4. What communicative behaviors does the infant elicit from the mother, and what is the effect of each on communication?

5. Explain why three interactions—joint reference, joint actions, and turn-taking—are particularly important for the development of early communication and trace briefly the development of each.

6. Explain the cultural and socioeconomic differences found in the interactions of caregivers and infants.

7

Language-Learning Processes in Young Children

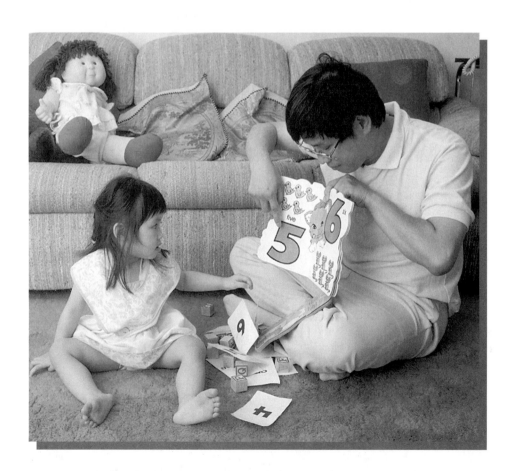

CHAPTER OBJECTIVES

It is difficult to explain language learning without discussing children's learning strategies and parents' teaching techniques. Although the relationship is not one of pupil and teacher, many of the elements of that relationship exist in a more subtle form.

Learning language is not just a process of accumulating language structures and content. Children use certain strategies to comprehend the language they hear and to form hypotheses about the underlying language rules. Caregivers also aid linguistic analysis by modifying the speech stream directed at children. When you have completed this chapter, you should understand

- the relationship between comprehension, production, and cognition.
- the role of selective imitation and formulas.
- universal language-learning principles.
- the characteristics of motherese or parentese.
- the types of parental prompting.
- the effects of parental expansion, extension, and imitation.
- the use of parental turnabouts.
- the importance of play.
- the effects of cultural variation on the language-learning process.
- the following terms:

bootstrapping	hypothesis testing
contingent query	interrogative utterances
evocative utterances	motherese
expansion	selective imitation
extension	turnabout
formula	

In Chapters 5 and 6 we discussed the bases for language development. These bases are inadequate, however, as an explanation of the extremely complicated process of language learning. Language development is not haphazard. Large, general changes occur in an orderly, predictable fashion, although there is great individual variation. The orderliness of development reflects underlying language-learning strategies, the linguistic complexity of the message, and cognitive-conceptual growth.

Even though adults do not attempt to teach language directly to normally developing children, we do adapt our language input to the child's level of attention and comprehension. In the process, we provide models of simplified language for the child. We also tend to react to the child's utterances in a way that increases the chance that the child will repeat the structures later. This reinforcement is not direct but instead includes such indirect behaviors as repeating and responding to the child's utterances. It is also important to remember the context of most language-learning exchanges. Children engage in conversations with their caregivers throughout the day while engaged in activities and routines that form the back-drop for communication.

In this chapter we examine issues related to language learning. We begin by explor-ing the relationship between comprehension, production, and cognitive growth. In addi-tion, child language-learning strategies and adult teaching strategies are explored. Finally, we discuss the conversational context in which the child's language develops and the mater-nal strategies for maintaining a conversation. Naturally, the strategies used by both the child and the adult differ with the language maturity of the child.

COMPREHENSION, PRODUCTION, AND COGNITIVE GROWTH

There is a strong link between comprehension, production, and cognition. The child's cog-nitive conceptual development is the primary tool for comprehension of the language that the child hears. Although conceptual development is both an enabler and a constraint on development, cross-linguistic studies indicate that the properties of individual languages also affect development (Weist, Wysocka, & Lyytinen, 1991).

Cognition and Language

Cognitive skills and language abilities are associated, but not causally. New and increased cognitive ability enables the child to function differently but does not cause change. Cog-nition and language are strongly related with underlying factors that pace the developmen-tal paths of each. Attainment of a skill may be evidenced first in either area (Gopnik & Meltzoff, 1986). In short, no overall relationship exists. Instead, specific relationships occur during development. For example, cognitive development in infants and toddlers is strongly related to increased memory and to ability to acquire symbols in many areas, including lan-guage and gestures (Fischer, 1980; Gopnik & Meltzoff, 1987). First words and recognitory gestures or gestural labels, such as sniffing flowers, appear at about the same age. At times, the correlation between language and cognition is strong; at others, it is not.

Piagetian stages of development are of little value in classifying corresponding cogni-tive and language development. Language skills seem to be more closely related to specific cognitive skills than to stages of cognitive development (Kelly & Dale, 1989). For example, a significant difference in the cognitive levels of play exists between children who use no words and those who use single words. Single-word users are more likely to engage in con-ventional play with "animate" objects. For example, children who do not produce words are more likely to play with toys such as blocks, while children who produce single words are more likely to play with dolls or action figures.

Both imitation and play differ for single-word users and those who are beginning to combine words. The significant change in imitation is the child's ability to imitate sounds not previously in his or her repertoire. The play of children beginning to combine words consists of combining two or more play sequences and/or performing the same action on a sequence of entities. Early combiners and those using the semantic rules also differ in means–ends abilities, with the rule users able to solve problems that require some level of foresight.

Cognitive growth may have a great influence on early word combinations. Many of the principles of cognitive learning can also be applied to language learning. These might include the following (Peters, 1986):

- Pay attention to perceptually salient stimuli.
- Discriminate stimuli along salient dimensions.
- Remember stimuli.
- Classify stimuli according to the results of the discriminations.

These principles correspond to the steps taken in information processing presented in Chapter 4.

The child is an active learner, forming hypotheses based on patterns in the incoming language stream. Data are tested and incorporated into the system or used to reorganize the system. Once the mind stores a certain number of bits of information, it tries to organize them based on perceived relationships.

Organization of longer utterances requires better short-term memory and knowledge of syntactic patterns, or frames and word classes. Hierarchical word-order organization develops, and individual words become "slot fillers" for various word classes.

Many grammatical constructions also reflect cognitive development. For example, the child's embedding of a phrase or clause within an utterance seems to follow the development of the ability to manipulate more than two objects. The child must be able to perform the operation cognitively before using it linguistically. For example, reversibility, or the ability to trace a process backward, is strongly related to acquisition of *before* and *after*.

Knowledge structures of two types are assumed to guide word acquisition: *taxonomic knowledge* and *event-based knowledge* (Sell, 1992). Taxonomic knowledge consists of categories and classes organized hierarchically. New words are compared categorically and organized for retrieval. Until a child has a label for a concept, he relies on overextensions, such as calling all men *Daddy*, or novel words, such as *go-boom* for gun.

Event-based knowledge or representation consists of sequences of events or parent–child routines. Used to separate events from nonevents, event-based knowledge is temporal or causal in nature and organized toward a goal; contains actors, roles, props, and options or alternatives; and may include embedded subevents (Fivush, 1984; Nelson, Fivush, Hudson, & Lucariello, 1983). The child uses this knowledge to form *scripts* for predictable interactional sequences. Scripts are sets of expectations about routine events that aid memory and enhance comprehension (Constable, 1986; Furman & Walden, 1989). Based on common experience, scripts possess wholeness or the totality of the event, thus giving the individual child a knowledge base for interpreting individual events (Nelson, 1986). Even very young children remember routine events in a highly organized fashion (Nelson et al., 1983).

Event-based knowledge influences vocabulary acquisition and may be the basis for taxonomic knowledge (Kyratzis, Lucariello, & Nelson, 1988). Words are learned within a social context; their meaning is found in event representations. Early words are first comprehended and produced in the context of everyday events (Nelson, 1986). Embedded within event scripts are the words that are part of the event. From repeated use, the words themselves become cues for the event. For example, the words *bath* and *soap* become cues for bathing, while *cookie* and *juice* represent snack. As the child acquires more words, *cookie*, *cracker*, *milk*, and *juice* become *things I eat* which later evolves into the category *food*. Preschoolers rely on event-based knowledge, while kindergarteners use more categorical script-related groupings such as *things I eat*. By age seven to ten, children are using taxonomic categories, such as *food* (Kyratzis et al., 1988; Sell, 1992).

Comprehension and Production

Linguists continue to argue, however, over the relationship between language comprehension and production. Comprehension prior to production was previously considered a universal of language acquisition. Data from young Thai children suggests, however, that they may employ a distributional (location and frequency) strategy for production of certain language forms before they comprehend these forms (Carpenter, 1991); in other words, produce frequently used words that appear in the same linguistic location repeatedly.

The relationship of comprehension to production is one of mutual dependence. Although its exact nature is unknown, the relationship is a dynamic one that changes with the child's developmental level and with each aspect of language. In other words, the relationship between comprehension and production changes because of different rates of development and different linguistic requirements made of the child.

Judgments of the comprehension of presymbolic infants are complicated by the strategies used by the child. Using a "context-determined" strategy, the infant may look where mother looks, act on objects that mother references, and imitate the actions of others. The infant relies on its event knowledge and on the interactive cooperation of the caregiver who interprets the child's behavior as meaningful.

In early phonological development, perception of speech-sound differences greatly precedes expression. The child can perceive speech sounds very early. Intonational patterns are also discriminated early, at around eight months of age.

First words pose a different problem. Obviously, the child does not fully comprehend the word before he or she produces it. Full comprehension would require a greater linguistic and experiential background than that of the year-old infant. Toddlers don't have adultlike word definitions. Instead, event-based knowledge scripts are used to form their responses based on their acquired expectations of repetitive adult behaviors (Paul, 1990). For example, when the caregiver says, "Let's read a book" and hands one to the child, the child responds by opening the book which is part of the book script. Later, preschoolers focus on linguistic factors to gain the information needed. Event knowledge continues to be important, however, even for adults, and comprehension is easiest within familiar events.

The toddler's comprehension is aided by the nonlinguistic context because most speech addressed to the child is associated with the here and now. In fact, adults may overestimate a child's comprehension unless they analyze all the paralinguistic cues and situational redundancies. Estimates of production may also be inflated (Elliot, 1981). The child may imitate others, either immediately or after some delay, and repeat stock phrases, songs, and rhymes. In comprehension, the child uses both linguistic and conceptual input plus his memory. In contrast, production also uses linguistic and conceptual input but relies on linguistic knowledge alone for encoding.

"The Original Word Game" (Brown, 1958) demonstrates the relationship between comprehension and production. After the mother labels an entity, the child forms hypotheses about its nature. In turn, the child tests these hypotheses by applying the label. The mother monitors the child's output to check the accuracy of fit between her and the child's underlying concepts. The mother improves the child's accuracy by providing evaluative feedback. Hence, the child's comprehension and production are fine-tuned essentially at the same time.

Even though a symbol signifies a particular referent, the meaning of the symbol goes beyond that referent. For example, the symbol or word *car* can be used to label a toy car or a limousine, but the meaning of *car* is quite different in each example. Meaning refers to a concept. The symbols used to convey that meaning are arbitrary.

Within the first fifty words, comprehension seems to precede production. As a group, children may understand approximately fifty words before they are able to produce ten. The range of comprehended words varies greatly. The distribution of syntactic types also varies between comprehension and production (Table 7.1). As children mature, the distribution changes. While action words may account for 50 percent of the first ten words understood, general naming words may account for only 14 percent. With increasing age, the percentage of action words drops and that of nominal words rises. The initial difference between the two word types is not reflected in production, where nominals outnumber actions by at least two to one.

Infant acoustic-phonetic comprehension of first words may be less specific than it seems (Walley, 1993). Initially, recognition and comprehension are holistic, such as grossly discriminating *dog* from *cookie*. Rather quickly, however, the infant acquires the detailed perceptual skill needed for more subtle distinctions, such as *hot* and *hit*. Over 50 percent of the

TABLE 7.1   Comprehension and Production of Single Words by Syntactic Category

	COMPREHENSION (FIRST 100 WORDS)	PRODUCTION (FIRST 50 WORDS)
Nominals (Nouns)		
Specific	17%	11%
General	39	50
Action	36	19
Modifiers	3	10
Personal-social	5	10

Source: Adapted from H. Benedict, "Early Lexical Development: Comprehension and Production," *Journal of Child Language*, 1979, 6, 183–200.

most common monosyllabic words spoken by one- to three-year-olds have three or more other words that differ by only one phoneme (Dollaghan, 1994). Actually, the increasing size of the child's lexicon probably necessitates such differentiation (Aslin & Smith, 1988; Walley, 1993).

During the second year of life, the child increases his or her vocabulary and begins to combine words within a single utterance. Gradually, the child realizes that a word refers not to a single referent or type of referent but to a related group of referents (Oviatt, 1982). If comprehension precedes production, we would expect the child to understand word combinations before using multiword utterances. Here the nonlinguistic context is an essential comprehension aid. In addition, comprehension of a sentence depends on recognition of highly meaningful words. The child need not know syntax if he or she knows the meanings of these words separately. The nonlinguistic context provides relational information. Yet, children seem to respond best to verbal commands that are slightly above their production level.

Toddlers rely on basic semantic relations, use of objects, and routines for comprehension, possessing little knowledge of syntactic relations. Two strategies may be used with objects, do-what-you-usually-do and act-on-the-object-in-the-way-mentioned, disregarding the agent mentioned. Using the first strategy, balls would be rolled, thrown, dropped, or passed back and forth no matter what the child heard. With the second, the child would throw the ball whether the caregiver said, "Now, you *throw* the ball" or "Remember how Johnny *throws* the ball in the baseball game?" While there is some limited linguistic processing, event knowledge is still very important.

As the child approaches two years of age, the comprehension–production discrepancy seems to decrease. Nevertheless, production still lags behind comprehension.

Young preschoolers use a "probable event" strategy (Paul, 1990). If there is no obvious probable action, the child responds randomly or uses basic syntactic relationships. By twenty-eight months, he or she can use word order for limited comprehension but may be easily influenced by other cues (Golinkoff, Hirsh-Pasek, Cauley, & Gordon, 1987; Roberts, 1983). Even though production can be characterized as observing word-order rules of construction, the child does not appear to use word order as a primary tool for comprehension until about the third year, or when the average length of his or her utterances reaches 4.0 morphemes. Verb comprehension may be acquired one verb at a time, moving from general verbs, such as *do*, to more specific verbs, such as *eat* and *sit*.

Even children with average utterance lengths of approximately 1.5 to 2.75 are more accurate in responding to adult linguistic forms than to child forms. These data suggest an early ability to comprehend adult forms.

By late preschool, children are using word order consistently for comprehension although they have no preferred strategy and may still revert to event knowledge (Bridges, 1980; Tager-Flusberg, 1989). Children may overrely on word order as noted previously and ignore such terms as *before* and *after*. It is not until age five or six that children begin to rely consistently on syntactic interpretation (Keller-Cohen, 1987).

With the development of metalinguistic skills and the shift from syntagmatic to paradigmatic semantic organization—both discussed in Chapter 11—there is a change in children's comprehension strategies. By age seven to nine, children are using language to acquire more language, such as word definitions, and are more sensitive to phrases and subordinate clauses and to temporal connectors, such as *before, after, during,* and *while.*

Summary

In the preschool years, the relationship between comprehension, production, and cognition becomes very complex. In general, linguistic developments parallel much of the cognitive growth of the preschool child. This is not a one-to-one relationship. Such heterogeneity suggests that development is very complex (Flavell, 1982). The relationship between the linguistic aspects of comprehension and production is less clearly defined, and it is no longer possible to make the blanket statement that comprehension precedes production. At the present time, we are not aware of all of the relationships between cognition, comprehension, and production. Further research is needed to understand these relationships more completely.

CHILD LEARNING STRATEGIES

Although there are many variations in the way in which children learn American English, there are ample similarities. These suggest underlying strategies used by most children to interpret and produce language. Naturally, these strategies differ with the language level of the child. In the following section, we consider the language-learning strategies most frequently associated with toddlers and preschoolers.

Toddler Language-Learning Strategies

To assume that toddlers merely produce what they comprehend is to oversimplify the acquisition of language. The child must use certain learning strategies to sort out relevant and irrelevant information. Speech and language in adult and sibling conversations are often poor. The child must decide which utterances are good examples of the language and must hypothesize about their underlying meanings and structures.

Receptive Strategies: When Is a Word a Word?

As toddlers mature, they become increasingly adept at acquiring new words under conditions that are not always ideal (Baldwin, 1993). Although fourteen- to fifteen-month-olds experience difficulty establishing stable symbol-referent associations even with caregiver assistance, eighteen- to nineteen-month-olds are able to establish these links even when the caregiver names entities to which the toddler is not attending.

Before children can recognize words, they gain a sense of how sounds go together to form syllables of the native language (Jusczyk, 1999). Armed with these structures, the child can more easily locate word boundaries. The seemingly endless speech stream becomes a series of distinct but meaningless words. For example, six- to ten-month-old children reared in English-speaking homes begin to develop a bias in favor of words with emphasis on the first syllable, such as *mommy, daddy, doggie,* and *baby*. Eleven-month-old infants are sensitive to the word boundaries and phonological characteristics of their native language (Myers, Jusczyk, Nelson, Charles-Luce, Wordward, & Hirsh-Pasek, 1996; Shafer, Shucard, Shucard, & Gerken, 1998).

Although adults modify the speech stream to highlight unit boundaries and to hold the child's attention, and although symbols map semantic and pragmatic functions previously established, these explanations alone are insufficient for describing the ways in which toddlers learn symbols. What do children bring to the task? What assumptions do children make about language they encounter? Linguists don't really know but can infer from the language behavior of toddlers that certain lexical principles or assumptions are being used.

Three assumptions of toddlers seem basic or fundamental: (1) people use words to refer to other entities, (2) words are extendable, and (3) a given word refers to the whole entity, not its parts (Golinkoff, Mervis, & Hirsh-Pasek, 1994). The first or *reference principle* assumes that people refer. Words do not just "go with" but actually "stand for" entities to which they refer. Therefore, the toddler must be able to determine the speaker's intention to refer, the linguistic patterns used to refer, and the entities to which they refer. Infants and caregivers are able to establish joint reference well before the appearance of first words. A subprinciple, the *mutual exclusivity assumption*, guides initial word learning by presupposing that each referent has a unique symbol. In other words, a referent cannot be both a *cup* and a *spoon*. Eventually, as the child gains multiple referents, this assumption will be overridden (Markman, 1992; Merriman & Bowman, 1989).

As you will recall from Chapter 1, words or symbols usually represent concepts, not unique referents. Using the second or *extendability principle*, the infant assumes that there is some similarity, such as shared perceptual attributes, that enables use of one symbol for more than one referent. Thus, *cup* can refer to the child's cup and to those that the child perceives to be similar.

There is still some ambiguity, however, because the word *doggie* could refer to the dog's fur, color, bark, four legs, or any number of similarities. The third or *whole-object principle* (Horton & Markman, 1980; Macnamara, 1982; Markman & Wachtel, 1988; Mervis, 1987) assumes that a label refers to a whole entity rather than to a part or attribute. In fact, object parts are rare in toddler lexicons (Mervis, 1990). Mothers aid this assumption of their children by providing general or basic-level terms (*cup*) before more restricted terms (*mug, glass, teacup*). Basic-level terms are often accompanied by pointing, while more restricted terms often require additional explanation or information. Parents seem to prefer basic-level nouns to adjectives or verbs (Ninio, 1980). Thus, parental teaching strategies seem to match children's learning preferences.

Three additional assumptions may be necessary to speed acquisition by enabling the toddler to form hypothetical definitions quickly and to use syntactic information. These are the categorical or taxonomic assumption, the novel name-nameless assumption, and the conventionality assumption (Golinkoff et al., 1994; Markman, 1992). The *categorical assumption* is used by children as young as eighteen months to extend a label to related entities (Markman & Hutchinson, 1984; Mervis, 1987). Classification is based not just on perceptual attributes, but on function, world knowledge, and communication characteristics, such as shortness of length and commonality. Unlike the extendability principle, which would apply *cup* to a limited sample, the categorical assumption goes beyond basic-level referents of the same kind to categories of entities. In this case, *cup* may be extended to all objects that hold liquid.

The *novel name-nameless assumption* enables the child to link a symbol and referent with very few exposures. In short, the child assumes that novel symbols are linked to previously unnamed referents. Use of this assumption seems to correspond to the vocabulary spurt experienced by many children at around eighteen months (Mervis & Bertrand, 1993). Caregivers aid the child by naming and pointing to, holding, or manipulating novel objects to further specify the referent (Masur, 1997). As children mature, they rely less on these gestural assists and more on the caregivers' language (Namy & Waxman, 1998).

Finally, the *conventionality assumption* leads the child to expect meanings to be expressed by others in consistent conventional forms (Clark, 1983). In other words, caregivers don't change the symbol with each use. A car is consistently called by that name. Conversely, because the child must use conventional forms in order to be understood, he or she is motivated to produce the forms used by the community.

We are not certain that children actually use these principles or make these assumptions. Toddlers must employ these or similar principles, however, in order to make sense of the speech stream directed at them. It cannot be overemphasized that this learning process is an active one (Tomasello, Strosberg, & Akhtar, 1996). Children actively attempt to understand adult language and to make word-referent associations.

Expressive Strategies

Young children use four metalinguistic strategies to gain linguistic knowledge: evocative utterances, hypothesis testing, interrogative utterances, and selective imitation (McLean & Snyder-McLean, 1978). **Evocative utterances** are statements the child makes naming entities. After the child names, the adult gives evaluative feedback that confirms or negates the child's selection of exemplars. As a result, the child either maintains or modifies his or her hypothesis. As expected, there is a positive correlation between the quantity of verbal input by adults at twenty months and vocabulary size and average utterance length of the child at twenty-four months.

Hypothesis testing and **interrogative utterances** are more direct methods of acquiring linguistic knowledge. When seeking confirmation of a hypothesis, the child may say a word or word combination with rising intonation, such as "doggie ↑ " or "baby eat ↑." A responding adult either confirms or denies the child's utterance. When unaware of an entity label, the child uses an interrogative utterance, such as "what?", "that?", or "wassat?" These requests for information can be found in the gestural-vocal behaviors that precede the appearance of the first word. *What* and its variants are found among the first words of many children, and at twenty-four months there is a positive correlation between the number of questions asked by children and their vocabulary size.

The nature and significance of the final strategy, **selective imitation**, have generated much research. Most linguists would agree that imitation is selective. Children do not imitate indiscriminately. Given that a child may imitate an utterance in whole or in part, he is free to select any utterance from another speaker. Yet the toddler will select short utterances of others for imitation. If imitation is a learning strategy, then surely the child is employing some criterion for selection.

Role of Selective Imitation. Imitation has been reported as a device used in the acquisition of words, morphology, and syntactic-semantic structures (Perez-Pereira, 1994; Speidel & Herreshoff, 1989). In general, imitation is defined as a whole or partial repetition of an utterance of another speaker within no more than three successive child utterances. Table 7.2 contains examples of selective imitation. It has been noted that much of what toddlers say—varying between 4 and 52 percent of their utterances—is an imitation of other speakers. Widespread differences across children may reflect methodological or situational variations.

Usually, imitations are just beyond the structural production capacities of children, indicating the use of imitation as a learning strategy (Speidel & Herreshoff, 1989). The role of imitation as an aid in the acquisition of language is very complex. For example, self-imitation, not imitation of others, seems to be important for the transition from single-word to multiword language production (Veneziano, Sinclair, & Berthoud, 1990).

The use of imitation as a learning strategy may also vary with individual children, although the overall amount decreases with age, especially after age two (Casby, 1986; Kuczaj, 1982; Masar, 1989; Owens & MacDonald, 1982; Snow, 1981). It appears that imitation's usefulness as a language-learning strategy decreases as language becomes more complex. Interestingly, children with delayed development may maintain the strategy long after it has ceased to be a viable learning tool (Owens & MacDonald, 1982).

TABLE 7.2 Examples of Selective Imitation

Adult:	Daddy home.
Child:	*Daddy home.*
Adult:	The doggie is sick.
Child:	*Doggie sick.*
Adult:	You want the baby?
Child:	No.
Adult:	Okay, mommy want baby.
Child:	*Want baby.*
Adult:	Throw ball.
Child:	No.
Adult:	But you just did. Now what?
Child:	*Throw ball.*

At the single-word level, imitation seems particularly important for vocabulary growth, although conceptual development seems to be central as well. The presence of the referent increases the likelihood of imitation. In turn, the child's ability to imitate an utterance depends on his or her understanding of its meaning. The best way for parents to teach a young child a new word is to provide the word and give a demonstration and explanation (Banigan & Mervis, 1988).

Many imitations and much early vocabulary growth take place within the context of daily routines which may contain predictable or repetitious language. Imitations may be immediate or may appear later in an altered form. For example, the child might repeat the last word of an utterance but change its function.

The ends of utterances seem to have particular perceptual importance for children. For example, when the child goes to the door, his mother may say, "Do you want to go out?" When next the child goes to the door, he or she may say, "Out." The word is the same, but the illocutionary function has changed. The function of the mother's speech may have a great effect upon imitation. The amount of child imitation seems to reflect the amount of maternal imitation.

It has been suggested that imitation may serve as a discourse device, enabling the child to relate his or her utterances to those of more mature language users. In the following exchange, note how the child uses imitation to tie utterances to those of the adult:

Parent:	See Johnny ride his bike?
Child:	Ride bike. Fall.
Parent:	No. He won't fall.
Child:	Fall. Go boom.

The form of the imitation is often determined by its function.

Development often proceeds from highly repetitious utterances to semantically diverse ones. In these diverse revisions, the child alters the preceding utterance in order to maintain discourse and semantic relations and to sustain the topic. The child uses two strategies of revision: *focus operations* and *substitution operations*. Focus operations, which predominate until about age three, require only minimal linguistic skills. The child focuses on one or more words and repeats them. For example, when the caregiver says, "Baby's going to sleep in her bed," the child might say, "Sleep bed." In a substitution operation, the child repeats only a portion of the utterance but replaces words. For example, in response to "Baby's going to sleep in her bed," the child might say, "Sleep blanket." The topic is maintained, but the semantic–syntactic structure is changed. This behavior increases with age and resembles the conversational replies found in more mature language use.

It is assumed that the child must store enough adult examples to allow him or her to abstract the relationship involved and to form a linguistic hypothesis. As children become more proficient with a structure in spontaneous speech, their imitation of it decreases. Although the exact role of imitation in language acquisition is unclear, it appears that children imitate most frequently items that they are in the process of learning or that have recently appeared. As such, imitation may serve young children as a modeling and stabilizing process for new structures. Imitation would thus reflect a child's developmental level and the teaching strategies of the adults around him or her.

Role of Formulas. A verbal routine or unanalyzed chunk of language often used in everyday conversation is called a **formula**. As memorized, automatized units, formulas function as a whole unit, often as an entire utterance. For example, I remember a young child who produced the Wendy's "Where's the beef?" commercial phrase frequently and without understanding as "Wa-a-bep?" Children's use of formulas is reported in several languages (Hickey, 1993; Perez-Pereira, 1994; Plunkett, 1993). Although they seem to be the result of deferred imitation, formulas have a purpose well beyond a repetitive or even referential one.

Use of formulas may represent a whole-to-parts learning strategy for some children (Hickey, 1993; Nelson, 1981a; Pine, 1990; Pine & Lieven, 1990). Many newly acquired forms may be learned initially as formulas (Elbers, 1990). The child gradually progresses from unit or whole learning to system or parts learning as he or she analyzes or segments formulas into their individual symbols.

Segmentation of formulas, in turn, coincides with the vocabulary spurt noted in children at approximately eighteen months (Plunkett, 1993). Thus, while formulas aid initial vocabulary growth, their nonsegmentation may constrain the development of large vocabularies.

Summary. Selective imitations and formulas function much as routines, providing a "scaffolding" for the child and reducing the language-processing load. Both aid linguistic analysis and are used meaningfully in conversation. Other strategies, such as the use of evocative and interrogative utterances and hypothesis testing, enable the child to further participate in conversation and to explore and test new words and structures.

Preschool Language-Learning Strategies

Obviously, the usefulness of selective imitation is limited when the child begins to acquire structures of more than a few words. This accounts for the rapid decline of the use of imitation at around thirty months of age, suggesting the use of other learning strategies.

In general, children use what they know about language to help them decipher what they don't know. For example, they may use semantics to decode syntax or syntax and context to figure out word meanings. This process is called **bootstrapping**. "To pull yourself up by your bootstraps" is to use the resources at hand to better yourself. This is what the child does when he or she uses knowledge in one area to enhance performance in another.

Using *semantic bootstrapping*, young language-learning children analyze syntax based on semantic structures previously acquired (Macnamara, 1982; Pinker, 1982, 1984). Persons and things form one category later indicated as nouns, actions indicate verbs, attributives indicate adjectives, and spatial relations and directions indicate adverbs and prepositions. Syntactic functions are formed similarly, with semantic agents indicating subjects, and so on (Matthei, 1987). While this early organization is limited—not all nouns are agents and objects, nor all verbs actions; and not all subjects are agents—it does provide a basis for the syntactic system.

In similar fashion, observable syntactic structures can be used to deduce word meanings (Gleitman, 1993). This process is called *syntactic bootstrapping*. Relationships between words can aid in identification of verbs or other parts of speech and their use. In practice, semantic and syntactic bootstrapping are complementary processes.

Language rules are learned gradually. Initially, the rule may be unanalyzed and used in situation-specific instances. Use will generally proceed sporadically until the child masters the rule.

We can assume that children begin by learning the basic sentence type, which in English is subject-verb-object. The model presented to young language-learning children may have this basic sentence type only 40 to 60 percent of the time. It seems that children pick the most frequently modeled order to represent the basic sentence type. Additional intonational and situational cues may serve to differentiate those utterances that differ from the basic sentence type. For example, interrogatives usually end in a rising intonation and accompany certain activities or routines.

Most likely, children determine the syntactic rules by using cues provided by the meaning of the adult's utterance. Thus, the child figures out the meaning of the adult's utterance based on nonsyntactic information. Mothers aid in this process by talking primarily about the present context.

From a cross-linguistic perspective, the development of syntactic and morphological features seems to progress through three stages (Berman, 1986). In the first stage, use of the feature is context based and depends on extralinguistic cues. The second stage is structure-based or grammatical, in which the child relates meanings to forms. In the third stage, the child acquires mature language use of the feature based on internalized rules.

The first stage is a universal one prior to the development of language-specific grammar. Regardless of the language being learned, toddlers produce similar content or meanings and uses or functions. Thus, we find children using similar semantic and illocutionary categories that include words without morphological markers. These forms are the unmarked building blocks for later development.

Regardless of the language, certain semantic distinctions are learned before others. For example, *red*, *blue*, and *yellow* are learned before *green*, *brown*, and *orange*; *in* and *on* before *behind*. Similarly, one-time actions, such as *fall* and *break*, are likely to appear first in past tense, while ongoing durative actions, such as *eat* and *play*, appear in the present tense. Regardless of the language, changes in question form generally occur in yes/no questions prior to *wh-* questions. Within *wh-* questions, those that ask *what* and *where* appear first, while *why* and *when* questions appear later. This is true in languages as different as Korean, Tamil, and English (Clancy, 1989; Vaidyanathan, 1988).

Children in the initial stage of language development also talk about the same general types of things, using a restricted set of semantic categories. Sentences always consist of animate agents and inanimate objects. Only later do children use inanimate subjects (*Ball* fall) and animate objects (Kiss *baby*).

Initially, the strategies for processing and acquiring language are similar across children learning different languages. One is the *plausible event strategy* of comprehension (Berman, 1986). Basically, this strategy is one in which language is interpreted based on the most commonsense understanding in a particular context. Children use their knowledge of routines and contexts to decode the meaning of the language they hear. A second strategy is *rote learning* for production (Peters, 1983). Initially, the child learns to use certain words in certain contexts through imitation.

Even though stage 2 learning, which is grammatical, obviously differs with the language being learned, some operating principles seem universal. First, the preschooler attempts to *pay attention to how and where semantic distinctions are marked*. For example, consonants and the inside of words are important in modern Hebrew, stems and word endings are important in Hungarian, and word and phrase relationships are important in English.

In addition to learning words and word meanings, the child learns the classes in which words belong. Language rules apply to word classes, not to individual words. Most likely the child hypothesizes that words are similar and thus belong together because of the way they are treated linguistically (Maratsos, 1988). For example, the child hears certain words receive *-ed* and *-ing* markers and begins to "chunk" these words together into what adults call *verbs*. Initially, words are learned individually and treated as if each is its own category. As the child discriminates similarities, words treated in the same manner are organized and stored together. New members are added as they meet the criteria for linguistic treatment. Although this explanation is somewhat simplified, it adequately describes an active process by the child that corresponds to our knowledge of information processing and hypothesis building by humans.

The second principle is to *recognize words with the same consonants as related*. Thus, *dog paddle* and *dog catcher* must have something in common. This strategy can backfire when older children encounter *dogma* and *dogwood*.

Third, *word order is important*. Initially, children rely on a few rigid formulas. In English, children become overdependent on the subject-verb-object sentence form. Later, they learn other forms and develop a flexible system that is adaptable to different discourse situations. The evolution from rigid to flexible systems has been reported in the development of languages as different as English, Chinese, French, modern Hebrew, Hungarian, and Turkish (Aksu & Slobin, 1985; Berman, 1985; Erbaugh, 1980; MacWhinney, 1985; Maratsos, 1983).

Universal Language-Learning Principles

After studying forty different languages, linguist Daniel Slobin (1978) noticed that there were patterns of development that suggested underlying universal learning strategies and operational principles of children (see Table 7.3). Although we do not know the exact strategies children use, we can infer their presence from consistent language behaviors of young children. The following sections address each of Slobin's seven principles.

Pay Attention to the Ends of Words. Across languages, the same semantic notion, such as a verb tense or temporal relation, may be produced linguistically at very different ages. If we assume that the concept can be learned by all children at the same age, then differences in age of production must reflect differences in the rate of acquisition of linguistic markers for this concept. In general, children acquire linguistic markers that occur at the ends of words (*-s, -er, -ed*) before those that appear at the beginnings of words (*un-, dis-, in-*). Similarly, English regular verb endings are acquired before auxiliary verb forms that precede

TABLE 7.3 Universal Language-Learning Principles

1. Pay attention to the ends of words.
2. Phonological forms of words can be systematically modified.
3. Pay attention to the order of words and morphemes.
4. Avoid interruption and rearrangement of linguistic units.
5. Underlying semantic relations should be marked overtly and clearly.
6. Avoid exceptions.
7. The use of grammatical markers should make semantic sense.

Source: Drawn from D. Slobin, "Cognitive Prerequisites for the Development of Grammar." In L. Bloom & M. Lahey (Eds.), *Readings in Language Development.* New York: Wiley, 1978.

the verb. A corollary could be stated as follows: *For any given semantic notion, suffixes or post-positions will be acquired earlier than will prefixes or pre-positions.* For example, the comparative *-er* and superlative *-est* endings are acquired before the alternative *more* and *most* markers. The child is thus more likely to learn *sweeter* than *more sweet.*

Many new or expanded grammatical structures initially occur at the end of sentences, suggesting that the final position in longer structures is also important for learning. Initial use of the verb in children's questions may also reflect attention to the ends of adult utterances. For example, after hearing his parent say, "I don't know where it is," the child may later produce the question form "Where it is?"

Phonological Forms Can Be Systematically Modified. Through experimentation, the child learns to vary pronunciation. Gradually, the child recognizes that various sound changes can reflect underlying meaning changes.

Pay Attention to the Order of Words and Morphemes. Word order is one of the earliest principles learned. The standard order of morphemes used in adult utterances is preserved in child speech. The child produces "charm*ingly*," not "charm*lying*." In English, general word order is maintained by preschoolers also, although there is some initial difficulty with negative and interrogative transformations. This ordering leads to another developmental universal: *Word order in child speech reflects word order in adult forms of the language.* This seems to be especially true in languages such as English, in which word order often reflects underlying meaning. In imitating tasks, the American child tends to retain word order.

A second developmental universal states that *in early stages of development, sentences that do not have standard word order will be interpreted using standard word order.* Two examples from English relate to interpretation of passive sentences and temporal ordering of joined sentences. The English-speaking preschooler interprets passive sentences as if they represent the more common subject-verb-object form. Any noun-verb-noun sequence is interpreted as agent-action-object. The child will therefore interpret "The cat is chased by the dog" as "The cat chased the dog." In compound or conjoined sentences the three-year-old child will ignore the conjunctions *before* and *after*, interpreting the relationship of the clauses as an order of occurrence. In other words, clause 1 occurred first, then clause 2. For example, the sentence "We'll go to Gran'ma's after the movie" may be interpreted as "Gran'ma's, then movie."

Avoid Interruption and Rearrangement of Linguistic Units. Interruption and rearrangement place a strain on the child's processing. Processing is most difficult with sentences that require the child to retain large amounts of information, such as interrupted units, in order to complete the task.

A related developmental universal states that *structures requiring rearrangement of elements will first appear in nonrearranged form* . In other words, a form that differs from the predominant subject-verb-object format will first appear in the subject-verb-object form. In some children's speech, the auxiliary or helping verb in questions (What *are* you eating?) appears originally in a noninverted form (What you *are* eating?) not found in adult queries. In addition, children have greater difficulty making subject-verb inversions for questions when there is a relative clause modifying the subject and thus separating the subject-verb elements of the sentence as in "The speaker *who came by plane* was three hours late" (Nakayama, 1987).

A second related universal states that *discontinuous morphemes are reduced to, or replaced by, continuous morphemes whenever possible*. In English, this universal is demonstrated in the progressive verb inflection *-ing*, which appears initially in children's speech without the auxiliary verb, as in "I eating ice cream."

There is a tendency, states a third universal, to *preserve the structure of the sentence as a closed entity by initial sentence-external placement of new linguistic forms*. In other words, new structures may be tacked on to the beginning or end of the sentence prior to moving within it. Early negatives are attached to the beginning and, occasionally, to the end of a sentence. Only later does the negative move next to the verb. Initial subordinate clauses and infinitive phrases also occur in the object position at the end of the sentence.

Finally, a fourth universal states that *the greater the separation between related parts of a sentence, the more difficult it is for the child to process adequately*. Several studies have shown that the difficulty of processing sentences is more closely related to the separation of elements than to the number of phrases or clauses embedded in it (Hakuta, de Villiers, & Tager-Flusberg, 1982). Thus, a sentence containing a phrase or clause is more difficult to interpret if the embedded portion interrupts the subject-verb-object format. A sentence such as "I saw the man *who fell down*" is easier for preschoolers to interpret than "The man *who fell down* ran away." In a sentence such as "The girl who stole the horse ran away," a young child is likely to interpret it as "The girl stole the horse and the horse ran away."

To produce reversals or interruptions, the preschooler must take some risks (Dale & Crain-Thoreson, 1993). Those preschoolers who use reversals less are also less likely to attempt other structures, such as pronouns.

Underlying Semantic Relations Should Be Marked Overtly and Clearly. As the child listens to and attempts to interpret speech, overt morphological markers may provide perceptually meaningful and consistent aids. With maturation, the child may be able to derive more and more semantic information from minimal cues. To some extent, children demonstrate the importance of these markers in their own speech. There is some evidence that small functor words (*the, of, and*) and other morphological markers may receive more emphasis in child speech than in adult speech.

Both the Tamil and Turkish morphological systems are learned early because of their regularity and clarity of marking (Raghavendra & Leonard, 1989). Each affix encodes only one feature, and by age two, most children are using them correctly. Compare this to English, in which three phonological shapes (/s, z, əz/) are used for plural, third person singular, and possessive marking.

A related universal states that *a child will begin to mark a semantic notion earlier if its morphological structure is more obvious perceptually*. As evidence, Slobin noted the development of the passive in Indo-European languages, such as English and in Egyptian Arabic. The concept of the passive form is not difficult for children to learn, but in English the linguistic marking is. Egyptian Arabic-speaking children learn the passive prefix *it-* rather early compared to the length of time required for English-speaking children. In English, a passive sentence requires several changes in the basic subject-verb-object format and may not be acquired fully until adolescence.

A second universal states that *there is a preference for marking even unmarked members of a semantic category*. This universal may account for some of the overextensions in English to unmarked words. For example, the clear *-ed* past-tense marker may be used with irregular verbs (*went*) that may appear to the child to have no marking (*wented*). Preference for marking may also be seen with the plural. For example, the word *some* may mean a portion of one or a few of many. The noun that follows may therefore be either singular or plural. It is not uncommon to hear a child say "I want some cakes," when he really desires a portion.

When a child first masters the full form of a linguistic entity that can be contracted or deleted, contractions or deletions tend not to be used. In other words, initially a child will use the full form of contractible or deletable forms. This universal has strong support in English. Young children may respond with "I will" when asked to imitate "I'll" in a sentence. Similarly, the verb *to be* first appears as "he *is*," although adults use *"he's"* more frequently. In an imitation task, children may replace optionally deleted forms that are not present in the model sentence.

Related to this finding is a final universal: *It is easier to understand a complex sentence in which optionally deleted material is not deleted*. This principle is demonstrated by the difficulty both children and adults experience with deletions.

Avoid Exceptions. There is a tendency among children to overgeneralize linguistic rules and to avoid exceptions to these rules. The rules for a larger class, such as past tense, are learned before those for a subclass, such as irregular past tense. One developmental universal of this principle outlines the stages of linguistic marking of semantic notions (Marchman & Bates, 1994; Marcus, Pinker, Ullman, Hollander, Rosen, & Xu, 1992):

1. No marking.
2. Appropriate marking in a small number of cases.
3. Overgeneralization of marking although limited and with a small number of examples.
4. Adultlike system.

For example, initially there is no marking of the English past tense. Next, some irregular past-tense verbs, such as *came* and *fell*, are formed correctly, but the regular past *-ed* is not used. Once learned, the regular past is overextended to irregular verbs, as in *comed* and *falled*, before full adult usage is acquired.

A second developmental universal states that *rules for larger classes are learned before rules for subdivisions, and general rules are learned before exceptions.* Most plural nouns, for example, can use the word *many* to indicate quantity, such as *many cookies* or *many blocks.* Children learn this rule quickly. Mass nouns, a smaller class—identifying liquids or granular substances, such as *sand* or *water*—require *much.* It takes children much longer to learn to use *much* with the appropriate nouns. Other examples of this principle are the overgeneralization of the regular past tense *-ed*, as in *eated*, and the regular plural *-s*, as in *mans.*

Overgeneralization or overextension of morphological or syntactic rules may be related to an increase in number of exemplars or units learned to which the rule applies (Marchman & Bates, 1994). Initial examples are learned most probably by rote memorization until such time as the number is large enough for the child to synthesize a general rule (Plunkett & Marchman, 1993). Overgeneralization or erroneous production begins at this point.

Grammatical Markers Should Make Semantic Sense.   Overgeneralization of rules is limited usually to the appropriate semantic category. Inflectional markers, such as *-s*, *-ed*, or *-ing*, and functor words, such as *a*, *the*, or *at*, are applied within grammatical classes. Thus, the *-ed* morphological marker is always applied to words in the verb class. Functor words, or smaller, less important words, are substituted for functors from the same class. For example, the child may use *in*, a preposition, incorrectly in place of *at*, another preposition, but he will not substitute *the* for *at*, because *the* is an article. Semantically defined classes take precedence in selection. In contrast, purely arbitrary rules are very difficult to master.

One universal of this principle states that *when selecting an appropriate marker from among a group performing the same semantic function, the child tends to rely on a single form.* For example, the selection of the /s/, /z/, or /əz/ phonological form of the plural is based on the ending consonant of the stem word. Initially, the child relies on one form of the plural where possible.

A second universal indicates that *the choice of the functor word is always within the given functor class and subcategory.* Although the child may confuse different words within a word class, such as prepositions, he or she rarely confuses words from different classes. Hence, an inappropriate preposition may be used, but it will not be confused with a pronoun. For example, a child may say, "Kerry is going *at* school" when he means "*to* school." He is unlikely, however, to say, "Kerry is going *when* school," since *when* is not a preposition.

Third, *semantically consistent rules are acquired early and are relatively error-free.* This universal was discussed earlier with reference to the progressive *-ing* ending. For the action words a two-year-old uses, there are no exceptions to the present progressive *-ing* rule.

Summary.   It must be stressed that Slobin's principles are theories that attempt to explain the order of acquisition. According to Slobin, the child has certain concepts, based on cognitive growth, that are expressed through the linguistic system. Using certain principles of acquisition, the child scans the language code to discover the means of comprehension and production.

Individual Differences

Children vary not only in the rate of language development but also in the route. Those developing normally may exhibit as much as thirty months' variation in language development at forty-two months of age (Wells, 1985). Individual developmental differences are related to differences in intellect, personality and learning style; ethnicity and the language of the home; socioeconomic status; family structure; and birth order. In general, these relationships are very complex, not simply cause and effect. Some factors, such as intelligence, may be much stronger than others. Socioeconomic factors alone, for example, may have little overall effect on rate of language development (Wells, 1985). There may be more differences within socioeconomic classes than between them. In contrast, birth order or position in the family has a significant effect on early language development. Single children have a greater opportunity to communicate with adults than do children with several siblings and thus develop language more quickly. Twins may spend a great deal of time talking to each other with resultant multiple phonological errors (Dodd & McEvoy, 1994).

The learning style of the child affects language learning to some extent. In general, the active, outgoing child is more likely to learn language more rapidly than the placid, retiring child (Wells, 1985). The former is more inclined to join in and to communicate with whatever means are available, fostering learning the language code.

Individual styles of learning are evident very early (Hampson & Nelson, 1993). Different types of maternal stimulation affect children in diverse ways. Some toddlers attend to symbols while others prefer paralinguistic and nonlinguistic elements. Maternal behaviors may be in response to these differences rather than a cause of them as is often assumed.

Comments on the rate of language learning may be invalid without accompanying information on route. Certain children may exhibit advances in expressive language use, while others who seem somewhat delayed in this area exhibit superior comprehension skills.

ADULT CONVERSATIONAL TEACHING TECHNIQUES

Adults engage in very little direct language teaching, but they do facilitate language acquisition by their behaviors. Although very little time is spent in direct instruction, many caregiving and experiential activities relate to language acquisition. Obviously, these parental techniques will vary with the language maturity of the child.

Adult Speech to Toddlers

Throughout the first two years of life, parents talk with the child, label objects and events, and respond to the child's communication. It would be simplistic, however, to assume that the child just applies the labels heard to his or her internal concepts. Meaning is also derived from the communication process (Levy & Nelson, 1994). Although words are constrained initially by the conversational context, they are later used more flexibly as the child encounters the word in other contexts and gradually modifies the meaning. Within the conversational context, parents aid acquisition by engaging in modeling, cueing, prompting, and consequating behaviors that affect the linguistic behaviors of their children.

Modeling: Motherese (Parentese)

Children's speech occurs in conversation and generally serves to maintain the exchange. As noted previously, conversational behavior is well established by the time the child begins to speak. Almost from birth, the child encounters a facilitative verbal environment that enables him or her to participate as a conversational partner.

As the child's communication behaviors develop, the mother unconsciously modifies her own behaviors so that she requires more child participation. The mother may not accept babbled responses once her child begins to use PCFs or single words. Instead, she responds to babbling with "What's that?"—a request for a restatement. When the child follows her pointing, the mother immediately asks a question. Whether the child responds with a gesture or a smile, the mother will supply a label. Once the child is able to vocalize, the mother "ups the ante" and withholds the label or repeats the question until the child vocalizes. Then mother gives the label.

Word learning depends on the establishment of joint reference, as noted in Chapter 6. As noted, mothers are very effective at following their child's line of regard, then labeling the object of the child's attention approximately 70 percent of the time (Harris, Jones, & Grant, 1983; Lueng & Rheingold, 1981; Masur, 1982). In general, the more time allotted to such joint attending, the larger the toddler's vocabulary (Akhtar, Dunham, & Dunham, 1991; Tomasello, Mannle, & Kruger, 1986; Tomasello & Todd, 1983). In short, the child is more likely to learn a symbol when focused on the referent (Tomasello & Farrar, 1986). As might be expected, mismatches between the child's attending and the adult's symbol occur frequently—approximately 30 to 50 percent of the time (Harris et al., 1983; Tomasello & Farrar, 1986; Tomasello & Mannle, 1985). When this occurs, the caregiver attempts to redirect the child who will use both nonverbal and verbal cues to redirect his focus (Baldwin, 1993). As a result, eighteen-month-old toddlers may learn some words from only one exposure.

Although first words express semantic knowledge and the child's conversational intent, they are learned within interactive contexts where the child learns to use the models for them. Data from English and Modern Hebrew demonstrate that nearly all the rules and utterances of young children mirror patterns used by their mothers. Those structures modeled most frequently by the mothers are most likely to be used by their children.

Although initially the mother provides object names, within a short time she begins to request labels from the child. By the middle of the second year, the mother is labeling and requesting at approximately equal rates and dialog is fully established. This dialog becomes the framework for a new routine. The mother begins to shape the child's speech by distinguishing more sharply between acceptable and unacceptable responses. The child's verbalizations are not immediate imitations but responses that fill specific slots within the dialog, usually following a question. Within the dialog, the mother provides consistency that aids learning. These consistencies include the amount of time devoted to dialog, the number of turns, the repetition rate, the rate of confirmation, and the probability of reciprocating (Bruner, 1978).

In addition, the mother makes other speech modifications that, taken together, are called **motherese** (Newport, Gleitman, & Gleitman, 1977) or *parentese*. The characteristics of motherese are listed in Table 7.4. Compared to adult–adult speech, motherese exhibits (a) greater pitch range, especially at the higher end; (b) lexical simplification characterized by the diminutive ("doggie ") and syllable reduplication (consonant-verb syllable repetition); (c) shorter, less complex utterances; (d) less dysfluency; (e) more paraphrasing and repetition; (f) limited, concrete vocabulary and a restricted set of semantic relations; (g) more contextual support; and (h) more directives and questions.

TABLE 7.4   Characteristics of Motherese Compared to Adult-to-Adult Speech

Paralinguistic

Slower speech with longer pauses between utterances and after content words

Higher overall pitch; greater pitch range

Exaggerated intonation and stress

More varied loudness pattern

Fewer dysfluencies (one dysfluency per 1,000 words versus 4.5 per 1,000 for adult–adult)

Fewer words per minute

Lexical

More restricted vocabulary

Three times as much paraphrasing

More concrete reference to here and now

Semantic

More limited range of semantic functions

More contextual support

Syntactic

Fewer broken or run-on sentences

Shorter, less complex sentences (approximately 50% are single words or short declaratives)

More well-formed and intelligible sentences

Fewer complex utterances

More imperatives and questions (approximately 60% of utterances)

Conversational

Fewer utterances per conversation

More repetitions (approximately 16% of utterances are repeated within three turns)

Although, as noted in Chapter 6, mothers use a short conversational style with infants, they use even shorter, less adult utterances with toddlers. The lowering of the mother's MLU, beginning in the second half of the child's first year, is positively related to better receptive language skills by the child at eighteen months of age (Murray et al., 1990). There seems to be no measurable effect on expressive language. Mothers aid *bootstrapping*, mentioned previously, by maintaining a semantic-syntactic correspondence (Rondal & Cession, 1990). For example, in utterances addressed to children, mothers use agents as subjects almost exclusively. The mother's behavior makes it easier for the child to decipher the syntax of mother's utterances.

As the child's language matures, the mother's speech directed to the child likewise changes. Motherese seems well-tuned to the child's language level.

The amount of maternal speech produced, partial repetitions of the child, and initiated statements commenting on child activity or eliciting attention vary with the child's overall language level. These dynamic elements appear to be strongly related to the child's subsequent development (Wells, 1980; Wells, Barnes, Gutfreund, & Satterly, 1983). Although language generally occurs in an action context, the dependence on nonlinguistic contextual cues, such as gestures, decreases with an increase in the child's linguistic abilities (H. Schaffer, Hepburn, & Collis, 1983; Schnur & Shatz, 1984).

Slow at first, the rate of change increases with age. The length and complexity of the mother's utterances change most between twenty and twenty-seven months, when the child's language changes most rapidly, although at any given time the syntax is fairly consistent (Bellinger, 1980; Wells et al., 1983). There seems to be little or no change in the structural complexity of motherese between eight and eighteen months. During this period there is also little corresponding change in the complexity of child speech, the changes consisting primarily of the addition of single words.

Not all elements differ with the language level of the child. For example, maternal use of the verb *to be* (copula), tense markers, and verbs and nouns does not change (Smolak & Weinraub, 1983). Overall use of imperatives or requests/commands and of initiations intended to elicit or provide information also remains consistent.

Mothers fine tune their language input to the child based primarily on the child's comprehension level. Other factors that influence the level of the mother's language are the conversational situation, the content, and different conversational acts (Snow, 1986). Overall, adults will simplify their input if the child does not seem to comprehend.

The amount of parental labelling or naming in both English and French varies with the age and development of the child, although a relationship exists between the amount of adult labelling and the child's subsequent vocabulary growth (Poulin-Dubois, Graham, & Sippola, 1995). Data from Mandarin, Korean, Italian, and English suggest that the initial parental emphasis on nouns is not universal (Choi & Gopnik, 1995; Gopnik, Choi, & Baumberger, 1996; Tardif, Shatz, & Naigles, 1997). Both gesturing and the use of noun labels in English decrease with development (Schmidt, 1996). Nouns are replaced by verbs describing the action performed by the object.

Undoubtedly, the influence of the child's characteristics on the interaction and on motherese also has an influence on the language input to which the child is exposed (Yoder & Kaiser, 1989). The toys that the child plays with also influence the amount and types of language produced by the parent (O'Brien & Nagle, 1987). In general, toys that encourage role play, such as dolls, elicit more language and a greater variety of language from parents.

If adults simplify their language in order to be understood, then these modifications must reflect cues coming from the child. Apparently, however, adults are not conscious of their modifications, nor are they attempting to teach language. Adult-to-child speech seems to be modified in response to the amount of child feedback and participation. Not only is much of the speech addressed to the child adapted for the child's linguistic level, but speech not adapted is simply ignored or not processed (Snow, 1986). In other words, children play an active role in selecting the utterances to which they will attend. A lack of response is important, for it informs the parent there has been a breakdown in communication that, in turn, necessitates linguistic changes by the parent. Although the exact nature of child feedback is unknown, the child seems to be the key to adult linguistic changes (Furrow & Nelson, 1984).

The pragmatic aspects of the mother's speech may be related to either the referential or the expressive style of the child. Referential children tend to name frequently while expressive children engage in more conversation. Mothers of referential children seem to use more descriptive words and fewer directives (Della Corte, Benedict, & Klein, 1983). In addition, these mothers use more utterances within a given situation than mothers of children with more expressive speech.

Nonlinguistic behaviors are also critical. Child linguistic behaviors alone are not sufficient to produce the adult changes. It is necessary for the adult to see the child in order to gain some information (Rembold, 1980). In fact, maternal linguistic modifications are different when the child is absent.

Since the child has already demonstrated some turn-taking ability, he or she is capable of engaging in some conversation with the caregiver. Despite linguistic inadequacies, the child can participate effectively because of the mother's ability to maintain the conversation. The steady, rhythmic flow of the dialog depends on the structural similarity of the mother's and child's utterances and on the correspondence of the mother's speech to events in the environment. She enables the child to participate through her use of turn-passing devices. She does not use turn-grabbing or turn-keeping behaviors, such as "well . . . ," "but . . . ," or pause fillers.

The mother maintains control, and the dialog is much less symmetrical than it may appear. After the child reaches age two, the mother slowly relinquishes her control of both sides of the dialog (Kaye, 1980). She maintains the interaction by (a) second-guessing the child's communication intentions, (b) compensating for the child's communication failures, and (c) providing feedback for those failures (L. Wilkinson & Rembold, 1982).

Within the interactional sequence, the mother analyzes, synthesizes, and abstracts language structures for her child (Moerk, 1985). Through modeling word equivalents, she aids the child's pattern learning. A sequence might be as follows:

> *Child:*   She running.
> *Mother:*   She's running fast. Oh, she's tired. Now she's running slowly. She's stopping. She's jumping slowly. Now she's jumping quickly.

Thus, the child is not a lone linguist attempting to learn the language code; much of analysis, synthesis, and abstraction is performed by the mother (Moerk, 1985).

Despite the name *motherese*, these speech modifications are not limited to mothers. Fathers and other caregivers modify their speech in very similar ways (Hladik & Edwards, 1984; Rondal, 1980). In fact, fathers may provide even more examples of simplified adult speech than mothers (Hladik & Edwards, 1984).

The range of vocabulary used by fathers and mothers with their young language-learning children is similar, but fathers use fewer common words (Ratner, 1988). In this way, fathers are more lexically demanding than mothers.

Although fathers make modifications similar to those of mothers, they are less successful in communicating with toddlers, as measured by the amount of communication breakdown (Tomasello, Conti-Ramsden, & Ewert, 1990). Fathers use more requests for clarification than mothers. In addition, the form of these requests is more nonspecific ("What?") than those of mothers ("You want what?"). Fathers also acknowledge their children's utterances less frequently. In return, children tend to persist less in conversation with their fathers than with their mothers. It is possible that fathers serve as a bridge for their children between communication with the mother and with other adults. The child learns to communicate with those less familiar with his or her style and manner.

Even children as young as four years of age make language and speech modifications when addressing younger language-learning children. Adult and peer language modifications differ somewhat. In general, peer speech to toddlers is less complex and shorter and contains more repetition than adult-to-toddler speech, although peers elicit fewer language responses than parents (Wilkinson, Hiebert, & Rembold, 1981). Peer interaction may provide a "proving ground" for trying new linguistic structures.

Children enrolled in daycare centers also encounter a variety of motherese that varies with the size of the group and the age of the children (Scopesi & Pellegrino, 1990). In general, the larger the group of children, the less individual adaptation by the adult. Larger groups force teachers to concentrate on keeping attention and control.

The presence of older siblings may also influence the language a younger child hears and produces (Wellen, 1985). For example, an older child will usually respond to more of the parent's questions, thereby reducing the number of responses made by the younger child. The younger child will often respond by imitating the older sibling. In this situation, the mother uses fewer rephrased questions, fewer questions with hints and answers, and fewer questions as expansions or extensions when the older child is present. (Expansions and extensions will be explained in more detail in the section on consequating behaviors in this chapter.) In addition, the mother uses more direct repetitions of questions.

Parents who use a more conversational style with less instructing are more likely to have children who learn language more quickly (Wells, 1985). In other words, children benefit more from language input when parents are more concerned with their mutual understanding and participation and less so with direct instruction.

The exact effect of motherese on language acquisition is unknown. The modifications made by mothers may (a) aid in language acquisition, (b) bring maternal utterances into the "processing range" of the child, or (c) merely increase the mother's chances of getting a correct response from the child (Wilkinson & Rembold, 1982). Since we find similar modifications in many cultures, we can assume that, at least, they somehow facilitate communication between adults and children.

The modifications of motherese seem to be maximally effective with the eighteen- to twenty-one-month-old child, although the acquisition of specific structures is not associated with its use (Gleitman, Newport, & Gleitman, 1984). Rather, the child attends selectively, focusing on the best examples of various structures. Thus, the greater the range of utterances—within limits—the more rapidly the child will discover the underlying rule system.

Prompting

Prompting includes any parental behaviors that require a child response. Three common types are fill-ins, elicited imitations, and questions. In fill-ins, the parent says "This is a. . . ." No response or an incorrect response from the child will usually result in additional prompts and recueing. In elicited imitations, the parent cues with "Say X." Young language-learning children respond to slightly over half of the elicited imitations addressed to them. Questions may be of the confirmational yes/no type, such as "Is this a ball?", or of the *wh*-variety, such as "What's that?" or "Where's doggie?" Unanswered or incorrectly answered questions are usually reformulated by the adult. Approximately 20 to 50 percent of mothers' utterances to young language-learning children are questions. The individual range varies greatly.

Children's nonverbal replies to their mothers' questions seem to be significantly affected by the gestural information accompanying the questions. There appears to be a strong link between maternal gestures and children's action responses. Maternal gestures serve as attention getters or prompts for action. Gradually, over the course of the first year, the link between maternal gestures and the child's verbal responses increases (Allen & Shatz, 1983).

In general, language-teaching utterances have a shorter average length than the majority of the utterances addressed to the child. Maternal yes/no interrogatives, such as "Are you going home?", appear to correlate with child language development gains in syntactic complexity, while intonational interrogatives, such as "You going home?", correlate with gains in the child's pragmatic ability. In contrast, maternal directives, such as "go get your coat," seem to correlate highly with child gains in utterance length and semantic–syntactic complexity (Wells et al., 1983), although they may slow vocabulary growth even when attention-directing in nature (Harris, Jones, Brookes, & Grant, 1986; Tomasello et al., 1986; Tomasello & Todd, 1983).

One interesting technique that parents employ to give the child an opportunity to produce two related single-word utterances is called the *vertical strategy* (R. Schwartz, Chapman, Prelock, Terrell, & Rowan, 1985). After the child produces a single-word utterance, the parent uses questions to aid the child in producing other elements of a longer utterance. The parent concludes by repeating the whole utterance. The following exchange is an example of the vertical strategy:

> *Child:*   Daddy.
> *Adult:*   Uh-huh. What's Daddy doing?
> *Child:*   Eat.
> *Adult:*   Yeah, *Daddy eat* cookie.

Although prompting and cueing are effective teaching techniques, their exact effect on language development is unknown. Several studies have demonstrated the effectiveness of these training techniques with children with language disorders.

Consequating Behaviors

Parents do not directly reinforce the syntactic correctness of children's utterances verbally. In fact, less than 10 percent of children's utterances are followed by verbal approval. Generally, such reinforcement is given for truthfulness and politeness, not for the correctness of the syntax.

Differential feedback by parents follows their children's language production (Bohannon & Stanowicz, 1988; Demetras, Post, & Snow, 1986; Furrow, Baillie, McLaren, & Moore, 1993; Hirsh-Pasek, Treiman, & Schneiderman, 1984; Moerk, 1991; Penner, 1987). Imitation, topic changes, acknowledgments or no response are more frequent following grammatically correct child utterances, while recasts or reformulations, expansions of the child's utterance, and requests for clarification are more likely following ungrammatical utterances. These responses may signal the child as to the acceptability of the utterance.

Recasts modify the child's utterance slightly by replacing and/or rearranging elements. For example, when the child says "Dat bes horsie," the adult might respond "Is that one?" Expansions, discussed in the next paragraph, are a more mature form of the child's utterance, as in "That's a horsie." Requests for clarification may take the nonspecific form of "What?" or "Huh?" or be more direct, as in "What was that?"

Some consequating behaviors seem to serve a reinforcing function. Approximately 30 percent of mothers' responses to eighteen- to twenty-four-month old children consist of expansions (R. Brown & Bellugi, 1964). An **expansion** is a more mature version of the child's utterance in which the word order is preserved. For example, if the child says "Mommy eat," Mother might respond with "Mommy is eating her lunch." As the child's average utterance length increases beyond two words, the rate of expansion by the mother decreases. Approximately one-fifth of the two-year-old's ill-formed utterances are expanded by the mother into syntactically more correct versions (Hirsh-Pasek et al., 1984). By producing the expanded version, the mother assumes that the child intends to communicate a certain meaning.

Children seem to perceive expansions as a cue to imitate (Scherer & Olswang, 1984). Nearly a third of adult expansions are in turn imitated by the child. These imitations are more likely to be linguistically correct than the child's original utterance. It is believed that spontaneous productions follow, and rules are generalized to conversational use. As spontaneous production of structures occurs, imitation of these structures decreases. Expansions may facilitate the learning of word classes and their combinations rather than the learning of specific lexical items (Scherer & Olswang, 1984). Expansion adds meaning to the child's utterance at a time when the child is attending to a topic he or she has established. In addition, expansion provides evaluative feedback. Expansions continue the topic of conversation and encourage the child to take his or her turn and, thus, to maintain the dialog (Scherer & Olswang, 1984).

The type of expansion used by the mother may have an effect on the particular form being learned by the child (Farrar, 1990). For example, reformulating the child's previous utterance by adding, substituting, or moving a morpheme may aid learning of plurals and progressives but has less effect on the past tense or copula, which seem to benefit from removal of morphemes and restatement of correct forms with embellishment of other aspects of the utterance.

Extension, a semantically related comment or reply on a topic established by the child, may be even more helpful as a facilitative device. For example, when the child says "Doggie eat," his partner replies, "Doggie is hungry." Thus, extension provides more semantic information. Its value lies in its conversational nature, which provides positive feedback, and in its *semantic* and *pragmatic contingency*. A semantically contingent utterance is one that retains the focus or topic of the previous utterance. A pragmatically contingent utterance concurs with the intent of the previous utterance; that is, topics invite comments, questions invite answers, requests invite responses, and so on. In short, contingency maintains the flow, which is inherently rewarding to almost all children.

The order of acquisition of grammatical structures is more a reflection of adult free speech than of the form of expansion. Maternal extending utterances also seem to correlate significantly with changes in the length of the child's utterances (Barnes, Gutfreund, Satterly, & Wells, 1983).

Finally, parents imitate their child's speech. A little over 20 percent of adult repetitions are imitated, in turn, by the child.

All three consequating behaviors—expansion, extension, and imitation—result in greater amounts of child imitation than adult topic initiation or nonimitative behaviors. Hence, expansion, extension, and imitation appear to be valuable language-teaching devices. Each consequates a child verbal behavior, and expansion and extension also provide models of more mature language. In addition, the adult utterance is semantically contingent upon the preceding child utterance. This characteristic decreases the linguistic processing load on the child because the adult utterance is close to the child's utterance in form and content. Parents do not consciously devise these teaching strategies; rather, they evolve within the conversational context of child–caregiver interactions.

Adult Conversations with Preschoolers

As noted in Chapter 6, caregivers alter their behavior to enable infants to engage in successful communication as early as possible. This process continues in the preschool years. Mothers provide opportunities for their children to make verbal contributions, draw them into conversations and provide a well-cued framework for the exchange, show the child when to speak, and thereby develop cohesiveness between the speaker and the listener. Mothers ask children to comment on objects and events within their experience, knowing

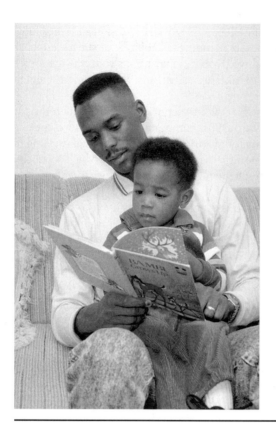

Adults in the child's environment structure conversations around many items and activities, such as reading.

that they can do this. They also expand information by talking about the same object or event in different ways or by adding new ideas and elaborating on them (Martlew, 1980). Moreover, these maternal modifications appear to be correlated with advances in the child's language abilities.

In general, the mother of a three- to four-year-old uses many techniques to encourage communication. Mothers use twice as many utterance prefixes, such as *well* and *now*, as their children do (Martlew, 1980). These signals, plus varied intonation, are used with responses and help the child understand by signaling that a response is coming. In addition, mothers use a high proportion of redundant utterances to acknowledge and reassure the child. The mother frequently acknowledges with "good" or "that's it," which add little additional information. The behavior fills a minimal turn, however, without being overly disruptive to the child's speech stream. Maternal repetition of the child's utterance seems to be for the purposes of emphasis and reassurance.

Mothers are not equally facilitative in all areas of language development. For example, mothers are not as facilitative with turn-taking as they are with other pragmatic skills (Bedrosian, Wanska, Sykes, Smith, & Dalton, 1988). Thus, mothers seem more interested in control than in facilitation.

Throughout the preschool years, mothers interrupt their children much more than their children interrupt them. When interrupting, mothers usually omit the politeness markers seen in adult–adult dialog. The frequency of these interruptions decreases with the child's maturity level.

When interrupted, children usually cease talking and reintroduce the topic. In contrast, mothers usually continue to talk when interrupted by their children and do not reintroduce the topic as often.

Teaching methods change as the child becomes a more mature language user. Expansion is not as effective a teaching tool with the preschool child as it is with the toddler. Instead, a mother's "partial-plus expansion" of her own prior utterances may be more important (Hoff-Ginsberg, 1985). Partial-plus expansion is characterized by a maternal self-repetition followed by an expansion, such as "Want big cookie? Does Tommy want a big cookie?" Thus, the mother assists the child in finding the structural similarity by a comparison of adjacent utterances.

Mothers also continue to facilitate the structure and cohesiveness of discourse by maintaining or reintroducing the topic (Wanska & Bedrosian, 1985). With increasing age and utterance length, the child takes a greater number of turns on each topic. The number of turns per topic is still low by adult standards and does not change radically until school age. Preschoolers also begin to use *shading*, or a change of topic focus, rather than a discrete transition to a new topic. For example, when discussing a birthday party, the child might say "My favorite birthday cake is chocolate," shifting the topic to a related or shaded one. A younger child might introduce an unrelated topic such as "My doggie is sick!"

Compared to her preschool child, the mother makes more demands and suggestions. As the child gets older, the mother uses more imperatives. The mother sustains her child's interest by the use of mild encouragement ("Oh, that's nice") and praise ("What a lovely picture") (Martlew, 1980).

Maternal speech to thirty-month-olds benefits syntactic learning by providing language-advancing data and by eliciting conversation (Hoff-Ginsberg, 1990). From the mother's point of view, it seems more important to engage the child in conversation than to elicit advanced forms from the child. Generally, such elicitation and feedback on the quality of the child's productions does little to contribute to development (Pinker, 1989). In contrast, conversation keeps the child's attention on language input and motivates the child to participate.

The effects of conversation, however, appear to be structure-specific. As might be expected, questions contribute to the development of auxiliary or helping verbs and the verb *to be*, because these forms are prominently placed at the beginning of the sentence, as in "*Did* you eat the cookies?" and "*Is* he happy or sad?" (Hoff-Ginsberg, 1986; Richards,

1986, 1987, 1990; Richards & Robinson, 1993). Mothers use yes/no questions to reformulate their children's utterances.

The mother invites child utterances, primarily through the use of questions, often followed by self-responses. This form of modeling is an effective teaching tool. For example, She might ask, "What color should we use?" followed by "I pick red."

Shared event knowledge is still important and provides scaffolding for new structures (Lucariello, 1990). Scripts that emerge from these events concentrate the child's attention, provide models, create formats, and limit the child's linguistic options, thus decreasing the amount of child cognitive processing and supporting the topic of conversation. This scaffolding is particularly important when discussing either nonpresent referents or topics. Approximately 85 percent of twenty-four- to twenty-nine-month-old children's information providing utterances on nonpresent topics occur in scripted contexts.

Turnabouts

The goals of adult–adult and adult–child conversations differ. In adult–adult conversations the goal appears to be to obtain a turn, whereas the adult goal in adult–child conversations is to get the child to take his turn. As with a younger child, the mother relies heavily on the questioning technique of elicitation. One variant of this technique has been called a *turnabout* (Kaye & Charney, 1981). A **turnabout** is an utterance that both responds to the previous utterance and, in turn, requires a response. Thus, a turnabout fills the mother's turn and then requires a turn by the child. By using turnabouts, the mother creates a series of successful turns that resemble conversational dialog.

With a child aged two to two-and-a-half, the mother is twice as likely to use a turnabout as the child (Kaye & Charney, 1981). Generally, a turnabout consists of some type of response to, or statement about, the child's utterance and a request for information, clarification, or confirmation that serves as a cue to the child. The mother often initiates a topic or an exchange with a question, thus gaining control. If asked a question, she regains control by responding with another question. Resultant dialogs consist of three successive utterances: the mother's first question, the child's response, and the mother's confirmation, which may include another question. For example, the mother might say, "Can you tell me what this is?" and then respond to the child's answer with "Um-hum, and what does it do?" Thus, the mother is now back in control. In general, the child is less likely to respond to the mother unless she requests a response, as in a turnabout (Kaye & Charney, 1981).

There are several types of turnabouts, shown with examples in Table 7.5. One type, the **request for clarification** or **contingent query**, is used by both adults and children to gain information that initially was not clearly transmitted or received. Its use requires that both the listener and the speaker attend to prior discourse in their production. Thus, its use may be related to the development of the ability to refer to what has come before. Children receive little negative feedback via contingent queries when they make language errors (Morgan & Travis, 1989). Parental requests for clarification are just as likely to be attempts to clarify genuine misunderstandings and miscommunications as to correct production errors.

TABLE 7.5   Turnabouts

TYPE	EXAMPLE
Tag	Child: *Baby's panties.* Mother: *It's the baby's diaper, isn't it?*
Clarification (contingent query)	*Huh?* *What?*
Specific request	*What's that?*
Confirmation	*Horse?* *Is that a hippopotamus?* (Hand object to partner and give quizzical
glance)	

Expansions
  Suggestions
  Corrections
  Behavior comment
	I want one.
	No, it's a zebra! (Expectant tone)
	You can't sit on that.

Expansive question for sustaining conversation	*What would the policeman do then?*

Source: Drawn from K. Kaye and R. Charney, "Conversational Asymmetry Between Mothers and Children," *Journal of Child Language*, 1981, 8, 35–49.

The contingent query consists of four components: the original utterance, the query, the response, and the utterance for resumption of the speaker's turn (Gallagher, 1981). These four components are illustrated as follows:

Original utterance	*Child:*	We saw mahmees.
Query	*Adult:*	What did you see?
Response	*Child:*	Monkeys.
Resumption	*Adult:*	Oh, did they do funny things?

Children aged three to five-and-a-half are able to produce and respond effectively to contingent queries with their peers, although younger children are more effective in their use with adults.

The three-year-old is able to respond appropriately to neutral queries such as "What?" and "Huh?" The child's primary strategy is to repeat what was said previously. With a second query about the same utterance, the three-year-old gets frustrated. In contrast, the five-year-old responds to a second query but employs the same repetition strategy as the three-year-old (Brinton, Fujiki, Loeb, & Winkler, 1986).

With two- to three-year-olds, mothers employ yes/no questions in turnabouts most frequently (Gallagher, 1981). This form requires a confirmation and is easy for children as young as eighteen months to process. Recall that maternal yes/no questioning may be positively correlated with the child's increased language abilities. If a child does not respond appropriately, the conversational expectations of the mother are not fulfilled, and she will ask fewer contingent queries.

It is clear that the caregiver's conversational behaviors reflect the feedback she receives from the child.

IMPORTANCE OF PLAY

It is easy to forget that much of the child's language develops within the context of play with an adult or with other children. Play can be an ideal vehicle for language acquisition for a number of reasons (Sachs, 1984):

- Since play is not goal oriented, it removes pressure and frustration from the interactive process. It's fun.
- Attention and the semantic domain are shared by the interactive partners, so topics are shared.

TABLE 7.6   Cognition, Play, and Language

APPROX. AGE (MOS.)	COGNITIVE DEVELOPMENT	PLAY DEVELOPMENT	LANGUAGE DEVELOPMENT
Below 12	Association of events with habitual actions	Recognition of objects and functional use	Presymbolic communication
12–15	Global representation of events	Self-pretend: Meaningful actions used playfully	Single words for global referent
15–21	Analysis of represented objects or events	Differentiated pretend play with dolls and other activities. Decentered play with reference to others	Reference to a range of entities, parts, and states
21–24	Juxtaposition of symbolic elements	Pretend combinations	Simple language combinations
24–26	Complete event stored with organized component parts	Planning and storage of symbolic goal while trying to accomplish. Combinatorial play episodes with two themes.	Store message while parts organized

Source: Bretherton, 1984.

- Games have reciprocal role structure and variations in the order of elements, as do grammars.
- Games, like conversations, contain turn-taking.

In languages as different as English and Japanese, levels of play and language development appear to be similar (McCune-Nicolich, 1986; Ogura, 1991). While play and language are different, they develop interdependently and demonstrate underlying cognitive developments. This relationship is presented in Table 7.6.

Initially, both play and language are very concrete and depend on the here and now. As cognition develops, however, they both become less concrete (Bates, MacWhinney, Caselli, Devescove, Natale, & Vanza, 1984). At about the time that children begin to combine symbols, they begin to play symbolically. One play object, such as a shoe, is used for another, such as a telephone. In like fashion, symbols represent concepts.

Children often attempt to involve their parents in this pretend play. As playmates, parents can show by example how to play. Often, parents contribute running narratives of the play as it progresses and provide children with the basic problem–resolution narrative or story model. Even two-year-olds can learn the basic problem–resolution format, as in "The baby cried; the Mommy picked it up" (Sachs, 1972). In general, the number of sequences in children's play is correlated with syntactic development (Bates, Bretherton, & Snyder, 1988).

Thematic role playing and accompanying linguistic style changes begin at around age three. By this age, children possess generalized sequentially correct scriptlike representations of familiar situations (Nelson, 1986). At first, the child's role represents himself or herself. Later roles are projected on passive persons and dolls. Eventually, an object or active person may play a reciprocal role (Bretherton, 1984).

By age four the child is able to role-play a baby, using a higher pitch, phonetic substitutions, shorter and simpler utterances, and more references to self. At about this time, the child begins to role play "Mom and Dad" differently. In general, mothers are portrayed as more polite, using more indirect requests, with a higher pitch and longer utterances. Role-played fathers make more commands and give less explanation for their behavior. Prosodic and rhythmic devices are the first stylistic variations used by children, followed by appropriate content and then syntactic regularities.

Although the language used in solitary play is not typical of the child's performance, social play is quite different. In social play, language is used explicitly to convey meaning because of the different realistic and imaginary meanings of props ("This'll be a phone.") and roles ("You be the daddy.") Language is used to clarify ("You can't say that if you're the baby.") and negotiate ("Okay, you can say it if you want to."). Play themes consist of sequential episodes whose organization increases with the child's age (Galda, 1984; Pellegrini, 1985).

The language used in play is influenced by the participants and the play context. In general, preschoolers prefer same-gender pairs with no adult present (Hartup, 1983;

Pellegrini & Perlmutter, 1989). While children of both genders prefer replica play, such as dolls, a pretend store, or dress-up, boys also prefer play with blocks.

Initially, preschoolers prefer very functionally explicit props. As children mature and participate in more frequent imaginative play, they use more ambiguous props (Pellegrini & Perlmutter, 1989).

Although the preschool child is too young for team games and is not cognitively ready to follow game rules, he or she does enjoy group activities. Language learning is enhanced by the songs, rhymes, and finger plays common among preschoolers. Within play, the child and his communication partner can participate in a dialogue free of the pressures of "real" communication. In addition, the child is free to experiment with different communication styles and roles.

CULTURAL AND SOCIAL DIFFERENCES

Obviously, not all children receive the sort of "idealized" language input reported in this chapter. In non-Western cultures, mothers use techniques other than conversation to gain and hold children's attention.

Middle-class American mothers talk *with* their children, not *at* them. Many maternal utterances consist of comments on topics established by the child through word or action. This tendency to follow the child's conversational lead is evidenced in maternal expansion and extension of the child's utterances. While these semantically related maternal utterances can enhance language acquisition, it has not been proven that they are crucial to the process. For example, not all cultures value verbal precocity in children or demonstrate the adult modifications seen in motherese. Among the Kipsigis of Kenya and rural African Americans in Louisiana, comprehension is more important than verbal production in young children; many of the utterances directed to them consist of directives and explanations. Kaluli parents in New Guinea and Samoan parents rarely follow their children's conversational leads (Ochs & Schieffelin, 1984). Language acquisition does not seem to be slowed or delayed in any way.

These mothers use other strategies that seem equally effective. For example, Kaluli mothers in Papua, New Guinea, and some Mexican American mothers provide models of appropriate language for specific situations and direct their young children to imitate them (Briggs, 1984; Schieffelin & Eisenberg, 1984). In situations with other adults, children are directed by their mothers in the appropriate responses. This recycling of appropriate utterances for recurring situations is presumably a language-learning device. Like semantically related adult utterances found in middle-class American homes, these predictable situational responses may be highly comprehensible to the child without complete grammatical knowledge (Snow, 1986).

Among deaf parents of deaf children with whom American Sign Language is being used, motherese is conveyed by sign and facial expression. Use of sign can present a potential problem because facial expression marks both affect and grammatical structures, such as questions. With only limited use of paralinguistic cues, such as higher pitch and exaggerated intonation and stress, the mother's facial expression takes on added importance as a conveyer of her intentions and as a device to hold the child's interest. Prior to the child's second birthday mothers use facial expression primarily for affect. There is a shift to more grammatical uses after that point (Reilly & Bellugi, 1996).

In middle-class American English families, parental behaviors differ based on the number and gender of the children, perceived differences in the children's abilities, and in two- or single-parent households. For example, the conversations of mothers with their twins are five times longer and elicit more turns from all speakers than conversations between mothers and a single child (Barton & Strosberg, 1997). Similar findings are reported for conversations between a mother, her infant, and an older sibling.

Parent-initiated communication with young American girls and boys also differs in both play and nonplay situations. Adults tend to emphasize useful domestic activities with young girls, while they emphasize more free-ranging exploratory manipulation with young boys (Wells, 1986). It is unclear whether these preferences represent desires of the parent or the child.

Mothers of premature children may continue to use linguistic strategies more appropriate for younger children even when their children are age four (Donahue & Pearl, 1995). In contrast, mothers of late-talking toddlers seem to use the same conversational cues as mothers of toddlers developing typically, although both highly controlling mothers and their late-talking children appear to have less conversational synchrony as measured by semantic relatedness and amount of responding (Rescorla & Fechnay, 1996).

Across all socioeconomic levels, preschoolers from single-parent homes appear to have better receptive and expressive language and to have fewer communication problems, especially when compared to children from households with married, working parents (Haaf, 1996). This difference may reflect the more intensive, one-on-one communication between the single parent and the children in these homes. In the absence of another adult, the single parent may spend more time talking to the child.

Socioeconomic and cultural factors result in many different child–caregiver interactive patterns reflecting (1) the role of children, (2) the social organization of caregiving, and (3) folk beliefs about how children learn language (Schieffelin & Eisenberg, 1984). We must also be careful not to assume that the way middle-class mothers in the United States interact with their children is the only way or the most correct way. In general, interactive patterns between children and their caregivers have evolved to fulfill the special needs of the populations and cultures in which they occur.

In the middle-class American family, the child is held in relatively high regard. This is also true among the Kaluli people. In contrast, the relatively lower standing of children reported in western Samoa and among some African Americans in rural Louisiana results in an expectation that children are to speak only when invited to do so (Ochs, 1982). It is important to remember that low status does not mean a lack of affection for the child. Within these same rural southern African American communities, the child is not expected to initiate conversation but to respond to adult questions in the shortest possible form. The child is not expected to perform for adults, and most of the child's requests for information are ignored. What expansion exists is an expansion by adults of their own utterances, not those of the child. It is believed in this culture that children learn by observation, not interaction.

The expectation of a quiet child does not necessarily reflect children's low status. Among the Apache Indians, it is a societal norm to value silence from all people. In general,

Japanese parents also encourage less talking by their children, although children are held in very high regard. Nonverbal behavior is more important in Japan than in the United States, and Japanese parents anticipate the child's needs more often, so the child has fewer reasons to communicate.

The social organization of caregiving also varies widely and reflects economic organization and kinship groupings. In some cultures, such as that of western Samoa, older siblings are more responsible for caregiving than in middle-class American homes. This arrangement is also characteristic of many inner-city households in the United States. There is no evidence, however, that children raised by older siblings learn language more slowly than those raised by adults.

Finally, folk "wisdom" on language acquisition varies widely and affects language addressed to the child. The Kipsigis of Kenya believe that the child will learn by himself or herself. Thus, there is no baby talk or motherese. The child is encouraged to participate in conversation through imitation of the mother's model of adult speech. The Kaluli of New Guinea also require imitation from the child in certain social rituals, even though the child does not seem to understand what he or she is saying (Schieffelin, 1982).

It should be noted that children also learn language from speech that is not addressed to them (Oshima-Takane, 1988). This may be especially true of some pronouns, which may be best learned by observing their use in various contexts.

Japanese and American mothers exhibit several maternal differences. While American mothers talk more with their children and encourage them to respond, Japanese mothers engage in more rocking, carrying, and "lulling." In responding to their infants, American mothers use more facial and vocal behaviors, while Japanese mothers are more nonverbal, responding with touch (Fogel et al., 1988). With toddlers, Japanese mothers employ more vocalizations similar to the American English uh-huh, which is not surprising given the importance of omoiyari, maintenance of harmony in that culture (Maynard, 1986; White, 1989). The intentions of American mothers are providing information and directing. In contrast, the Japanese mother exhibits less of these behaviors, preferring to use nonsense words, sound play, and emphatic routines, such as discussing feelings (Morikawa et al., 1988). Her productions are usually very easy for her child to imitate.

In general, Japanese mothers are less likely to label and talk about objects; when they do, it is often without the use of an adult label. Although both American and Japanese mothers use questions frequently, American mothers use them more in the context of labeling. It is not surprising, therefore, that American toddlers have larger noun vocabularies while Japanese toddlers have more social expressions (Fernald & Morikawa, 1993; Hess, Kashiwagi, Azuma, Price, & Dickson, 1980).

Still, similarities exist across languages. Both American and Japanese mothers use linguistically simple forms when addressing young language-learning children, repeat frequently, and use intonation to engage the infant (Fernald & Morikawa, 1993). The common motivation for these changes seems to be an intuitive sense of the developmental level of the child.

Children are not limited to direct language input. They can also learn language by indirect means, such as conversational exchanges between other individuals. Television can also provide some input with systematic viewing (Lemish & Rice, 1986). Unlike conversations directed to the child, television does not require a response. In addition, the language provided by television is not related to the ongoing events within the child's interactive context. Children acquire language-based knowledge by drawing upon a range of experiences.

With all this variety, children from other cultures still learn their native languages at about the same rate as middle-class American children. In general, in the United States, most adults treat the child as a communication partner. The language-learning American child is raised primarily by his or her parent(s) or paid professionals or paraprofessionals who model and elicit language. Even within the United States, however, there is no definitive pattern.

Of most importance among children in the United States are maternal stimulation and the overall quality of the home. For example, among African American families, a strong correlation exists between maternal sensitivity, responsiveness, stimulation, and elaborativeness and a child's cognitive and communicative skills at age one (Wallace, Roberts, & Lodder, 1998). Although socioeconomic differences exist within the African American community, there is strong evidence of these maternal behaviors among all African American mothers.

CONCLUSION

Language learning is a complex process that involves linguistic processing and child and adult language-learning strategies. Different cultures exhibit different strategies.

Comprehension and imitation by the toddler seem to be particularly important. Both appear to be at the cutting edge of language development, although the exact relationship is unknown and seems to change with the child's functioning level.

We do not know the exact language-learning strategies used by young children. These strategies and their underlying cognitive abilities are inferred from the child's behaviors. Consistency in the child's language suggests the presence of underlying rule systems. At present, linguists are unsure of the process of rule construction. Undoubtedly, though, comprehension and production are interrelated. This dynamic relationship changes with the level of development and with the structure being learned. The order of acquisition of structures for expressing complex relationships reflects the child's cognitive growth. The child must understand the concept of the relationship and the linguistic forms used to express that relationship before he or she can use this relationship in his or her own language.

Environmental influences strongly affect language development. Adult modeling and consequating behaviors are very important with toddlers. Adult–child language provides a simplified model. Certain consequating behaviors also reinforce the child's communication attempts.

Although a direct conditioning explanation of language development is inadequate, there is a strong indication that modeling, imitation, and reinforcement are central to the learning process. Those elements of maternal speech that change to reflect the child's overall language level seem to be most significant for later language development. The process is much more subtle than that employed in direct language training.

Although diminished, the role of significant caregivers in language development is still critical with preschoolers. Caregivers continue to manipulate the conversational context to maximize language learning by the child. This context and play are important sources of language modeling and use for preschool children.

DISCUSSION

In this chapter, we've seen how children approach the learning of language, how they decide what a word is, how they try to decipher the sequential code by applying certain rules to breaking down language, and how they are helped by the environment. If you assume that you are in another culture in which English is never used, you begin to appreciate what the child and caregivers do in order to be understood and to help the child's learning. Look at the child learning strategies again. Wow, what a great way to try to understand this other language and to attempt to use it! Now look at the adult teaching strategies. We could only hope that those speakers of that other language would be so kind as to use some of these strategies with us until we understand their language.

It is important to recall that caregivers do not decide to teach language. The so-called teaching strategies mostly flow from a desire to be understood. Are they all applicable to intervention with the child with a language impairment? Each SLP and teacher must decide for himself or herself how to best use this developmental knowledge.

We must also remember that just as language is culturally based, so are the teaching strategies demonstrated by middle-class mothers in the United States. The French-speaking Haitian mother of a toddler or preschooler with a language impairment may interact very differently. Again the SLP must decide if the mother's interactions are appropriate given her culture and the severity of the child's impairment. The goal is not to create a carbon copy of the middle-class American mother. Remember, that even mothers who exhibit the best "motherese" can have children with language problems. All professional interactions must be mindful of and sensitive to cultural variability.

REFLECTIONS

1. Describe the complex relationship between comprehension and production as it relates to the young language-learning child.

2. After noting similarities in children's structures in several languages, Slobin proposed a set of universal principles of language learning. State the main principles and give an example of each.

3. Describe the role of imitation for toddlers and the development from repetitious utterances to semantically diverse ones.

4. Mothers and fathers talk very differently to their young child than they do to other adults. What are the characteristics of motherese or parentese?

5. List the various types of prompts parents use to encourage their children to speak.

6. Though parents may not directly reinforce their young language-learning children, they do expand, extend, and imitate. Describe the differences between these three behaviors and explain the effects of these behaviors on the child.

7. What is a turnabout and how is it used by caregivers?

8. Describe the importance of play for language development.

9. Children in the United States and in other cultures receive a variety of linguistic inputs and are expected to communicate in numerous ways. What are the factors that affect parent–child interaction? What effects do these factors have on language development?

8

A First Language

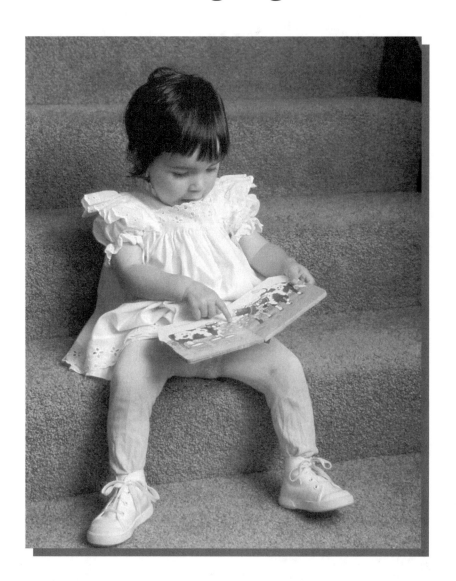

CHAPTER OBJECTIVES

Children's initial language consists of more than the mere accumulation of single words. As with all language, children's initial attempts reflect rule-governed patterns of production. When you have completed this chapter, you should understand

- the most frequent categories and syllable constructions in first words.
- the intentions of early vocalizations/verbalizations.
- the bases for early concept development.
- the bases for extensions and overextensions.
- the two-word semantic rules of toddlers.
- the common phonological rules of toddlers.
- the following terms:

action relational words	possession relational words
agent	presupposition
associative complex hypothesis	prototypic complex hypothesis
attribution relational words	reduplication
consonant/cluster reduction	reflexive relational words
diminutive	relational words
functional-core hypothesis	semantic-feature hypothesis
location relational words	semantic-syntactic rules
object	substantive words
open syllable	underextension
overextension	

This is it, the place where language is said to begin. But don't expect a change overnight. Words will appear gradually and may be mixed with jargon in long, incomprehensible strings. The child is still experimenting with sounds. Speech may be suddenly interrupted by shrieks or a series of babbles. As a result, a child may talk a great deal without seeming to say much. (In that way, children resemble some adults I know.) One sound pattern may represent several concepts, or inconsistent production may result in several sound patterns for one word. Words may be changed by deletion of syllables or modification of stress patterns. Whole phrases may be used as single words. If it sounds confusing, it is; but what a wonderful time for the excited family.

The point at which language is said to begin is arbitrary and depends on your definition of *language*. For our purposes, we shall assume that language begins at around the first birthday with the appearance of the first word. To be considered a true word, the child's utterance must have a phonetic relationship to some adult word. In addition, the child must use the word consistently. Consistent use in the presence of a referent implies an underlying concept or meaning. Therefore, a babbled "dada" would not qualify because there is no referent. Likewise, phonetically consistent forms do not approximate recognizable adult words. (See Chapter 3 for a description of PCFs.)

The emergence of first words or verbalizations does not signal the end of vocalizations, such as babbling, jargon, and PCFs. All three continue to be produced by the child throughout the second year of life (Robb, Bauer, & Tyler, 1994). Individual children exhibit very different patterns of vocalization-verbalization use. A sample of the speech and language of a 12-month-old child is presented on track five of the CD that accompanies this text. Words emerge slowly and often are accompanied by gestures. Note that babbling and jargon also continue to occur.

Before you begin this chapter, take a few minutes to think about the twelve- to eighteen-month-old child and what he or she knows. Soon the child will begin talking about the world. Jot down a short list of words that he or she might say. Try it; you'll be surprised how much you already know. Much of the child's pronunciation will not mirror adult language. For that reason, you might write possible child pronunciations after applicable words. For example, *water* will probably be spoken as "wawa."

Once you have completed your list, imagine how these words might be used in conversation. Examine your list for patterns. You probably know more about language development than you realize. What types of words—nouns, verbs, and so on—predominate? What speech sounds are used most frequently? What syllabic constructions—CV, VC, CVCV-reduplicated, CVCV, CVC, and so on—are most frequent? It is also important to consider the contexts in which first words occur. The child's primary communication partner, mother, sibling, or other caregiver, engages the child in *protoconversations* within familiar activities and routines. These events form the backdrop for communication and provide a script for what is said. The child's first words occur as requests for information, or for objects or aid, or as comments. The child's intentions, previously expressed through gestures and vocalizations, are now expressed through words. There is carryover of pragmatic functions from presymbolic to symbolic communication. As we progress through this chapter, you may be surprised by the accuracy of your responses.

SINGLE-WORD UTTERANCES

The toddler's first meaningful speech consists of single-word utterances, such as "doggie," or single-word approximations of frequently used adult phrases, such as "thank you" ("anku") or "what's that?" ("wasat?"). At this point, "words" are phonetic approximations of adult words that the child consistently uses to refer to a particular situation or object. The meaning of the word may be very restricted at first and may apply to only one particular referent. For example, "doggie" (usually "goggie" or "doddie") may refer only to the family's pet but not to other dogs. Early meanings may have very little in common with those generally used by mature speakers. As a result of linguistic and nonlinguistic, or sensory, experience, the child will gradually modify the definition. At some point, the child's definition will approximate the generally shared notion of the word's meaning. Remember that a word signifies a referent but that the referent is not the meaning of the word. Meaning is found in language users' concepts or mental images, not in objects.

In general, the toddler talks about the world he or she knows and will not comment on inflation, unemployment, politics, or nuclear holocaust. Instead, the toddler may request toys, call people, name pets, reject food, ask for help with clothing, and discuss familiar actions or routines.

Pragmatic Aspects of a First Language

In order to explain early child language fully, we must consider the uses to which these utterances are put. As we noted in Chapter 6, communication is well established before the first word appears. The child develops the ability to communicate meanings before acquiring any language. Language "maps" or processes these early meanings within the established communication system of the child and caregiver. In many ways, the transition from presymbolism to symbolism can be best understood by considering this communication context.

Both the repetitiveness of certain daily verbal and nonverbal routines and the mother's willingness to assign meaningful intent to the child's speech aid language development. Parent responses also foster word–meaning associations by providing feedback to the child that the intended meaning was or was not comprehended.

In addition, the social functions of the child's early utterances are important in the actual words the child will select for his or her lexicon or personal dictionary. Early words develop to fulfill the social functions originally conveyed by gestures. Novel words may be learned through actual use (Nelson, 1991; Nelson, Hampson, & Shaw, 1993). The child may use a word in a context where it "sounds right." The responses of others confirm or deny the particular usage.

There is a strong relationship between first words and the frequency of maternal input of these words (Harris, Barrett, Jones, & Brooks, 1988). Many of the words are used in the same context in which the mother used them previously, such as "bye-bye" while waving and "choo-choo" while playing with a toy train. Not all words are used this way, however, and a significant number are also used to name or label entities.

Before we continue, return to the fictitious list of first words you generated at the beginning of this chapter. Pause for a moment and consider how these words might be used socially, that is, to attain information, fulfill needs, provide information, and so on.

Development

In Chapter 6 we examined the illocutionary functions or intentions of early gestures. Initially, intentions are signaled by gestures only. To these the child adds vocalizations and then words. Many early words, however, can be interpreted only with consideration of the accompanying gesture. Gradually, the child learns to express intentions in more grammatically correct ways.

Gestures. Gestural development continues along with verbal growth. Not all gestures are of equal developmental importance. Pointing, for example, accompanies many early utterances with a variety of meanings. Young children's early use of pointing is a good predictor of early language performance.

During the second year, gestures and verbalizations become more coordinated for specific intentions. Reaching increasingly signals a request or demand, while pointing

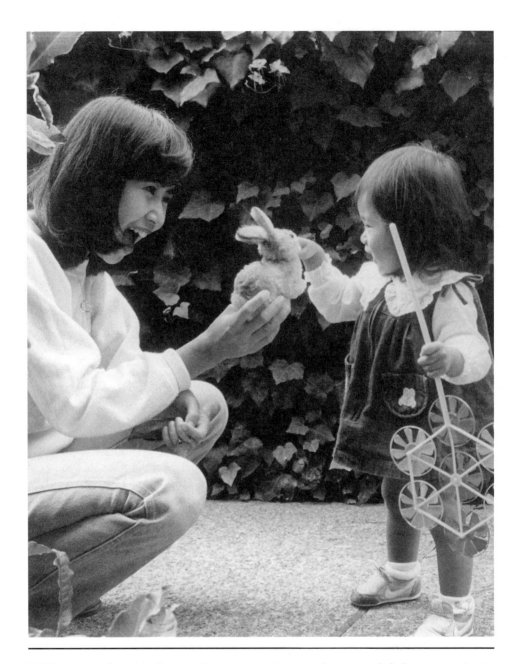

Toddlers use words to describe, to ask, to request, to name, and to accomplish their communicative goals.

signals a declaration or a reference to something in the environment (Franco & Butterworth, 1996). Between one year and eighteen months, a subtle shift in looking at the partner occurs with pointing. Initially, the child looks after the gesture for both pointing and reaching. Gradually, the child changes so that the look occurs before the pointing gesture only, indicating knowledge on the child's part that a speaker must have the listener's attention before referring to something.

Symbolic gestures, such as panting like a dog, appear at about the same time as first words and development is parallel for several months (Acredolo & Goodwyn, 1988, 1990; Bates et al., 1988). Children will use symbolic gestures along with presymbolic gestures (pointing, showing, etc.) for communication purposes (Caselli, 1990). Some children rely more on gestures, while others prefer speech. Gestures can be used as a backup for speech or as an assist for words that are lacking. Almost all toddlers use gestures spontaneously with speech (Morford & Goldin-Meadow, 1992). In addition, young toddlers may rely on caregiver gestures for comprehension (Boswell, 1988; Goldin-Meadow & Morford, 1985; Zinober & Martlew, 1985).

Vocabulary production in eighteen- to twenty-eight-month-olds appears to be correlated with production of functional gestures (Thal & Bates, 1988; Thal, Tobias, & Morrison, 1991). Functional gestures depict objects through actions demonstrating the object's function, such as pretending to eat from an empty spoon.

The development of multiword utterances seems to be correlated with the production of gestural combinations (Brownell, 1988; McCune-Nicolich, 1981; McCune-Nicolich & Bruskin, 1982; Shore, 1986). The lengths of sequences in the two are similar (Shore, O'Connell, & Bates, 1984).

From age twelve to eighteen months, a progression toward production of coordinated, dual-directional signals in which the child gestures and verbalizes while looking at her communication partner exists. Initially, the child merely gestures but may not look at her partner. The child then progresses to a gesture and verbalization plus a gaze toward the communication partner rather than toward the object of the gesture. This dual directionality may be an important transition to the ability to consider two communication aspects— the topic and the listener—simultaneously (Masur, 1983). Finally, the child is able to look at the partner while performing two coordinated gestures in sequence or a gesture plus a conventional verbalization or word.

Primitive Speech Acts. There appear to be patterns in young children's vocalizations and gestures used to express intentions. Since these behaviors frequently lack words or depend on gestures to convey intent, we consider these patterns to be precursors to adultlike speech acts and label them *primitive speech acts* (PSAs) (Dore, 1974). A PSA is a single gesture or single vocal/verbal pattern that conveys intention. For example, when requesting an action, a child may use a sound and gesture while attending to the object followed by attending to the adult. The most common PSAs are presented in Table 8.1. At this age, the child's utterances are unifunctional. Each carries only one social function. PSAs are similar to the intentions expressed in children's speech in the second year of life (Owens, 1978; Wells, 1985). This continuity suggests differentiation with maturity. Not surprisingly, the range of early intentions seems to be universal (Roth & Davidge, 1985).

TABLE 8.1   Primitive Speech Acts

PRIMITIVE SPEECH ACT	CHILD'S UTTERANCE	CHILD'S NONLINGUISTIC BEHAVIOR
Requesting action	Word or marked prosodic pattern	Attends to object or event; addresses adult; awaits response; most often performs gesture
Protesting	Word or marked prosodic pattern	Attends to adult; addresses adult; resists or denies adult's action
Requesting answer	Word	Addresses adult; awaits response; may make gesture
Labeling	Word	Attends to object or event; does not address adult; does not await response
Answering	Word	Attends to preceding adult utterance; addresses adult
Greeting	Word	Attends to adult or object
Repeating	Word or prosodic pattern	Attends to preceding adult utterance may not address adult; does not await response
Practicing	Word or prosodic pattern	Attends to no specific object or event; does not address adult; does not await response
Calling	Word (with marked prosodic contour)	Addresses adult by uttering adult's name loudly; awaits response

Source: Adapted from J. Dore, "Holophrases, Speech Acts and Language Universals," *Journal of Child Language,* April 1975, 2(1), p. 33.

Intentions in Words. First words fulfill the intentions previously expressed through gestures and vocalizations. Initially, different, often very diverse verbal forms may develop to express different functions. This phase may last until about sixteen months of age. At first, specific words or PCFs are used with each function. Gradually, functions fulfilled by words emerge. As words and functions increase, words and utterances become more flexible and multifunctional. The disappearance of specific symbol–function relationships usually occurs from sixteen to twenty-four months, corresponding to the beginning of multiword combinations.

Six pragmatic categories describe the general purposes of language: control, representational, expressive, social, tutorial, and procedural (Wells, 1985). Speakers use the control function to make demands and requests, to protest, and to direct others. The representational function is used to discuss entities and events and to ask for information. In contrast, the expressive function is not necessarily for an audience. The child may use language to accompany play, to exclaim or to express feelings and attitudes. The social function includes greetings, farewells, and talk routines. For young children, the tutorial function

TABLE 8.2   Early Illocutionary Functions

BROAD PRAGMATIC CATEGORIES (Wells, 1985)	PRIMITIVE SPEECH ACTS (PSAS) (Dore, 1974)	EARLY VERBAL INTENTIONS (Owens, 1978; Wells, 1985)	EXAMPLES
Control	Requesting action	Wanting demands	*Cookie* (Reach)
		Direct request/commanding	*Help* (Hand object to or struggle)
	Protesting	Protesting	*No* (Push away or uncooperative)
Representational	Requesting answer	Content questioning	*Wassat?* (Point)
	Labeling	Naming/labeling	*Doggie* (Point)
		Statement/declaring	*Eat* (Commenting on dog barking)
	Answering	Answering	*Horsie* (in response to question)
		Reply	*Eat* (in response to "The doggie's hungry."
Expressive		Exclaiming	Squeal when picked up
		Verbal accompaniment to action	*Uh-oh* (With spill)
		Expressing state or attitude	*Tired*
Social	Greetings	Greeting/farewell	*Hi* / *Bye-bye*
Tutorial	Repeating/practicing	Repeating/practicing	*Cookie, cookie, cookie*
Procedural	Calling	Calling	*Mommy*

*This table represents a combination of the work of several researchers and an attempt to remain true to the intended purposes of child speech.

consists mostly of practice with language forms. Finally, the procedural function is used to maintain communication by directing attention or by requesting additional or misinterpreted information.

Early toddler utterances fulfill aspects of all functions. There is a continuity from PSAs to early verbal intentions. Table 8.2 illustrates the relationship of PSAs to later pragmatic categories and offers examples of early verbal illocutionary functions or intentions.

Along with the development of single words and word combinations, the child develops sound patterns for specific intentions. (Galligan, 1987) These pattern-intention relationships appear to be true for both relatively nontonal languages, such as English, and tonal languages, such as Latvian, Thai, and Lao that have varied intonational patterns (Ruke-Dravina, 1981). These patterns are used most often by two-year-olds when talking to a conversational partner rather than in monologs, although these pitch patterns are not the same as those found in adult speech (Furrow, 1984).

Beginning with a falling contour only—similar to that used by adults for statements—children first develop a flat or level contour for naming or labeling, usually accompanied by variations, such as use of falsetto or variations in length or loudness. Between thirteen and fifteen months, children develop a rising contour to express requesting, attention getting, and curiosity and a high falling contour, which begins with a high pitch that drops to a lower one, to signal surprise, recognition, insistence, or greeting (Marcos, 1987). Next, children use a high rising and a high rising-falling contour to signal playful anticipation and emphatic stress, respectively. Finally, at around eighteen months, children use a falling-rising and a rising-falling contour for warnings and playfulness, respectively.

By fifteen months, most children are naming or labeling favorite toys and foods and household pets, exclaiming, and calling to attract attention (Wells, 1985). Within another three months, the average child adds wanting demands (*I want. . . .*). By two years of age, 50 percent or more of all children have added verbal requesting or commanding, content questioning, unsolicited statements or declarations, verbal accompaniments to play (*Whee!*), and expressions of states and attitudes, most frequently, "I tired" (Wells, 1985). Other early illocutionary functions include protesting (*no*), answering, greeting, and practice or repeating.

As children mature, the frequency of pragmatic functions changes (Wells, 1985). At fifteen months, over 75 percent of all utterances are representational, expressive, and procedural, with the illocutionary functions of naming/labeling and calling predominating. By twenty-one months, control functions increase markedly, while expressive functions are reduced by nearly half. Throughout this period, social and tutorial functions occur infrequently. Some early illocutionary functions, such as wanting demands, naming/labeling, calling, and practice, decrease rapidly as a percentage of overall intentions from twenty-four to thirty-six months. Other relatively later-developing functions, such as direct requesting/commanding and statement/declaration, gradually increase.

During the one-word stage, my own sons gave a striking exhibition of requesting/commanding. Both boys had stayed with their grandmother during their mother's hospitalization for their sister's birth. While visiting with "Gran'ma," they learned to chase two particularly pesky stray tomcats with "Skat!" Later, when in a room alone with their newly arrived, sleeping sister, the two boys looked through the bars of her crib and ordered "Skat! Skat!" Fortunately, she didn't follow orders well even then.

Initially, speech emerges to accompany action, such as requests to perform some "ritual" possibly as simple as *notice me*. The child's first words may accompany pointing and be used to display a wish or to express displeasure. The child may draw attention first (*Mommy*), then make a request (*up*). The child may use *look* for control or *there* to complete a task. As he or she matures, the child may attend to an object and the action associated with it. Thus, the child may use *eat* when referring to a cookie being eaten. Later, he or she notes object relations or comments on the event, such as asking for a repetition with *again* and *more*. Thus, the child is not just acquiring a stack of meanings. Rather, the child is making meanings known to a conversational partner by using them to build a communication system with that partner.

Two-word speech represents more complete speech acts because the content can be communicated completely without dependence on nonlinguistic channels (Chalkley, 1982). It is important to remember, however, that grammatical form is not the determiner of communication function. A single illocutionary function can be realized in a variety of grammatical forms. A child can express a request with "Gimme cookie," "Cookie me," or "Cookie please." Conversely, one form can serve a variety of functions. For example, an utterance such as "Daddy throw" can serve as a descriptor of an event, a request for action, or even a request for information (question).

At around age two, the child begins to combine language functions within a single utterance. For example, on spying some fresh-baked cookies, the child might say, "Mommy, cookies hot?" Even though she is attempting to attain information, she also hopes to attain a cookie. Thus, we have a request for information and a request for an entity within the same utterance.

Conversational Abilities

Even at the single-word stage, the child has some knowledge of the information to be included in a conversation. For example, the child gives evidence of using **presupposition**, that is, the assumption that the listener knows or does not know certain information that the child must include or delete from the conversation. For example, as an adult, when you are asked, "How do you want your steak?" you might reply, "Medium rare." There is no need to repeat the redundant information, "I would like my steak. . . ." You omit the redundant information because you presuppose that your listener shares this information with you already. In contrast, you would call your listener's attention to new, different, or changing circumstances that may be unknown to the listener ("Did you know that . . . ?" "Well, let me tell you about . . .").

Toddlers seem to follow certain rules for presupposition (Greenfield, 1978):

1. An object not in the child's possession is uncertain. The child's first utterance will label the object.
2. An object in the child's possession, while undergoing change, is relatively certain. The child's utterance will encode the action or change.
3. Once encoded, an object or action/state change becomes more certain and less informative. If the child continues, she will encode the other aspect that has not been stated.

The order of successive single-word utterances reflects the interplay of these rules. Therefore, the presuppositional rules may, in part, explain the variable order of successive single-word and early two-word utterances. With the onset of two-word utterances, the child learns that a word-order rule overrides informational structure as a determinant of word order.

Since children often encode the here and now, it is relatively easy for adults to interpret an utterance in a manner similar to that of the child. This does not imply, however, that

TABLE 8.3   Representative List of Early Words

juice (/dus/)	mama	all gone (/ɔdɔn/)
cookie (/tʊti/)	dada	more (/mɔ/)
baby (/bibi/)	doggie (/dɔdi/)	no
bye-bye	kitty (/tldi/)	up
ball (/bɔ/)	that (/da/)	eat
hi	dirty (/dɔti/)	go (/d oʊ/)
car (/tɔ/)	hot	do
water (/wʌwʌ/)	shoe (/su/)	milk (/mʌk/)
eye	hat	
nose (/n oʊ/)		

the child is able to adopt the listener's perspective. Luckily, the ability to establish joint reference develops prior to the appearance of first words as noted in Chapter 6.

Initial Lexicons

Initial individual vocabularies or *lexicons* may contain some of the words listed in Table 8.3. Although there are many variations in pronunciation, some of the common forms are included in parentheses. (See the appendix for an explanation of the International Phonetic Alphabet.) How does this sample compare with the one you devised? As we note other patterns, check them against your list.

Most first words contain one or two syllables. Syllabic construction is usually VC (vowel-consonant), CV, CVCV-reduplicated, or CVCV. For example, in our list in Table 8.3 we find VC words, such as *eat* and *up*; CV words, such as *no* and *car* (/tɔ/); CVCV-reduplicated words, such as *mama*, *dada*, and *water* (/wʌwʌ/), and CVCV words, such as *doggie* (/dɔdi/). How does your list compare? There are very few CVC words, and many of these are modified in production. The final consonant may be omitted or followed by a vowel-like sound approximating a CVCV construction. For example, a word such as *hat* might be produced as *hat-a* (/hatʌ/) approximating a CVCV construction. Front consonants, such as /p, b, d, t, m/, and /n/, and back consonants, such as /g, k/ and /h/, predominate. No consonant clusters, such as /tr/, /sl/, or /str/, appear.

The first words of Spanish-speaking children demonstrate some of the same characteristics. CV, VC, and CVCV syllable structures predominate (Jackson-Maldonado, Thal, Marchman, Bates, & Gutierrez-Clellen, 1993). The phonemes /p, b, m/, and /n/ are also used frequently, plus /g/ and /k/. As a group, these sounds can be found in 70 percent of the most frequent words of Spanish-speaking children.

The child's first lexicon includes several categories of words. The most frequent words among the child's first ten words generally name animals, foods, and toys. First words usually apply to a midlevel of generality (dog) and only much later to specific types (spaniel, boxer) and larger categories (animal). Even at this midlevel, however, the child often uses the word at first to mark a specific object or event. The list in Table 8.3 contains animals (*doggie* and *kitty*), foods (*juice* and *cookie*), and toys (*ball*). How about your own list?

Initial lexical growth is slow, and the child may appear to plateau for short periods. Some words are lost as the child's interests change and production abilities improve (McLaughlin, 1978). In addition, the child continues to use a large number of vocalizations that are consistent but fail to meet the "word" criterion. At the center of the child's lexicon is a small core of high-usage words. The lexical growth rate continues to accelerate as the child nears the fifty-word mark. The second half of the second year is one of tremendous vocabulary expansion, although there is much individual variation.

By eighteen months of age, the toddler will have a lexicon of approximately fifty words. The most frequently produced categories of words and examples of each are listed in Table 8.4. Noun words predominate. Most entries are persons and animals within the environment or objects the child can manipulate. Not all noun types are represented; individual objects and beings are most frequent. There are no collections, such as *forest*, or abstractions, such as *joy* (Gentner, 1982).

Again, many of these characteristics are also found in the first words of Spanish-speaking toddlers. *Mama* and *papa* are popular, along with labels for toys, body parts, foods, the names of people, *more* (*mas*), and *yes/no* (*si/no*) (Jackson-Maldonado et al., 1993).

Between eighteen and twenty-four months, most children experience a "vocabulary spurt," especially in receptive vocabulary (Harris, Yeeles, Chasin, & Oakley, 1995; Mervis & Bertrand, 1995). Words that are learned only in specific contexts and those that are relatively context-free tend to retain these characteristics. Specific words learned are determined by a combination of factors, including their relevance for the child and the cultural significance of the referent (Anglin, 1995a).

When the first fifty words are classified according to grammatical category and as a percentage of the child's vocabulary, the prominence of nouns is apparent (Table 8.4). Nouns account for 60 to 65 percent of the words that the child produces. In contrast, action words account for less than 20 percent of the total. In the list in Table 8.3, nouns account for approximately 60 percent of the total.

TABLE 8.4 Grammatical Classification of First 50 Words Produced

GRAMMATICAL FUNCTION	PERCENTAGE OF VOCABULARY		EXAMPLES
	BENEDICT (1979)	NELSON (1973)	
Nominals			
General	50	51	milk, dog, car
Specific	11	14	mama, dada, pet names
Action words	19	14	give, do, bye-bye, up
Modifiers	10	9	mine, no, dirty
Personal-social	10	9	no, please
Functional	—	4	this, for

These percentages change with development (Bates, Marchman, Thal, Fenson, Dale, Reznick, Reilly, & Hartung, 1994; Marchman & Bates, 1991). There is an initial increase in nouns until the child has acquired approximately 100 words. At this point, verbs begin a slow proportional rise with a proportional decrease in nouns. Other word classes, such as prepositions, do not increase proportionally until after acquisition of approximately 400 words. The proportional increase, then decrease, in nouns is also found in the lexicons of Spanish-speaking toddlers, but it is not universal (Heath, 1983; Jackson-Maldonado et al., 1993; Ochs & Schiefflin, 1984). For example, Korean children's earlier and proportionally higher use of verbs may reflect the maternal tendency to use single-word verbs and the SOV organization of the Korean language which places verbs in a prominent position at the end of the sentence (Gopnik & Choi, 1990). In fact, Korean children exhibit a "verb spurt" in their vocabulary that is not seen in English (Choi & Gopnik, 1995).

Children initially produce referential nouns (R. Schwartz & Leonard, 1984). This finding seems to be universal (Gentner, 1982), although there may be some minor differences across languages. Individual children exist along a continuum from a referential style in which they use many nouns ("noun lovers") to an expressive style in which they use few ("noun leavers"), preferring interactional and functional words, such as *hi*, *bye-bye*, and *no*, and unanalyzed wholes or formulas. Children with a referential learning style tend to elaborate the noun portion or noun phrase of their sentences, whereas those with an expressive style prefer to elaborate the verb phrase.

Children with a high proportion of nouns—70 percent or more—exhibit a rapid increase in the number of words in their lexicons between fourteen and eighteen months of age. In contrast, children whose lexicons have more balance between nouns and other word types tend to have a more gradual increase in word acquisition. These differences may indicate two acquisition strategies: (1) naming "things" and (2) encoding a broad range of experiences (Goldfield & Reznick, 1990).

More than just a high or low proportion of nouns, the referential-expressive continuum represents a difference in learning style that affects language development. Children with a referential style seem to have more adult contacts, use more single words, and employ an analytic, or bottom-up, strategy in which they gradually build longer utterances from individual words (Hampson, 1989; Nelson, 1981a). In contrast, children with an expressive style have more peer contacts, attempt to produce longer units, and employ a holistic, or top-down, strategy in which longer utterances are broken into their parts. Although the referential style is usually associated with a faster rate of development, other factors, such as gender, birth order, and social class, seem to be more important (Bates et al., 1994; Lieven & Pine, 1990).

The effects of maternal speech may also vary with the child's learning style. In general, referential children benefit from maternal labeling, imitating the child's speech, and describing the environment, while expressive children benefit from appropriate utterance use in context and from paralinguistic modifications (Hampson & Nelson, 1993).

There are several possible explanations for the early predominance of nouns in the speech of toddlers learning American English. First, the child may already have a concept of objects within his or her world knowledge (Dromi, 1987). Much of the child's first year was spent in social interaction around objects and in object exploration.

Second, nouns may predominate because they are *conceptually simpler* and *perceptually/conceptually distinct*. The "things" that nouns represent are more perceptually cohesive than events or actions, in which perceptual elements are scattered. Therefore, the child can determine the referent more easily. It is easier for the child to learn a new label that refers to a referent that is perceptually dissimilar from a label already in the child's vocabulary (Diesendruck & Shatz, 1997). The names for things are provided by the adult language that surrounds the child. Prelinguistic infants perceive objects as coherent and stable.

Third, it is also possible that the *linguistic predictability* of nouns makes them easier to use and accounts for their early predominance. Nouns represent specific items and events and thus relate to each other and to other words in specific, predictable ways.

Fourth, the frequency of adult use, adult word order, the limited morphological adaptations of nouns, and adult teaching patterns seem to affect children's production. Learning may be made easier by clear parental referencing within context. Maternal naming of objects accompanied by gesturing is most frequent about the time that the first word appears. After that time there is a subtle shift to more action words and gestures referring to those actions (Schmidt, 1996). Although the frequency of noun appearance in adult-to-adult speech is low, nouns occur more frequently in adult-to-child speech, receive more stress than other words, are often in the final position in utterances, and have few morphological markers (Goldfield, 1993; Nelson et al., 1993). The proportion of nouns in adult-to-child speech varies with the context and the child's developmental level (Barrett, Harris, & Chasin, 1991; Goldfield, 1993). Nouns are more frequent in toy play and in short maternal utterances. Verbs are more frequent in nontoy or social play and in conversations. It is important to note that object-naming games are culture-based and not found in all cultures (Tomasello & Cale Kruger, 1992). Mothers also prompt their children to produce nouns often. Although a strong correlation exists between the frequency of use in maternal speech and the child's initial lexicon, this relationship is very weak by the time the child has acquired approximately forty words (Harris et al., 1988).

Although word order varies across languages, nouns form a substantial, although not predominant, part of most initial lexicons. Mothers may violate word order to place nouns in more prominent positions. In Turkish, mothers may violate the SOV order to place nouns last (Aslin, 1992). In Mandarin, caregivers tend to emphasize verbs over nouns, consistent with the higher proportion of verbs in the initial lexicon of Mandarin-speaking toddlers (Tardif et al., 1997).

In English, nouns have few morphological adaptations, only the addition of the plural -*s* (Goldfield, 1993). Hence, the child hears the root word more often than with verbs, which are highly inflected. However, this distinction is not true for other languages, and still, initial lexicons tend to be dominated by nouns in most languages.

Noun teaching is also nonuniversal. In some cultures, there is very little direct language teaching of any sort. In most cultures, children learn words within natural social interactions. Nouns still persist, although the proportion may be lower than in the first lexicons of American English-speaking toddlers..

Modifiers and verblike words, such as *down*, appear soon after the first word. True verbs, such as *eat* and *play*, occur even later (Gentner, 1982). Verbs and other words serve a relational function; they bring together items or events. In addition, unlike objects, actions are not permanent; so verbs may not be accompanied by any consistent maternal gesturing (Schnur & Shatz, 1984). Thus, a child learning language is less able to guess their meanings after only a brief opportunity to make the symbol–referent connection.

Verb learning presents a different situation than noun learning. As many as 60 percent of the verbs in maternal speech refer to impending or future action. This presentation of verb followed by action seems to facilitate comprehension and production for fifteen- to twenty-one-month-olds (Tomasello & Cale Kruger, 1992). The reverse process, action followed by the verb, also facilitates production. In contrast, noun learning is best in an ongoing condition, when the child can focus on the adult and still maintain the object within the visual field. Given the transient nature of actions, simultaneous gazing at the event and the adult may not be possible.

Although parents engage in very little direct language training, as noted in Chapter 7, they do modify their speech with young children to emphasize content words such as nouns. It is possible, therefore, that nouns are learned before other categories of words because of perceptual salience, frequency of appearance in adult speech to toddlers, and patterns of production.

Meaning of Single-Word Utterances

The toddler initially uses language to discuss objects, events, and relations that are present. She or he has spent a year or more organizing the world, making sense of, or giving meaning to, experiences. A word refers to a stored concept rather than to an actual entity. The child's exact word meaning—what is mapped on the word—is unknown. The child's early lexicon until about eighteen months of age seems to follow a rule of mutual exclusivity mentioned in Chapter 7. Stated simply, *if the word means X, it can't mean Y or Z.*

The child may use two different processes to form internal representations (Barrett, 1986). Some symbols may be context-bound, or attached to a certain event, and, thus, only used in that context. Many of these word definitions will modify and become decontextualized. Other words may be used to designate entities, actions, and relationships in several contexts. The definitions may broaden with maturity. In general, context-bound words are less likely to appear as the child approaches age two (Barrett et al., 1991; Dromi, 1987).

The child's communication partner generally interprets the child's utterance with reference to the ongoing activity and to the child's nonlinguistic behavior. Adults often paraphrase the child's utterance as a full sentence, thereby implying that the child encoded the full thought. This assumption is probably erroneous. The child is operating with several constraints of attention, memory, and knowledge. In particular, the child has some difficulty with the organization of information for storage and retrieval.

The child's comprehension or receptive vocabulary precedes her production or expressive vocabulary. Although there is wide individual variation, the receptive vocabulary may be four times the size of the expressive vocabulary between ages twelve to eighteen months (Griffiths, 1986). Some meanings will be shared with adults, while others will be private or idiosyncratic. Private meanings have little effect on communication because no one understands them except the child.

More frequently, the child's meaning encompasses a small portion of the fuller adult definition. For example, the child might hear a mature speaker say "No touch—hot!" as the child approaches the stove. Subsequently, the child may use the phrase as a general prohibition.

Concept Formation

When a toddler uses the word *dog* for a horse but not for a poodle, it is difficult to determine the concept of *dog* that underlies the child's word. Naturally, adults might conclude that the child is using perceptual characteristics. This explanation is insufficient, however, for the meaning of nonnoun words, such as *more* and *here*.

Several hypotheses have been proposed to explain concept formation and word learning. These include the semantic-feature hypothesis (E. Clark, 1973a, 1973b, 1975), the functional-core hypothesis (Nelson, 1974, 1977), and the associative (Vygotsky, 1962) and prototypic complex hypotheses (Bowerman, 1978). Each theoretical position assumes that the child organizes word concepts in a certain manner based on recognition of certain aspects of the referent.

Before we examine the concepts that underlie early words, we must state some seemingly obvious, but easily forgotten, points. As adults, we do not really know what a given word or statement means to a child. We can only infer the child's meaning from the linguistic and nonlinguistic contexts. When linguists perform this type of contextual analysis, it is called a *rich interpretation*. For example, a child might say "Open." Noting that she is struggling to get her shoe on and that she has responded to your query, "What's the problem?", an adult concludes that the child wants help. The linguist interprets "Open" as a general request for aid.

Semantic-Feature Hypothesis. The **semantic-feature hypothesis** proposes that all referents can be defined by a universal set of semantic features, such as animate/inanimate or human/nonhuman. The child establishes meaning by combining features that are present and perceivable in the environment. These perceptual features are the attributes of the referent, such as shape, size, and movement. Shape may be the most salient of the perceptual features. Color does not appear to be particularly important to young children. Not all perceptual features are visible; children can also recognize entities by taste, smell, and hearing. For example, the child might shout "doggie" when she hears a dog bark.

The child's definition of *doggie*, therefore, may include features such as four legs, fur, barking, and tail. When she encounters a new example of the concept *doggie*, or one that is close, such as a bear, the child must apply the perceptual attribute criteria to determine the name of this new being. Since we occasionally encounter three-legged, hairless, nonbarking, or tailless dogs, the child may use a subset of the criteria, such as three out of four characteristics. As the child matures, it adds or deletes features, and the concept becomes more specific, thus more closely resembling the generally accepted meaning. Initially, the child may actually think that the label for the referent is a characteristic of that referent. In my own family, my children had always known me with a beard and called me "daddybob." When I shaved off the beard, my daughter began to call me "Bob." As one of her toddler brothers explained, "You not daddy; now you bes Bob."

The major disadvantage of the feature approach is that it fails to explain the holistic nature of meaning or to discriminate between features to determine the most relevant ones (Palermo, 1982). In short, even a three-legged, hairless, nonbarking, tailless dog is a dog, if a somewhat shopworn one. There is a totality to any definition that transcends the individual features of an object. The perception of the features alone is not the same as the concept.

The feature hypothesis is also inadequate as an explanation of nonobject concepts, such as *more*, *all gone*, and *up* that apply across many situations and involve a relationship between objects or events or between object or event states. Frequently, the objects involved have very few, if any, similar features.

Functional-Core Hypothesis. In the functional-core hypothesis, it is the motion features, rather than the static perceptual features, that are salient and from which the child derives meaning. Concept formation begins with the formation of a functional-core or object-use meaning to which perceptual features may be added.

The child begins meaningful speech by naming objects that embody a high degree of movement or that she can manipulate. These are the entities to which young children attend. The functional-core hypothesis is appealing because it relates to just such aspects of early child development. For example, Piaget observed that infants investigate object functions through manipulation and demonstrate early object knowledge by using an object for its intended purpose. A brush used in a certain accepted manner indicates that the infant has a notion or concept of "brushness." Thus, early experience provides the basis for concept learning. In addition, functional concepts are relational in that they describe an entity's use in relation to other entities, such as the relationship of brush to hair. These relationships could explain the concepts underlying many early two-word utterances.

To some extent, children's early spoken definitions lend support to an underlying functional concept. Stop for a moment and compose your own definition of *apple*. You would probably say that it is "a red, round fruit grown on trees in moderate climates" or something similar. In contrast, a child's definition might be "something you eat." A *dog* becomes "something that lives in your yard and sleeps outside in a little house." Children's definitions have a strong element of function or action.

The concept of static perceptual features may be too analytical for very young children (Nelson, 1974). Rather, concepts may be defined in terms of logical relationships or logical acts.

While the functional-core hypothesis has appeal, it is difficult to find extensive use of shared function in child utterances. For example, young Eva (Bowerman, 1978a) used the word *moon* for the moon, a half grapefruit, a lemon slice, a circular chrome dial, a ball of spinach on her plate, and so on. Although the action or use of these entities is very dissimilar, the shapes are all spherical or crescent. In addition, the word *moon* was uttered when the objects were static and at a distance.

Associative and Prototypic Complexes. Theories built around one type of similarity, whether perceptual or functional, may be too restricted. The child may use words "complexively," shifting from one feature to another with each use. This shifting might indicate a loosely defined criterion for the concept. In fact, there seems to be little difference in the learning of labels whether the features are functionally or perceptually based (R. Schwartz & Leonard, 1984).

According to the **associative complex hypothesis**, each successive use of the word shares some feature with a central instance or core concept (Vygotsky, 1962). For example, a child may produce the word *baby* in the presence of a younger infant, extend it to self, to pictures of himself or herself, and to books with pictures.

This notion has been expanded to a **prototypic complex hypothesis** in which the child's underlying concept includes a central reference or prototype, usually the referent most frequently used with the adult speech model and the first referent for which the word was used. Thus, the child has a highly specific, stored mental representation of the concept. The closer the new instance is to the prototype, the more likely it is to be labeled by that symbol. Originally, Eva produced the word *kick* when she propelled a ball with her foot. Subsequently, she used the word for a moth and for the "hitting of a bicycle with her kid-dicar." The moth was similar in limb movement, and the kiddicar incident duplicated the striking of an object (Bowerman, 1978).

The prototypic complex hypothesis has much appeal. The nonlinguistic categories of seven- to nine-month-old children may be organized around prototypes as well, since exposure to prototypes facilitates category formation (Roberts & Horowitz, 1986). In addition, if children's meanings are based on a central referent, there appears to be a continuum from infancy to adulthood in which many semantic categories are organized this way.

Some adult concepts are finite, while other concept boundaries, especially those of categorical terms, are fuzzy. Some examples are always included in the concept, others only in certain contexts. For example, the prototype for the concept *furniture* probably does not represent any one piece of furniture (Figure 8.1). There is no one best exemplar at the center of the concept. Some items, such as a table or a sofa, are good examples of the concept. Others, such as a footstool or a cot, are less so. A lamp, although considered to be furniture, is even further from the central concept (see Figure 8.1). A second example is the concept *bird*. Some examples, such as a robin and a sparrow, are prototypic. Others, such as an ostrich and a penguin, are not. The degree to which a particular instance is considered to be prototypic of the concept is related to the number of features the example has in common with other referents of the concept. The most prototypical examples share the most features. Obviously, some features are more central than others.

Older children and adults seem to analyze a concept into its essential features, which are used to determine the "goodness-of-fit" of new exemplars (Greenberg & Kuczaj, 1982). We are not sure of the process used by young children. They may use a holistic-based comparison encompassing both perceptual and functional information (Greenberg & Kuczaj, 1982).

The mother aids the child's referential process by supplying categorical names to the most typical examples of the concept. Typical dogs are labeled *doggie*. Atypical dogs are labeled by less frequently used breed names, such as *chihuahua* or *afghan* (Whitehurst, Kedesdy, & White, 1982). Larger categories, such as *animal*, have fewer perceptual or functional similarities and are avoided. During maternal labeling, the child makes a preliminary identification of the attributes and features that characterize the prototypic referent (Barrett, 1982). Therefore, meaning consists initially of the prototypic referent and a small group of

FIGURE 8.1   Possible Prototypic Concept of Furniture

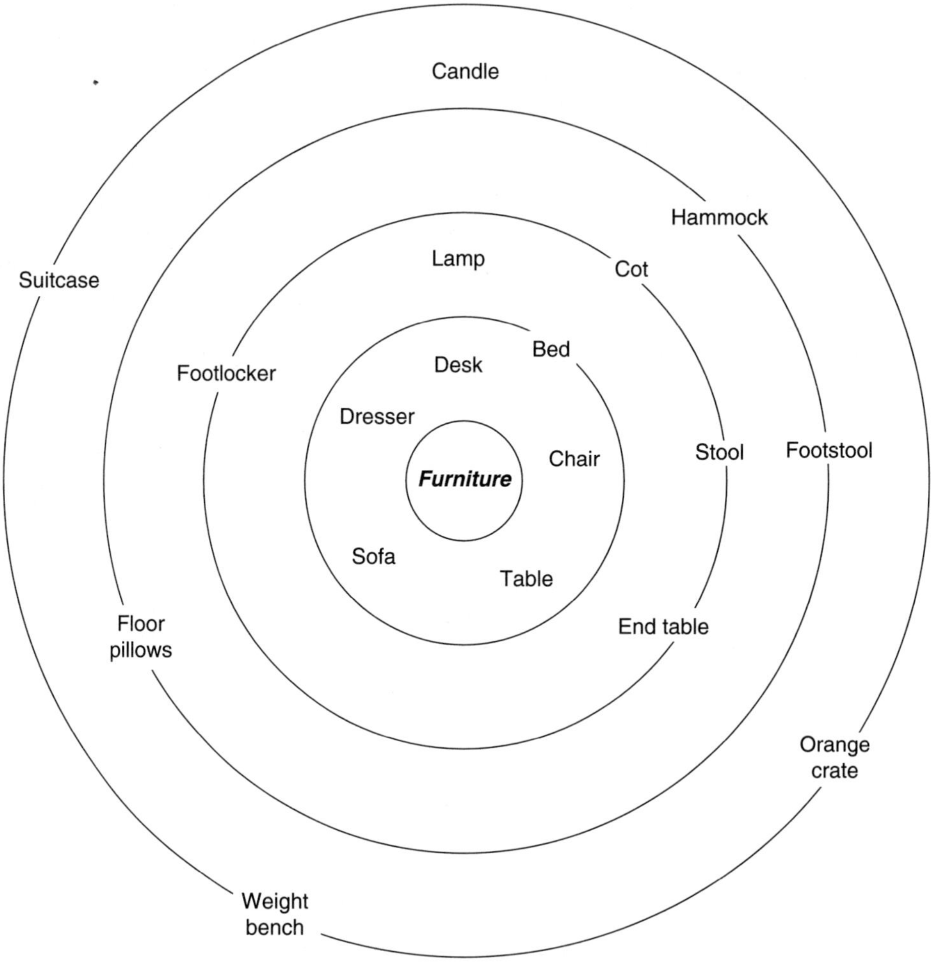

features. These features can be recognized independently when they do not occur together. Hence, the child is able to extend the word to other exemplars.

The child's meaning may lack some features critical to the adult concept but may include other features that are not. It is important to note that it is the child who determines the related features; adults generally provide only the label.

The child now assigns the word to a particular semantic group based on the identified features (Barrett, 1982). The word's referent is grouped with other referents that have similar features. For example, the referent may be identified as a mover or causer of action and hence may be classed with other causative agents. Obviously, some features have more "definingness" than others.

The final step is to identify the features that distinguish the prototypic referent of this word from those of other words within the same semantic field. For example, toys and foods are both receivers of action and fill a semantic function called *object*, discussed later in this chapter, but the two concepts are very different. Thus, meaning consists of the prototypic referent, a set of features that define the word's semantic field, and a set of features that differentiate the prototypic referent from the referents of other words in the same semantic field.

Initial prototypes will vary across children, reflecting different experiences. The concept prototypes change as well; concepts are modified as a result of experience. Concept formation and refinement is an ongoing process. Even among adults, subtle concept changes occur with experience and, as a result, meanings are refined.

Initial concept formation is based on holistic inclusion of prototypic exemplars. Decisions of relatedness, however, are determined by the similarities between the prototype and the new instance or example.

Extension: Under, Over, and Otherwise

In the process of refining meanings, the child forms hypotheses about underlying concepts and extends current meanings to include new examples. Through this extension process, the child gains knowledge from exemplars and nonexemplars of the concept. Occasionally concepts are very restricted; others are widely extended. Overly restricted meanings that contain fewer exemplars than the adult meaning are called **underextensions**. Using "cup" for only a "Tommy Tippee cup" is an example of underextension. In contrast, **overextensions** are meanings that are too broad, containing more exemplars than the adult meaning. Calling all men "Daddy" is an example of overextension. Note that these terms are used in reference to the adult meaning. As for the child, he or she is applying the hypothesized meaning, not the adult's meaning. It is also important to note that children usually do not overgeneralize or overextend in their comprehension of words (Fremgen & Fay, 1980). Children often comprehend the adult meaning but use their own meaning in expression.

The child receives implicit and explicit feedback about the concept extensions. Implicit feedback can be found in the naming practices of others, to which the child attends. In contrast, explicit feedback includes direct correction or confirmation of the child's extensions by more mature language users. As the child extends the meaning of *cup* from "Tommy Tippee," he or she may include bowls and pots in addition to coffee mugs and tea cups. In the course of daily events, more mature speakers will call bowls and pots by their accepted names and correct the child's attempts more directly.

It may be incorrect to assume that the criteria used for extension are those used in formation of the initial concept. Other factors, such as a lack of specific words in the child's lexicon, may account for behavior that appears to adults to be overextension. If the child could verbalize the situation, he or she might say, "I know that that thing is not a dog, but I don't know what else to call it, and it is like a dog, so I'll call it a dog" (L. Bloom, 1973, p. 79). It is possible for the child to underextend and overextend a word at the same time

(Greenberg & Kuczaj, 1982). For example, the child may use the word *dog* to refer to a sheep but not a Newfoundland.

As the child gains experience, he or she uses fewer and fewer overextensions and underextensions. In addition, the child broadens categories to include more and more disparate but similar examples. Adult feedback to children can help them adjust their overextensions. An adult demonstration of the important attributes that make X an X is more helpful than providing the correct label or correcting the child's overextension error (Mervis & Mervis, 1988).

Underextensions are common in both receptive and expressive language. In contrast, overextension is usually limited to expressive language, although there is considerable individual variation (Rescorla, 1980). At this early stage of acquisition, toddlers comprehend many more words than they produce. The child who is able to point to a motorcycle, bike, truck, plane, and helicopter may label all of them *car*. When overextension does occur in comprehension, it is usually based on perceptual similarities (Behrend, 1988).

Overextensions are common among toddlers in all languages, including those acquiring American Sign Language (Siedlecki & Bonvillian, 1998). Most overextensions fall into three general types: categorical overinclusions, analogical overextensions, and predicate statements. Most overextensions are categorical overinclusions in which children use a word to label a referent in a related category. For example, the child may use *baby* for all children, *hot* for cold, or *dada* for mother. The largest number of generalizations are within the people category.

Analogical overextensions include the use of a word to label a referent not related categorically. Rather, the inferred similarity is perceptual, functional, or affective. For example, children may use *ball* to refer to round objects or *comb* to label a centipede.

With predicate statements, children note the relationship between the object and some absent person, object, property, or state. For example, a child might say "doll" when seeing the empty bed or "door" when requesting adult assistance with opening or closing some object. Unlike the other two types, predicate statements are relational and therefore may represent presyntactic productions. Types of predicate overextensions are shown in Table 8.5.

TABLE 8.5   Predicate Overextensions

STATEMENT TYPE	EXAMPLE
Former or unusual state	*Cookie* for empty plate
Anticipations	*Key* while before door
Elements	*Water* for turned-off hose
Specific activity	*Peepee* for toilet
Pretending	*Nap* while pretending to sleep

Source: Adapted from Thomson, J., & Chapman, R., Who is "Daddy" revisited: The status of two year extensioned words in use and comprehension. *Journal of Child Language*, 1977, *4*, 359–375.

When we examine both extensions and overextensions of the first seventy-five words, perceptual similarity seems to account for nearly 60 percent of both (Rescorla, 1980). Most perceptual similarities seem to be visual. Action or functional similarity accounts for about 25 percent of children's extensions. Thematic or contextual association of an object with the event in which it is used seems to account for only about 12 percent of extensions. For example, a child may use the word *nap* when referring to a blanket. Finally, a very small number of extensions are based on affective or emotional similarity. More than half of these extensions involve prohibitive or frightening words, such as *hot* or *bad*.

The majority of children seem to use words correctly (Rescorla, 1980). Most words are used for generalized referents rather than for a single referent. Within one month of acquisition, more than three-fourths of words are generalized to more than one referent. Of the remainder, most are names for specific entities, such as *Mama*. Words acquired during initial lexical growth are more likely to be overgeneralized than words acquired later; however, the overgeneralization does not occur at once, but rather during the period of rapid vocabulary growth preceding early multiword utterances. Early words are also more likely to exhibit underextension and associative complexes.

Approximately a third of the first seventy-five words seem to be overextended (Rescorla, 1980). Some categories, such as letters, vehicles, and clothing, are overextended at a greater rate than others. Many children overextend words such as *car, truck, shoe, hat, dada, baby, apple, cheese, ball, dog,* and *hot*. Words are not usually overextended to label referents for which the child has already acquired the correct symbol (Barrett, 1982).

In summary, it appears that extension and overextension are aspects of the same word-acquisition process. Overextension seems to serve a dual function: as a device for expressing categorization and concept formation and as a presyntactic means to convey relationships. Overextension usually ends when the child begins to use the acceptable adult meaning, probably because of adult unwillingness to accept the child's overinclusiveness.

Semantic Class Distinctions

Children organize their early words by semantic categories. (See the psycholinguistic-semantic/cognitive section of Chapter 2.) At the two-word stage, children follow simple word-order patterns of construction based on semantic distinctions. It has been assumed, therefore, that these distinctions are present prior to the appearance of two-word utterances, suggesting a continuity from single-word to multiword structures.

Different types of knowledge may be required for the use of single-word and multiword utterances. Children at the single-word stage may refer to the total situation, both entities and dynamic states. For example, a child observes Daddy throwing a ball and says "ball" to describe the entire event. Behavior at the two-word stage indicates the cognitive ability to separate entities from dynamic states and relationships. At this point, a child may say "Daddy throw" or "Throw ball." Since the single-word stage represents limitations in processing and production as well as in memory, we cannot be sure of the child's underlying referencing abilities. Children may be separating entities and dynamic states but may be unable to encode more than one element.

Substantive and Relational Categories. Variation can be found in the semantic structure of early child utterances. In general, early single-word utterances can be classified as either of two large semantic categories, *substantive* or *relational*, depending on the words used and their intended meaning (L. Bloom & Lahey, 1978).

Substantive words refer to specific entities or classes of entities that have certain shared perceptual or functional features. Much of the early section of this chapter was devoted to a discussion of this category. Examples include *mama, dada, doggie, cup,* and *hat.*

Early word combinations indicate that children classify substantive words on the basis of action. One class, **agents**, is the source of action; the other, **objects**, is the recipient of action. These noun-type words appear alone and in the singular, rather than plural, form.

Relational words refer to relations that an entity shares with itself or with other entities. In relation to itself, an entity can exist or not exist, disappear and reappear. For example, when an entity exists or is present, the child might point and say "that." In contrast, when it disappears, she might say "all gone." Other entities may share static states (possession and attribution), dynamic states (actions), or locations.

Relational words make reference across entities. As such, they express relational meanings that transcend the individual objects involved. For example, the utterance "all gone" can apply to an empty glass or bowl or to a vacant dog house. Use of relational words is evidence that the child is able to conceptualize and encode the dynamic state separately from the entity. This ability represents notions of object permanence, object constancy, and causality. The most common relational categories are reflexive, including existence, nonexistence, disappearance, and recurrence; action; location; possession; and attribution.

The most frequent relational words in early speech are reflexive in that they relate the object to itself. **Reflexive relational words** mark existence, nonexistence, disappearance, and recurrence (see Table 8.6). The relations are expressed by words such as *this, there, uh-oh, gone,* and *nuther.* For some children, these reflexive relational terms are the predominant

TABLE 8.6   Reflexive Relational Words in Children's Single-Word Utterances

TYPE	EXPLANATION	EXAMPLES
Existence	Child's attention gained by an entity, especially a novel one: notes that it exists	May point and say "this," "that," "here," or "what's that?"
Nonexistence	Child notes that an entity is not present though expected	"No" or "gone" or name of object with a rising intonation
Disappearance	Child notes that an entity that was present has disappeared	"Gone," "all gone," "away," "bye-bye" ("all gone" may be used as a request that an entity disappear or as a notice that it has moved)
Recurrence	Child notes that an object appears after an absence or that another object replaces an absent one	"More," "again," or "another" (may be used to request reappearance or to note additional entities)

forms found in their early lexicons. Relational words conveying visual displacement, such as *bye* and *uh-oh*, occur in sensorimotor stage V, when these cognitive skills have been attained. Absent-relational terms, such as *all gone* and *more*, convey invisible displacement and occur later in stage VI (Tomasello & Farrar, 1984).

A second group consists of **action relational words**. The predominant concept in children's early speech is the way that different objects relate through movement or action. Early meanings center on action. Although nouns dominate as a percentage of many children's vocabularies, they do not dominate in frequency of use even in languages as different as English and Japanese.

Very few of the child's action words are true action verbs. Instead, the child uses words such as *in* to accompany putting one object into another or *off* to describe separation. These types of words, called *protoverbs*, are the first action-type words to develop (Barrett, 1983). Although terms such as *in, out, off, up, down, no, on here, inside, there, get down, bye-bye*, and *ni-night* are not verbs, they are used by the child in verblike contexts (Barrett, 1983).

Children also use *here* and *there* to accompany action sequences (McCune-Nicolich, 1981). *Here* is often used to accompany exchange games. When a child passes an object to her partner, she may accompany that action with the word *here*, in imitation of mother's behavior. *There* follows the completion of an action. A child may use both terms in this manner for several months before using them as location words.

Following the development of protoverbs, several kinds of action-type words appear, including general-purpose, deictic, object-related action-specific, and intransitive action-specific (Huttenlocher, Smiley, & Charney, 1983). General-purpose action words, such as *do, put*, and *make*, do not refer to any specific action and must be interpreted from the context. Deictic action words, which must be interpreted from the perspective of the speaker, include words such as *lookit* and are used to direct the listener's attention. Object-related action-specific words, such as *push* and *drink*, refer to precise actions performed on objects. Finally, intransitive action-specific words represent precise non-object-related actions, such as *walk*.

Location relational words describe the directional or spatial relationship of two objects. Dynamic locative events are acquired before, and occur more frequently than, static spatial relationships. Thus, the child is more likely to comment on a knock at the door ("door") than on a shoe residing on a chair ("chair").

Finally, state relations include possession and attribution. **Possession relational words** recognize that an object is associated with a particular person. Initially, possessives are used to mark alienable possessions, such as food, clothing, and toys, rather than body parts or relatives. The possessive relationship may be one of the few features of the object that the child knows. For example, the child may say "Juan" to note brother's soccer gear but know little else about the equipment. In addition to names of other people, the child may use his or her own name or say "mine."

Attribution relational words mark the attributes, characteristics, or differences between similar objects, such as *big, little, dirty, hot, funny*, and *yukky*. Attributes seem to be used more as names than as properties of objects . As a class, attributes are rare in single-word and early multiword utterances.

One additional category may be *mismatch* (McCune-Nicolich, 1981), in which conditions conflict with the child's expectations, desires, or efforts. The child may respond with a protesting "no" or with a startled "uh-oh." Parents use both words in similar situations, the latter often accompanied by a high-low musical contour that may be learned before the actual phonetics.

Although substantive and relational words develop during the single-word period, the onset of relational words is "somewhat abrupt" (McCune-Nicolich, 1981). In contrast, use of substantive words has a more linear growth. Relational words are also less likely to occur as imitations, which lends support to the idea that the child has a sensorimotor knowledge base for the concepts expressed. The supposedly universal nature of sensorimotor thought may account for the widespread appearance of these early semantic categories. Variation in the specific topics children "discuss" reflects the different experiential background of each child.

Order of Appearance. For most children, initial words may be "pure performatives"; that is, the word itself performs the act named (such as *hi* and *bye-bye*). These precede operations of reference, including nomination of substantive words, existence, nonexistence, disappearance, recurrence, and negation. The action function develops next, coincident with the agent and object functions for substantive words. These are followed by the attribution, location, and possession functions.

Not all children will adhere to this order of appearance of semantic categories. The frequency of appearance of a semantic function may depend on the child's frequency of experience with the objects and events. Later, the frequency of use probably reflects the communication value of the semantic functions for the child.

EARLY MULTIWORD COMBINATIONS

When children begin to combine words into longer utterances at about eighteen months of age, they do so in predictable patterns that appear to be universal. With increasing memory and processing skills, the child is able to produce longer utterances by recombining these early patterns. Language learning in much of the latter half of the second year involves these combinations. It is important to keep in mind, however, that the child still produces a great many single-word utterances.

Transition: Early Word Combinations

Prior to the appearance of two-word utterances is a period in which the child produces sequences of words, sounds, and gestures in seeming combination and in a variety of forms. In any gesture-rich culture, such as Italy, children may make early transitional combinations of a word plus a representational gesture, such as putting a fist to the ear to signal *telephone* or flapping the arms for *bird* (Capirci, Iverson, Pizzuto, & Volterra, 1996). A larger number of such combinations is related to greater verbal production in the later multiword stage.

A verbal-vocal transitional form consists of a CV syllable preceding or following a word. The phonology of the extra syllable is inconsistent and has no referent. For example, the child might say the following on several different occasions:

ma baby
te baby
bu baby

Other forms may be more consistent but still have no referent. Empty forms include a word plus a preceding or following sound in which the word, rather than the nonreferential element, varies. Examples of empty forms are as follows:

beda cookie
beda baby
beda doggie

A third form consists of reduplications of a single utterance, such as "Doggie doggie." Other seeming combinations may actually consist of two words learned as a single unit, such as "daddybob." In general, the child does not use the two words independently as single words nor in combination with others. Common examples of single-unit words include:

all-gone
go-bye
so-big
go-potty

Finally, some children reportedly produce successive single-word utterances. In these successive utterances, each word occurs with terminal falling pitch and relatively equal stress, and there is a pause between words. To understand the terminal falling pitch contour, try a little experiment. Say "Mommy" in a matter-of-fact manner. Note that you drop your pitch at the end of the word.

Mommy.↓

Now say "laugh." Again, there should have been a drop in pitch.

Laugh.↓

The next part is more difficult. Say the two words in succession, with a momentary pause between them. Since "Mommy" + "laugh" approximates a mature sentence form, it may be difficult to drop your pitch after each word. It may help if you reverse the order.

Mommy↓   Laugh↓   or   Laugh↓   Mommy↓

Compare this pitch contour to the utterance "Mommy laugh." In the two-word combination, the drop in pitch occurs only at the end of the utterance.

Mommy laugh↓

The word order of successive single-word utterances is variable, unlike that of two-word combinations.

Initial successive single-word utterances may exhibit a terminal falling pitch with each word as mentioned. The child soon modifies pitch contours to resemble those of short adult utterances, although the child still uses a somewhat longer pause. Such a progression might be expected, given the well-documented ability of young children to adopt adult intonational patterns. Finally, at about eighteen months of age, the pitch, pause, and word-order characteristics approximate those of the adult. At this point, most child specialists credit the child with multiword utterances.

Two-Word Combinations

Children seem to comprehend two-word utterances before they produce them, although children may key into certain words or to context rather than to word order. Just what the child comprehends is difficult to say.

In the initial period of word combination, the child may experiment with a variety of rules. Individual differences in the actual words chosen and in the combination forms used are great (Goldfield & Snow, 1985) and may reflect individual strategies for rule acquisition. Some children seem to focus on individual words and their combinations, whereas others focus on small groups of words classed according to meaning (B. Brown & Leonard, 1986). By twenty-four months, however, the average child is using two-word utterances frequently (Wells, 1985).

Some words are used without any positional consistency. In this *groping pattern* (B. Brown & Leonard, 1986) the child uses a word regardless of semantic class. For example, the child might say "Eat cookie" or "Cookie eat" without regard for word order or position. A second form, the *positional associative pattern* (Braine, 1976), is characterized by consistent word order but reflects patterns heard in adult speech, such as "Stop that" and "Come here," and does not appear to be a creative rule system.

Finally, a third strategy, the *positional productive pattern* (Braine, 1976), is characterized by consistent word order and creative combinations. One variety of this strategy focuses on individual words and the ways in which they're used by adults (Lieven, Pine, & Baldwin, 1997). Children may hypothesize positional rules for words based upon repeated hearing of those words in specific locations in adult speech. The child then uses these words repeatedly in the first or second location in combination with another word. It has been suggested that positional rules rather than semantic rules are the basis for early multiword utterances and, indeed, some 60 percent of multiword utterances can be analyzed in this manner (Pine & Lieven, 1993).

Most linguists believe that children eventually begin to use creative word-order rules based on semantic categories, such as action + object. Using this rule, the child might create "Eat cookie," "Throw ball," "Up me," "Drink juice," and so on. Other possible semantic rules are presented in Table 8.7.

Simple word-order rules relative to the child's semantic categories provide an adequate system for elaborating upon meanings and for interpreting adult utterances beyond the information contained in the words themselves. The child goes beyond the words alone,

TABLE 8.7 Two-Word Semantic Rules

SEMANTIC-SYNTACTIC RULE (L. Bloom, 1973; R. Brown, 1973; Schlesinger, 1971)	EXAMPLES
Modifier + head	
Attributive + entity	*Big doggie*
Possessor + possession	*Daddy shoe*
Recurrent + X	*Nuther cookie*
	More up
Negative + X	
Nonexistence or disappearance	*No juice*
	Allgone (ba)nana
Rejection (of proposal)	*No bed* (when told it's bedtime)
Denial (of statement)	*No baby* (when referred to as such)
Demonstrative (this/that) + entity	*This cup*
X + locative	*Doggie bed*
	Throw me
X + dative	*Give mommy*
	Cookie mommy
Agent + action	*Daddy eat*
	Mommy throw
Action + object	*Eat cookie*
	Throw ball
Agent + object	*Daddy cookie*
	Mommy ball

*This table represents a combination of the work of several researchers and an attempt to remain true to the meanings of early child utterances.

expressing relationships between them. In fact, in languages such as English in which word order is important, the earliest rules used relate to ordering.

The child's earliest two-word combinations probably reflect rules that he or she has constructed for the specific words involved. One early rule seems to be *the/a/some* + *X*, in which *X* can be almost anything (Nelson et al., 1993). Before long, these rules proliferate and become cumbersome. There appears to be a developmental order in the child's acquisition of two-word phrases. Words used in positional productive patterns (consistent word order as heard in adult speech) are acquired before those used in the other two patterns, groping and associative (B. Brown & Leonard, 1986), possibly because the child has had more time to become familiar with the semantic aspects of these earlier words. A sample of the speech and language of an eighteen-month-old child is presented on track six of the CD that accompanies this text. Word combinations will emerge slowly at first but will increase in speed with each new addition. Compare this sample to that of the 2-year-old on track seven. A transcript of the speech of a 20-month-old child is presented in Table 14.1 of this text.

Semantic Rules

One of the results of the Semantic Revolution of the early 1970s was that linguists attempted to describe the two-word linear or word-order rules of young children. The motivation was to describe the rules for word combination that children seemed to be following and to find similarities in the language of young children that might suggest universal meaning categories. The resultant rules, combined in Table 8.7, may account for as much as 70 percent of the multiword utterances of English-speaking children.

The early combination rules can be described as **semantic-syntactic**—semantic because the bases for combination are meaning relations and syntactic because word-order rules and relationships pertain. Initially, word order varies, but it stabilizes shortly before the child begins to use grammatical markers, such as possessive -'s (Chi-Minh's toy) and past tense -ed (walked). Use of these markers would seem to indicate that the grammatical functions they serve are present earlier but marked by other means, such as word order.

Reflexive two-word semantic expansions, such as "More milk" or "Allgone juice," represent a combined meaning of little more than the individual words. Neither word's meaning changes as a result of the combination. The linear order of combination is relatively constant, and initial two-word utterances usually are of this type. Other expansions, such as those involving an action word, do not have a constant word order. The word order depends on the semantic relationship of the words involved. The relationship is not simply linear but represents the relationship of verbs to different types of nouns. Some types of nouns precede the verb; others follow it. Action expansions, possessives, and locatives develop after the reflexive expansions.

The reflexive functions include nomination (this/that + nominative), recurrence (recurrent + X), and nonexistence (negative + X). A two-word nomination consists of the demonstrative (this, that) plus some entity, as in "That ball." If the child initiates the utterance, he or she accompanies it with a pointing gesture. In contrast, the child usually does not point when responding to a question.

Recurrence is used initially as a request, such as "Nuther (another) cookie" or "More jump." Later, such forms will also be used to comment on a situation. Although children seem to make little distinction between more and another, they usually do not use another with verbs, as in nuther jump.

Nonexistence/disappearance is the predominant type of negative. It is often used with the expectation that the entity will return. As with recurrence, nonexistence/disappearance may be used to comment or request. Negative forms can also be used for rejection, as when the child pushes away a bowl of strained peas with a "No" or "No peas." A third form of negative is denial, often found in the word games of parents and children. To the parent's question "Is this a book?", asked while holding a cup, the child responds "No book."

In several different languages, denial appears around twenty to twenty-five months (Choi, 1988; Pea, 1980; Vaidyanathan, 1991). Cognitively, the child must be able to hold two mental models for comparison, the child's perceptual model and that described by the adult (Hummer, Wimmer, & Antes, 1993).

Nearly all children are using reflexive semantic functions before fifteen months of age (Wells, 1985). This category dominates, accounting for approximately 70 percent of single-word and two-word utterances, until almost two years of age. By thirty-six months, reflexive functions may account for as little as 10 percent of children's utterances (Wells, 1985).

The primary "relational types" consist of *X + locative*, in which *X* may be almost any word, *possessor + (possession)*, *attributive + entity*, *agent + action*, *action + object*, and *agent + object*. Usually, the locative function is signaled in two ways: *entity + locative*, which develops first, and *action + locative*. *Entity + locative* constructions include a stationary entity and its location or an entity moving or being moved plus the direction of movement (*up*) or the location. In general, the static entity develops prior to the moving one (Wells, 1985). In the *action + locative* type, the child names the action and direction of movement in relation to some location (*Throw me*). By twenty-one months, the average child is using locative functions (Wells, 1985).

Two-word locative utterances (*X + locative*) and possessive (*possessor + possession*) begin to appear at about the same time as the object-related utterances but take longer for most children to learn (Wells, 1985). By age two, 90 percent of children are using these constructions. As we have seen, the use of agents or objects in locatives precedes the use of action words. Children also encode static locations and possessions before directional movement or changing possession.

Generally, the *possessor + possession* construction is used for alienable possessions, such as clothes or toys, as in the single-word phase. Inalienable entities, such as body parts, do not appear with possessor words initially because the owner is obvious. Very few possessive pronouns are used, except *my*.

Attributive two-word utterances (*attributive + entity*) and *agent + action* and *action + object* are used by some children at around 18 months but take even longer than the other categories for most children to learn (Wells, 1985). Although the average child is using the attributive construction by twenty-four months, all three types of construction are not used by 90 percent of children until thirty months. Initially, attributive words describe physical characteristics, such as "big." In English, the *attributive + entity* construction may vary in word order. English-speaking adults may say "blue book" or "the book is blue." At this stage, however, the attribute generally precedes.

The action categories initially take the two-word forms *agent + want* and *want + object*. Some studies have found very few true action words in early constructions (Wells, 1985). Action words appear later in two-word utterances, initially as unspecific actions or protoverbs, such as "do," or as particles of verbs, such as *off*, *on*, and *away*.

The child's initial notion of agent words is probably restricted to animate entities (*mommy*, *doggie*, *baby*). Nonagentive words, such as *cup* and *ball*, usually do not appear in this position in child utterances, although these can fulfill the subject function in adult sentences. The child probably does not have the abstract notion of subject. While agents cause action, objects are the recipients of the action. The *agent + object* construction has a very low incidence and is not found universally.

Stress Patterns and Meaning. At the two-word level, a child's meaning is often difficult to interpret. Small words, such as articles and prepositions, are omitted. In general, more mature language users employ a rich interpretation using the linguistic and nonlinguistic contexts to determine the child's meaning. The child's word order is a clue to meaning, but it may be ambiguous. Suppose that the child says "doggie bed." Is he or she commenting on the dog's new cushion (*possessor + possession*) or warning that Fido still prefers to sleep on Mommy's bed (*entity + locative*)? The child may aid this interpretive process.

Children use stress, or emphasis, to indicate meaning. As shown in the hierarchy of stress (Figure 8.2), a child could be expected to stress the action term in *agent + action* and the object in *action + object* utterances. Applying the hierarchy to "doggie bed," interpretation becomes easier. A comment on the dog's new bed would be "*doggie* bed," while a warning of the dog's location would be "doggie *bed*." New information receives the most stress, as we might expect, since it is novel to the conversation. The newness criterion is seen throughout the hierarchy. We can assume, for instance, that a pronoun object is old information, because pronouns are used to refer to previously identified entities. In contrast, noun objects would represent newer information.

The child's meaning thus may be interpreted from a number of indicators. The ongoing events and the preceding utterances establish the nonlinguistic and linguistic contexts. Word order and stress help us interpret the semantic categories produced.

Longer Utterances

When approximately half of the child's utterances contain two words, he or she begins to use three-word combinations. The most common three-word utterances are *agent + action + object*, such as "Mommy eat cookie," and *agent + action + location*, such as "Mommy throw me" (to me) or "Mommy sleep chair." These and other three-word utterances consist of two types: recombinations and expansions. Action relations, such as *agent + action* and *action + object*, recombine and the redundant term is deleted.

[agent + action] + [action + object] = agent + action + object
Daddy   throw   Throw   ball   Daddy   throw   ball

FIGURE 8.2   Hierarchy of Stress in Toddler's Two-Word Utterances

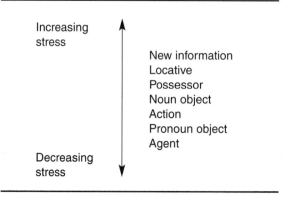

Increasing stress

New information
Locative
Possessor
Noun object
Action
Pronoun object
Agent

Decreasing stress

This process is also seen in the locative functions.

[entity (agent) + locative] + [action + locative] = agent + action + locative
Mommy   chair   Sit   chair   Mommy   sit   chair

In contrast, other semantic relations expand from within to express attribution, possession, or recurrence. The noun term is expanded. For example, within the recurrent "more cookie," the noun portion could be expanded to "big cookie," resulting in "more big cookie." Other examples are as follows:

[action + object] → [action + (attributive + entity)]
Eat   cookie   Eat   big   cookie
[action + locative] → [action + (possessor + possession)]
Sit   chair   Sit   baby   chair

Four-word or four-term utterances are expanded in the same way. No new relations are learned while the child develops a skill with longer word combinations. The average child is producing some four-word utterances by age two.

PHONOLOGICAL PATTERNS

During the first two years, children learn that sound sequences can carry distinct meanings. These sequences and meanings are associated in the brain. Categorization and storage are based initially on the entire phonological pattern or auditory image of the word rather than on the individual phonemes involved.

With first words, the child shifts to greater control of articulation. Babbling requires less constrained production, but when the child adds meaning to sound, he or she needs some phonological consistency to transmit messages. After the onset of meaningful speech, there is much individual variation in the pattern and rate of vocabulary growth, the use of invented words, and the syllable structure of the words acquired.

Single-Word Utterances

As noted previously, nearly all of the initial words are monosyllabic CV or VC units or CVCV constructions. Labial (/p, b, m, w/) and alveolar consonants (/t,d/), mostly plosives (/p, b, t, d, g, k/), predominate but there are occasional fricatives (/s,f/) and nasals (/m,n/). Vowel production varies widely among children and within each child, but the basic triangle of /a/, /i/, and /u/ is probably established early. Within a given word, the consonants tend to be the same or noncontrasting, such as *baby, mama, daddy, dawdie (doggie)*. It is the vowels that initially vary. Consonant contrasts occur more frequently in CVC constructions, such as *cup*.

The child begins to construct his or her own production capacity with the words selected to produce. Some words are actively avoided, even though the child recognizes and understands them. Two possible selection patterns for initial words are (a) the size and complexity of the syllable structure and (b) the sound types included. The child may choose to produce words that contain only certain sounds. Generally, these phonological constraints on lexical choices have disappeared by age two (Dobrich & Scarborough, 1992).

Different children exhibit different "favorite sounds" and use these in selecting the first words that they will produce. Thus, vocabulary expansion occurs at the expense of phonological differentiation. Although there is a wide range of individual differences (Grunwell, 1981), certain language-based phonetic tendencies are seen in most children, including a preference for monosyllables over longer strings, and stops (/p, b, t, d, k, g/) over all other types of consonant production (Locke, 1983). Preferences for particular speech sounds at age one year do not correspond to mastery of these speech sounds at age three years (Vihman & Greenlee, 1987). Relationships are more subtle. In general, the greater the proportion of true consonants in babbling and true words at age one, the more advanced the phonological development of the child at age three (Vihman & Greenlee, 1987).

Phonological organization may exist along a continuum from those who are very cautious or systematic to those who are exploratory. More systematic children operate with strong phonetic and structural constraints that are relaxed gradually. In contrast, exploratory speakers have a loose, variable phonological organization and attempt words well beyond their capabilities. This variability at age one tends to become inconsistent production of sounds at age three (Vihman & Greenlee, 1987).

Phonological rules or processes are systematic procedures for making adult words pronounceable. The patterns and systemicity enable children to produce an approximation of an adult model. In other words, for the child, phonological processes are a way of getting from an auditory model to speech production. In other words, phonological processes are a method of achieving a goal of production. For example, the child familiar with CV words may adopt a CV strategy for CVC words, producing /kʌ/ for *cup* (/kʌp/).

During the period from twelve to eighteen months of age, children generally do not exhibit phonological rules. These evolve slowly as each child's lexicon grows and each child attempts to say more words. Instead, children follow two rather broad strategies of sound production: selection and modification (Menyuk, Menn, & Silber, 1986). Following a selection strategy, a child decides to avoid certain words and to exploit or favor others based on the sounds contained in those words. Thus, the child's lexicon is shaped, in part, by the presence of certain phonemes. There are no rules as such other than those used with each word. In other words, rules are word-specific. Modification is the slow expansion and change of the child's phonological system as rules are created and new words are modified to fit the child's existing sound patterns. In this process, two or more similar words may initially exist separately but may then be collapsed into one sound pattern.

Phonological patterns are not easy to reproduce. The child's initial attempts at word production involve trial and error and may be very unstable.

In addition to being complex, phonological processes exhibit tremendous individual variation for several reasons (Ingram, 1986). First, the entire system of each child is constantly changing. Initially, the child may have one phonemic form for several adult words or several forms for the same word. Thus, *baba* may be used for *baby*, *bottle*, and *rabbit*, or *doddie* and *goggie* may be used for *doggie*. Gradually, the child develops processes that enable him or her to distinguish between similar adult words. Word production strategies may even precede the development of selection patterns. For example, a child with the rule CV = /d/V may produce *no*, which becomes *do* (/dou/), and *key*, which becomes *dee* (/di/).

Second, some words are produced consistently, while others vary greatly. Within a given word, there may be "trade-offs": the acquisition of one part of a word may, in turn, distort another part, which the child produced correctly in the past.

Third, phonological variation may be the result of toddlers' use of differing, although similar, phonological production patterns or processes, such as reduplication, diminutives, open syllables, and consonant cluster reductions (Table 8.8). **Reduplication** occurs when the child attempts a polysyllabic word (*daddy*) but is unable to produce one syllable correctly. The child compensates by repeating the other syllable (*dada*). In contrast, the **diminutive** is an /i/ added to the end of a word, frequently a CVC (*dog*), to produce a CVCV (*doggie*).

Multisyllabic words or words with final consonants are frequently produced in a CV multisyllable form. For example, *teddybear* becomes /tedibɛ/ (CVCVCV). **Open syllables**—those that end in a vowel—predominate in multisyllabic words. Thus, *dirty* may become /dɔti/ and *blanket* may become /bæki/. Closed syllables—those that end in a consonant—occur only at the ends of early words.

Consonant/cluster reduction results in single-consonant production, as in *poon* for *spoon*. Other phonological rules of preschool children are found in Chapter 10. Differences exist across languages as to which sound—first or second—is usually omitted. For example, German-speaking children tend to keep the first consonant, while Spanish-speaking children tend to prefer the second. Differences reflect the different sound combinations allowable in each language and that languages rules for syllabification (Lleo & Prinz, 1996). Other phonological rules of preschool children are found in Chapter 10.

The child produces those parts of words that are perceptually most salient. Auditory saliency is related to relatively low pitch or frequency, loudness, and long duration. For similar reasons, children often delete weak syllables, resulting in *nana* for *banana*.

Fourth, variation may reflect multiple processes within the same word. The result may only vaguely resemble the target word. For example, *tee* may be used for *treat*. In this example,

TABLE 8.8 Common Phonological Rules of Toddlers

TYPE	EXAMPLES
Reduplication (CVCV)	
Same syllable	*Water* becomes *wawa* (/wɑwɑ/)
	Mommy becomes *mama* (/mɑmɑ/)
	Baby becomes *bebie* (/bibi/)
Same consonant	*Doggie* becomes *goggie* (/gɔgi/) (diminutive)
	Candy becomes *cacie* (/kæki/)
CVCV construction	*Horse* becomes *hawsie* (/hɔsi/)
	Duck becomes *ducky* (/dʌki/)
Open syllables	*Blanket* becomes *bakie* (/bæki/)
	Bottle becomes *baba* (/bɑbɑ/)
Cluster reduction	*Stop* becomes *top* (/tɑp/)
	Tree becomes *tee* (/ti/)

the child has deleted the final consonant and simplified the consonant cluster. In similar fashion, suppose that the child has one rule that says that clusters reduce to a front consonant, a second that all initial sounds are voiced, and a third that words with a closed syllable ending receive a final vowel. If the target word is *treat*, it might change as follows:

Target	Treat
Apply rule 1 (cluster = front C)	Peat
Apply rule 2 (initial C = voiced)	Beat
Apply rule 3 (CVC = CVCV)	Beatie (/biti/)

Of course, this is neither a conscious nor a step-by-step process for the child. The child reduces the complexity of the adult model to a form he or she can produce.

The child may even produce the same form for two different words. She or he may interpret adult words as having identifiable and unidentifiable portions to which different rules apply. For example, suppose that the child produces both *spoon* and *pudding* as *poo* (/pu/). Consonant clusters, such as *sp*, may be reduced to the plosive—in this case—and final consonants, such as *n*, are omitted. Thus, *spoon* becomes *poo*. If the child also omits unfamiliar sounds, such as -*ing*, *pudding* would become *pud*, which, in turn, with omission of the final consonant, might be reduced to *pu* (/pu/).

Finally, individual phonological variation may reflect each child's phonological preferences as well. Such preferences might involve different articulatory patterns, classes of sounds, syllable structures, and location in words. Particular words may conform to the child's production patterns. As the child learns different phonological patterns, he or she applies them to the production of words.

The most frequent phonological process found in children under thirty months of age is consonant cluster reduction, although there is a dramatic drop in the use of this process after twenty-six months (Preisser, Hodson, & Paden, 1988). Overall, phonological processes decrease rapidly just prior to the second birthday.

Multiword Utterances

When the child begins to combine words, he or she continues to use phonological processes to produce single words. Familiar words appear in succession just as syllables appeared in CVCV words. Words and sentences with repeated elements are used frequently as a particular structure is being assimilated into the child's phonological system. With maturity, the number of repetitive elements gradually decreases and differentiation increases. It appears that at least some of the multiword constructions produced may have a phonological as well as a semantic–syntactic base.

Learning Units and Extension

Most likely, individual speech sounds are not the units of development. Rather, the whole word functions as a phonetic unit. Only later does the child become aware of speech-sound contrasts. The child's "word" is a representation of its adult model. The primacy of words over individual phonemes may be reflected in (a) the wide variation in pronunciation of individual words, (b) the difficulty of establishing phonemic contrasts within the wide range of word pronunciations, and (c) movement of sounds within but not between words.

The child's earliest words are very limited in the number and type of syllables and in the phoneme types. These restraints are gradually relaxed, resulting in greater structural complexity and phonetic diversity. In this progression, the child frequently generalizes from one word to another. Thus, phonological development occurs with changes in the pronunciation of individual words. Some changes result in improved identification of structures and sounds, others in new skills of production, and still others in the application of new phonological rules governing production.

While constructing his or her own phonological system, the child will extend rule hypotheses to other words. As a result, some child "words" will change to versions that are closer to the adult pronunciation, and others will become more unlike the model. In these cases, the rules or segments have been overextended. These changes reflect the acquisition of underlying phonological rules rather than word-by-word or sound-by-sound development.

It appears, then, that the child's first language is governed by phonological rules in addition to those for pragmatics, semantics, and syntax. The child invents and applies a succession of phonological rules reflecting increasing phonological organization via a problem-solving, hypothesis-forming process.

CONCLUSION

First language acquisition offers an informative look into the organizational world of the child. In order to understand this world, adults have categorized and subdivided the child's language in adult terms. But there is some danger in doing this. As adults, we may assume that children must be expressing either one of the intentions or meanings that an adult can express. This implies that children conceptualize the world and language as an adult does, and that children's motivation or communicative intent to use language is also adultlike. Actually, we don't know the child's meanings or purposes. We cannot assume that the salient features of an event that we might encode also have meaning for the child. In fact, as adults, we may be describing merely the products of the child's rule system and not analyzing the actual rules the child uses. For example, "the 'boy' in the utterance 'boy push truck' may be simply the first element in a perceived physical event" (McLean & Snyder-McLean, 1978, p. 37), rather than an agent.

The child's utterances are the result of a complex process that begins with the referents involved. In single-word utterances, the child's selection of lexical items seems to be strongly influenced by the pragmatic aspects of the communication context and by the concepts she can encode. Many words represent the child's very limited repertoire of phonetic elements. In addition, longer utterances follow simple ordering rules that express meaning. This rule system is independent of pragmatic rules and illocutionary functions but is strongly influenced by both in actual use.

During the second year of life, the child becomes more efficient in regulating social interactions through language; communication becomes more easily interpretable (Dunst &

Lowe, 1986; Wetherby, Cain, Yonclas, & Walker, 1988). By twenty-four months, the child can truly engage in conversations, initiating and maintaining topics, requesting information, and predicting and describing states and qualities (Bates et al., 1988). The child is more independent, secure, and autonomous and takes greater responsibility for communication interactions.

Although the child's language is different from the adult's, it is nonetheless a valid symbolic system for the child. It works for him or her within his or her world. First language acquisition is an important initial step in language development. Many of the relations the child has learned to express via a combination of gestures, vocalizations, single words, and word order are now ready for more adultlike linguistic forms.

DISCUSSION

Finally, the first word! You probably thought I'd never get to it. But don't worry, there's lots of book left.

Were you surprised by how much you knew about first words? If you went to the trouble to create your own fictitious list as I suggested, undoubtedly you had many of the same words as me. If you had other words, most probably you still had the same characteristics I outlined for sounds and syllable structure. Were you surprised by the similarities across languages?

Remember that toddlers talk about what they know. Choice of words is also constrained by the toddler's phonological repertoire, context, and culture. It only seems logical that the child's definitions would be different from your own, if for no other reason than that you have had so much more experience. What about the child with very little experience? What does he or she talk about? Sometimes children with severe handicapping conditions are sheltered from the world by well-meaning caregivers. Might the job of an SLP, psychologist, or teacher include experiential enhancement?

Because learning a word is more than just saying it, early meanings are very important and probably form the basis for early grammar. The semantic rules mentioned in Chapter 2 are once again seen in this chapter. Likewise, early pragmatic skills such as intentions, turn-taking, and presupposition are also important.

REFLECTIONS

1. First words follow predictable patterns. List the most frequent categories of first words and give some explanation for the things children talk about. Describe the syllable structure of first words.

2. Describe the various intentions toddlers express in their early vocalizations and verbalizations.

3. Compare the three hypotheses that have been advanced as explanations of early concept formation: semantic-feature, functional-core, and prototypic complex.

4. Children extend early words to novel examples. Describe the bases for most over- and underextensions and explain the possible uses of extensions by children.

5. List the linear word-order rules, based on semantic categories, that children follow when they begin to combine words, and give examples of each.

6. Three common phonological rules of toddlers are reduplication, open syllables, and consonant cluster reduction. Explain each and give an example.

7. Define the terms *agent* and *object*.

9

Preschool Pragmatic and Semantic Development

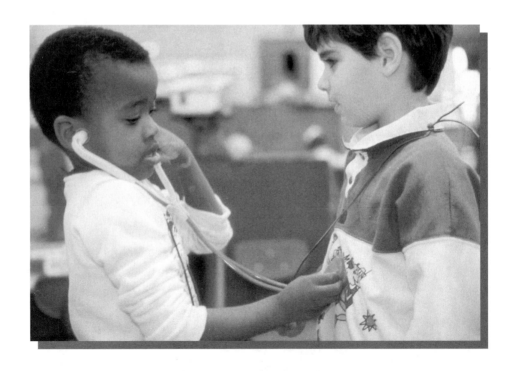

CHAPTER OBJECTIVES

Preschool language development is characterized by rapid changes in the use, content, and form of language. Children become real conversational partners and use their language to create context. In addition to learning new words, children learn the meaning of word relationships. When you have completed this chapter, you should understand

- conversational abilities of the preschool child.
- narrative development.
- lexical growth.
- development of relational terms.
- the following terms:

anaphoric reference	fast mapping
centering	narrative
chaining	narrative level
contingent query	register
deixis	script
ellipsis	topic
event structure	

The speed and diversity of language development during the preschool years are exciting. Within a few short years, the child moves from using simple multiword utterances to using sentences that approach adultlike form. This development is multidimensional and reflects the child's cognitive and socioemotional growth.

All aspects of language are related, and changes in one part of this complex system affect others. For example, increased vocabulary enables the preschooler to express a wider range of intentions.

Although we will not attempt to explain every detail of preschool language development, we will highlight in this chapter the major achievements within pragmatics and semantics. First, we will examine the social context of language development and the use of language within that context. Special attention will be given to conversational abilities and narrative development. Then we will explore semantic development, especially vocabulary and relational terms. These changes will be discussed as they relate to cognitive development.

PRAGMATIC DEVELOPMENT

In general, children learn language within a conversational context. For most children, the chief conversational partner is an adult, usually a parent. As children broaden their social networks to include those beyond the immediate family, they modify their self-esteem and self-image and become more aware of social standards (Cicchetti, 1989; Rutter, 1987). Their language reflects this larger network and the need for increased communicative clarity and perspective (Bretherton & Beeghly, 1982; Greenspan, 1988).

During the preschool years, the child acquires many conversational skills. Still, much of the child's conversation concerns the here and now, and he or she has much to learn about the conventional routines of conversation. Even though the child has learned to take turns, conversations are short and the number of turns is very limited. These skills will be refined during the school years.

Much of the child's conversation still occurs within the mother–child dialogue. This linguistic environment has a significant influence on language learning. Even though the child is becoming a fuller conversational participant, mother is still very much in control, creating and maintaining a semblance of true dialog (Kaye & Charney, 1981). This conversational asymmetry continues throughout the preschool period.

Conversational formats and routines provide a scaffolding or support for the child that frees cognitive processing for more linguistic exploration and experimentation. In part, scaffolding and increased cognitive abilities and knowledge enable the child to talk about nonpresent referents. This more decontextualized language emerges around eighteen to twenty-four months (Eisenberg, 1985; Sachs, 1983). When the mother discusses past or future events, she tends to rely on their shared knowledge of known, routinized, or scripted events. This event knowledge is the topic over 50 percent of the time. With their two- to two-and-a-half-year-olds, mothers talk about specific past events, such as going to the zoo, and future routine events, such as the upcoming bathtime (Lucariello, 1990)

In addition to conversation, the child engages in monologues. These self-conversations, with no desire to involve others, may account for 20 to 30 percent of the utterances of four-year-olds (Schober-Peterson & Johnson, 1991). Monologues can serve many purposes for preschoolers, such as self-guidance accompanying activity.

The presleep monologues of many children are rich with songs, sounds, nonsense words, bits of chitchat, verbal fantasies, and expressions of feelings. Some children engage in presleep self-dialog in which the child takes both parts.

Gradually, the child's monologues become more social. First, the child engages in them when others are nearby; later he or she will share a topic with a listener.

In general, throughout the preschool years, audible monologue behavior declines with age, but inaudible self-talk increases. Self-talk decreases after age ten but doesn't disappear. As adults, most of us still talk to ourselves occasionally, especially when we believe we are alone.

In the following sections, we shall explore the conversational context of preschool language development and the child's conversational abilities and describe the development of narration or storytelling.

The Conversational Context

In general, the two-year-old is able to respond to his or her conversational partner and to engage in short dialogs of a few turns on a given topic. The child can also introduce or change the topic of discussion. The young language-learning child is limited in the topics he or she can discuss. In addition, the two-year-old has limited conversational skills, although he or she learned turn-taking as an infant. Within mother–child conversations, the child begins to learn to maintain a conversational flow and to take the listener's perspective. The child is aided by mother's facilitative behaviors. In general, mother and child each engage in roughly 30 percent opening and 60 percent responding behaviors (Martlew, 1980). Initiating behaviors include introductions of a new topic, referrals to a previous one for the purpose of shifting the topic, and deliberate invitations for the partner to respond, such as a question. Responding behaviors include acknowledgments (*I see, uh-huh*), yes/no responses, answers, repetitions, sustaining or reformulated responses, and extensions. Mothers appear to be in control, however, and maneuver the conversation by inviting verbal responses (Martlew, 1980).

Child Conversational Skills

The young child is very good at introducing new topics in which interested but has difficulty sustaining that topic beyond one or two turns. Frequent introduction of topics results in few contingent responses by the child. Contingent speech is influenced by and dependent on the preceding utterance of the partner, as when one speaker replies to the other. Fewer than 20 percent of the preschooler's responses may be relevant to the partner's previous utterance (George & Krantz, 1981). This percentage increases with the child's age.

Taking a turn or building a bridge for the next and previous speaker's turns is especially difficult. By age three, the child can engage in longer dialogs beyond a few turns, although spontaneous speech is still easier than the contingent or connected speech found in conversations. Contingent speech is influenced by, and dependent on, the preceding utterance of the partner. With increased age, the child gains the ability to maintain a topic, which in turn results in fewer new topics being introduced within a given conversation. Nearly 50 percent of 5-year-olds can sustain certain topics through about a dozen turns. Whether or not they do depends on the topic, the partner, and the function of the child's talking. A sample of the speech and language of a three-year-old child is presented on track eight of the CD that accompanies this text. Compare this sample to the transcript of the speech of a thirty-three-month-old child presented in Table 14.2 of this text.

There is a large increase in the amount of verbal responding between ages twenty-four and thirty months. The thirty-month-old is, in addition, very successful at engaging the listener's attention and responding to listener feedback. There is an increase in overall talkativeness at around thirty-six months of age (Wells, 1985). Many three-year-olds and even more four-year-olds chatter away seemingly nonstop. The largest proportion of the speech is socially directed.

The two-year-old considers his conversational partner only in small measure by providing descriptive details to aid comprehension. He or she uses pronouns, however, without previously identifying the entity to which they refer, as in initiating a conversation with "I not like *it*." Between ages three and four, the child seems to gain a better awareness of the social aspects of conversation. In general, utterances addressed to conversational partners are clear, well-formed, and well-adapted for the listener. By age four, the child demonstrates a form of motherese when addressing very young children. This use of register or style is evidence of a growing awareness of conversational roles.

Becoming more aware of the listener's shared assumptions or presuppositions, the three- to four-year-old child uses more *elliptical* responses or responses that omit shared information. The child need not repeat shared knowledge contained in the partner's questions. If his mother asks, "What are you doing?" the child responds, "Playing," the *I am* being redundant information.

The two-year-old's language is used in imaginative ways and in expression of feeling, often "I'm tired." By age four, the child uses twice as many affective utterances as the child of three, discussing feelings and emotions (Martlew, 1980). My children constantly amazed me with their affective responses. Once, my four-year-old son Todd comforted an elderly neighbor at Christmas by stating, "I hope our lights will make you happy."

There is also a related shift in verb usage with less use of *go* and *do*. By age five, the child uses *be* and *do* predominantly (Bennett-Kaster, 1986). This change indicates that the child is speaking more about state, attitude, or feeling and less about action.

The preschool child appears to be aware of the conventions of turn-taking but does not use as many turnabout behaviors as adults. Although simultaneous vocalizations are common among infants and their mothers, by age two simultaneous talking has decreased significantly and the more mature alternating pattern found in conversations is predominant (Elias & Broerse, 1996). Conversational turn-taking between mothers and their two-to two-and-a-half-year-old children is very smooth (Kaye & Charney, 1981). Less than 5 percent of the turns of either participant are interrupted by the other partner. As the three-year-old becomes more aware of the social aspects of discourse, he or she acknowledges the partner's turn with fillers, such as *yeah* and *uh-huh*. Preschool children learning languages as different as Japanese and English find it easier to follow maternal linguistic cues to turn-taking, such as questions, than paralinguistic or phonetic cues (Miura, 1993).

Throughout the preschool period, about 60 percent of the child–partner exchanges are characterized by the child's attempts to control the partner's behavior or to relay information. Preschool boys are more likely than girls to use the word *no* to correct or prohibit a peer's behavior (Nohara, 1996). Girls use *no* more to reject or deny a playmate's proposition or suggestion. By kindergarten age, the child is able to cloak intentions more skillfully and to use indirect requests. The exchange of information has gained in importance throughout the preschool years, however, and by age four is clearly the most important function, accounting for nearly 40 percent of these exchanges (Wells, 1985). Other exchanges serve functions such as establishing and maintaining social relations, teaching, managing and correcting communication, expressing feelings, and talking to self. A sample of the speech and language of a four-year-old child is presented on track nine of the CD that accompanies this text. A transcript of the speech of two forty-eight-month-old children is presented in Table 14.3 of this text. Note the conversational interaction in this transcript. A five-year-old child is presented on track ten.

Register. By age four, children can assume various roles, especially in their play. Roles require different styles of speaking called **registers**. *Motherese*, discussed in Chapter 7, is a register. Children as young as age four demonstrate use of register when they use a form of motherese to address younger children.

Competence with different registers varies with age and experience (E. Anderson, 1992). The family register exhibited in the ability to play various family roles, such as mother or baby, appears early in play. Roles outside the family require more skill, possibly even technical-sounding jargon, as when playing a nurse, teacher, or auto mechanic. My five-year-old daughter loved to play beauty parlor using all the terms that accompanied that activity and using me as the customer. Younger children prefer familiar roles.

Pitch and loudness levels are the first variations used by children to denote differing roles (E. Anderson, 1992). For example, louder voices are used for adult males. Later variations include the average or mean length of the utterances and the choice of topics and vocabulary.

There are some gender differences. Girls assume more roles, speak more, and modify their register more to fit the roles. Due to socialization, boys may be more conscious of assuming gender roles that might be interpreted as inappropriate (E. Anderson, 1992).

One aspect of register is politeness, achieved by using polite words (*please, thank you*), a softer tone of voice, and more indirect requests (*May I have a cookie please?* instead of *Gimme a cookie*). Use of these devices varies with the conversational partner and with the age of the child. For example, two- to five-year-olds use more commands with other preschoolers and more permission requests (*Can I . . . , May I . . .*) with older children and adults. Imperatives also may be used with superiors, but their compliance, followed by a sly smile, indicates that the child knows he has scored a coup. Although even two-year-olds are capable of using *please* and a softer tone, it is not until age five that children recognize that indirect requests are more polite (McCloskey, 1986). This recognition occurs in other languages with indirect forms, such as Italian, at about the same age.

Contingent Queries. Young children use questions and contingent queries, or requests for clarification ("What?," "Huh?," "I don't understand"), to initiate or continue an exchange, but not to the extent that adults do when addressing young children. Approximately one-fourth of the contingent queries of two-year-olds are nonverbal, such as showing a confused expression (Gale, Liebergott, & Griffin, 1981). Nonverbal methods decrease as the primary means of communicating confusion as children mature.

Although two-and-a-half-year-olds are able to respond to requests for clarification, they do not respond consistently and do not resolve the breakdown at least 36 percent of the time when they do (Shatz & O'Reilly, 1990). Young preschoolers are more likely to respond, and with more success, to requests for clarification that follow their own requests for action rather than to those that follow their assertions or declarations. In general, these children are more motivated to have something happen than to be understood. They probably understand little about communication breakdown, but they recognize the need to maintain the conversational flow (Shatz, 1987).

Approximately one-third of preschoolers' clarification requests seek general or nonspecific information ("What?," "Huh?"). The child may lack the ability to state what is desired, however, in part because he or she has difficulty determining what is misunderstood. It is not until mid-elementary school that the child develops the ability to make well-informed specific requests for clarification.

The preschooler is not always successful in getting the message across because of difficulty detecting ambiguity. The preschooler is unable to reformulate the message in response to a facial expression of noncomprehension and must be specifically requested to clarify. The most common clarification strategy among preschoolers is a simple repetition, especially if the request is nonspecific, such as "Huh?" or "What?" The abilities to clarify and to organize information more systematically also do not develop until mid-elementary school.

Topic Introduction, Maintenance, and Closure. A topic can be defined as the content about which we speak. Topics are identified by name as they are introduced. You might say, "I had escargots last night," in an attempt to establish the topic of eating snails. I might reply, "Oh, did you like them?" We are sharing a topic. My reply was an agreement to accept the topic. Not all topics are as direct, and the listener may have to identify the topic by noting the central focus or central concern of the utterance. For example, the utterance "Well, what did you think of the rally last night?" might be used to establish several different topics, depending upon the manner in which it is stated.

In a larger sense, a topic is also the cohesion in the conversation. Through skillful manipulation, we as participants can make a conversation successful or unsuccessful (Maynard, 1980). For example, the topic of professional sports will work in conversation with many adult males; needlepoint, French cuisine, and American folk art may not. There are conversational partners, however, who could converse on any of these topics for hours.

Once introduced by identification, the topic is maintained by each conversational partner's commenting on the topic with additional information; altering the focus of the topic, called *shading*; or requesting more information. The topic is changed by introducing a new one, reintroducing a previous one, or ending the conversation. Obviously, topic development evolves in the context of conversations (Foster, 1986).

At first, the infant attracts attention to self as the topic. By age one, the child is highly skilled at initiating a topic by a combination of glances, gestures, vocalizations, and verbalizations, although he or she is limited to topics about items that are physically present. Typically, topics are maintained for only one or two turns at this age. Only about half of the utterances of children below age two are on the established topic. Child utterances on the topic usually consist of imitations of the adult or of new related information. Extended topic maintenance beyond a turn or two seems to be possible only within well-established routines. These routines, such as bathing or dressing, provide a structure for the discourse, thus relieving the young child of the (for now) nearly impossible task of conversational planning (Andersen & Kekelis, 1983).

By age two, the child is capable of maintaining a topic in adjacent pairs of utterances. These utterances follow a pattern, such as question/answer. The mature language partner usually offers the toddler choices, as in "Do you like candy or ice cream best?"; asks questions; or makes commands or offers. In this way, the mature partner interprets events for the child and scaffolds or structures the conversation for coherence (Foster, 1981; Kaye & Charney, 1981).

Between ages two and three, the child gains a limited ability to maintain coherent topics (Foster, 1986). By age three-and-a-half, about three-fourths of the child's utterances are on the established topic. Topics may last through more turns when children are enacting familiar scenarios or engaging in sociodramatic play, describing a physically present object or an ongoing event, and problem solving (Schober-Peterson & Johnson, 1989). Shorter topics may occur when capturing someone's attention, establishing a play situation, and ensuring cooperation while assigning toys or roles.

Repetition is one tactic used by preschoolers to remain on a topic. In the following conversation, the child imitates the adult skillfully:

> *Adult:* Later, we'll go to the store for daddy's birthday present.
> *Child:* Go store for daddy's present.
> *Adult:* Um-hum, should we get him a new electric razor?
> *Child:* Yeah, new razor.

Even five-year-olds continue to use frequent repetition to acknowledge, provide cohesion, and fill turns. Still, topics change quickly, and five-year-olds may discuss an average of fifty different topics within fifteen minutes (Brinton & Fujiki, 1984).

Presuppositional: Adaptation to the Listener's Knowledge. Presupposition, as we mentioned earlier, is the process whereby the speaker makes background assumptions about the listener's knowledge. This occurs on several levels. The speaker needs to be aware of the listener's word meanings, as well as his knowledge of the social context and the conversational topic. You and I can't have a meaningful conversation if you don't understand either the words I'm using or the topic. Every one of us has had to stop a speaker—usually someone close to us—at some time and say, "I don't have any idea what you're talking about." We didn't identify the topic.

In general, the preschool child becomes increasingly adept at knowing what information to include, how to arrange it, and which particular lexical items and linguistic forms to use. This ability emerges gradually on a usage-by-usage basis rather than as a single linguistic form (DeHart & Maratsos, 1984). Nonetheless, some linguistic forms are used as presuppositional tools. These include articles, demonstratives, pronouns, proper nouns, some verbs, *wh-* questions, and forms of address. The definite article (*the*), pronouns, demonstratives (*this, that, these, those*), and proper names refer to specific entities that, it is presupposed, both the speaker and the listener can identify. In addition, demonstratives and some pronouns must be interpreted from the speaker's physical location. For example, *I* always refers to the speaker and *you* to the listener(s). The speaker must presuppose that his listener understands this process.

The form of address used is based on presuppositions relative to the social situation. As speakers, we address only certain people as *dear* or *honey* or by their nicknames. These forms are not used with strangers or with people in positions of authority over us.

The choice of topic itself is based on an assumption of participant knowledge or at least interest. Once the topic is introduced, each participant generally presupposes that the other knows what the topic is, so there is no need to keep restating it. New topics or information are generally introduced in the final position or near the end of a sentence, marked with the indefinite article *a* or *an*, and emphasized to signal the listener.

Acquiring presuppositional skills requires learning to use many linguistic devices. Thus, the acquisition process extends well into school age.

Prior to age three, most children do not understand the effect of not providing enough information for their listener. By age three, however, they are generally able to determine the amount of information the listener needs (Bretherton & Beeghly, 1982; Shatz, Wellman, & Silber, 1983). Children usually mention the most informative items first, as in the following example:

> Adult: What happened yesterday?
> Child: I went to the doctor and got a needle. (Rather than "I got up, had breakfast, then brushed my teeth, and . . . ")

Three-year-olds are able to adjust their answers based on decisions of what the listener knows and does not know. Thus, the more knowledgeable listener receives even more information and more elaborate descriptions while receiving less redundant information.

Most three-year-olds also can distinguish between definite (*the*) and indefinite (*a, an*) articles. At this age, they use the articles with approximately 85 percent accuracy. If the preschooler makes errors in usage, it is usually because he or she has assumed erroneously that the listener shares the referent. For example, the child might say, "I liked *the* popsicle," without ever having mentioned it before. Thus, the definite article is used without first identifying the referent. This same error of assuming a shared referent is also evident in the use of pronouns. Even older preschool children will point to the referent rather than identify it verbally (VanHekken, Vergeer, & Harris, 1980). The referent may be even more ambiguous if it is not present.

Some verbs, such as *know* and *remember*, when used before a *that + clause* construction, presuppose the truthfulness of the clause that follows. In the following sentences, the speaker is conveying a belief in the truthfulness of the ending clause:

> I know that you have a red dress.
> I remember that the cat was asleep in this chair.

Not all verbs presuppose the truth of the following clause, such as in the case of "I think. . . . " In this instance, the speaker is not as certain as when he says, "I know. . . . "

Verbs such as *know, think, forget*, and *remember* are used correctly as presuppositional tools by age four. Prior to age four children use *think* and *know* to regulate an interaction (*You know how*) not to refer to a mental state (*I know my letters*). Children's use reflects that of their mothers (Furrow, Moore, Davidge, & Chiasson, 1992). By age five or six, the child understands the use of other verbs, such as *wish, guess*, and *pretend* (Moore, Harris, & Patriquin, 1993). These verbs presuppose that the following clause is false. Thus, when I say "I wish I had a pony," it is assumed that I do not. Verbs such as *say, whisper*, and *believe* are not comprehended by most children until age seven (Abbeduto & Rosenberg, 1985; DeHart & Maratsos, 1984; Moore et al., 1993).

Questions are used to gain more information about a presupposed fact stated in the clause. In the example "What are you eating?" it is presupposed that the listener is eating.

In "Where is the party?" the speaker presupposes that there is one and that the listener knows its location.

The presuppositions that accompany *wh-* questions seem to be learned with each *wh-* word. Children seem to be able to respond to specific *wh-* words even though they use these words infrequently in their own speech (Gallagher, 1981).

Through a process called **ellipsis**, the speaker omits redundant information that has been previously stated, thereby assuming that the listener knows this information. For example, in response to "Who is baking cookies?" the speaker says "I am," leaving out the redundant information "baking cookies."

The use of other devices, such as word order, stress, and ellipsis, also changes with age. At the two-word level, children initially place new information first, as in "Doggie eat," establishing *doggie* as the topic. This practice declines with longer, more adultlike utterances in favor of the more widely used last position, as in "Wasn't that a great picnic?", establishing *picnic* as the topic. Children use stress at the two-word stage to mark new information for the listener. With age, the child becomes even more reliable in his use of this device. In general, ellipsis is used more selectively and with greater sophistication as the child's language and conversations become more complex throughout the preschool years.

Directives and Requests. The purpose of directives and requests is to get others to do things for the speaker. Examples include:

Stop that! (direct)
Could you get the phone? (indirect, conventional)
Phew, it's hot in here. (indirect, nonconventional)

In the first example, the goal is clearly stated or direct. In the second, the form appears to be a question, although the speaker is not really interested in whether the listener has the ability to perform the task; the ability is assumed. Finally, in the third, an indirect nonconventional form, the goal is not mentioned and cannot be identified by strict syntactic interpretation.

By two years of age, the child is able to use some attention-getting words with gestures and rising intonation; however, he or she is usually unsuccessful at gaining attention (Ervin-Tripp, O'Connor, Rosenberg & O'Barr, 1984). The child tends to rely on less specific attention-getting forms, such as "Hey," often ignored by adults. Request words such as *more, want,* and *mine,* problem statements such as *I'm tired* and *I'm hungry,* and verbal routines are common (Newcombe & Zaslow, 1981). Two early directive types are the need statement ("I want/need a . . .") and the imperative ("Give me a . . ."). Few, if any, indirect forms are used. The child refers to the desired action or object. These requests become clearer with age, and the child identifies all elements of the request, not just what is desired.

Two- to three-year-olds make politeness distinctions based on the age or size, familiarity, role, territory, and rights of the listener. Often young children will use *please* in a request, especially if the listener is older or bigger, less familiar, in a dominant role, or possessor of an object or privilege desired (Ervin-Tripp & Gordon, 1986).

Action requests addressed to the child are likely to be answered with the action even when information is sought. Thus, when Grandma says, "Can you sing?" and is seeking a simple "yes" response, she may get a tuneful rendition that she didn't really want. Interpretation seems to be based on past experience and on the child's knowledge of object uses and locations, activity structures, and roles.

At age three, the child begins to use some modal auxiliary verbs in indirect requests ("*Could* you give me a . . . ?"), permissive directives ("*Can/may* I have a . . . ?"), and question directives ("*Do* you have a . . . ?"). Modals are auxiliary or helping verbs that express the speaker's attitude toward the main verb and include *may, might, must, could, should,* and so on. These forms reflect syntactic developments and the child's increasing skill at modifying language to reflect the social situation. These changes, especially the use of auxiliary verbs within interrogatives, enhance the child's skill at politeness and the use of requests.

The four-year-old is more skilled with indirect forms although still unsuccessful more than half of the time at getting someone else's attention (Ervin-Tripp et al., 1984). Only about 6 percent of all the requests by forty-two- to fifty-two-month-olds are indirect in nature. There is a sharp increase in the use of this form at around age four and a half (James & Seebach, 1982; L. Wilkinson, Calculator, & Dollaghan, 1982). Examples include "Why don't you . . . " and "Don't forget to. . . . " The child also offers more explanations and justifications for requests. At around age four, the child becomes more aware of the partner's point of view and role, and of the appropriate form of request and politeness required (D. Gordon & Ervin-Tripp, 1984). The four-year-old is able to respond correctly to forms such as "You should . . . ," "Please . . . ," and "I'll be happy if you . . . " (Carrell, 1981).

A desired goal may be totally masked in the five-year-old's directive. The form of the request may be very different from the child's actual intention. For example, desiring a glass of juice, the child might say, "Now, you be the mommy and make breakfast." Such inferred requests or other nonconventional forms are very infrequent, however, even in the language of five-year-olds. In general, the child relies on conventional, ritualized forms and the use of markers such as *please* (Ervin-Tripp & Gordon, 1986). The five-year-old continues to increase use of explanations and justifications, especially when there is a chance of noncompliance by the listener. Often the justifications are self-contained statements, such as "I need it" or "I want it," but they may refer to rights, reasons, causes, or norms. Justifications are initially found in children's attempts to stop an activity. My daughter gained neighborhood notoriety for her very precise "Stop it, because I do not like it!"

Although he has made tremendous gains, the preschooler is still rather ineffectual in making requests or in giving directives. He or she needs to become more efficient at gaining a potential listener's attention, more effective in stating the goal, more aware of social role, more persuasive, and more creative in forming requests. The increased complexity of the school-age child's social interactions and the new demands of the school environment require greater facility with directive and request forms.

Deixis. In ancient Greek, **deixis** means indicating or pointing. Deictic terms may be used to direct attention, to make spatial contrasts, and to denote times or participants in a conversation from the speaker's point of view. Thus, correct use of these terms indicates the child's pragmatic and cognitive growth. It is not easy for young children to adopt the perspective of another conversational participant. In this section, we discuss the development of *here/there*, *this/that*, and personal pronouns. As many as 30 percent of seven-year-olds may have difficulty comprehending some deictic contrasts, even those used in their own speech production.

The development of *this*, *that*, *here*, and *there* illustrates the difficulties inherent in learning these terms (Wales, 1986). Mothers use *that* and *there* more frequently than the other two, although children use all four more equally. Mothers use these terms most frequently in directing the child's attention. It is not surprising, then, that children use *that* and *there* for directing attention. *There* is also used to note completion.

Later, children use *this* and *here* for directing attention but make little differentiation based on the location of the object of interest. The child's comprehension is aided by the gestures used by adults.

Gradually, children begin to realize that these terms denote a contrast in location relative to the speaker. Adult gestures are no longer depended on for interpretation. Children still experience difficulty with the actual size of the area covered by terms such as *here*. This is made more difficult by the fact that this term can be used for a variety of references, from "Come *here*," meaning this very spot, to "We have an environmental problem *here*," meaning on the entire earth.

There are three problems in the acquisition of deictic terms: point of reference, shifting reference, and shifting boundaries. The point of reference is generally the speaker. Hence, when you use the term *here*, you are speaking of a proximal or near area. The child must learn two principles in order to understand the point of reference (E. Clark & Sengul, 1978). These principles—the *speaker principle* and the *distance principle*—also relate to the problem of shifting reference and boundaries. First, the speaker principle states that the speaker is the point of reference. This introduces a potential problem, since the reference point, each new speaker, creates a new *I*. Terms that shift most frequently seem to be the hardest to learn. The *I* shifts to each new speaker, although this is limited usually to one person at a time. The *you* refers to any other conversational partner(s), and the *he* or *she* to any third party, a seemingly endless choice. This hierarchy describes the developmental sequence *I* before *you*, followed by *he* and *she*. Even the initial use of *he* and *she* may be based more on gender than on the deictic role fulfilled (Brener, 1983).

Pairs such as *this/that* and *here/there* contrast distance dimensions. The boundaries of these dimensions shift with the context and are not generally stated by the speaker. For example, the term *here* has very different boundaries in the following two sentences:

Put your money here, please.
We have a democratic form of government here.

At least one deictic term—*here*, *there*, *this*, or *that*—is usually present in the first-fifty-word lexicon of most children. Adverbs such as *here* and *this* are proximal to the speaker, while *there* and *that* may be anywhere else. The distance principle states that proximal terms should thus be easier to learn.

Some pronoun contrasts develop prior to spatial deictic terms. The contrasts *I/you* and *my/your* develop relatively early. The two-and-a-half-year-old can comprehend and produce *I*, *you*, and *he* (Tanz, 1980). These terms may be easier to learn than spatial contrasts because of the relatively distinct boundaries. The pronoun meaning is integral to the concept of person (Tanz, 1980).

There appear to be three phases of acquisition of deictic terms (E. Clark & Sengul, 1978). In the initial phase, there is no contrast between the different dimensions. As previously discussed, terms such as *here* and *there* are used for directing attention or for referencing. In other words, deictic terms are used nondeictically. Among two-and-a-half-year-olds, deictic words seem to be used indiscriminately, with a gesture to indicate meaning. Because there are no definitive boundaries between terms such as *here* and *there*, it is difficult to determine the child's concept. No difference between the use of *this* and *that* may be found as late as age four. In the no-contrast phase, children tend to employ one of four possible strategies of comprehension (E. Clark & Sengul, 1978). All deictic terms are interpreted as being (a) near the speaker, (b) far from the speaker, (c) near the child, or (d) far from the child. Children seem to prefer to use themselves or a near point as reference.

The second phase is characterized by a partial contrast. The child frequently uses the proximal term (*this*, *here*) correctly but overuses it for the nonproximal (*that*, *there*). An alternative pattern is characterized by correct child use only in reference to self or to some inconsistent point.

In the final phase, the child masters the full deictic contrast. The age of mastery differs for the various contrasts, and many children continue to produce deictic errors beyond age four. In general, mastery of *here/there* precedes mastery of *this/that*, possibly because the concept of *here/there* is an integral part of the latter pair. Even a large number of seven-year-olds have difficulty comprehending some deictic contrasts, although they use them in their speech. In contrast, terms such as *in front of* and *in back of* are mastered by age four (Tanz, 1980). Less precise terms, such as *beside* and *behind*, develop later. Mastery of the adult system of deixis requires several years.

Intentions

As might be expected from the preceding sections, the child's language intentions are increasing in number and diversity. By about thirty months, the relative frequency of the six large pragmatic categories (Wells, 1985)—representational, control, expressive, procedural, social, and tutorial, found in Table 8.2—stabilizes throughout the rest of the preschool period. The control and representational functions account for 70 percent of all child utterances. Table 9.1 lists the major intentions mastered by preschoolers.

The representational category is dominated by the *statement* function, which gradually increases to 50 percent of all representational utterances and roughly 20 percent of all utterances by age five. The earlier dominance of *naming* in toddler language no longer exists, and these utterances, as might be expected, account for very few representational utterances by age five. Other representational functions used by at least 90 percent of five-year-olds include *content questions* ("What . . . ?", "Where . . . ?"), *content responses* or answers, and *yes/no questions* ("Is this a cheeseburger?") (Wells, 1985). Among thirty-month-olds, statements or assertions may outnumber direct requests by as much as three to one (Golinkoff, 1993).

TABLE 9.1   Intentions Exhibited by 90 Percent of Children

INTENTION	AGE AT WHICH 90% OF CHILDREN USE INTENTION (IN MONTHS)
Exclamation and call	18
Ostention (naming)	21
Wanting, direct request, and statement	24
Content question	30
Prohibition, intention, content response, expressive state, and elicited repetition	33
Yes/no question, verbal accompaniment, and contingent query	36
Request permission	45
Suggestion	48
Physical justification	54
Offer and indirect request	57

Source: Adapted from Wells (1985).

Within the control function, there is great diversity. The *wanting* function that domi-nated in toddler language decreases rapidly after twenty-four months of age. In contrast, *direct requesting* continues a slow increase until around thirty-nine months, when its fre-quency levels off at 25 percent of all control utterances and remains the dominant control function throughout the preschool years. Other control intentions or illocutionary functions used by at least 90 percent of five-year-olds include *prohibition* ("Don't do that"), *intention* ("I'm going to put it in"), *request permission* ("Can I have one?"), *suggestion* ("Should we have ice cream?"), *physical justification* ("I can't 'cause the dollie's there"), *offer* ("Do you want this one?"), and *indirect request* ("Will you pour the juice?") (Wells, 1985).

Expressive functions used by at least 90 percent of five-year-olds include *exclamation*, *expressive state*, and *verbal accompaniment*, all noted previously in toddler language. Proce-dural functions used by at least 90 percent of five-year-olds include *call*, *contingent query*, and *elicited repetition*, in which the child repeats the speaker's utterance with a rising into-nation ("Daddy will be home soon?"↑). Finally, the *social* and *tutorial* functions together account for less than 4 percent of the child's utterances at age five.

Narratives

Oral narratives are an uninterrupted stream of language modified by the speaker to capture and hold the listener's interest. Unlike a conversation, the narrator maintains a social mono-logue throughout, producing language relevant to the overall narrative while presupposing the information needed by the listener. **Narratives** include self-generated stories, telling of familiar tales, retelling of movies or television shows, and recounting of personal experiences. Most conversations include narratives of this latter type, often beginning with "You'll never believe what happened to me on the way to work. . . . " Common in the conversations of preschoolers, narratives aid children in constructing their own autonomous selves as portrayed in their stories (Wiley, Rose, Burger, & Miller, 1998).

Although conversation and narratives share many elements, such as a sense of purpose, relevant information, clear and orderly exchange of information, repair, and the ability to assume the perspective of the listener, they differ in very significant ways. Conversations are dialogues, while narratives are essentially decontextualized monologues. *Decontextualization* means that the language does not center on some immediate experience within the context.

Narratives contain organizational patterns not found in conversation. In order to share the experience, the speaker must present an explicit, topic-centered discussion that clearly states the relationships between events. Thus, events are linked to one another in a predictable manner.

Narratives usually have an agentive focus, which means that they concern people, animals, or imaginary characters engaged in events (Longacre, 1983). Conversations usually involve activities in the immediate context.

Other differences include the narrative use of extended units of text; introductory and organizing sequences that lead to a narrative conclusion; and the relatively passive role of the listener, who provides only minimal informational support in our culture (Roth, 1986). The narrative speaker is responsible for organizing and providing all of the information in an organized whole (Roth & Spekman, 1985). It is not surprising, therefore, that narratives are found more frequently in the communication of more mature speakers.

Possibly even more than conversations, narratives reflect the cultures from which they emerge. Within the United States, middle-class children are encouraged to elaborate on their own experiences and to express opinions on these experiences. In contrast, working-class children are also encouraged to tell personal narratives but are not automatically given the right to express their own views or opinions (Wiley, et al., 1998).

Japanese and American children differ in the length of personal narratives. Japanese children tend to speak succinctly about collections of experiences, while children from the United States were more likely to elaborate on one experience (Minami & McCabe, 1991). A possible link may be found in maternal speaking styles. Japanese mothers request less information from their children, give less evaluation, and show more verbal attention (Minami & McCabe, 1995). In response, the conversational turns of Japanese children are shorter than those of children from the United States.

Development of Narratives

Before the appearance of first words, children have some understanding of familiar events and of the positions of some actions at the beginning, middle, and end of sequences (DeLemos, 1981). Although two-year-olds possess basic patterns for familiar events and sequences, called *scripts*, they are not able to describe sequences of events accurately until about age four (Karmiloff-Smith, 1981; Peterson & McCabe, 1983). Nonetheless, children as young as age two to three-and-a-half talk about things that have happened to them. These early *protonarratives* have five times as much evaluative information ("I didn't like it," "It was yukky," "I cried," "I hate needles.") as their regular conversation. Between ages two and two-and-a-half, the number of these protonarratives doubles, and children begin to sequence events with very little help from others (P. Miller & Sperry, 1988).

The overall organization of a narrative is called the **narrative level**. In general, children use two strategies for organization: centering and chaining. **Centering** is the linking of entities to form a story nucleus. Although causal links are not present, sequential ones may be. Links may be based on similarity or complementarity of features. *Similarity* links are formed using observable attributes, such as actions, characteristics, scenes, or situations. *Complementary* links consist of conceptual bonds based on abstract, logical attributes, such as members of a class or events linked by cause-and-effect bonds. **Chaining** consists of a sequence of events that share attributes and lead directly from one to another.

Children begin to tell self-generated, fictional narratives between two and three years of age (Sutton-Smith, 1986). Most of the stories of two-year-olds are organized by centering. The stories usually center on certain highlights in the child's life and may have a vague plot. The theme is usually some disquieting event in the child's life. Frequently, children tell of events that they find disruptive or extraordinary. Considering the listener only minimally, the child demonstrates little need to introduce, to explore with, or to orient the audience. Thus, these stories often lack easily identifiable beginnings, middles, and ends.

By age three, however, nearly half of the children use both centering and chaining. This percentage increases, and by age five, nearly three-fourths of the children use both strategies.

Initially, identification of the participants, time, and location may be nonexistent or minimal. Although these elements improve with maturity, even children of three-and-a-half may not identify all story participants (Peterson, 1990). In part, this may result from the fact that most stories involve individuals well-known to the child and to most listeners, thus there is no need to identify them. A sense of time frame is also vague or nonexistent initially but improves with the use of terms such as *yesterday* or *last year*, even though these terms may be used inaccurately. Location is more commonly identified, especially when the narrative events occurred in the home. With maturity, children become better able to identify out-of-home locations.

The organizational strategies of two-year-olds represent centering *heaps* or sets of unrelated statements about a central stimulus, consisting of one sentence added to another. The statements provide additional information or identify aspects of the stimulus. Although there is no overall organizational pattern, there may be a similarity in the grammatical structure of the sentences:

> The doggie go "woof." The cow go "moo." The man ride tractor—
> "Bpt-bpt-bpt."

There is no central focus, no story line, no sequencing, and no cause and effect. The sentences may be moved anywhere in the text without changing the overall meaning. Heaps may also be used to describe a scene.

Somewhat later, children begin to tell narratives characterized as centering *sequences*. These include events linked on the basis of similar attributes or events that create a simple but meaningful focus for a story. The organization is additive, not temporal or time-based, and sentences may be moved without altering the narrative:

> I ate a hamburger (Mimes eating). Mommy threw the ball, like this. Daddy took me swimming (Moves hand, acts silly). I had two sodas.

In these early stories, there is a dominance of performance and textual qualities, such as movement, sound production, and prosody (Scollon & Scollon, 198; Sutton-Smith, 1986). Gradually, between ages three and seven years, children's narratives increase in the use of prose and plots.

Temporal or time-based event chains emerge between ages three and five years. Events follow a logical sequence. *Primitive temporal narratives* are organized around a center with complementary events:

> We went to the parade. There was a big elephant. And tanks (Moves arm like turret). The drum was loud. There was a clown in a little car (Hand gestures "little"). And I got a balloon. And we went home.

Although there is sequencing, there is no plot and no cause and effect or causality.

Event description, such as explaining how to make cookies, involves more than describing single events in a sequential order. To describe sets of event sequences called **event structures**, the speaker must be able to describe single events and event combinations and relationships and to indicate the significance of each event within the overall event structure.

Event structures or descriptions of entire events are based on a framework of scripts. Scripts based on actual events form an individual's expectations about sequences and impose order on event information (Johnston, 1982). These familiar activity sequences or scripts consist of ordered events within routine or high-frequency, regularized activities. As such, scripts influence interpretation and telling of events and narratives. By age three, children are able to describe chains of events within familiar activities, such as a birthday party (Nelson, 1981b). Theoretically, scripts are similar across members of the same culture based on their common experiences.

The speaker must have knowledge of both single events and connected event sequences, the linguistic knowledge of the method for describing events, and the linguistic skill to consider the listener's perspective (Duchan, 1986). Linguistic devices that speakers use include marking of event beginnings and endings, marking of perfective and imperfective aspect, and modal verbs. Beginnings can be marked by words or phrases such as *once upon a time, guess what happened to me, let's start at the beginning,* and so on. Endings include *the end, all done,* and *and that's how it happened.* Aspect and modal verbs will be explained in detail in Chapter 10.

The elements of event knowledge are seen in the narratives of four-year-olds. Underlying every story is an *event chain.* Events include actions, physical states such as possession and attribution, and mental states such as emotions, dispositions, thoughts, and intentions that are causally linked as motivations, enablements, initiations, and resultants in the chain. Causal explanations contain many of these same features.

Narratives characterized as *unfocused temporal chains* lead directly from one event to another while other attributes—characters, settings, and actions—shift. This is the first level of chaining, and the links are concrete. As a result of the shifting focus, unfocused chains have no centers:

> The man got in the boat. He rowed. A big storm knocked over the trees—
> whish-sh, boom. The doggie had to swim. Fishies jumped out of the water.
> He had warm milk. And then he went to bed.

Temporal chains frequently include third-person pronouns (*he, she, it*); past-tense verbs; temporal conjunctions such as *and, then,* and *and then*; and a definite beginning and ending.

Focused temporal or causal chains generally center on a main character who goes through a series of perceptually linked, concrete events:

> There is this horsie. He eats—munch, munch—hay for breakfast. He runs
> out of the barn. Then he plays in the sun. He rolls in the warm grass. He
> comes in for dinner. He sleeps in a bed (Mimes sleep).

Causal chains, in which one event causes or has caused another, are infrequent until age five.

By the time children begin school, most have acquired the basic elements of narratives and can recount sequentially familiar or significant events. These narratives form much of the content of the conversations later encountered in older children and adults.

Summary

Although there is a considerable difference among families in the overall amount of talking, there are certain overall patterns. The amount of talking is a function of the energy level of the child and his conversational partners. Therefore, the largest proportion of talking occurs in the morning shortly after breakfast (Wells, 1985). The amount of talking is also related to the activity in progress. Most speech accompanies solitary play or play with others or occurs within activities devoted primarily to conversation. The amount of talking within these latter activities increases throughout the preschool years. In contrast, very little talking occurs while either game or role playing, looking at books or television, or doing chores (Wells, 1985). In general, preschool boys play more alone, talking to themselves and calling bystanders to notice this play. In contrast, girls engage more in household activities and are drawn into talk while organizing the task at hand (Wells, 1985). The conversational context is dynamic, influencing what is said and, in turn, being influenced by it.

Throughout the preschool years, the child learns to become a truer conversational partner, using a greater variety of forms to attain desired ends. In addition, the child expands presuppositional skills and is better able to take the perspective of the other participant. Although he or she takes conversational turns without being prompted with a question, the child still tends to make more coherent contributions to the conversation if discussing an ongoing activity in which engaged at the time. The child is more aware of social roles at age five than at age two and can adjust his or her speech for younger children (Shatz & Gelman, 1973) or for role playing, but lacks many of the subtleties of older children and adults. As he or she begins to attend school, the child will be under increasing pressure by both teachers and peers to use language even more effectively.

SEMANTIC DEVELOPMENT

The preschool period is one of rapid lexical and relational concept acquisition. There is even some indication that preschoolers with larger vocabularies are more popular with their peers (Gertner, Rice, & Hadley, 1994). It is estimated that the child adds approximately five words to his or her lexicon every day between the ages of one and a half and six years. Word meanings are inferred without direct teaching by adults.

It is possible that the preschool child employs a **fast-mapping** strategy that enables him or her to infer a connection between a word and its referent after only one exposure (Pinker, 1982). How much the child stores through fast mapping is unknown, but initial acquisition may be receptive rather than expressive in nature (Dollaghan, 1985; Holdgrafer & Sorenson, 1984). Obviously, only a small portion of the overall meaning will be available for mapping into the child's memory. The information actually mapped is affected by both the world and word knowledge of the child.

Fast mapping may be the first in a two-step process of lexical acquisition. First, the child roughs out a tentative definition connecting the word and available information. This step may be followed by an extended phase in which the child gradually refines the definition with new information acquired on subsequent encounters. Comprehension and production are achieved separately (Dollaghan, 1985). Retrieval may be affected by the nature of the referent, the frequency of exposure to the word, the form and content of the utterance in which it occurs, and the context (Crais, 1987; Dickinson, 1984).

Verbs may be initially mapped based on the types of morphological endings applied (Behrend, Harris, & Cartwright, 1995). Children tend to use the -ing ending on action verbs and -ed on verbs denoting results of events. In order to generalize verb meanings, chidren must be able to dissociate the verb itself from the agent and to extend the verb to other outcomes and manners of action (Forbes & Poulin-DuBois, 1997).

Most likely, young children learn single words as unique units, each with its own meaning, probably unrelated to other word meanings. Although these word meanings lack relationship, the system is simple and easy to use.

Children may use two operating principles to establish meanings: *contrast* and *conventionality* (E. Clark, 1990; Gathercole, 1989). Contrast is the assumption that every form—morpheme, word, syntactic structure—contrasts to every other in meaning. A speaker chooses a form because it means something other than what some other expression means. In other words, it contrasts to other options. Conventionality is the expectation that certain forms will be used to convey certain meanings.

Taken together, the two principles predict that, whenever possible, speakers will use established forms with conventional meanings that contrast clearly to other forms. Difficulty occurs when a well-established form has a meaning similar to that of a newly learned form. Thus, it may be easier for children to have unrelated unique meanings initially.

Preschoolers' noun definitions often include physical properties, such as shape, size, and color; functional properties or what the entity does; use properties, and locational properties, such as *on trees* or *at the beach*. Often missing are superordinate categories, as in *a car is a vehicle*; relationships to other entities, as in *a mouse is much smaller than a cat*; internal constituents, as in *an apple has seeds inside*; origins, as in *hatch from eggs*; and metaphorical uses, as in *suspicious things are called "fishy"* (Anglin, 1985). Adult and older school-age children's definitions contain all these elements.

Preschool verb definitions also differ from those of adults or older children. The preschooler can explain who or what does the action, to what or whom it's done, and where, when, and with what it's done. Usually missing is how and why it's done and a description of the process.

New word meanings come from both the linguistic and nonlinguistic contexts (Au, 1990) and from the surrounding syntactic structure (Naigles, 1990). Let's assume that a child hears the following sentence: "Bring me the *chromium* tray, not the red one" (Gathercole, 1989, p. 694). He might proceed through the following steps to differentiate the meaning:

1. Assume that Mommy is trying to communicate with me.
2. Unknown word used in reference to trays as descriptor.
3. Only observable difference between the trays is color.
4. Chromium must be a color.
5. One tray is red.
6. Must not have wanted red tray or would have asked for it.
7. Therefore, must want other than red tray, which is chromium in color.

Children also expand their vocabularies through parental storybook reading. Especially helpful for children are the contextual discussions that accompany the narrative (Senechal, 1997). Even low levels of language participation, such as naming and describing, as well as reasoning and making inferences, can have a positive effect on the child's subsequent language use (van Kleeck, Gillam, Hamilton, & McGrath, 1997).When gaps exist in preschoolers' vocabularies either because they've forgotten or never knew a word, children invent words (E. Clark, 1981). For example, verbs might be created from nouns to produce the following:

I'm *spooning* my cocoa. (Stirring)
You *sugared* your coffee. (Sweetened)

In the preschoolers' defense, English allows this practice with some nouns, as in *paddling a canoe*, *shoeing a horse*, and *suiting up*, to name a few. Production of invented words seems to follow from children's construction of compound words, as in *doghouse*, *birdhouse*, and *fishhouse* (aquarium) (E. Clark, Gelman, & Lane, 1985). Production demonstrates recognition of word formulation.

Most invented words reflect adult practices, that is, *fisherman* and *policeman* are reflected in *cookerman* (chef) and *pianoman* (pianist), or overgeneralization, that is, *house-houses* extended to *mouse-mouses*.

As the child's lexicon expands, the need for better organization increases and some semantic networks or interrelationships are formed. Relationships may consist of words for referents found in the same context, such as *spoon, bowl, cup,* and *table,* or word associations, such as *stop and go, rise and shine,* and *red, white, and blue.* Preschoolers demonstrate these relationships in their inappropriate use of words and in word substitutions, such as using *spoon* to refer to a fork.

Relational Terms

The acquisition of relational terms, such as those for location and time, is a complex process. In general, the order of acquisition is influenced by the syntactic complexity, the amount of adult usage in the child's environment, and the underlying cognitive concept. We shall briefly consider interrogatives or questions, temporal relations, physical relations, locational prepositions, and kinship terms.

Interrogatives

Children's responses to different types of questions and their production of these same types have a similar order of development. Early question forms include *what* and *where,* followed by *who, whose,* and *which,* and finally by *when, how,* and *why.* Most of the later forms involve concepts of cause, manner, or time. Their late appearance can be traced to the late development of these concepts. In other words, the child must have a concept of time in order to comprehend *when* or to answer *when* questions. Occasionally, however, the child responds to or asks questions without fully understanding the underlying meaning. The child may be employing the following two answering strategies (Tyack & Ingram, 1977):

1. If you have already acquired a particular question word, answer with an appropriate subject.
2. If you have not acquired the word, answer on the basis of the semantic features of the verb.

Observing the first principle, the child would respond to "When are you going to eat?" with some temporal comment. Unaware of the meaning of *when,* the child might use the second strategy and respond, on the basis of the verb, "A cookie!"

Semantic features of the verb are particularly important for certain types of child responses. For example, the verb *touch* is more likely to elicit a response focusing on what was touched, where it was touched, and for what reason. Other verbs elicit different responses, with little regard for the *wh-* question form employed.

Recognition of the general type of information requested may precede the ability to give acceptable and accurate answers (Parnell, Patterson, & Harding, 1984). Even young school-age children have difficulty answering some forms of *wh-* questions.

Causal questions may be especially difficult for the child because of the reverse-order thinking required in the response. The three-year-old child experiences difficulty reversing the order of sequential events. Yet it is this type of response that is required for the *why* interrogative. For example, "Why did you hit Randy?" requires a response explaining the events that preceded the fist fight. It is not unusual to hear a three-year-old respond " 'Cause he hit me back," demonstrating an inability to reverse the order.

Temporal Relations

Temporal terms such as *when*, *before*, *since*, and *while* can convey information on the order of events, duration, and simultaneity. The order of acquisition of these terms is related to their use and to the concept each represents. In general, words of order, such as *after*, *before*, *since*, and *until*, precede words of duration, such as *since* and *until*, used with the progressive verb tense (*eating, running, jumping*). These, in turn, precede terms of simultaneity, such as *while* (Feagans, 1980). This hierarchy reflects a sequence of cognitive development. Preschool children gain a sense of order before they have a sense of duration. Five-year-olds understand *before* and *after* better than simultaneous terms such as *at the same time* (see Table 9.2).

Temporal terms are initially produced as prepositions and then as subordinating conjunctions. Thus, the child will produce a sentence such as "You go *after* me" before he says "You can go home *after* we eat dinner." It is not uncommon for six-and-a-half-year-olds to have difficulty with some of the syntactic structures used with *before* and *after* to link clauses (Tibbits, 1980).

When the meaning of a temporal term is unknown, the child tends to use two strategies of interpretation. He or she will (1) rely on the order of mention and (2) interpret the main clause as the first event. The first strategy reflects the ease of interpretation of sequences that preserve the actual order of events (E. Clark, 1971; L. French & Brown, 1977; Hatch, 1971; H. Johnson, 1975). Employing this strategy, a three-year-old will interpret the following sentences as all having the same meaning:

> Before you go to school, stop at the store.
> Go to school before you stop at the store.
> After you go to school, stop at the store.
> Go to school after you stop at the store.

Note that the desired order of occurrence of events is the reverse of the word order stated in the first and last examples.

TABLE 9.2 Summary of Comprehension of Locational and Temporal Relationships

AGE (MONTHS)	RELATIONSHIPS UNDERSTOOD
24	Locational prepositions *in* and *on*
36	Locational preposition *under*
40	Locational preposition *next to*
48 (approx.)	Locational prepositions *behind*, *in back of*, and *in front of*; difficulty with *above*, *below*, and *at the bottom of*; kinship terms *mother*, *father*, *sister*, and *brother* (last two are nonreciprocating)
60	Temporal terms *before* and *after*
60+ (school-age)	Additional locational prepositions in temporal expressions, such as *in a week*; most major kinship terms by age ten; more precise locational directives reference the body (*left* and *right*)

The second interpretive strategy reflects a syntactic approach. Difficulties of interpretation with *before* and *after* may reflect syntactic difficulties in processing subordinate clauses. Thus, the child adopts a strategy in which the main clause becomes the first event. For example, the sentence "After he arrived home, Oz bought a paper" would be interpreted as "Oz bought a paper, then he arrived home." The main clause precedes the subordinate in a temporal sequence. Subordinate clauses are discussed in more detail in Chapter 10.

When all else fails, the child relies on knowledge of real-life sequences. This strategy of comprehension works as long as the utterance conforms to the child's experiential base.

Children three-and-a-half to five years of age often omit one of the clauses when following directives. This behavior may be more common than order reversal and may reflect the cognitive-processing load. Preschoolers generally do not follow multiple directions well.

Physical Relations

Relational terms such as *thick/thin*, *fat/skinny*, *more/less*, and *same/different* are frequently difficult for preschool children to learn. In general, the child first learns that the terms are opposites, then the dimensions to which each term refers. The order of acquisition may be based on semantic–syntactic relations and the cognitive relations expressed. Terms such as *big* and *little* refer to general size on any dimension and would be acquired before more specific terms, such as *deep* and *shallow*. In other words, less specific terms are usually learned first.

The positive member, such as *big* or *long*, of each relational pair, as in *big/little* and *long/short*, represents the presence of the entity that it describes (size and length, respectively) and is learned first. There may be a conceptual basis for the prominence of the positive element. For example, the presence of size is *big*, the positive term. The negative aspect or the absence of size is *little*. A general order of acquisition is presented in Table 9.3.

The child seems to learn by accumulating individual examples of each term. Hence, understanding may be restricted to specific objects even if it appears to be more adultlike. General terms may also become more restricted as the child learns more specific ones.

Learning and interpretation of descriptive terms is dependent on context. For example, two-year-olds understand *big* and *little* used in comparing the size of two objects or

TABLE 9.3   Order of Acquisition of Physical Relationships

Hard/soft
Big/little, heavy/light
Tall/short, long/short
Large/small
High/low
Thick/thin
Wide/narrow
Deep/shallow

judging an object's size for a particular task. It is more difficult for the child to recall the size of a stored mental image.

Terms such as *more/less* and *same/different* pose a different problem for the preschool child. There may be an underlying concept for *more/less* in which the child interprets both terms to mean amount. When presented with a selection task, preschoolers tend to pick the larger grouping, whether cued with *more* or with *less*. In general, the child's concept of relative number appears to be based on varied criteria.

Conceptual development seems equally important for the acquisition of *same* and *different*. The ability to make same/different judgments seems to be related to development of *conservation*, the ability to attend to more than one perceptual dimension without relying strictly on physical evidence.

Locational Prepositions

The child understands different spatial relations before beginning to speak about them. The exact nature of that comprehension is unknown, since a child as old as three-and-a-half still relies on gestures to convey much meaning (Tfouni & Klatsky, 1983). The first

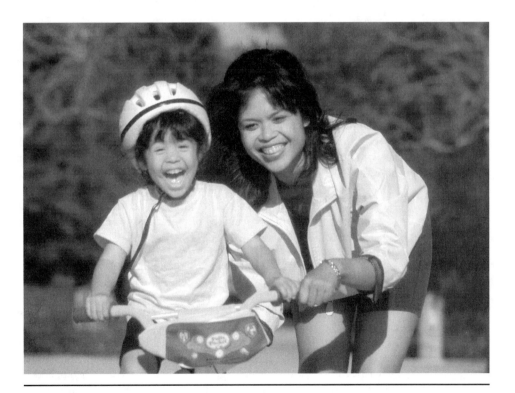

Interactions while riding a trike can teach the child spatial concepts, such as on, off, up, and down; *adjectives, such as* fast *and* slow; *verbs, such as* balance; *and the names of common objects.*

English prepositions appear at around two years of age. When a child does not comprehend a preposition, he or she seems to apply a few general interpretive strategies (E. Clark, 1973a):

> *Rule 1:* If B is a container, A belongs inside it.
> *Rule 2:* If B is a supporting surface, A belongs on it.

Rule 1 takes precedence since containers, whatever their orientation, always seem to be treated as containers. Using a "probable event strategy," children may respond in relation to the objects mentioned rather than the prepositions used. Other possible interpretive cues may be the word order of adult utterances and the context. Using these rules, children respond in predictable ways.

Children eighteen months of age base their hypotheses about word meanings on Rules 1 and 2. As a result, they act as if they understand *in* all the time, *on* with surfaces but not containers, and *under* not at all. By age three, most children have figured out the meanings of all three prepositions. When three- and four-year-olds are faced with more complex prepositions such as *above, below, in front of,* or *at the bottom of,* however, they tend to revert to strategies based on Rules 1 and 2.

Vertical alignment, however, does not result in the confusion found with other spatial relations. Terms such as *next to* or *in front of* offer special problems. For example, *next to* includes, but is not limited to, *in front of, behind,* and so on. In turn, these terms differ in relation to the locations to which they refer. With fronted objects, such as a chair or a television set, locational terms take their reference from the object. For example, *in front of the TV* means *in front of the screen.* With nonfronted objects, such as a saucer, the term takes its location from the speaker's perspective. Interpretation requires a certain level of social skill on the part of the listener, who must be able to adopt the perspective of the speaker. *Next to* is usually learned at about forty months, followed by *behind, in back of* and *in front of* by about forty-nine months (Johnston, 1984) (see Table 9.2). Children seem to use fronting and the height of the object as cues for initial interpretation.

Movement between locations seems to be interpreted using a locational rule. A three-year-old child interprets most prepositions of movement to mean *toward.* This preference can be characterized as follows:

> *Rule 3:* If A and B are related to each other in space, they should be touching.

Hence, the child at first favors *to* over *from, into* over *out of,* and *onto* over *off.*

Applying these rules, we can predict that *in* is easier for the child than *on,* which in turn is easier than *under.* Terms that signal movement *toward* should be easier than their opposites. These predictions reflect the acquisitional order seen in young children.

Syntactic form may also affect acquisition. Prior to age four, *in, on,* and *over* often are used predominantly as prepositions for object location while *up, down,* and *off* are used as verb particles. A *verb particle* is a multiword grammatical unit that functions as a verb, such as *stand up, sit down,* and *take off.*

TABLE 9.4   Order of Acquisition of Kinship Terms

Mother, father, sister, brother
Son, daughter, grandfather, grandmother, parent
Uncle, aunt, cousin, nephew, niece

Kinship Terms

The preschooler gains a very limited knowledge of kinship terms that refer to family members, such as *dad*, *sister*, and *brother*. At first the child treats the term as part of the person's name. For a short time, my children called me "daddybob." In this stage the child does not possess the components of the kinship term. Terms are described in relation to specific individuals and with reference to the child's personal experience (Benson & Anglin, 1987).

Next, the child gains some features of the definition of the person but not of the relationship. For example, "A grandmother is someone who smells like flowers and wears funny underwear" (an actual child's definition).

The child gains a few of the less complex relationships first (Table 9.4). Complexity may be thought of as the number of shared features. For example, *father* has the features *male* and *parent*, but *aunt*, a more complex term, has *female*, *sister*, and *parent* of whom she's the sister. After *Mommy* and *Daddy*, the child learns *brother* and *sister*. Roughly, the meanings are *brother* = *related boy* and *sister* = *related girl*. By age four, the child may understand what a brother or sister is but doesn't realize that he can also be a brother to someone else. In other words, the term is not used reciprocally. Eventually, the child will understand all features of the kinship terms and reciprocity. Most of the major kinship terms are understood by age ten.

INTERDEPENDENCE OF FORM, CONTENT, AND USE: PRONOUNS

Learning the English pronominal system is a very complex process. Although a pronoun is a simple device that enables one word to be the equivalent of one or several other words, the listener must understand these equivalences. Speakers use **anaphoric reference**, or referral to what has come before. We can thus decipher *his* and *it* in the sentence, "The boy was watching *his* television when *it* caught fire."

Pronouns offer a special situation in which it is easy to see the complex relationship between form, content, and use. Some pronouns appear around age two, whereas others emerge much later. (See Table 9.5 for the general order of pronoun acquisition.) The actual order is variable with each child. Initially, children use labels or pronouns that can signal notice, such as *that*, as in "*That* a doggie." As a group, subjective pronouns, such as *he*, *she*, and *they*, are acquired before objective pronouns, such as *him*, *her*, and *them*. These are followed by possessive pronouns, such as *his*, *her*, and *their*, and finally, around age five by reflexive pronouns, such as *himself*, *herself*, and *themselves*.

TABLE 9.5   Development of Pronouns

APPROXIMATE AGE IN MONTHS	PRONOUNS
12–26	*I, it* (subjective and objective)
27–30	*My, me, mine, you*
31–34	*Your, she, he, yours, we*
35–40	*They, us, hers, his, them, her*
41–46	*Its, our, him, myself, yourself, ours, their, theirs*
47+	*Herself, himself, itself, ourselves, yourselves, themselves*

Source: Adapted from Haas & Owens (1985); Huxley (1970); Morehead & Ingram (1973); Waterman & Schatz (1982); and Wells (1985).

The child begins with *I* and *it* and then adds *you* (Chiat, 1986). From there, children exhibit great individual diversity. Initial use tends to be sporadic and stereotypic. For example, *it* first appears in unanalyzed phrases, such as *stop it* and *look it*.

Children's production of nouns and pronouns suggests a number of use strategies (Haas & Owens, 1985):

- When in doubt, use a noun.
- Look for regularity. After learning the *her* (objective)/*hers* (possessive) relationship, the child may produce *him/hims*. Similarly, *her/herself* may generalize to *his/hisself*.
- Simplify complex pronominal forms. Reflexives may be reduced to objective case. For example, the child might say, "You looked in the mirror and saw *you*," rather than *yourself*. Plural pronouns may also be broken into their singular components. For instance, *they* may become *he* and *she*, and *we* may become *you* and *me*.
- Use previously learned pronominal forms to aid in the production of unlearned forms. Thus, children may use subjective forms for objective, objective forms for possessive, and possessive forms for reflexive. The following examples illustrate these substitutions:

"I gave it to *he*." (subjective for objective)
"It's *hims*" or "It *them* toy." (objective for possessive)
"He sees *his* self." (possessive for reflexive)

By thirty-six months, children have mastered nearly all subjective and objective pronouns and the two demonstrative pronouns *this* and *that* (Wells, 1985). By age five, nearly all children have mastered the subjective, objective, and possessive pronouns. They still must learn reflexive pronouns and the plural demonstrative pronouns *these* and *those*.

In part, the lengthy acquisition period for pronouns reflects the complex interaction of form, content, and use. Pronouns fill syntactic and semantic roles; make semantic distinctions based on gender, person, and number; and act as cohesive discourse devices. The preschooler's usage, however, may reflect learning of only one component of the pronoun's complex definition. Children seem to acquire one feature of the definition at a time. In general, the distinction of conversational role (*I/you*) is acquired before the semantic gender distinction (*he/she*), which is followed by the distinction of conversational participant-nonparticipant (*I, you/he, she*) (Brener, 1983; Charney, 1980). The general developmental order of first person (I), followed by second person (you), the third person (he, she, it), is found in both English and French (Girouard, Ricard, & DeCarie, 1997). Data from Spanish-speaking Puerto Rican children and Italian children demonstrate objective pronouns developing before subjective, reflecting grammar and use differences in these languages (Anderson, 1998; Leonard, Sabbadini, Volterra, & Leonard, 1988).

The appearance of the first person singular pronoun *I* is quickly followed by the use of *you*. The child learns early to make the distinction between the roles of speaker and listener. Although children make errors within type, such as *I* for *me*, most children do not make errors between types, such as *I* for *you*. *You* is first used in the imperative sentence form, as in the command "*You* shut door." Use of *you* reflects syntactic and pragmatic learning.

The child follows a general strategy in which *I* is used if it is the first word in the sentence and *me* if it is not. This strategy very gradually evolves into a subjective/objective (*I/me*) semantic case distinction. Not all children progress through the often-reported stages of referring to themselves by name, then by *me*, and finally by *I*. In general, parents of toddlers avoid pronouns and refer to the child by name or as "Baby."

Other pronouns also cause some semantic case confusion. *He* and *she* are often confused with the possessive pronouns *his* and *her*. The child's developing phonological system no doubt contributes to the overlapping use of *he*, *his*, and *him*, as in *he's book* and *him's coat*. Similar errors are seen with *she*, *her*, and *hers*. The possessive pronouns *my* and *your* do not appear to be overgeneralized to other cases and are usually mastered by age two and a half.

It has been theorized that the child forms a phonetic core for first and third person. If /m/ is for first person (*me, my, mine*) and /h/ for third person (*him, her, he, his*), it explains, in part, why *I* and *she* usually are not overextended and *me, him, he, his*, and *her* are (Rispoli, 1994).

Morphological distinctions related to possession may also pose a problem for the child. Inconsistent use of the possessive marker ('s), present in "Mommy's hat" but not in "her hat," may result in confusion. It is not uncommon to hear utterances such as "This is *hers* hat," in which the child adds the possessive marker to subject and object pronouns.

In general, the deictic function of pronouns is acquired before the anaphoric one. In other words, children use pronouns initially to mark the spatial relationship of persons and things to the speaker (*I, me* vs. *you* vs. *it*), and only later to mark nouns previously identified (*Mary* becomes *she*) (Wales, 1986). (See discussion on page 285.)

As a conversational device, pronouns provide cohesion between old and new information. As we discussed earlier, new information is first identified by name. Then, once identified, it becomes old information and can be referred to by a pronoun. The pronoun refers to what came before or makes anaphoric reference to it. When there is possible confusion, preschool children often use pronominal apposition, as in "My mother, she. . . ." Unless it is a dialectal characteristic, pronominal apposition begins to disappear by school age.

It is easy to see why pronouns are so difficult for some children to learn. The pronoun system is very complex and combines elements of all aspects of language. Surprisingly, confusion between pronouns is rare (Chiat, 1986; Haas & Owens, 1985). Although children may overuse nouns in place of pronouns, the reverse is almost nonexistent.

CONCLUSION

By kindergarten, the child is able to uphold his or her end of the conversation. Although the preschooler does not have the range of intentions and subtle conversational abilities or vocabulary of a school-age child, he or she can participate and make valuable conversational contributions. As the child matures socially and cognitively, communication skills and language reflect these developments.

Within a conversational context, the preschool child has progressed from two-, three-, and four-word sentences to longer utterances that reflect adultlike form and content rules. Caregivers continue to treat the child as a conversational partner, and the child's contribution increases in meaningfulness in addition to skill of formation. Increased vocabulary and relational terms enable the child to sustain a conversation on limited topics and to relate action narratives of past and imagined events.

Adults, especially parents, are still the primary conversational partners, although others, such as preschool or daycare friends or siblings, are becoming more important. As the child plays with other children and interacts with adults, he or she learns to modify language for the listener and becomes more flexible. This aspect of language will change greatly throughout the school years.

DISCUSSION

Although turn-taking develops early, it is a big jump from taking turns to becoming a good conversational partner. The preschool child is learning to begin and end conversations, to introduce, maintain, and change topics, and to decide on the right amount of information to provide. In addition, he or she is introducing narratives into the conversation, recalling past events for the conversational partner. It will be many years before conversational and narrative skills reach that of an adult, but we have a beginning.

New words and word relationships are also being added to the preschooler's expanding vocabulary. Relational terms, such as *better than* and *in front of* are especially difficult. Terms, such as conjunctions,(*and, because, so*), that link sentence elements will also take more time to develop. These and other terms will be added to the child's lexical storage.

At the end of the chapter is the development of pronouns. The importance of that development for us is in its illustration of the interdependence of the different areas of language. Pronouns might seem simple, but little in language development really is.

In practice, the SLP cannot ignore these aspects of language. To program only for the child's language form is to miss the importance of that form's use within the environment. Training structures for which the child has no use is insuring that the structures will not generalize.

REFLECTIONS

1. Briefly describe the conversational skills of the preschool child.

2. Describe the development of preschool narratives.

3. Explain the process of vocabulary expansion among preschool children.

4. Summarize the development of relational terms. Explain the principles in operation.

5. Explain the order of pronoun acquisition based on the unique semantic, pragmatic, and syntactic aspects of pronouns.

10

Preschool Development of Language Form

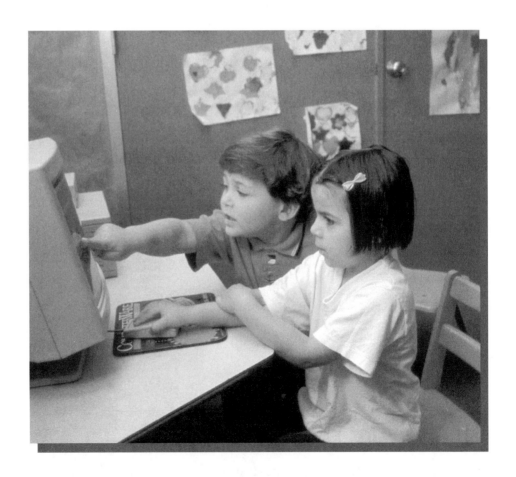

CHAPTER OBJECTIVES

The preschool years are a time of tremendous growth in all aspects of language, especially language form. From two- and three-word utterances, the child progresses to sentences that approximate adult language in their complexity. When you have completed this chapter, you should understand

- how to compute the mean length of utterance.
- the major characteristics of the stages of syntactic development.
- preschool morphological development.
- the acquisition order for negative and interrogative sentences.
- the differences between embedding and conjoining and their acquisitional order.
- the major phonological processes observed in preschool children.
- the following terms:

aspect	modal auxiliary
clause	object noun-phrase complement
complex sentence	phrasal coordination
compound sentence	phrase
conjoining	relative clause
copula	sentential coordination
embedded *wh-* question	sibilant
embedding	simple sentence
epenthesis	subordinate clause
main clause	tense
mean length of utterance (MLU)	

During the preschool years, there is a tremendous growth in language form in a very brief period. Much of adult morphology, syntax, and phonology has begun to appear by the time a child goes to kindergarten. This chapter will explain this process and help you understand the course and method of these incredible changes.

In general, the child observes the regularized patterns of language use in the environment and forms hypotheses about the underlying rules. These hypotheses are then tested in production. Over time, the rules change to reflect the child's greater sophistication in producing and using the linguistic code in conversation. Many months or years may be required before the child has complete control of a linguistic element in all contexts.

In this chapter we shall first discuss stages of language development that will help you relate developments in one area of language to those in others. Next, we shall explore the changes that occur in morphology, syntax, and phonology during the preschool years. You may find it helpful to refer to Chapter 7 for an explanation of the developmental process and to the glossary for unfamiliar terms.

STAGES OF SYNTACTIC AND MORPHOLOGIC DEVELOPMENT

Characteristic periods of preschool language development correspond to increases in the child's average utterance length, measured in morphemes. This value, the **mean length of utterance (MLU)**, is a moderately reliable predictor of the complexity of the language of English-speaking young children. For English-speaking preschoolers, MLU relates well to age, is reliable, and is a good predictor of language development, especially clausal complexity (Blake, Quartaro, & Onorati, 1993; Rondal, Ghiotto, Bredart & Bachelet, 1987). Up to an MLU of 4.0, increases in MLU correspond to increases in utterance complexity. Above an MLU of 4.0, complexity of utterances relates more to the context, and utterance length is not necessarily increased (D'Odorico & Franco, 1985).

At best, MLU is a crude measure that is sensitive only to those language developments that increase utterance length. For example, the movement of elements within the utterance may result in more mature utterances but will not increase the MLU. Although there is a positive correlation between MLU and age, MLU may vary widely for children with the same chronological age (J. Miller, 1981; J. Miller & Chapman, 1981; Wells, 1985). It is also important to note that although MLU is a rough estimate of language complexity for English-speaking preschoolers, it is not so for users of other languages such as modern Hebrew, in which complexity does not necessarily result in longer utterances (Dromi & Berman, 1982).

From age eighteen months to five years, MLU may increase by approximately 1.2 morphemes per year, although there is some indication of a decreased rate after forty-two months (Scarborough, Wyckoff, & Davidson, 1986). MLU is a gross developmental index that itself provides no information on specific structural complexity or grammatical competence, even among children with the same MLU (Klee & Fitzgerald, 1985). We use it here because of its conceptual simplicity for discussion.

Computing MLU

In general, 50 to 100 utterances are considered a sufficient sample from which to generalize about a speaker's overall production. An utterance may be a sentence or a shorter unit of language that is separated from other utterances by a drop in the voice, a pause, and/or a breath that signals a new thought. Once transcribed, each utterance is analyzed by morphemes; the total sample is then averaged to determine the speaker's MLU.

When analyzing the language of young children, several assumptions about preschool language must be made. Let's use the past tense as an example. The regular past tense includes the verb stem plus -ed, as in *walked* or *opened*. Hence, the regular past equals two morphemes, one free and one bound. In contrast, the irregular past is signaled by a different word, as in *eat/ate* and *sit/sat*. As adults, we realize that *eat* plus a past-tense marker equals *ate*. It could thus be argued that *ate* should also be counted as two morphemes. It seems, however, that young children learn separate words for the present and the irregular past and are not necessarily aware of the relationship between the two. Therefore, the irregular past counts as one morpheme for young children. A similar logic exists for words such as *gonna* and *wanna*. As adults, we can subdivide these words into their components: *going to* and *want to*. Young children, however, cannot perform such analyses. Therefore, *gonna* counts as one morpheme for the child, not as the three represented by *going to*.

Although we may not agree with this rationale, we must adopt it if we are to discuss language development within this framework. Guidelines for counting morphemes are presented in Table 10.1 (R. Brown, 1973). Applying these rules, we would reach the following values:

> *Daddy bring me choo-choo-s.* = 5 morphemes
> *Mommy eat-ed a-a-a sandwich.* = 5 morphemes
> *Doggie-'s bed broke baboom.* = 5 morphemes
> *Smokie Bear go-ing night-night.* = 4 morphemes
> *He hafta.* = 2 morphemes

Once the morphemes for each utterance are counted, they are totaled and then divided by the total number of utterances. The formula is very simple:

$$\text{MLU} = \frac{\text{Total number of morphemes}}{\text{Total number of utterances}}$$

TABLE 10.1 Brown's Rules for Counting Morphemes

RULE	EXAMPLE
Count as one morpheme:	
Reoccurrences of a word for emphasis	*No! No! No!* (3 morphemes)
Compound words (two or more free morphemes)	*Railroad, birthday*
Proper names	*Billy Sue*
Ritualized reduplications	*Night-night, choo-choo*
Irregular past tense verbs	*Went, ate, got, came*
Diminutives	*Daddie, doggie*
Auxiliary verbs and catenatives	*Is, have, do, gonna, hafta*
Irregular plurals	*Men, feet*
Count as two morphemes (inflected verbs and nouns):	
Possessive nouns	*Tom's, daddie's*
Plural nouns	*Doggies, kitties*
Third-person singular, present-tense verbs	*Walks, eats*
Regular past-tense verbs	*Walked, jumped*
Present progressive verbs	*Walking, eating*
Do not count:	
Dysfluencies, except for most complete form	*C-c-c-candy, bab-baby*
Fillers	*Um-m, ah-h, oh*

Source: Adapted from R. Brown, *A First Language: The Early Stages.* Cambridge: Harvard University Press, 1973.

Thus, if the total number of morphemes for a 100-utterance sample is 221, the MLU will equal 2.21 morphemes per utterance. Remember that this is an average value and does not identify the length of the child's longest utterance. In other words, an MLU of 2.0 does *not* mean that the child uses only two-word utterances.

MLU and Stage of Development

The focus of development changes with increased MLU. Major developments occur that can characterize certain MLU phases or stages. These stages are presented in Table 10.2 (R. Brown, 1973).

Stage I is characterized by single-word utterances and by the word-order rules of early multiword combinations. Chapter 8 described this stage in some detail. Stage II is characterized by the appearance of grammatical morphemes, which mark many of the relations expressed previously by the child with word order in stage I. By stage III, the child exhibits simple sentence forms and begins to modify these forms to mirror more adultlike forms for different sentence modalities, such as yes/no questions, *wh-* questions, negatives, and imperatives. Stage IV is marked by the beginning of embedding of phrases and clauses within a sentence. For example, the clause *who laughed* can be embedded in the clause *the boy is funny* to produce "The boy *who laughed* is funny." Finally, stage V is characterized by conjoining or by compound sentences. For example, the clauses *Mary washed* and *John dried* can be combined to form "Mary washed and John dried." Although each stage has some characteristic linguistic modifications, it should be noted that other, less obvious changes are also occurring.

MORPHOLOGIC DEVELOPMENT

Several morphological developments begin in stage II but continue well into the school-age years. In fact, the period of greatest acquisition is from four to seven years. Since many morphemes are redundant or have alternative forms of expression, it is difficult to determine

TABLE 10.2 Characteristics of Brown's Stages of Language Development

STAGE	MLU	APPROXIMATE AGE (MONTHS)	CHARACTERISTICS
I	1.0–2.0	12–26	Linear semantic rules
II	2.0–2.5	27–30	Morphological development
III	2.5–3.0	31–34	Sentence-form development
IV	3.0–3.75	35–40	Embedding of sentence elements
V	3.75–4.5	41–46	Joining of clauses
V+	4.5+	47+	

Source: Compiled from Brown (1973).

their age of acquisition. Even as adults, we are not aware of many morphological differences, such as the difference between *data* and *datum* or between **uninterested** and **disinterested**. Only the most commonly used morphemes will be discussed in the following section.

Stage II: Brown's Fourteen Morphemes

Stage II can be described by the appearance of morphemes that signify the semantic relations specified in stage I through word order. R. Brown (1973) isolated fourteen morphemes for study. Selection was based on obligatory use. If use is obligatory rather than optional, then, it is reasoned, absence of the morpheme would indicate nonacquisition, not choice.

The fourteen selected morphemes, presented in Table 10.3, have the following characteristics:

1. They are phonetically minimal forms. In general, they include simple phonemic additions or changes, such as the addition of an *s*.
2. They receive only light vocal emphasis.
3. They belong to a limited class of constructions, as opposed to the larger number of nouns and verbs.
4. They possess multiple phonological forms and can vary with the grammatical and phonetic properties of the words to which they are attached. For example, the *s* in *cats* is pronounced /s/, whereas the *s* in *dogs* is pronounced /z/.
5. Their development is very gradual.

Each morpheme emerges in stage II, but most are not fully mastered (used correctly 90 percent of the time) until later. The order presented in Table 10.3 reflects the order of mastery, not of initial appearance.

Present Progressive -ing

The present progressive verb tense is used in English to indicate an activity that is currently in progress and is of temporary duration, such as I *am swimming*. The form consists of the auxiliary or helping verb *to be* (*am, is, are, was, were*), the main verb, and the *-ing* verb ending. Children initially express this verb tense with only the *-ing* ending. For example, a child might say "Doggie swimming" or "Mommy eating." The present progressive verb tense without the auxiliary is the earliest verb inflection acquired in English and is mastered within stage II for most verbs used by young children (R. Brown, 1973; J. Miller, 1981).

The present progressive can be used with action verbs in English but not with verbs of state, such as *need, know,* and *like*. Young children learn this distinction early, and few overgeneralization errors result. The child probably learns the rule one verb at a time by applying it to individual verbs to determine whether they are "*-ingable*." Later the child abandons this strategy as too cumbersome and adopts an *-ing* rule.

State verbs are not capable of expressing the present progressive meaning of temporary duration. When a child says "I eating," it is assumed that she'll stop soon. The action is temporary. On the other hand, adults don't say "I am knowing" because with *know* or

TABLE 10.3   Brown's Fourteen Morphemes

MORPHEME	EXAMPLE	AGE OF MASTERY* (IN MONTHS)
Present progressive -ing (no auxiliary verb)	Mommy driving.	19–28
In	Ball in cup.	27–30
On	Doggie on sofa.	27–30
Regular plural -s	Kitties eat my ice cream. Forms: /s/, /z/, and /ɪz/ Cats (/kæts/) Dogs (/dɔgz/) Classes (/klæsɪz/), wishes (/wɪʃɪz/)	27–33
Irregular past	Came, fell, broke, sat, went	25–46
Possessive 's	Mommy's balloon broke. Forms: /s/, /z/, and /ɪz/ as in regular plural	26–40
Uncontractible copula (verb to be as main verb)	He is. (response to "Who's sick?")	27–39
Articles	I see a kitty. I throw the ball to daddy.	28–46
Regular past -ed	Mommy pulled the wagon. Forms: /d/, /t/, /ɪd/ Pulled (/pʊld/) Walked (/wɔkt/) Glided (/g l aɪ d i d/)	26–48
Regular third-person -s	Kathy hits. Forms: /s/, /z/, and /ɪz/ as in regular plural	26–46
Irregular third person	Does, has	28–50
Uncontractible auxiliary	He is. (response to "Who's wearing your hat?")	29–48
Contractible copula	Man's big. Man is big.	29–49
Contractible auxiliary	Daddy's drinking juice. Daddy is drinking juice.	30–50

*Used correctly 90% of the time in obligatory contexts. Adapted from Bellugi & Brown (1964); R. Brown (1973); and J. Miller (1981).

other verbs, such as *possess* and *love*, it is assumed that this state is of some duration. Thus, a child learns some general rule of application that enables her or him to generalize the progressive form while not overgeneralizing to inappropriate verbs.

Early learning may also reflect a difference between the progressive and many other morphological inflections. There are no irregular progressive forms, resulting in less confusion for the child. Forms that are overgeneralized by children, such as the regular past tense -ed, have both regular (*walked*) and irregular (*ate*) forms.

Prepositions

In and *on* are the only two prepositions that occur frequently enough to be considered as acquired within stage II (R. Brown, 1973; J. Miller, 1981). Often, the child relates the preposition to the object itself. For example, you can put something *in* a cup but rarely *on* it. Other early prepositions include *away*, *out*, *over*, and *under*. Simple topographic or locational relations, such as *in*, *on*, and *under*, appear to be easier for the child to comprehend than dimensional spatial relations, such as *behind*, *beside*, *between*, and *in front of*. Cognitive and pragmatic skills relative to other locational prepositions have been discussed in Chapter 9.

Plural

In English there is no morpheme to indicate the singular form of a noun; thus, a singular noun is called *uninflected* or *unmarked*. The regular form of the plural, marked in writing by -*s*, is acquired orally within stage II (R. Brown, 1973; J. Miller, 1981). Learning of irregular forms, such as *feet* and *mice*, takes considerably longer and largely depends on how frequently these forms are used in the preschooler's environment.

The regular plural appears in short phrases first, then in short sentences, and finally in longer sentences. In addition, there appear to be four phases of development. Initially, there is no difference between the singular and plural, and a number or the word *more* may be used to mark the plural. In other words, the child might say "Puppy" for one or more than one, or she might say "Two puppy" or "More puppy" to indicate plural. Next, the plural marker will be used for selected instances, probably on plural words that are used frequently. In the third phase, the plural generalizes to many instances, some of which are inappropriate. Thus, we get such delightful forms as *foots* and *mouses*. Finally, the regular and irregular plural are differentiated. The amount of overgeneralization to irregular past forms is relatively low, suggesting that children prefer the correct form to an overgeneralized rule (Marcus, 1995).

Acquiring the English plural involves phonological learning as well. Three different speech sounds are used with the plural: /s/, /z/, and /ɪz/ or /əz/. If a word ends in a voiced consonant (see the appendix for an explanation), the voiced plural marker /z/ is used, as in *beds* (/bɛdz/). In contrast, voiceless consonants are followed by the voiceless /s/, as in *bets* (/bɛts/). These rules do not apply if the final consonant is similar to the /s/ and /z/. The /s/, /z/, /ʃ/, /ʒ/, /tʃ/, and /dʒ/ are called *sibilant sounds*, or **sibilants**. If a word ends in a sibilant, the plural marker is /ɪz/ or /əz/, as in *bridges* (/brɪdʒɪz/). The /s/ and /z/ rules are learned first, followed by the rule for /ɪz/. The child may be in stage V or beyond before these phonological rules are acquired. This distinction is especially difficult for children with hearing impairments because of the relatively high frequency or pitch and the complexity of sibilant sounds.

Irregular Past

Irregular past-tense verbs, those that do not use the -*ed* ending, such as *ate*, *wrote*, and *drank*, are a small but frequently used class of words in English. Not all of the approximately 200 irregular verbs in English occur with the same frequency. A small subset of these verbs appears in single-word utterances and is acquired in stage II, probably learned individually by rote rather than as the result of rule learning and application (Bybee & Slobin, 1982; Shipley & Banis, 1989). These include *came, fell, broke, sat*, and *went*. Although the child acquires these forms early, he or she may later use the regular *-ed* marker to produce *goed/wented* or *falled/felled*. A relationship exists between the vowels in the base word and the overgeneralized *-ed* (Stemberger, 1993). The irregular past of common verbs is produced correctly by stage V, although many irregular verbs are not learned until school age. Table 10.4 presents the ages at which 80 percent of preschoolers correctly use certain irregular verbs (Shipley, Maddox, & Driver, 1991). Given the lack of rules for irregular past tense verbs, it's surprising that preschool children actually make so few errors (Xu & Pinker, 1995). Most errors seem to be based on attempts to generalize from existing irregular verbs.

Even some adults have difficulty with irregular verbs such as *lie*, and *lay*. I avoid writing or saying them whenever possible. Like adults, children may generalize from a known form to one being learned. Thus, knowledge of *sing/sang* may yield the incorrect *bring/brang*. Likewise, knowledge of *drink, drank, drunk* may result in *think, thank, thunk*.

Possessive

The possessive is originally marked with word order and stress; the use of the possessive marker ('s) appears relatively late. Initially, the possessive is attached only to single animate nouns, such as *Mommy* or *doggie*, to form *Mommy's* or *doggie's*. The earliest entities marked for possession are alienable objects, such as clothing, rather than inalienable entities, such as body parts. The morphological form is mastered by stage III. Phonological mastery takes much longer, however, and is similar to the plurals /s/, /z/, and /Iz/.

Uncontractible Copula

The verb *to be* (*am, is, are, was, were*) may serve as a main verb or as an auxiliary, or helping, verb. As a main verb it is called the **copula** and is followed by a noun, an adjective, or some adverbs or prepositional phrases. For example, in the sentences "He *is* a teacher,"

TABLE 10.4   Age of Development of Irregular Past-Tense Verbs

AGE (IN YEARS)*	VERB
3–3 1/2	Hit
	Hurt
3 1/2–4	Went
4–4 1/2	Saw
4 1/2–5	Gave
	Ate

Source: Taken from Shipley, Maddox, & Driver (1991).

*Age at which 80% of children use verb correctly in sentence completion task.

"I *am* sick," and "They *are* late," the verb *to be* is the only verb and hence the main verb. All of these sentences contain the copula, followed by a noun, *teacher*; an adjective, *sick*; and an adverb, *late*, respectively.

The copula appears initially in an uncontractible or full form (R. Brown, 1973). The notion of uncontractibility is based on those adult uses of the copula in which it is not permissible to form a contraction. In the sentence "She *is* angry," we can contract the copula to form "She's angry." Thus, the copula is contractible. It is not permissible to contract the copula when the answer to a question omits known or redundant information, leaving only the verb *to be*. For example, in response to the question "Who is hungry?", it is only acceptable to say "I *am*," not "I'm." In addition, the copula may not be contracted when it is the first or last word in a question ("*Is* he ill?" or "Do you know where she *is*?") or appears in negative sentences in which *not* is contracted (*n't*), as in "He isn't a lawyer." It would be incorrect to say "He'sn't a lawyer." Finally, the copula may not be contracted in the past tense, as in "She *was* here." "She's here" is clearly present tense and would thus be incorrect because it changes the tense of the sentence.

In general, the copula, both uncontractible and contractible, is not fully mastered until stage V (J. Miller, 1981). It takes some time before the child sorts through all the copular variations for person and number (*am, is, are*) and tense (*was, were, will be, been*).

Articles

The articles *the* and *a* appear in stage II but take some time to be mastered. Initial use is probably undifferentiated, and it is sometimes difficult to ascertain from the child's pronunciation which article is being used. For adults, the indefinite article *a* is used for non-specific reference and the definite *the* denotes specific reference. As noted in Chapter 9, pragmatic considerations also influence article use. New information is generally marked with *a*, whereas old information is signaled by *the*. For example, you might introduce a new topic with "I need *a* new car." The subject of an automobile is new information, and the specific vehicle has not been identified. In your next sentence you might say, "*The* red one I saw last night was beautiful." Since *car* has already been mentioned, it is old information, and you have now identified a specific automobile. For both reasons, *the* is appropriate.

Articles are first acquired in a nominative, or naming, function, as in "See the puppy." Initially, the indefinite article *a* tends to predominate, as in naming expressions such as "That's *a* kitty." As the child begins to use articles for reference, he or she uses the definite article *the* predominantly, as in "*The* kitty go meow" even when it hasn't been identified as a specific "kitty." Use of the indefinite article in referencing expressions is acquired later (Emslie & Stevenson, 1981).

The age of article acquisition varies widely. Three-year-olds generally observe the indefinite–definite distinction, although they tend to overuse the definite article. This overuse, discussed under presuppositional skills in Chapter 9, may reflect the child's egocentric assumption that the listener knows more. By age four, the child is more capable of making complicated inferences about the listener's needs (Emslie & Stevenson, 1981; J. Miller, 1981). In addition, the four-year-old knows to use *some* and *any* rather than *a* and *the* with nouns, such as *sand* and *salt*, called *mass nouns* because the name denotes no specific quantity (Gordon, 1982). Some children as old as nine years will continue to overuse the definite article.

Regular Past

Few regular past inflected verbs appear at the single-word level. Once the child acquires the regular past-tense rule, it is overgeneralized to irregular past-tense verbs, producing forms such as *comed*, *eated*, and *falled*. Like other morphemes, the regular past has several phonological variations. The voiced /d/ follows voiced consonants, as in *begged* (/bɛgd/), and the unvoiced follows unvoiced consonants, as in *walked* (/wɔ kt/). The third variation, /ɪd/ or /əd/, follows words ending in /t/ or /d/, such as *sighted* (/saɪtɪd/). The /əd/ form is acquired later than the voiced–voiceless /d–t/ distinction, which may explain why this ending only occasionally overgeneralizes to irregular verbs ending in /t/ or /d/, such as *heard*, *told*, and *hurt*.

Third Person Singular Marker: Regular and Irregular

The person marker on the verb is governed by the person (I, you, he/she) and number (I, we) of the subject of the sentence. In English, the only present-tense marker is an *s* on the third person singular verb, as in "That dog barks too much" or "She runs quickly." All other forms are uninflected or unmarked, as in *I run*, *you dance*, *we sit*, and *they laugh*. The third person singular marker is redundant in most instances, since the subject generally expresses person and number. Only a few English verbs, such as *do* and *have*, are irregular. Although the regular and irregular forms appear in stage II, they are not mastered until stage V, and there is a long period of inconsistent use.

Uncontractible Auxiliary

In general, the auxiliary or helping verb *to be* develops more slowly than the copula. Brown did not report on other helping verbs, such as *do* and *have*. Unlike the copula, the auxiliary *be* is followed by a verb, as in "She is singing," which is a present progressive form. The uncontractible auxiliary is most frequent in the past tense, in which contraction of "He *was* eating" to "He's eating" would change the meaning. Like the copula, the uncontractible auxiliary *to be* is also used when it is the first or last word in a sentence, when the negative is contracted or when redundant information is omitted, as in "He *is*" in response to the question "Who's painting?" The uncontractible auxiliary is mastered by stage V (J. Miller, 1981).

Contractible Copula

The contractible copula is mastered in late stage V or afterward (J. Miller, 1981). The copula is contractible if it can be contracted, whether or not it is actually contracted. Therefore, "Mommy *is* tall" and "Mommy's tall" are both examples of the contractible copula.

The copula may take many forms to reflect person and number. In general, the *is* and *are* forms develop before *am*. The *is* form tends to be overused, contributing to singular–plural confusion, such as "He *is* fast" and "They *is* big" or "We *is* hungry." The overlearning of contractions, such as *'s* and *'re*, also seems to add to the confusion. Contracted forms are short, often unemphasized, and therefore easily undetected when used incorrectly.

There is considerable variation with *it's*. Initially, young children use *it's* and *it* interchangeably, the copula appearing only very gradually.

Contractible Auxiliary

The development of the auxiliary is similar to that of the copula in the contractible form. The auxiliary *is* and *are* forms precede the *am* form, as in the copula. The contractible auxiliary is mastered after stage V.

Determinants of Acquisition Order

The cognitive relationship between the semantic and syntactic complexity of these morphemes is the key to developmental order, not the frequency of use in adult speech. Syntactic and semantic complexity become more evident when we note the order of acquisition in other languages. For example, the concept underlying plural—one and more than one—is quite simple and is learned early. Plural marking is very complex in Egyptian Arabic, however, and there are many exceptions to the plural rule. In contrast to English-speaking preschoolers, many Egyptian teenagers still have difficulty with the plural.

Distinctions of gender can also be difficult. In English, as in French, there are only two genders, male and female, although most English words are not marked for gender. Fulani, a Niger-Congo language, contains about a dozen genders. These forms are semantically and syntactically complex, so children learn them more slowly and over a longer period of time than children learning English gender markers.

Initial morphological development of verb markers may be related to the underlying semantic aspects of the verb (Bloom, Lifter, & Hafitz, 1980). The child begins by developing a few protoform verbs that are general and nonspecific, such as *do*, *go*, and *make*. Once these general forms are developed, the verb markers for these forms appear quickly, suggesting that initial morphological learning may be on a word-by-word basis. In contrast, more specific verbs may be unmarked.

The underlying temporal concept of the verb seems to be a factor in marking. For example, the present progressive *-ing* first appears on verbs that display a discrete end, such as *drive*, but not on verbs that describe a discrete event, such as *hit* or *drop*. In contrast, the past-tense marker is more likely to appear on verbs that describe a discrete event. Thus, initially the child is more likely to say "Daddy is *driving* the car" and "I *dropped* my cup." Initial morphological use is limited.

Morphological learning requires that the child correctly segment words into morphemes and correctly categorize words into semantic classes. If the child undersegments, she or he won't break the word or phrase into enough morphemes. The result is a creation such as "He *throw-uped* at the party" or "I like *jump-roping*." Most of us learned the alphabet as ". . . J, K, Elemeno, P, Q, . . . ," another good example of undersegmenting. In oversegmenting, the child uses too many morphemes, as in "Daddy, you're *interring-upt* me!" My son Todd referred to grownups as *dolts*, having oversegmented *adult* into the article *a* and *dolt*. Judging from some of the adults I know, maybe my son was more observant than we gave him credit for being!

Morphemes are not treated the same way by all language-learning children. In polymorphemic languages such as Mohawk, a northern New York and southern Quebec Native language, in which words consist of many morphemes, children initially divide words by syllables rather than morphemes (Mithum, 1989). Children are more likely to note and produce stressed syllables than morphemes. In English, however, morphological development is more important.

Morphological rules apply to classes of words. Hence, *-ing* is used only with action verbs. If the child miscategorizes a word, errors may result. He or she may use inappropriate morphological prefixes and suffixes, as in the following:

> I'm *jellying* my bread. (Using a noun as a verb, although we do say
> "buttering my bread")
> I got *manys*. (Using a pronoun as a noun)
> He runs *fastly*. (Using an adjective as an adverb)

Often these errors reflect the child's limited descriptive vocabulary. One of my favorites came from my son Jason who, after a fitful sleep, announced, "I hate *nightmaring*." Undercategorization occurs when the child applies a category rule to subcategories, such as the regular past *-ed* on irregular verbs. Other examples include the following:

> I saw too many *polices*. (Using the plural *s* inappropriately on a mass noun)
> I am *hating* her. (Using the present progressive *-ing* inappropriately
> on a state verb)

Finally, in overcategorization the child applies a limited morpheme to other words, as in *unsad* and *unbig*. Many of the humorous utterances that young children produce reflect errors in segmentation or categorization.

Other Early Morphemes

Other morphemes appear and develop within Brown's stages but were not studied in detail by Brown. As a consequence, less is known about their acquisition.

Auxiliary Verbs

Auxiliary, or helping, verbs in English can be classified as primary, such as *be*, *have*, and *do*, or as secondary or modal, such as *will*, *shall*, *can*, *may*, and *must*. In general, auxiliary verbs are the only verbs that can be inverted with the subject to form questions or that can have negative forms attached. Examples of auxiliary forms include the following:

> *Are* you running in the race? (Inverted from the statement "You are
> running. . . .")
> What *have* you done? (Inverted from the statement "You have done. . . .")
> I *can't* help you. (Negative form)
> I *may* not be able to go. (Negative form)

The copula (*to be*) is an exception to this rule, since it can also be inverted and made into a negative form, as in *Is she sick?* or *This isn't funny*.

In addition, auxiliary verbs are used to avoid repetition in elliptical responses that omit redundant information and for emphasis. For example, when asked "Who can go with me?", a respondent avoids repetition by the elliptical reply "I *can*." To affirm a statement emphatically, a speaker might say, "I *do* like to dance."

Wide variation exists in the acquisition of auxiliary verbs. Table 10.5 presents the ages by which 50 percent of children begin to use selected auxiliary verbs. Most children use the auxiliaries *do*, *have*, and *will* by forty-two months.

Noun and Adjective Suffixes

During the preschool years, the child masters a few additional suffixes for nouns and adjectives. These include the adjectival comparative -*er* and the superlative -*est*. By adding these to descriptive adjectives, the child can create forms such as *smaller* or *biggest*. Children understand the superlative by about three-and-a-half years of age; the comparative somewhat later, at age five. Correct production follows shortly. Specific forms, such as *better* or *best*, which are exceptions to the rule, usually take longer to master.

The derivational noun suffix -*er*, added to a verb to form the name of the person who performs the action, is also understood by age five and mastered in production within a short time. For example, the person who *teaches* is a *teacher*; the one who *hits* is a *hitter*, and so on. One reason for the late appearance of this marker may be its ambiguous nature. The -*er* is used for the comparative (*bigger*) and for noun derivation (*teacher*). In addition, several other derivational noun suffixes, such as -*man*, -*person*, and -*ist*, can also be used. Two-year-olds tend to rely on the -*man* suffix, often emphasizing it, as in *fisherman*, which

TABLE 10.5 Auxiliary Verb Use by 50 Percent of Children

AGE (IN MONTHS)	AUXILIARY VERB
27	*Do*
	Have + V-*en*
30	*Can*
	Be + V-*ing*
	Will
33	*Be going to*
36	*Have got to*
39	*Shall*
42	*Could*

Source: Adapted from G. Wells, "Learning and Using the Auxiliary Verb in English." In V. Lee (Ed.), *Language Development.* New York: Wiley, 1979, p. 258.

contains both the -er and the -man. Other more creative examples are *busman*, *storewomen*, and *dancerman*.

Morphological Rule Learning and Other Aspects of Language

Morphological rule learning reflects phonological and semantic rule learning as well. Morphological rules are learned at an early age, beginning with rules that apply to specific words and continuing through sound-sequence rules. Initial learning may occur on a case-by-case basis. Higher-order rules require more complex integrative learning. Through lexical generalizations, the child learns that a concept may have more than one form and that forms originally construed to be morphologically distinct, such as *big* and *bigger*, are actually alternatives of the same concept.

Later, morphophonemic rules are required to account for commonalities. For example, the /f/ turns to /v/ preceding a plural, as in *knife/knives* and *wolf/wolves*. This rule is not true for all words ending in /f/, though, such as *cough* or *laugh*. The child recognizes regularity but must sort out the exceptions. Each of us has heard a small child say a word such as *knifes* (/n aI fs/) during this phase.

At the highest level, sound sequence rules may cross several morphological variations to govern sound sequences. The plural, possessive, and third-person markers all follow the same "both voiced or voiceless" rule [dogs (z), cats (s)] discussed earlier.

In fact, phonological variations may influence early morphological use. The child may not recognize the common morpheme beneath variations. For example, the child may not realize that the ending sound on *cats*, *dogs*, and *bridges* signals the same morphological change, pluralization. Morpheme recognition is easier if the semantic and phonological variations are minimal, as with *teach–teacher* rather than *good–better–best*.

In addition to phonological considerations, the underlying semantic concept may influence morphological development. For example, cognitive and semantic distinctions may be reflected in the order of acquisition of auxiliary verbs. Initially, the child learns auxiliary verbs concerned with the agent in actual events (*do, have, will*), then with the agent as potential doer (*can, have got to, have to, must, should, had better*), then with a likelihood of events (*might, may*), and finally with inferences about events not experienced (*could*). Thus, the child progresses from a more concrete action orientation to an abstract reference. Early morphological development focuses on more concrete relationships, such as plural and possession. Abstract relationships such as person and number markers on the verb tend to take longer to master. The progression from concrete to abstract is also reflected in the developing child's cognitive processing.

SENTENCE-FORM DEVELOPMENT

By the time the child enters stage III, at around thirty months, he or she has mastered the basic subject-verb-object (*Ramona eats vegetables*) and subject-copula-complement (*Byung is big*) forms of the English sentence (Wells, 1985). Children learning other language, such as Portuguese, also demonstrate early acquisition of the noun and verb elements (Valian & Eisenberg, 1996).

Recall that the most basic of Chomsky's phrase-structure rules is that a sentence consists of a noun phrase and a verb phrase. The only required syntactic elements are the noun (subject) and the verb (predicate). Therefore, the child has acquired both elements of simple adult declarative sentences by late stage II to early stage III. Once these are acquired or in the process of being acquired, the child begins to experiment with and to modify the basic pattern. Thus, development occurs at two levels: within sentence elements and at the sentence level. The result is the internal development of noun and verb phrases and the development of declarative, interrogative, and imperative sentence types and the negative forms of each. A sample of the speech and language of a four-year-old child is presented on track nine of the CD that accompanies this text. A transcript of the speech of two 48-month-old children is presented in Table 14.3 of this text. Note the sentence form in this transcript. Although the content is very child-based, the sentence structure seems more mature. For contrast, note the transcript of a thirty-two-month-old in Table 14.2 and the sample of a five-year-old child on track ten of the accompanying CD.

Sentence Elements

Before we look at different sentence forms, we should examine internal sentence development. Of interest are development of noun and verb phrases.

Noun-Phrase Development

Singular nouns form the largest syntactic class represented in children's first fifty words. Although combined with other words in stage I, nouns are generally elaborated only when they occur alone. Initially, elaboration includes the addition of the indefinite article (*a*) or the demonstrative *that* to the noun. The average child is forming these combinations by twenty-one months (Wells, 1985). Thus, the child is likely to say such phrases as "A kitty" or "That candy." Later noun-phrase expansions include the addition of possessive nouns (*Daddy's* shoe), quantifiers (*Some* cookie), and physical attributes (*Big* doggie) to the noun. Multiple modifiers are rare in stage I; the child is not yet likely to say "My big doggie." The list of early modifiers is generally small and only gradually expands.

In stage II, nouns that appear alone and in the object position are modified. For example, the child might say "Daddy throw *big ball*" (objective) but rarely "*Big doggie* go 'ruff'" (subjective). In addition, the child uses a limited set of pronouns in the noun position, including *I*, *it*, and *that*. The two-year-old child is thus capable of achieving coherence by introducing new noun phrases and marking their given or old status later with pronouns (Bennett-Kaster, 1983). Pronoun confusion occurs most frequently in *noun + verb + noun* formats and in imitation (Dale & Crain-Thoreson, 1993).

Children seem to acquire a general rule that adjectives precede nouns in English very early. In addition, they learn that adjectives do not precede pronouns and proper nouns (P. Bloom, 1990). Usually, it is not acceptable for mature English speakers to say *little he* or *old Juan*. Two-year-olds rarely use this form. Possibly, they make a semantic distinction between nouns, which can take descriptors, and pronouns and proper nouns, which do not.

Elaboration occurs in both the subject and object positions by stage III, with both articles and modifiers preceding the noun (Wells, 1985). Both singular and plural nouns are elaborated. Demonstratives and articles may include *this, that, these,* or *those* and *a* or *the,* respectively. Modifiers include quantifiers, such as *some, a lot,* and *two;* possessives, such as *my* and *your;* and adjectives.

By stage IV, the child demonstrates by production that he or she knows that a noun or pronoun subject is obligatory or required for a sentence. Nouns dominate until thirty-three months, when they decrease as pronouns increase sharply. At thirty-nine months, nouns level off at 30 percent and pronouns increase in more than 40 percent of all noun phrases (Wells, 1985). Modifiers may include *some, something, other, more,* and *another.* The most frequent noun-phrase elaborations still involve only one element preceding the noun, such as "A girl eated *my* cookie." Only gradually does the child learn the different noun-phrase elements and the rules for sequential ordering. For example, as mature language users, you and I intuitively know that the words in the phrase *my big red candy apple* are in the correct order but that those in *red big candy my apple* are not. The ordering of elements of the mature noun phrase is illustrated in Table 10.6.

The first postnoun modification appears early in stage IV with short phrases, such as in "That *there*" and "The one *with the collar.*" By the end of stage IV, nouns appear with both prenoun and postnoun modifiers (Wells, 1985).

With the appearance of relative clauses—subordinate or dependent clauses that modify nouns, such as *who lives next door*—the child begins in stage V to use *clausal postnoun modifiers* as well, such as in "The dog *who lives next door* is big." Neither phrasal nor clausal postnoun embedding is widely used by children until school age.

Between ages four and five, the child makes dramatic changes in ability to use several noun phrases in succession (Bennett-Kaster, 1983). Thus, the child's stories become denser and longer. Five-year-olds can introduce noun phrases throughout a narrative and weave events relevant to these noun phrases. The result is that younger children tell stories about a relatively limited number of characters and events, while older children spin episode after episode with "mini" narratives for nearly all noun phrases within the larger narrative (Bennett-Kaster, 1983).

Verb-Phrase Development

Verb phrases may be of three types: *transitive, intransitive,* and *stative* (Table 10.7). In mature language, transitive verbs take a direct object and include words such as *love, hate, make, give, build, send, owe,* and *show.* With few exceptions—verbs such as *have, lack,* or *resemble*—transitive verbs can be changed from active to passive voice by exchanging the positions of the two noun phrases.

Active Voice	**Passive Voice**
Mary sent a letter.	A letter was sent by Mary.
Sue loves Fran.	Fran is loved by Sue.

TABLE 10.6 Elements of the Noun Phrase

INITIATOR	+ DETERMINER	+ ADJECTIVE	+ NOUN	+ MODIFIER
Only, a few of, just, at least, less than, nearly, especially, partially, even, merely, almost	Quantifier: *All, both, half, no, one-tenth, some, any, either, each, every, twice, triple* Article: *The, a, an* Possessive: *My, your, his, her, its, our, your, their* Demonstratives: *This, that, these, those* Numerical term: *One, two, thirty, one thousand*	Possessive Nouns: *Mommy's, children's* Ordinal: *First, next, next to last, last, final, second* Adjective: *Blue, big, little, fat, old, fast, circular, challenging* Descriptor: *Shopping, (center), Baseball, (game), hot dog, (stand)*	Pronoun: *I, you, he, she, it, we, you, they, mine, yours, his, hers, its, ours, theirs* Noun: *Boys, dog, feet, sheep, men and women, city of New York, Port of Chicago, leap of faith, matter of conscience*	Prepositional Phrase: *On the car, in the box, in the gray flannel suit* Adjectival: *Next door, pictured by Renoir, eaten by, Martians, loved by her friends* Adverb: *Here, there* Embedded clause: *Who went with you, that you saw*
Examples:	*all the one*			*attending the*
Nearly	*hundred*	*old college*	*alumni.*	*event*
Almost all of	*her thirty*	*former* . . . . *brother's*	*clients*	
Nearly	*half of your*	*old baseball*	*uniforms*	*in the closet*

In contrast, intransitive sentences do not have a passive form, nor do they take direct objects. Examples include *swim, fall, look, seem,* and *weigh.* Although we say "She swam the river," it is awkward to say "The river was swum by her." Some verbs may be both transitive and intransitive:

> I *opened* the door slowly. (Transitive: *door* is direct object)
> The door *opened* slowly. (Intransitive: no direct object)

Overall, transitive verb phrases are more common in English than in other languages.

Stative verbs, such as the copula *to be,* are followed by a *complement,* an element that sets up an equality with the subject. In "She is a doctor," *doctor* complements or describes what *she* is.

TABLE 10.7   Elements of the Verb Phrase

MODAL AUXILIARY +	PERFECTIVE AUXILIARY +	VERB TO BE +	NEGATIVE* +	PASSIVE +	VERB +	PREPOSITIONAL PHRASE, NOUN PHRASE, NOUN COMPLEMENT, ADVERBIAL PHRASE
May, can, shall, will, must, might, should, would, could	Have, has, had	Am, is, are, was, were, be, been	Not	Been, being	Run, walk, eat, throw, see, write	On the floor, the ball, our old friend, a doctor, on time, late

Examples:
Transitive (may have direct object)

May . . . . .have. . . . . wanted . . . . . . .a cookie

Should . . . . .not . . . . throw . . . . .the ball in the house

Intransitive (does not take direct object)

Might . . . . .have . . . . .been . . . . .walking . . . . . to the inn

Could . . . . .not . . . . talk . . . . .with you

Equative (verb *to be* as main verb)

. . . . .is . . . . .not . . . . .a doctor

. . . . .was . . . . .late

. . . . .were . . . . .on the sofa

May . . . . .be ill

*When modal auxiliaries are used, the negative is placed between the modal and other auxiliary forms, for example, *might not have been going*.

Many verbs appear in the single-word phase of development. At this time, both *transitive* and *intransitive* verbs are produced, but the child does not observe the adult rules for each. Obviously, the child using only single-word action, such as *eat* and *throw*, or *want* utterances will be using verbs without direct objects.

In stage II, the child begins to use the morphological modifications discussed previously. The present progressive tense -*ing* marker is mastered within this stage. In addition, the child begins to use semi-infinitive forms such as *gonna*, *wanna*, and *hafta* (J. Miller, 1981). *Infinitives* consist of *to verb*, as in *to go*. When we say "I'm gonna go" we include the infinitive in our meaning "I'm going *to go*." These early forms may be used with a main verb, as in "I *gonna* eat," or alone, as in a response such as "I *hafta*." Auxiliary or helping verbs, such as *can*, *do*, and *will/would*, first appear in their negative form in later stage II. Every parent can attest to the appearance of forms such as *can't*, *don't*, and *won't*.

True auxiliary or helping verbs appear in late stage III, including *be, can, do,* and *will.* The verb *to be* may not correctly reflect the verb tense or the number and person of the subject. Thus, the child may produce "He *am,*" "You *is,*" and so on, although initially may overuse *is.* In addition, the stage III child will usually begin to overextend the regular past -*ed* marker to irregular verbs, thus producing *eated, goed,* and so on.

A strong correlation exists between the variety, but not the frequency, of maternal verb usage and the child's development of verbs (J. de Villiers, 1985). The child seems to learn verbs as individual items rather than as categories of words. As the child acquires each new verb, he or she observes similarities of syntactic use across items and uses these similarities to predict novel combinations.

By stage IV, the modal auxiliaries *could, would, should, must,* and *might* appear in negatives and interrogatives or questions. Semantically, **modal auxiliaries** are used to express moods or attitudes such as ability (*can*), permission (*may*), intent (*will*), possibility (*might*), and obligation (*must*).

The child still overextends the regular past in stage IV. A sentence may be doubly marked for the past, producing sentences such as "I *didn't* throw*ed* it." In this example, the child applies the past-tense marker to the main verb, even though the auxiliary verb takes the tense marker.

By stage V, the child has mastered both the regular and the irregular past tense in most contexts, as well as other morphemic inflections, such as the third person singular and the contractible copula (J. Miller, 1981). Auxiliary verbs and sentence subjects are inverted appropriately in questions ("What *is* she doing?"), and *do* is inserted when no auxiliary is present ("What *do* you want for your birthday?"). For example, the statement "Mother is eating a cookie" forms a question when the subject and the auxiliary verb are inverted, resulting in "Is mother eating a cookie?" When no auxiliary is present, as in "Joey wants a cookie," a *do*, called the *dummy do*, is inserted before the subject to form "*Does* Joey want a cookie?"

Many verb forms are still to be mastered after stage V. These include many of the forms of the verb *be*, past-tense modals and auxiliaries, and the passive voice.

Time and Reference. In English, time and reference to that time are marked by both verb tense and aspect. **Tense**, such as past or future, relates the speech time, which is in the present, to the event time, or the time when the event occurs. **Aspect** concerns the dynamics of the event relative to its completion, repetition, or continuing duration. The development of tense and aspect reflects both cognitive development and linguistic differences. Not all languages use tense and aspect. For example, Mandarin Chinese uses only aspect, and modern Hebrew uses only tense. The appearance of the linguistic markers for tense and aspect depends on the relative difficulty of acquiring these markers in each language. In English, tense and aspect, which are intertwined, are acquired later than in Japanese, in which there are distinct suffixes for each (Weist, 1986).

Children's sense of time and reference to it go through phases of development during the preschool years. These are noted in Table 10.8 (Weist, 1986). Initially, the child talks about things that are occurring now. The event time is the same as the speech time. There is no tense or aspect marking, although verbs have various pragmatic functions (Wells, 1985). In many different languages, children use the imperative form for requests ("Want

TABLE 10.8   Development of Production of Time and Reference

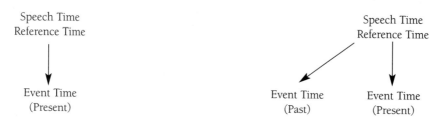

Event time and speech time are the
same initially.
Both are in the present.

By age 1½ to 3, children are able to speak
of events in the past as well as the present.

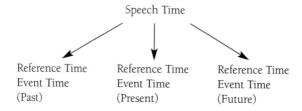

Around age 3 to 3½, the child develops a reference other than the present. Thus, an event may be described in a
limited manner from the reference of the past, present, or future.

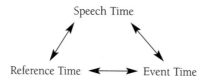

By age 3½ to 4, the child develops a flexible system that enables her to describe events in the past, present, or
future from the perspective of all three times.

Source: Adapted from Weist (1986).

juice") and the indicative form to comment ("Doggie run") (Berman, 1985; Clancy, 1985;
Erbaugh, 1982).

Between the age of eighteen months and three years, children speak about the past or
present, although the reference point is always in the present. Although children are capable of distinguishing aspect, these markers are not combined with tense. In many languages
as different as Turkish, Japanese, and Brazilian Portuguese, children can distinguish past
from nonpast, complete from noncomplete, continuative from noncontinuative, and future
from nonfuture (Aksu & Slobin, 1985; Clancy, 1985; E. Clark, 1985; DeLemos, 1981; Eisenberg, 1982).

Around age three to three-and-a-half, the child gains a sense of reference other than the present. This occurs at about the same age in very different languages (E. Clark, 1985; Weist, 1986). The notion of referent points can be explained with the following two examples:

> Kim drove yesterday.
> We had hoped to go yesterday.

In the first, the action was completed in the past but we are describing it from the reference point of the present. In the second, the event is clearly in the past but the reference is some time even earlier, prior to yesterday. Initially, children use adverbs of time such as *yesterday* and *tomorrow*. Only later do they use terms such as *before* and *after*.

Finally, between age three-and-a-half and four, the child acquires a flexible reference system. This development allows free reference to different points in time. For example, the child might say, "Yesterday, Gran'ma asked, 'Would you like to go to the zoo next week?'" A flexible reference system evolves at about the same time that the child acquires the cognitive skills to arrange things in a series and to reverse this sequential order.

Sentence Types

Within stage III, the child begins to use more adult sentence types to express basic relationships, such as *declarative*, *interrogative*, and *imperative* and the *negative* forms of each (Table 10.9). Initial development of each appears early, but the emergence of adult forms takes some time. The majority of children, however, possess the basic sentence types in English by age five (Wells, 1985).

In general, preschool sentence development can be gauged by an increase in the number of sentence elements and in the diversity of sentence forms. Description of this process becomes increasingly difficult, as complexity reflects internal movement of elements and diversity results in many forms, each occurring only infrequently. Increases in the number of elements usually occur in declaratives before occurring in other sentence types, probably because of the extra processing demands required for interrogatives and negative (Wells, 1985). Likewise, changes in verbs occur later in the copula than in other verbs, probably owing to the many variations of *to be* (*am*, *is*, *are*, *was*, *were*).

Declarative-Sentence Form

Declarative sentences or statements gradually increase in complexity and in number of elements or constituents throughout the preschool years. Beginning with the *agent + action* and *action + object* semantic relationships, the child develops the basic *subject + verb + object* sentence format by about thirty months. Additionally, acquired lexical items enable the child to form transitive, intransitive, and stative clauses.

By stage III, the child has added the auxiliary verb forms *do*, *have*, *can*, *be*, and *will*. The *subject + auxiliary + verb + object* form ("Mommy *is* eating ice cream"; "I'll drive that") appears before the *subject + auxiliary + copula + complement* form ("Daddy *will* be here"), which occurs in late stage III or early stage IV (Wells, 1985). Declaratives with double auxiliaries, as in "You *will have* to do it" (Wells, 1985), appear in late stage IV.

TABLE 10.9 Acquisition of Sentence Forms within Brown's Stages of Development

STAGE	AGE (IN MONTHS)	DECLARATIVE	NEGATIVE	INTERROGATIVE	EMBEDDING	CONJOINING
Early I (MLU: 1–1.5)	12–22	Agent + action; Action + object	Single word—*no, all gone, gone; negative + X*	*Yes/no* asked with rising intonation on a single word; *what* and *where*		Serial naming without *and*
Late I (MLU: 1.5–2.0)	22–26	Subj. + verb + obj. appears	*No* and *not* used interchangeably	*That + X; what + noun phrase + (doing)?* *Where + noun phrase + (going)?*	Prepositions *in* and *on* appear	*And* appears
Early II (MLU: 2.0–2.25)	27–28	Subj. + copula + compl. appears				
Late II (MLU: 2.25–2.5)	28–30	Basic subject-verb-object used by most children	*No, not, don't,* and *can't* used interchangeably; negative element placed between subject and predicate	*What* or *where* + subj. + pred. Earliest inversion appears with copula in *What/where + copula + subj.*	*Gonna, wanna, gotta,* etc. appear	
Early III (MLU: 2.5–2.75)	31–32	Subj. + aux. + verb + obj. appears; auxiliary verb forms *can, do, have, will,* and *be* appear				*But, so, or,* and *if* appear
Late III (MLU: 2.75–3.0)	33–34	Auxiliary verb appears with copula in subj. + aux. + copula + X	*Won't* appears	Auxiliary verbs *do, can,* and *will* begin to appear in questions; inversion of subject and auxiliary verb appears in yes/no questions		

Stage		Structure	Negation	Questions	Embedding	Conjoining
Early IV (MLU: 3.0–3.5)	35–37		Negative appears with auxiliary verbs (subj. + aux. + neg. + verb)	Inversion of auxiliary verb and subject in wh- questions	Object noun-phrase complements appear with verbs such as *think, guess,* and *show;* embedded *wh-* questions	Clausal conjoining with *and* appears (most children cannot produce this form until late stage V); *because* appears
Late IV (MLU: 3.5–3.75)	38–40	Double auxiliary verbs appear in subj. + aux. + aux. + verb + X	Adds *isn't, aren't, doesn't,* and *didn't*	Inversion of copula and subject in yes/no questions; adds *when* and *how*	Infinitive phrases appear at the ends of sentences	
Stage V (MLU: 3.75–4.5)	41–46	Indirect object appears in subj. + aux. + verb + ind. obj. + obj.	Adds *wasn't, wouldn't, couldn't,* and *shouldn't;* negative appears with copula in subj. + copula + neg.	Adds modals; stabilizes inverted auxiliary; some adultlike tag questions appear	Relative clauses appear in object position; multiple embeddings appear by late stage V; infinitive phrases with same subject as the main verb	Clausal conjoining with *if* appears; three-clause declaratives appear
Post-V (MLU: 4.5+)	47+		Adds indefinite forms *nobody, no one, none,* and *nothing;* has difficulty with double negatives	Questions other than one-word *why* questions appear; negative interrogatives beyond age 5	Gerunds appear; relative clauses attached to the subject; embedding and conjoining appear within same sentence above an MLU of 5.0	Clausal conjoining with *because* appears with *when, but,* and *so* beyond an MLU of 5.0; embedding and conjoining appear within the same sentence above an MLU of 5.0

*Based on approximately 50% of children using a structure.

327

Finally, in stage V, the child acquires indirect objects. The *subject + verb + indirect object + object* form ("He gave *me* the ball") appears prior to the *subject + verb + object + to + indirect object* form ("He gave the ball *to me*") (Wells, 1985). Other later developments include embedding, conjoining, and the internal development of the noun phrase.

Interrogative-Sentence Form

Through the use of intonation, children learn to ask questions very early. By age four, the child, according to many parents, seems to do nothing else. Questioning is a unique example of using language to gain information about language and about the world in general. I recall my own sense of loss when I replied "I used to" to my daughter's query "Do you ever talk to the trees?"

There are three general forms of questions: those that assume a yes/no response, those that begin with a *wh-* word and assume a more complex answer, and those that are a statement to which agreement is sought by adding a tag, such as ". . . isn't he?" Yes/no questions seek confirmation or nonconfirmation and are typically formed by adding rising intonation to the end of a statement, as in "You're eating snails?"↑; by moving the auxiliary verb from its position in a declarative sentence (You *are* eating snails) to form "*Are* you eating snails?"; or by adding the auxiliary verb *do* to a position in front of the subject, as in "Do you like snails?" Typical *wh-* or constituent questions use words such as *what, where,* and *who.* The verb and subject are inverted, as in yes/no questions, and the *wh-* word appears before the subject (What do you want?) unless it is the subject, as in *who* questions (Who is here?). In tag questions, a proposition is made, such as "He loves sweets," then negated in the tag: "He loves sweets, doesn't he?" An equally acceptable reverse order might produce "He doesn't love sweets, does he?"

Questions are prevalent in the speech adults address to children. Although the amount of questioning doesn't change much in the first eighteen months for each parent–child pair, the types of questions and the topics do. At first, questions are used to comment on what the child is gazing at or to direct the child's attention to the mother's activity. By eighteen months, the questions are mostly tutorial or genuine requests for information.

Children begin to ask questions at the one-word level through the use of rising intonation ("Doggie?"↑), through some variation of *what* ("Wha?", "Tha?", or "Wassat?"), or through a phonetically consistent form (see Chapter 3). There appear to be three phases of question development in young children (Table 10.9). The first phase, which corresponds to an MLU of 1.75 to 2.25, is characterized by the following three types of question form:

Nucleus + intonation	That horsie?
What + noun phrase + (*doing*)	What that?
	What doggie (doing)?
Where + noun phrase + (*going*)	Where ball?
	Where man (go)?

These questions are confined to a few routines in which the child requests the names of objects, actions, or locations. The child neither comprehends nor asks other *wh-* questions appropriately, although *why* may be used as a turn filler to keep the conversation going. *What* and *where* may appear early because they relate to the child's immediate environment. *What* is used to gain labels; *where*, to locate lost objects. In addition, both are heavily used by parents to encourage the child's performance and are related to the semantic categories of nomination and location.

During the next phase, which corresponds to late stage II and early stage III, the child continues to ask *what* and *where* questions but uses both a subject and a predicate. Examples include "What doggie eat?" and "Where Johnnie is?" Other questions, such as the yes/no type, are still identified by rising intonation alone, as in "Daddy go work?"↑.

The first subject-verb inversion occurs at the end of this phase in *wh-* interrogatives with the copula (*wh-* + *copula* + *subject* as in *Where is daddy?*) (Wells, 1985). Inversion may occur in this form first because of its simplicity. As might be expected, the first *wh-* words in this construction are *what* and *where*.

In the third phase, the child begins to use the auxiliary forms required in adult question form. This phase corresponds to late stage III and stage IV (MLU, 2.75 to 3.5). It is during this stage that the child is developing the auxiliary verb in other sentence types, and there is carryover to interrogatives. Although rising intonation continues to be an alternative form for asking yes/no questions, the auxiliary begins to be inverted, as in the adult form. At about the same time or shortly after the child inverts the auxiliary in yes/no questions appropriately, he or she begins to invert within *wh-* and yes/no copular interrogative constructions (Wells, 1985). Some children may begin to use auxiliaries in the properly inverted form (Klee, 1985).

In *wh-* questions, the type of *wh-* word used may influence whether the auxiliary is inverted. In general, the earlier the *wh-* word is acquired, the more likely the verb is to be inverted. Hence, the child would be more likely to invert the verb in *what* questions than in *why* questions. Inverted forms, whether in yes/no or *wh-* questions, are not mastered for some time. These forms require the child to learn the following three rules:

1. The auxiliary verb is inverted to precede the subject.

   She can play house. *Can* she play house?
   Tom is eating candy. What *is* Tom eating?

2. The copula is inverted to precede the subject.

   They are funny. *Are* they funny?
   Mary is in school. Where *is* Mary?

3. The dummy do is inserted before the subject if no copula or auxiliary exists.

   Todd loves Joannie. *Does* Todd love Joannie?
   Mike drank a soda. What *did* Mike drink?

By the end of stage IV, the child has attained the basic adult question form. In addition, *who, when,* and *how* interrogatives appear, although the child still has some difficulty with the temporal aspects of the last two (Kuczaj & Maratsos, 1975). This difficulty was discussed in relation to cognitive growth in Chapter 9.

The general order of acquisition of *wh-* question types may relate to the elements in the sentence that each *wh-* word replaces. Words such as *what, where,* and *who* are pronoun forms for the sentence elements they replace. For example, in the sentence "Mother is eating ice cream," we can substitute *what* for *ice cream*. The resultant question is "What is mother eating?" In contrast, words such as *how* and *when* are used to ask for semantic relations within the sentence. These semantic relations are more difficult than simple noun substitutions; they develop later and usually cannot be replaced by a single word. The late development of *why* interrogatives can be explained in similar fashion. Unlike the other *wh-* types, *why* interrogatives affect the entire clause rather than sentence elements or relationships.

The ability to respond to *wh-* questions is also related to semantics and to the immediate context (Parnell et al., 1984). In general, preschool children are more successful in giving appropriate and accurate responses when the question refers to objects, persons, and events in the immediate setting. Recognition of the type of information sought, such as an object or a location, seems to precede the ability to respond with the specific information requested, such as the name of the object or location.

As in negation, stage V interrogative development is mainly concerned with tensing and modals. In addition, the child stabilizes the use of the inverted auxiliary. The adult tag question form doesn't appear until stage V because of its relative complexity and its infrequent usage in American English (Klee, 1985). Less complex forms—using tags such as *okay*, *huh*, and *aye*, as in "I do this, okay?"—develop earlier. These forms are more commonly used among English-speaking populations of Canada and Australia in sentences such as "Nice day, aye?"

Three phases have been identified in the development of tag questions (Reich, 1986). At first, grammatically simple tag forms, such as *okay* and *right*, are used. Truer tags are added later, but with no negation of the proposition (Mills, 1981; Richards, 1988; P. Todd, 1982; Weeks, 1992). For example, the child might ask, "You like cookies, *do* you?" Finally, the full adult tag, as in "You like cookies, *don't* you?" or "You don't like cookies, *do* you?", is acquired during early school age. Mature tags require complex syntax, so simple tags predominate until age five (Berninger & Garvey, 1982).

American English-speaking children acquire the adult form later than do British and Australian children because of its infrequent use in American English. Canadian children may also be somewhat late in mastering the full adult form because of the colloquial use of *aye*, as in "You bought a new suit, *aye*? Just right for this weather, *aye*?" (Dennis, Sugar, & Whitaker, 1982). I usually tease my Canadian students that it is impossible for them to make a declaration because they always attach *aye* to the end of every sentence.

Negative interrogatives appear after age five. In general, negative interrogatives, such as "Aren't you going?", are first acquired almost exclusively in the uninverted form, as in "You aren't going?" (Erreich, 1984).

Imperative-Sentence Form

Adult imperative sentences appear in stage III. In the imperative form the speaker requests, demands, asks, insists, commands, and so on that the listener perform some act. The verb is uninflected and the subject, *you*, is understood. Examples include the following:

Gimee a cookie, please.
Throw the ball to me.
Pass the peas, please.

It is somewhat difficult to recognize the imperative in English because there are no morphological markers. In addition, stage I children will produce early forms that mirror imperative sentence form, such as "Eat cookie." These are not true imperatives, however, because young children often omit the subject from sentences clearly intended to be declarative. Omission reflects processing limitations. There is no unequivocal marking of younger children's imperative forms. This is not meant to imply that toddlers cannot demand of or command others. Even at a prelinguistic level, infants are very adept at expressing their needs.

Negative-Sentence Form

Five adult forms of the negative exist: (1) *not* and *-n't* attached to the verb; (2) negative words, such as *nobody* and *nothing*; (3) the determiner *no* used before nouns or nounlike words, as in "*No* cookies for you"; (4) negative adverbs, such as *never* and *nowhere*; and (5) negative prefixes, such as *un-*, *dis-*, and *non-*. Rejection of, or opposition to, a proposition is the first type of negation to emerge, possibly because the child is expressing attitudes toward events and entities that are within her sensorimotor knowledge.

The side-to-side head shake to indicate negation appears at ten to fourteen months. The child uses this gesture to express rejection of an event, object, or activity that is being proposed or to self-reprimand for attempting some prohibited activity.

The earliest symbolic negative to appear is the single-word form *no*, which is frequently found within the first fifty words. The order of emergence of negative types is not the same for nonverbal and verbal modes (J. de Villiers, 1984). In contrast to the initial nonverbal use of negative as rejection, in the verbal mode the child expresses nonexistence first, then rejection, and finally denial (Clancy, 1985).

Syntactic negation appears in two-word utterances, generally as "negative + *X*," although the reversal may also be seen. In this period, *no* and *not* are used interchangeably. The *X* is usually less complex than an entire sentence. For example, the child might say "Baby eat ice cream," but when negating would produce "No eat ice cream" rather than "No Baby eat ice cream." Thus, the negative element appears prior to the verb, as in adult negation, and utterances such as "No Daddy go bye-bye" appear less frequently.

The full *negative + sentence nucleus* form is usually seen in rejection of a proposed or current course of action. For example, if the father were in the process of leaving and the child objected, he or she might state, "No Daddy go bye-bye." Other negative utterances use the *negative + verb* format, such as "No go bye-bye" when describing Daddy's return from putting something in the car or "No eat ice cream," mentioned previously.

The specific negative element(s) the child uses seems to reflect parental use with the child. Some parents prefer to control behavior with *no*; others employ *don't*. In general, children prefer to use certain forms to fulfill specific functions. Since this is an individual preference, there is great variety.

Within stage II, the child may also use the negative in nonsyntactic statements such as "No Daddy." These can be explained only as a conversational or discourse device (Bellugi, 1967). The child may produce "*No/not* + an affirmative statement" in response to a previous utterance. For example, if the mother says "Mommy pick you up," the child may respond with "No Daddy." While the surface interpretation appears to negate any help from father, the child may mean "*No*, Mommy, *Daddy* will do it."

There seem to be three periods of syntactic development of negation (Table 10.9) which do not correspond exactly to Brown's stages. The first period, discussed earlier, occurs in stage I and early stage II up to an MLU of 2.25. In the second period, which corresponds to late stage II and early III, the child uses the contractions *can't* and *don't* interchangeably with *no* and *not*. The child does not differentiate these forms, and their positive elements, *can* and *do*, appear only later. Hence, the sentences "I don't eat it" and "I can't eat it" may mean the same thing. *Won't* appears in late stage III and, for a brief period, may also be used interchangeably with *no*, *not*, *don't*, and *can't*. Within a sentence, the negative structure is placed between the subject and the predicate or main verb.

In the final period, an MLU of 2.75 to 3.5, the child develops other auxiliary forms. This period corresponds roughly to Brown's stage IV. The child develops the positive elements *can*, *do*, *does*, *did*, *will*, and *be*, which may be used with *not* followed by a verb, as in "She *cannot* go." Contracted forms also continue to occur. It will be some time, however, before the child correctly uses all the morphological markers for person, number, and tense with auxiliary verbs. Because use of auxiliaries is a relatively new behavior, the child may continue to make errors, such as double tense markers, as in "I didn't did it."

By late stage IV, the child's negative contractions include *isn't*, *aren't*, *doesn't*, and *didn't* (J. Miller, 1981). This development of negative forms continues in stage V with the addition of the past tense of *be* (*wasn't*) and modals such as *wouldn't*, *couldn't*, and *shouldn't*. These forms appear infrequently at first. In addition, the *copula + negative* form, as in "She *is not* (*isn't*) happy," appears in stage V (Wells, 1985).

The period of most note for negation is around stage III, when the child begins to vary the negative in form and to insert it between the subject and predicate (main verb). Thus, negative utterances move from the *negative + X* form to a *subject + negative + predicate* form. These changes are obvious adaptations toward the structure used by adults to express negation. Hence, the development of negation appears to be one of the significant aspects of stage III.

It would be incorrect to assume, however, that children master the negative within the preschool period. Negative interrogatives do not appear until after age five. In addition, indefinite forms, such as *nobody*, *no one*, *none*, and *nothing*, prove troublesome even for some adults. It is not uncommon to hear

> I don't want none.
> Nobody don't like me.
> I ain't scared of nothing.
> I didn't get no cookies.

Some of these double negatives occur so frequently in the speech of children and some adults that they almost seem acceptable.

EMBEDDING AND CONJOINING

Sentences are strings of related words or larger units containing a noun subject and a verb or predicate. For example, the sentence "She ate cookies" is a string of words related in a certain way. *She* has acted on *cookies*. Other strings can be in a series, one following another. We have all heard a child's sentence similar in form to this one:

I ate popcorn, cotton candy, hot dogs, soda, ice cream, pretzels, and threw up.

Here the subject acts on several serial objects.

The units within sentences are composed of words, phrases, and clauses. A **phrase** is a group of related words that does not include a subject and a predicate and is used as a noun substitute or as a noun or verb modifier. For example, the phrase *to fish* can take the place of a noun. In the sentence "I love candy," *to fish* can be substituted for *candy*, a noun, to form "I love to fish." Other phrases modify nouns, as in "The man *in the blue suit*," or verbs, as in "Loren fought *with a vengeance*." The phrase is said to be embedded within a sentence.

In contrast to a phrase, a **clause** is a group of words that contains both a subject and a predicate. A clause that can stand alone as grammatically complete is a **simple sentence**. Thus, "Jesus wept" is a simple sentence. Occasionally, a sentence may contain more than one clause. When a sentence is combined with another sentence, they each become **main clauses**. A **compound sentence** is made up of two or more main clauses joined as equals, as in "*Mary drove to work*, and *she had an accident*." Both "Mary drove to work" and "She had an accident" are simple sentences serving as main clauses in the larger compound sentence. Main clauses may be joined by conjunctions, such as *and*, *but*, *because*, *if*, and so on. This process is called **conjoining** or coordinating.

Some clauses, such as *whom we met last week*, cannot stand alone even though they contain a subject and a predicate. In this example, *we* is the subject and *met* is the predicate, or main verb. Such clauses, called **subordinate clauses**, function as nouns, adjectives, or adverbs in support of the main clause. For example, *she is the girl*, a simple sentence, or main clause, can be joined with the subordinate clause above to form "She is the girl whom we met last week."

A sentence such as this, made up of a main clause and at least one subordinate clause, is called a **complex sentence**. The subordinate clause is said to be *embedded* within the main clause. In general, subordinate clauses are introduced by subordinating conjunctions, such as *after*, *although*, *before*, *until*, *while*, and *when*, or by relative pronouns, such as *who*, *which*, and *that*. For example, the sentence "He doesn't know when it began to rain" contains the subordinate clause *when it began to rain*, which serves as the object of the verb *know*. In "the man who lives here hates children," *who lives here* is a subordinate clause modifying *man*.

In the following sections, we shall discuss the development of both embedding within a sentence and conjoining. As you can imagine, multiple embeddings may result in very complicated sentences.

The emergence of embedding is one of the primary characteristics of stage IV. Most children use some form of embedding within this stage (J. Miller, 1981). Conjoining characterizes stage V, although early conjoining may begin in stage IV. In **embedding**, a phrase or sentence becomes a grammatical element of a sentence, such as acting as an adverb or postnoun modifier. Although conjoining also combines clauses, these clauses each serve as a main clause.

Phrasal Embedding

Phrases can be formed in four ways: (1) with a preposition, (2) with a participle, (3) with a gerund, and (4) with an infinitive. A prepositional phrase contains a preposition, such as *in, on, under, at,* or *into,* and its object, along with possible articles and modifiers, as in *on the roof* or *at the school dance.* These forms have developed throughout stages II through V, beginning with the appearance of *in* and *on.* Development continues throughout the school-age years. Children begin adding prepositional phrases to the ends of sentences at around age three.

A participial phrase contains a participle (a verb-derived word ending in *-ing, -ed, -t, -en,* or a few irregular forms) and serves as an adjective. Examples of participles include the *setting* sun, a *lost* cause, a *broken* promise, and a *fallen* warrior. In the sentence "The boy riding the bicycle is athletic," *riding the bicycle* is a participial phrase describing or modifying *boy.*

In contrast, a gerund, which also ends in *-ing,* functions as a noun. Gerunds may be used as a subject ("*Skiing* is fun"), as an object ("I enjoy *skiing*"), or in any other sentence function that may be filled by a noun.

Finally, an infinitive phrase may function as a noun but also as an adjective or adverb. An infinitive consists of *to* plus a verb, as in "He wanted *to open* his present." The entire phrase *to open his present* is an infinitive phrase serving as the object of the sentence. The *to* may be omitted after certain verbs, as in "He helped *clean up the mess*" or "He dared not *speak aloud.*"

Infinitive Embeddings

At around age two-and-a-half the child develops semi-infinitives such as *gonna* and *wanna.* Occasionally, these forms are followed by a verb, as in "I want (or *wanna*) eat cookie," but at this age, they usually are used alone, as in "I wanna" (Wells, 1985). The word *to* is first used at about this time, but as a preposition indicating "direction toward," as in "I walked *to* the store," not as an infinitive (Bloom, Tackeff, & Lahey, 1984). By stage IV, forms such as *gonna, wanna, gotta, hafta,* and *sposta* are being used regularly with verbs to form infinitive phrases, usually in the object position. Examples include "I got*ta go* home" and "I wan*na play.*" The semiauxiliary and the verb share the same subject.

More complex infinitives also begin to appear, usually at the ends of sentences. For example, the child develops *wh-* infinitives, such as "I know *how to do it*" and "Show me *where to put it.*" The child also begins to use unmarked infinitive phrases following verbs such as *help, make,* and *watch,* as in "She can help me *pick these up.*" This form is more difficult for the child because the infinitive is not clearly marked.

In stage V, the child begins to use infinitives with nouns other than the subject. For example, the child may say "This is the right way *to do it*" or "I got this *to give to you.*"

Most post-stage V children (MLU of 4.5 to 5.0) continue to use simple but true infinitives with the same subject as the main verb (J. Miller, 1981). Infinitives are initially learned and used with a small set of verbs, such as *see*, *look*, *know*, *think*, *say*, and *tell*, as in "I want *to see it*" or "I don't have *to tell you*" (Bloom et al., 1984).

Gerund Embeddings

In general, gerund development follows that of infinitives (Table 10.9). Gerunds appear after stage V. They first appear in the object position at the end of the sentence. Gerunds are one of the first forms of derivational suffixes acquired, using -*ing* to change a verb to a noun.

Subordinate Clause Embedding

Embedding of subordinate clauses appears at about the same time as true infinitives (Table 10.9). In general, we find three types of embedding: (1) object noun-phrase complements, (2) indirect or embedded *wh-* questions, and (3) relative clauses. Although object noun complements and embedded *wh-* questions appear first, by age four-and-a-half to five, these types of subordination account for less than 15 percent of all two-clause utterances (Tyack & Gottsleben, 1986).

Object noun-phrase complements consist of a subordinate clause that serves as the object of the main clause. For example, we could say "I know *X* (something)" in which *X* is the object. We could replace *X* with a noun phrase (*a story*) or with a subordinate clause, such as (*that*) *I like it* to form "I know (*that*) *I like it*." An early form such as "I want *that*" may initially appear in stage III (Wells, 1985). The fuller clausal object noun-phrase complements first appear in stage IV. These subordinate clauses generally have the form of simple sentences, as in

I know *that you can do it.*
I think *that I like stew.*

In general, the subordinate clause fills an object role for transitive verbs, such as *think*, *guess*, *wish*, *know*, *hope*, *like*, *let*, *remember*, *forget*, *look*, and *show*. The verb in the main clause is most often *think*. By stages IV and V, these types of embedding account for over 85 percent of all two-clause utterances (Tyack & Gottsleben, 1986). By late state V, the child may omit the conjunction *that*. A similar construction following the copula, as in "that is what I know," develops after stage V (Wells, 1985).

Indirect or **embedded *wh-* questions** are similar to object noun-phrase complements. In the following sentences, the *wh-* subordinate clause fills the object function, as in "I know *X*":

I know *who did it.*
She saw *where the kitty went.*

Initial subordinating words include *wh-* words such as *what*, *where*, and *when*, with *what* being used most frequently (Scott, 1988). Since this form appears at about the same time that the child begins to acquire the adult interrogative form, some confusion may exist. Resultant forms may include

I know *what is that.*
Tell me *where does the smoke go.*

Relative clauses are subordinate clauses that follow and modify nouns. Rather than take the place of a noun, these clauses are attached to a noun with relative pronouns, such as *who*, *which*, and *that*. The earliest relative pronouns are *that*, *what*, and *where* (Scott, 1988; Wells, 1985). At first, these clauses modify empty or nonspecific nouns—*one*, *kind*, *thing*— or abstract adverbs—*place*, *way*—to form sentences such as "This is the one (*that*) *I want*" or "This is the way (*that*) *I do it*" (Wells, 1985). In these examples, the object of the sentence is *one* or *way*, and the subordinate clause specifies *which one* or *which way*. Later, relative clauses are used to modify common nouns, as in "Chien Ping has the book (that) I bought."

Full relative clauses appear in Stage V, close to the fourth birthday, although partial forms may appear earlier. They develop gradually, accounting for less than 15 percent of the two-clause utterances of four-and-a-half- to five-year-olds (J. Miller, 1981; Wells, 1985). As with other types of embedding, expansion begins at the end of the sentence, as in the following:

This is the kind *what I like.*
This is the toy *that I want.*

In these examples, the relative clause is attached to and modifies the object of the sentence. Some examples of relative clauses attached to the subject include

The one *that you have* is big.
The boy *who lives in that house* is a brat.

Relative clauses attached to the subject do not develop until after five years of age (Wells, 1985). These forms are still rare by age seven.

Many connective words used to join clauses are first learned in nonconnective contexts. For example, *what* and *where* appear in interrogatives prior to their use as relative pronouns. The connective *when* is an exception. *When* is used as a connector to mark temporal relations before the *when* question form develops. Thus, children are likely to produce "I don't know *when* he went" before "*When* did he leave?" Most preschool errors involve use of the wrong relative pronoun as in the following examples (McKee, McDaniel, & Snedeker, 1998, p. 587):

The potato what she's rolling.
Those plates why the elephants are eating them.
The chairs who are flying.

Mature English speakers can omit some relative pronouns, such as *that*, without changing the meaning of the sentence. At first, the child needs these pronouns in order to interpret the sentence. By stage V, however, she or he can comprehend a sentence that omits the subordinate conjunction. The child begins to omit some relative pronouns in production in late stage V, although this form is rare in the speech of preschool children:

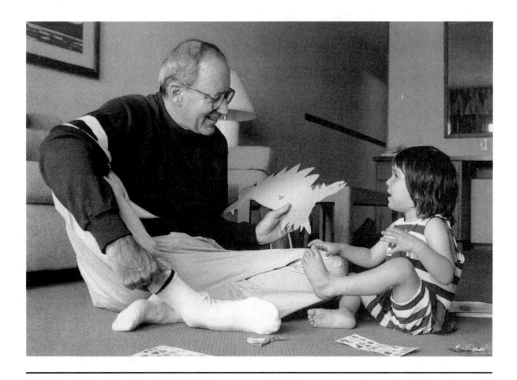

Coloring, cutting, and pasting projects can provide valuable input about sentential relationships, such as embedding and conjoining. An example is, Put the paste on the one that have in your hand, then put it on the paper.

This is the candy *that* Hasan likes. (relative pronoun present)
This is the candy Hasan likes. (relative pronoun omitted)

By late stage V, most children can produce multiple embeddings within a single sentence, although such forms are rare even throughout the early school years (J. Miller, 1981). For example, a child may combine a subordinate clause (italicized) with an infinitive (underlined) to produce

I think *we <u>gotta go home now.</u>*

Later forms also include conjoined clauses and embedding in the same sentence.

Clausal Conjoining

In stage I, the child may produce two-word or three-word utterances that consist of a series of objects, such as "Coat hat" or "Cookie juice." No relation seems apparent other than a naming sequence. The child may omit the conjunction *and* which is, however, the first conjunction to appear, usually by late stage I. Most children have appropriate production of *and* between twenty-five and twenty-seven months of age (Bloom, Lahey, Hood, Lifter, & Fiess, 1980; Lust & Mervis, 1980). Characteristically, the child lists entities or produces compound objects, such as "You got *this* and *this*." Such listing reflects cognitive growth. Cognitively, children are able to form collections of things before they can form an ordered series. Individual sentences within a series may begin with *and*, as in the following:

> And I petted the dog. And he barked. And I runned home.

In this example, *and* fills a temporal function meaning *and then*.

In stage IV, the conjunction *because* appears, either alone or attached to a single clause, as in the following examples:

> *Adult:*   Scott, why did you do that?
> *Child:*   Because.
>
> *Adult:*   Scott, why did you do that?
> *Child:*   Because Roger did.

Utterances with *because* are particularly interesting. Since the three- or four-year-old child has difficulty recounting events nonsequentially, she or he will respond to event queries with a result response rather than a causal one (see the discussion of four-year-olds in Chapter 3). In response to "Why did you fall off your bicycle?" the child is likely to respond "'Cause I hurted my leg"—a result, not a cause.

The first clausal conjoining occurs with the conjunction *and* in stage IV (Table 10.9). For example, the child might say "I went to the party *and* Jimmie hit me." It is not until late stage V, however, that most children can use this form (Lust & Mervis, 1980; J. Miller, 1981). In general, *and* is used as the all-purpose conjunction (Bloom et al., 1980; Scott, 1988). For example, *and*, which is additive, will be used for temporal, causal, and adversative functions in place of *when*, *then*, *because*, and so on, as in the following:

> We left *and* mommy called. (meaning *when*)
> We had a party *and* we saw a movie. (meaning *then*)
> She went home *and* they had a fight. (meaning *because*)

Depending on the child, *and* may be used five to twenty times as frequently as the next most common conjunction in the child's repertoire (Scott, 1988). Even in the narratives of five-year-olds and school-age children, *and* is the predominant connector of clauses (Bennett-Kaster, 1986; Scott, 1987).

Clausal conjoining with *if* appears in late stage V, *because* in post-stage V, and *when*, *but*, and *so* even later, beyond an MLU of 5.0 morphemes. Most children are capable of conjoining clauses with *if* during this latter period (J. Miller, 1981). These are not usually complicated sentences; they are more likely to be of the "I can *if* I want to" form. Initially, the causal relationship may be signaled by *that's why*, as in "They're running; that's why they broke the window" (Wells, 1985). The order of conjunction acquisition reported for American English seems to be true for other languages as well and may reflect the underlying cognitive relationship.

The conjunctions *because* and *so* are initially used to mark psychological causality or statements of people's intentions (H. Johnson & Chapman, 1980). For example, use of *because* might explain "He hit me *because he's mean*" rather than "The bridge fell *because the truck was too heavy*." If the child were to discuss the bridge falling, he or she might explain, "The bridge fell *because it was tired*," using feeling or intention to explain the event. Young children tend to talk about the present or the future, although there is a trend toward recounting the past as children get older and, as noted, narratives become more causally related (McCabe & Peterson, 1985). With this recounting, there is a greater necessity to discuss the intentions preceding behaviors.

At around age four, the child may begin to exhibit conjoining and embedding within the same sentence. Most children are using this type of structure, although rarely, by age five. Such multiple embedding might result in the following:

*Sally wants **to stay on the sand** and Carrie is scared of crabs.*

Three-clause sentences, both embedded and conjoined, appear at about the same age. The child might join three main clauses, as in the following:

Julio flew his kite, I ate a hot dog, and papa took a nap.

Another variation might include the embedding and conjoining of three clauses, as in the following:

*I saw Star Wars, and Claritta saw the one **that had Tarzan**.*

Although both multiple embedding and three-clause sentences are rare in the speech of the typical kindergartener, they do occur occasionally. By age four-and-a-half to five, multiple embeddings and three-clause sentences may account for about 11 percent of all child utterances.

Conjoining may include whole clauses or clauses with deleted common elements, called **phrasal coordination**, as in "Mary ran and fell." In full clausal or **sentential coordination**, such as "Mary ran and Mary fell," *Mary* is redundant and may be deleted, as in the first example. Obviously, sentential coordination, such as "Mary ran and John fell," does not lend itself to such shortening. Conjoining by children is relatively independent of the length of the two units to be conjoined, although, obviously, the very young child is not capable of producing long utterances (Lust & Mervis, 1980). Initially, sentential coordination seems to be used for events that occur at different times in different locations, while phrasal coordination is used for simultaneous or near-simultaneous events in the same location.

In phrasal coordination, forward reductions are more common and appear earlier than backward reductions (Lust & Mervis, 1980). In *forward reductions*, the full clause is stated first, followed by a conjunction, plus the nonredundant information. "Reggie made the cookies by himself and ate them before dinner" is an example of forward reduction. *Reggie* is redundant in the second clause. Conversely, in *backward reductions* the full clause follows the conjunction, as in "Reggie and Noi baked cookies." Ease of processing may be more closely related to the amount of information the child is required to hold than to the direction of reduction (Hakuta, et al., 1982). Preschool children have great difficulty with a sentence such as "The sheep patted the kangaroo and the pig the giraffe" because of the amount of information that must be held in short-term memory while deciphering this sentence.

Pragmatic and semantic factors seem to affect conjoining as well. Clausal conjoining occurs where two referents must be clearly distinguished. The child encodes only what he or she presupposes the listener needs to interpret the sentence (P. de Villiers, 1982). The complexity of semantic relations expressed by conjoining is also a factor (Bloom, Lahey et al., 1980). Although the forms of these compound sentences are all *clause + conjunction + clause*, the relations between the clauses, as expressed in the conjunction, form a hierarchy that affects the order of acquisition. These might be additive, causal, or contrastive. Initial clausal conjoining is additive; no relationship is expressed, as in "Tom went on the hike and Bob was at Grandma's." Next, conjoining is used to express either simultaneous or sequential events, as in "Diego went to school and he went shopping after dinner."

Causal relationships with *and* appear next, as in "*X and* [led to] *Y*." Later *because* is used for causality.

Finally, the child expresses a contrasting relationship, usually with the use of *but*. The late appearance of the conjunction *but* in clausal conjoining is probably related to the complex nature of such propositions. The expectation that is set up in the first clause is not confirmed in the second, as in "I went to the zoo, but I didn't see any tapirs."

Summary

The syntactic development of the preschool child is rapid and very complex. The interrelatedness of both syntactic structure and syntactic development makes it difficult to describe patterns of development. In general, the preschool child tries to discover and employ syntactic regularity. She or he uses the predominant subject-verb-object sentence structure and depends on order of mention for sequencing. Newly acquired structures, such as the negative and embedded phrases and clauses, are initially attached to either end of the sentence and only later integrated into it. These and other language-learning principles were discussed in detail in Chapter 7.

PHONOLOGICAL DEVELOPMENT

Many of the morphological and syntactic changes noted in the preschool years are related to phonological development and reflect the child's underlying phonological rule system. In addition to developing the phonetic inventory described in the appendix, the preschool child is also developing phonological rules that govern sound distribution and sequencing. Examples of distribution and sequencing are given in Chapter 1.

As with other aspects of language, the child's phonological development progresses through a long period of language decoding and hypothesis building. The child uses many rule forms, presented in Table 10.10, that will be discarded or modified later. These rules reflect natural processes that act to simplify adult forms of speech for young children. Much of the child's morphological production will depend on her ability to perceive and produce

TABLE 10.10 Phonological Processes of Preschool Children

PROCESSES	EXAMPLES
Syllable structure	
Deletion of final consonants	*cu* (/kʌ/) for *cup*
Deletion of unstressed syllables	*nana* for *banana*
Reduplication	*mama, dada, wawa* (water)
Reduction of clusters	/s/ + consonant (*stop*) = delete /s/ (*top*)
Assimilation	
Contiguous	
Between consonants	*beds* (/bɛdz/), *bets* (/bɛts/)
Regressive VC (vowel alters toward	
some feature of C)	nasalization of vowels: *can*
Noncontiguous	
Back assimilation	*dog* becomes *gog*
	dark becomes *gawk*
Substitution	
Obstruants (plosives, fricatives, and	
affricatives)	
Stopping: replace sound with a	*this* becomes *dis*
plosive	
Fronting: replace palatals and velars	*Kenny* becomes *Tenny*
(/k/ and /g/) with alveolars (/t/ and /d/)	*go* becomes *do*
Nasals	
Fronting (/ŋ/ becomes /n/)	*something* becomes *somethin*
Approximants replaced by	
Plosive	*yellow* becomes *yedow*
Glide	*rabbit* becomes *wabbit*
Another approximant	*girl* becomes *gaul* (/gɔl/)
Vowels	
Neutralization: vowels	
reduced to /ə/ or /a/	*want to* becomes *wanna*
Deletion of sounds	*balloon* becomes *ba-oon*

Source: Drawn from D. Ingram, *Phonological Disability in Children*. London: Edward Arnold, 1976.

phonological units. During the preschool years, the child not only acquires a phonetic inventory and a phonological system, but also "develops the ability to determine which speech sounds are used to signal differences in meaning" (Ingram, 1976, p. 22).

Some adult sounds and rules are more difficult to perceive and produce. This is evidenced by the long acquisitional process, which continues into early elementary school. It appears that perception of speech sounds precedes production but that the two aspects are not parallel.

Phonological Processes

We will discuss the phonological processes of the preschool child, summarized in Table 10.10, in some detail. Additional descriptive information and examples will also be presented. Most of these processes are discarded or modified by age four.

Syllable Structure Processes

Once the child begins babbling, the basic speech unit used is the CV syllable. During the preschool years, the child frequently attempts to simplify production by reducing words to this form or to the CVCV structure.

The most basic form of this process affects the final consonant. The final consonant may be deleted, thus producing a CV structure for a CVC—*ba* (/bɔ/) for *ball*—or followed by a vowel to produce a CVCV structure—*cake-a* (/k eI kə/) for *cake*. This process of vowel insertion is termed **epenthesis**. The child may also lengthen the vowel that precedes the final consonant or may substitute a glottal stop or plosive (/h/) for the consonant. These three behaviors—addition of a final vowel, lengthening of the preceding vowel, and glottal stop substitution—are usually the first steps in the acquisition of final consonants. Nasal sounds are some of the first to appear as final consonants. Final-consonant processes usually disappear by age three (Grunwell, 1981).

In addition, the child may delete unstressed syllables to produce, for example, *way* for *away*. Initially, any unstressed syllable may be eliminated, although the child gradually adopts a pattern of deleting only initial unstressed syllables. Syllable reduction may be more complex than simply deleting the unstressed syllable and may reflect the interaction of syllable stress, location within the word, and phrase boundaries (Snow, 1998). This deletion process continues until age four. Development of syllables, word shapes, and consonant cluster types are presented in Table 10.11.

Reduplication is a third process for simplifying syllable structure in which one syllable becomes similar to another in the word, resulting in the reduplicated structure, as in *wawa* for *water*. It appears that reduplication is a step in the acquisition of final consonants; thus, it should not surprise us that this process disappears for most children before thirty months of age (Grunwell, 1981).

TABLE 10.11 Phonological Development

AGE IN MONTHS	SYLLABLE STRUCTURE	NUMBER OF SYLLABLES
24	CV, VC CVC	2
36	CV, VC, CVC, CC____, ____CC	2
48	CV, VC, CVC, CC____, ____CC, CC____CC	3
60	CV, VC, CVC, CC____, ____CC, CC____CC	3+

Adapted from Shriberg, L.D. (1993). Four new speech and prosody voice measures for genetics research and other studies of developmental phonological disorders. *Journal of Speech and Hearing Research, 36,* 105–140.

Several factors influence reduplication processes in polysyllabic words (H. Klein, 1981). An interaction of syllable stress and order seems to be most significant. The final syllable is usually deleted or changed, as in *wawa*. Otherwise, the clearly stressed syllable is most often reproduced, while gradations of stress result in a less clear reproduction pattern. The final position is not particularly important for preschoolers unless it is preceded by an unstressed syllable, as in *elephant* or *ambulance* (H. Klein, 1981). The reduplication of stressed final syllables may reflect (a) the increased duration of the final syllable when it follows an unstressed syllable or (b) the reduced vowel quality of the unstressed syllable to a middle or neutral vowel, such as /ə/. This occurs in the second syllable of *elephant* (/ɛləfɪnt/). In this case, the final syllable receives more emphasis, and the child is likely to produce something such as "ehfafa" (/ɛfʌfʌ/), reduplicating this syllable.

Finally, preschoolers reduce or simplify consonant clusters, usually by deleting one consonant. Cluster reduction is one of the most common phonological processes seen in the speech of Spanish-speaking Puerto Rican preschoolers (Goldstein & Iglesias, 1996). While deletions differ based on the parent language and the individual child, we can predict with some certainty how preschoolers will simplify many clusters. The following are a few examples from English:

Cluster	Deletion	Example
/s/ + plosive	/s/	*stop* becomes *top*
plosive or fricative + liquid or glide	liquid or glide	*bring* becomes *bing*
	swim becomes *sim*	

Nasal clusters are more complex. If a nasal plus a plosive or fricative is reduced, younger children will delete the nasal. Thus, *bump* becomes *bup*. Older preschoolers will delete the plosive if it is voiced. Employing this rule, the child reduces *mend* to *men*. The child may also exhibit epenthesis, producing both consonants with a vowel between them. Thus, *tree* becomes *teree*. This vowel-insertion process is infrequent. The specific strategy used and the speed of consonant cluster development vary with the sounds involved (Grunwell, 1981; Vihman & Greenlee, 1987). Most children stop using the cluster-reduction process by age four.

Assimilation Processes

Assimilation processes simplify production by producing different sounds in the same way. In general, one sound becomes similar to another in the same word. Assimilation processes may be contiguous or noncontiguous and progressive or regressive. Contiguous assimilation occurs when the two elements are next to each other; noncontiguous assimilation, when apart. Progressive assimilation occurs when the affected element follows the element that influences it; regressive assimilation, when the affected element precedes. For example, children generally produce two varieties of *doggie*. One, *doddie*, exemplifies progressive assimilation, while the other, *goggie*, is regressive.

Regressive contiguous assimilation is exhibited in both CV and VC syllables. The consonant in CV structures may be affected by the voicing of the vowel, as when the voiceless *t* in *top* is produced as a voiced *d*, resulting in *dop*. In regressive VC assimilation, the vowel alters toward some feature of the consonant, as in the nasalized vowels in *can* and *ham*. Progressive contiguous assimilation is much less common.

The most common type of noncontiguous assimilation is back assimilation, in which one consonant is modified toward another that is produced farther back in the oral cavity. The *d* in *dark*, for example, may become a *g* to produce *gawk* (/gɔk/).

Substitution Processes

Many preschoolers substitute sounds in their speech. These substitutions are not random. Specific substitutions are usually in one direction. The /w/ is often substituted for /ɹ/, for example, but only rarely does the opposite occur. In addition, when the child masters a phoneme, it does not overgeneralize to words in which the substituted sound is the correct sound. For example, the child may say *wabbit* and *wooster* until mastering /ɹ/. At that point, the child can produce *rabbit* and *rooster*, but the /ɹ/ does not overgeneralize to the /w/ in *what* and *wanna*, in which /w/ is correct.

In general, the types of substitutions can be described according to the manner of production of the target sound. Obstruant sounds, which include fricatives and affricates, may experience *stopping*, in which a plosive is substituted. Stopping is most common in the initial position in words, as in *dat* for *that* or *dis* for *this*. This process decreases gradually as the child masters fricatives, although stopping with *th* sounds (/ð,θ/) may persist until early school age (Grunwell, 1981). Early production of nasal sounds may also be accompanied by stopping. This denasalization, similar to "head cold" speech, substitutes a plosive from the similar position in the oral cavity for a nasal (*Sam* becomes *Sab*).

Another process is *fronting*, a tendency to replace palatals and velars with alveolar sounds. Thus, /t/ and /d/ are substituted for /k/ and /g/, producing *tan* for *can* and *dun* for *gun*. As many as 23 percent of three-year-olds demonstrate fronting. This percentage decreases rapidly, so that by age four-and-a-half only about 3.5 percent of children still exhibit this behavior (Lowe, Knutson, & Monson, 1985). Fronting is also evident in nasal sounds. The /n/ may be substituted for /ŋ/, as in *sinin* for *singing*.

Approximants, /l/ and /ɹ/, may also experience stopping initially but are generally replaced by another approximant. *Gliding*, in which /j/ or /w/ replaces /l/ or /ɹ/, evolves only slowly and may last for several years. I recall one example of gliding that occurred after I had broken my leg in a bicycling accident. Out of concern, one of my children inquired, "How your yid?" (leg). Not only does this demonstrate gliding on the /l/; the /g/ is fronted as well.

Syllabic nasals and liquids may also be replaced. Frequently, a vowel is substituted for the syllabic unit. For example, *flower* becomes *fawa*. In contrast, glides and vowels are not difficult for most children. There is a tendency, however, for vowels to be neutralized or reduced to /ə/ and /a/.

Multiple Processes

In actual practice, it may be difficult to decipher the phonological rules a young child is using. Often, several processes will be functioning at once. For instance, my children all called our family dog "Peepa" (/pipə/). Her real name was Prisca (/pɹɪskə/). We see reduction of the *pr* cluster (in a *stop* + *liquid* cluster, the liquid is deleted). The second cluster, *sc*, may also experience reduction; but even more importantly, it demonstrates progressive non-contiguous assimilation, becoming a /p/. Finally, the first vowel, /I/, is replaced by /i/, which may be the result of the vowel's altering toward some feature of /p/, another assimilation effect.

Perception and Production

Although several infant studies have demonstrated that very young children can discriminate phonemes, all this research was accomplished in a nonlinguistic context. Sounds were presented individually or in isolated short words with no meaning attached.

More symbolic perceptual skills develop relatively late. Although three- and four-year-olds can be taught to separate the sounds in words, these skills are very limited. Children do not perform well when asked to make judgments of the appropriateness of sounds. For instance, when K.C., the child of a friend, was in kindergarten, he drew a painting with streaks of bright color and put a big W on it. His mother was delighted. "Is that 'W' for 'Whalen'?" (his last name). He looked at her with scorn. "No silly, wainbow!"

Preschool children probably do not perceive spoken language as containing phoneme-size units. Yet they seem able to make different speech sounds. Children may know that words are different or similar before they know the basis of those differences and similarities. Through slow evolution from relatively pure sound play, speech sounds gradually change into more deliberate productions that focus on phonological segments and their relationships (Hakes, 1982).

Another important factor in perception and production is phonological short-term or working memory. Preschoolers with good phonological memory skills tend to produce language that contains more grammatic complexity, a richer array of words, and longer utterances than preschoolers with poor memory skills (Adams & Gathercole, 1995).

Summary

The preschool child follows a set of phonological rules or processes that provide for consistent speech performance. Gradually, these rules change and evolve as the child develops better production skills. Because the child's perception does not mirror that of the adult, initial production also differs.

It may be that the child has two representations, or models, of production: the adult model and the child's own (Kuczaj, 1982). The child considers the adult model to be the correct one and monitors both productions for comparison.

During the preschool years, the child also acquires much of his or her phonetic inventory but does not master all English speech sounds until about age seven. In addition, there are many phonological rules related to morphological acquisition that are not mastered until school age.

Even at age three, however, there are wide differences in rate of development, phonological processes used, and phonological organization. The processes of assimilation, and of consonant and syllable deletion, are very common. Cluster reduction is determined, at least in part, by the sounds involved.

It's important to recall that all aspects of language and language development are intertwined and interdependent. Development in one area affects all the others. For example, among some two-year-olds the accuracy of phonemic production decreases as word combinations become more complex (Nelson & Bauer, 1991).

CONCLUSION

By age five, the child uses most of the major varieties of the English sentence. Language forms that will be mastered within the school years and adulthood have already begun to appear. The order of acquisition of these forms reflects patterns of underlying cognitive and social growth, as well as learning strategies. Resultant forms often reflect the use environment and the child's attempt to simplify complex forms.

During the school years, knowledge of language use increases, and use begins to influence form more decisively. Having acquired much of the *what* of language form during the preschool years, the child turns to the *how* of language use.

DISCUSSION

Long chapter? Congratulations for finishing. Language form is the area of language development expanding most rapidly during the preschool years.

In trying to visualize this chapter, separate the computation of MLU from the rest. I had to include that information for those of you planning on becoming SLPs. It represents a separate bit of information and should be studied as a unit.

Now, we're left with development of form. Brown's fourteen morphemes offer a good explanation for why words and suffixes develop the way they do. Notice the interdependence of suffixes with phonological rules. It's difficult to separate the two. Remember these are not the only morphemes developing and that they take a long time to be mastered by children.

Sentence development is a long process. Believe it or not, we have just skimmed the surface. Take a look at Table 10.9 again. I tell my students not to worry about what happens when. That will come with time. Instead, try to understand the sequence. What comes first? What next? Why? Look for similar developments, especially with auxiliary verbs, across sentence types.

Finally, with phonological rules, remember that these are process used by children to simplify words that they cannot pronounce. In this way they are like the shortened versions of adult sentences that children produce. Assume that the basic building block is CV and that the easiest words are CV and CVCV-reduplicated and everything else makes sence.

Can you imagine trying to decide what to teach a preschool child with language impairment? So many possibilities exist. Luckily, teachers will have SLPs to help them decide. SLPs will use a myriad of testing and sampling procedures, plus a strong dose of clinical intuition in deciding the best language features to target. Within time, the development of language form by preschoolers will be second nature and you'll find yourself listening to children and trying to determine which structures they do and do not have. Pity your poor nieces and nephews, not to mention your own children.

REFLECTIONS

1. MLU, the average length of the child's utterances, is a good predictor of the child's functioning level. How does one compute the MLU?

2. Roger Brown described five stages of language development based on the MLU. What are they and what are the main characteristics of each?

3. Stage II is characterized by morphological changes. List the fourteen morphemes that Brown studied and explain each briefly.

4. Describe the acquisition order of negative and interrogative sentences.

5. Stages IV and V are characterized by embedding and conjoining. Describe each of these processes and briefly explain their order of acquisition.

6. Language is a rule-governed behavior. Preschool children follow rules for sound placement and production. What are the phonological processes observed in the language of preschool children?

11

School-Age and Adult Pragmatic and Semantic Development

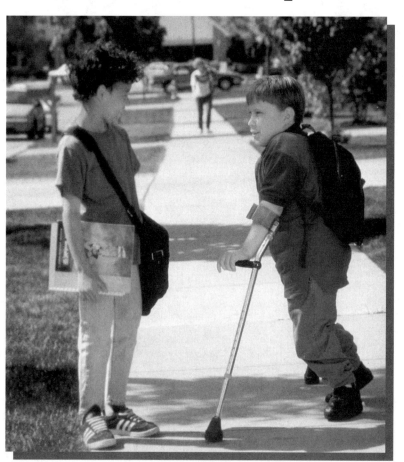

CHAPTER OBJECTIVES

The school-age and adult years are a very creative period for language development. Emphasis shifts from language form to content and use. The adult speaker is versatile and able to express a wide range of intentions. When you have completed this chapter, you should understand

- the conversational abilities of school-age children.
- language differences between genders.
- story grammar development.
- the syntagmatic-paradigmatic shift.
- development of figurative language.
- the following terms:

account	nonegocentrism
critical period	recount
decentration	story
eventcast	story grammar
genderlect	syntagmatic-paradigmatic shift
metaphoric transparency	

The preschool years have been viewed as the **critical period** for language learning. It is assumed that, by school age, the brain has lost much of the organic plasticity found in young children. Thus, with age, the brain becomes "fixated," and the various functions cannot be assumed as easily by other, related segments of the brain. In children as young as four years, there is evidence that the hemispheres of the brain process symbolic communication differently, with left-hemisphere dominance in speech and language. In adults, this phenomenon is even more pronounced. Older adults are less able to recover functions lost through brain injury than are children. It is reasoned that the optimum or critical period for language growth must be the early years of childhood. Although the early years do appear to be very important, there is little empirical support for the critical-period notion.

In fact, throughout school-age and adult years there is an increase in the size and complexity of the child's linguistic repertoire and in the use of that repertoire within the context of conversation and narration. The early school-age period is one of tremendous linguistic creativity filled with rhymes, songs, word games, and those special oaths and incantations passed along on the "underground" from child to child. Each small gang of children attempts to adopt its own special secret language. Children learn to pun and to find humor in word play. Special terms are invented, such as *bad* or *phat*, which means "really good," and *dweeb* or *geek* to note those to be excluded. There are also oaths children consider as binding as any adult legal code:

Finders keepers.
Cross your heart.
Dibs or Call it.
No call backs.
Pinky swear.

For those who break the rules or who, for some other reason, earn a child's enmity, there is that special area of school-age cruelty, the taunt or tease:

Fatty, fatty, two-by-four . . .
Hey, metal mouth.
Liar, liar, pants on fire.

The list of taunts, which are often based on physical characteristics, can go on for longer than any of us care to recall.

In its literary forms, the creative language of school-age children can be heard in camp songs, nursery rhymes, jump-rope rhymes, and jokes or read in autograph book inscriptions and graffiti. Those of us who grew up in inner-city areas experienced an especially rich heritage of urban rhymes and rumors, not to mention graffiti, such as my favorite paraphrase of Descartes:

I think, therefore, I am . . .
. . . a figment of my own imagination.

Such creativity is mirrored in overall language development.

The school-age, and to a lesser degree the adult, years are characterized by growth in all aspects of language, although the development of pragmatics and semantics seems to be the most prevalent (Table 11.1). In addition to mastering new forms, the child learns to use these and existing structures to communicate more effectively. Overall, language development slows, but individual differences are great. A lexical difference as great as 6,000 words may separate average from poor students (Scott, Nippold, Norris, & Johnson, 1992).

One of the main differences between young children and adults may be in the development of narration and of special styles of communicating found only in adulthood (Obler, 1985). Prior to age five, narratives are a collection of utterances rather than a single structured unit. In mature narratives, each utterance becomes constrained by the manner in which it advances the overall theme and purpose of the narrative.

Language development continues, albeit at a slower pace, throughout the life span. Although lexical recognition and comprehension seem unaffected by aging (Bayles, Tomoeda, & Boone, 1985; Bowles & Poon, 1985; Howard, 1983), longer units of language may alter subtly.

TABLE 11.1 Summary of School-Age Children's Pragmatic and Semantic Development

AGE IN YEARS	PRAGMATIC	SEMANTIC
5	• Uses mostly direct requests • Repeats for repair • Begins to use gender topics	
6	• Repeats with elaboration for repair • Uses adverbial conjuncts *now, then, so, though*; disjuncts rare	
7	• Uses and understands most deictic terms • Narrative plots have beginning, end, problem, and resolution	• Uses *left/right, back/front* • Shifts from single-word to multiword definitions
8	• Sustains concrete topics • Recognizes nonliteral meanings in indirect requests • Begins considering others' intentions	
9	• Sustains topics through several turns • Addresses perceived source of breakdown in repair • Produces all elements of story grammar	• Has generally completed most of syntagmatic-paradigmatic shift • Begins to interpret psychological states described with physical terms (*cold, blue*) but misinterprets
10		• Comprehends *in* and *on* used for temporal relations • Comprehends most familial terms
11	• Sustains abstract topics 20% of narrative sentences still begin with *and*	• Creates abstract definitions • Has all elements of conventional adult definitions • Understands psychological states described with physical terms
12	• Uses adverbial conjuncts (4/100 utterances) *otherwise, anyway, therefore*, and *however*, disjuncts *really* and *probably*	
13–15		• Comprehends some proverbs • Comprehends *at* used for temporal relations
16–18	• Uses sarcasm and double meanings • Makes deliberate use of metaphors • Knows partner's perspective and knowledge differ from own	• Approximately 80,000 word meanings

PRAGMATIC DEVELOPMENT

The area of most important linguistic growth during the school-age and adult years is language use, or pragmatics (Table 11.1). It is in pragmatics that we see the interaction of language and socialization (Stephens, 1988).

A preschool child does not have the skill of a masterful adult storyteller or even of a junior high student who wants something. No adult is fooled by the compliment, "Gee, Mom, those are the best-looking cookies you've ever made," but both parties understand the request, however indirect it may be.

Preschool children frequently begin a conversation assuming that *here* for them is *here* for everyone or without announcing the topic. Once, in imaginative play, my preschool daughter shifted characters on me with no announcement. As the Daddy, I was being told to go to my room! When I balked, she informed me that now I was a child—an abrupt demotion. It had not occurred to her to prepare me for the shift in conversation.

Throughout the school years, the cognitive processes of nonegocentrism and decentration increase and combine to enable the child to become a more effective communicator. **Nonegocentrism** is the ability to take the perspective of another person. In general, as the communication task becomes more complex or difficult, the child is less able to take the speaker's perspective. Thus, as the child gains greater facility with language structure, he or she can concentrate more on the audience. Not even adults can be totally nonegocentric, but being able to shift perspective enables the speaker and listener to use deictic terms and lets the speaker consider what the listener knows when constructing a conversation.

Decentration is the process of moving from rigid, one-dimensional descriptions of objects and events to coordinated, multiattributional ones, allowing both speaker and listener to recognize that there are many dimensions and perspectives to any given topic. Five- to six-year-olds are less able to communicate information than older children. In general, younger children's descriptions are more personal and do not consider the information available to the listener. Their accuracy depends on what is being conveyed, with abstract information being communicated least accurately by children.

In this section, we shall consider two aspects of language use: narratives and conversations. Finally, we shall explore *genderlect* or the styles of talking of men and women.

Narratives

Narratives reflect the storyteller's experience and, as such, are sense-making tools (Stephens, 1988). The scripts formed by experiences are the foundations for narratives. The ability to relate well-formed narratives affects the judgments others make about a speaker's communicative competence.

Five- and six-year-olds produce many different types of narratives. Anecdotal narratives of a personal nature predominate, possibly accounting for as many as 70 percent of all narratives (Preece, 1987). In contrast, fantasy stories are relatively rare.

Children learn about narratives within their homes and their language communities. The emerging narratives reflect different cultures (Heath, 1986b). Although every society allows children to hear and produce at least four basic narrative types, the distribution, frequency, and degree of elaboration of these types vary greatly. The four genres include three factual types called *recounts*, *eventcasts*, and *accounts*, and fictionalized *stories* (Stein, 1982).

The **recount**, common in school performance, tells about past experiences in which the child participated or observed or about which the child read. Usually, an adult who has shared this experience asks the child to speak.

The **eventcast** is an explanation of some current or anticipated event. Children may use eventcasts to direct others in imaginative play sequences, as in the following:

> You're the daddy. And you pretend to get dressed. You're going to take the baby to the zoo.

Eventcasts enable the child to consider and analyze the effect of language on others.

Accounts are spontaneous narratives in which children share their experiences ("You know what?"). Unlike recount narratives, the listener usually does not share the accounted experience. Children initiate this narrative form, rather than reporting information requested by adults. This gives accounts their highly individualized form.

In contrast, **stories**, although fictionalized and with seemingly endless content variation, have a known and anticipated pattern or structure. Language is used to create the story, and the listener plays a necessary interpretive function. The usual pattern is one in which the main character must overcome some problem or challenge.

In middle- and upper-class school-oriented families in the United States, the earliest narratives are **eventcasts** that occur during nurturing activities, such as play, and reading. Within these activities, caregivers share many accounts and stories. By age three, children are expected to appreciate and use all forms of narration. Parents invite children to give recounts. These invitations decrease as the child gets older.

By the time most children begin school, they are familiar with all four forms of narration. In the classroom, children are expected to use these forms. This expectation may be unrealistic given the experiences of some minority or bidialectal children. For example, Chinese-American children are encouraged to give accounts within their families, but not outside the immediate household.

In some white working-class Southern communities, recounts are tightly controlled by the interrogator and seem to be the predominant form during the preschool years. Accounts do not begin until children attend school. Children and young adults also tell few stories, a form predominantly used by older, higher-status adults (Heath, 1983).

In contrast, Southern African American working-class children produce mostly accounts or eventcasts and have minimal experience with recounts. This may relate to the general difficulty children in this environment have gaining adult attention. Societal expectations for children are different from those found in the majority culture.

When these minority or bidialectal children go to school, they may be at a disadvantage for narration and reading (Heath, 1986a). The expectations of educational institutions are usually those of the majority culture. Children are expected to be familiar with all narrative types. By enabling children to perform, narratives help children maintain a positive self-image and a group identification within their families and communities.

Development of Narratives

Most six-year-olds can convey a simple story or recount a movie or television show, often in the form of long, rambling sequential accounts. During the school-age period, these narratives undergo several changes, primarily in their internal structure.

As noted in Chapter 9, children gradually learn to link events in linear fashion and only later, with causal connectives. Generally, by age six, children's narratives become causally coherent as well (S. Kemper, 1984). These narratives require the child to manipulate content, plot, and causal structure. Causality involves descriptions of intentions, emotions, and thoughts and the use of connectives, such as *because*, *as a result of*, and *since*, to name a few.

To some degree, use of causality requires the speaker to be able to go forward and backward in time. While two- and three-year-olds can sequence in a forward direction, they have great difficulty with the reverse. The stories of these preschoolers consist predominantly of actions, with few initiations or causes of events and few motivations for characters' actions. Even so, the conjunction *and* continues to be used as frequently in the narratives of nine-year-olds as it was in those of preschoolers (Peterson & McCabe, 1987). The purpose seems to be cohesion (*And then . . . And then . . .*) rather than coordination (clause + *and* + clause).

Although two- and three-year-olds have mastered some causal expressions, they are unable to construct coherent causal narratives (S. Kemper & Edwards, 1986). Causality can be seen, however, in two- and three-year-olds' use of plans, scripts, and descriptions of their own behavior and thoughts (S. Kemper & Edwards, 1986). A *plan* is a means, or series of actions, intended to accomplish a specified end. Thus, a plan is an intention or a model of causality. Many of children's first words refer to intentions and consequences, such as *all gone*, *there*, *uh-oh*, and *oh dear*. *Scripts* are dialogs that accompany familiar routines in the child's everyday environment. Children incorporate these into their narratives. By age two-and-a-half, the child has acquired the words to describe perceptions (*see*, *hear*), physical states (*tired*, *hungry*), emotions (*love*, *hate*), needs, thoughts (*know*), and judgments (*naughty*) (Bretherton & Beeghly, 1982).

Between ages two and ten, children's stories begin to contain more mental states and more initiations and motivations as causal links (S. Kemper & Edwards, 1986). Initially, psychological causality, such as motives, is more frequently used than physical causality or the connection between events (McCabe & Peterson, 1985). At around age four, children's stories begin to contain more explicit physical and mental states. By age six, children's stories describe motives for actions.

In mature narratives, the center develops as the story progresses. Each incident complements the center, follows from previous incidents, forms a chain, and adds some new aspect to the theme. Causal relationships move toward the ending of the initial situation called the *climax*:

> There was a girl named Ann. And she got lost in the city. She was scared. She looked and looked but couldn't find her mommy and daddy. She slept in a cardboard box by the corner. And one day the box got blowed over and a police lady found her sleeping. She took her home to her mommy and daddy.

Mature narratives may consist of a single episode, as above, or of several episodes. An episode contains a statement of the problem or challenge, and all elements of the plot are directed toward its solution.

Although the conversations of four- and five-year-olds contain many elements of narration, such as plans and scripts, they lack the linguistic skill to weave a coherent narrative. Between ages five and seven, plots emerge consisting of a problem and some type of resolution. Gradually, these simple plots are elaborated into a series of problems and solutions or are embellished from within.

Both adults and children prefer stories directed toward a goal, such as the overcoming of an obstacle or problem (Stein & Policastro, 1984). Narratives of the seven-year-old typically involve a beginning, a problem, a plan to overcome the problem, and a resolution.

The development of causal chains within episodes is a very gradual process. Initially, the narrative may be truncated so that the problem is solved, but it is unclear how this happened. This occurs in the following:

> And there was this bad guy with a—"k-k-k-k" (gun noise)—death ray. And he was gonna blow up the city. So, the Power Rangers snuck in to his house and stopped him. The end.

In another early form, the problem is resolved without the intervention of the characters in the story. A common device is to have the main character awaken from a dream, resulting in the disappearance of the problem:

> . . . He was in the middle of all these hungry lions. And he lost his gun. He couldn't get away. And then he woke up. Wasn't that funny?

By second grade, the child uses beginning and ending markers (*once upon a time*, *lived happily ever after*, *the end*) and evaluative markers (*that was a good one*). Story length increases and becomes more complex with the aid of syntactic devices such as conjunctions (*and*, *then*), locatives (*in*, *on*, *under*, *next to*, *in front of*), dialog, comparatives (*bigger than*, *almost as big as*, *littlest*), adjectives, and causal statements. Although disquieting events are still central to the theme, characters tend to remain constant throughout the narrative, and distinct but similar episodes have been replaced by a multiepisodic chronology. The plot is still not fully developed.

The sense of plot in fictional narratives is increasingly clear after age eight (Peterson & McCabe, 1983; Sutton-Smith, 1981, 1986). Now there is definite character-generated resolution of the central problem. The narrative presentation relies largely on language rather than on the child's use of actions and vocalizations. Like a good storyteller, the child manipulates the text and the audience to maintain attention.

In general, older children's narratives are characterized by the following (Johnston, 1982):

1. Fewer unresolved problems and unprepared resolutions.
2. Less extraneous detail.
3. More overt marking of changes in time and place.

4. More introduction, including setting and character information.
5. Greater concern for motivation and internal reactions.
6. More complex episode structure.
7. Closer adherence to the story grammar model.

These changes represent the child's growing awareness of story structure and increasing understanding of the needs of the audience. The internal organization can be described by story grammar.

Two later developing narrative abilities are drawing inferences and summarizing. Even ten-year-olds have difficulty making inferences from a narrative (Crais & Chapman, 1987). Summarizing may involve (1) comprehending propositions, (2) establishing connectives between these propositions, (3) identifying the structure of the story, (4) remembering information, (5) selecting information for summarizing, and (6) formulating a concise, coherent representation (Johnson, 1983). The last two skills are refined in the upper elementary grades (Johnson, 1983).

Story Grammar Development. Narratives are organized in predictable, rule-governed ways that differ with culture. The structure of the narrative consists of various components and the rules underlying the relationships of these components. These components and rules, collectively called a **story grammar**, form a narrative framework, the internal structure of a story.

Formed from reading and listening to stories and from participating in conversations, story grammars can aid information and narrative processing, as well as narrative interpretation and memory (Johnston, 1982; Snyder & Downey, 1983; Stein & Glenn, 1979; Whaley, 1981). Components may help the listener anticipate content. The competent storyteller constructs the story and the flow of information to maximize comprehension.

The typical story in English involves an animate or inanimate protagonist in a particular setting who faces some challenge to which he or she responds. The character makes one or more attempts to meet the challenge and, as a consequence, succeeds or fails. The story usually ends with the character's emotional response to the outcome. This outline contains the main components of a story grammar in English.

A story grammar in English consists of the setting plus the episode structure (*story grammar = setting + episode structure*) (Johnston, 1982). Each story begins with an introduction contained in the setting, as in "A long, long time ago, in a far off galaxy . . ." or "You'll never guess what happened on the way to work this morning; I was crossing Main Street. . . ." An episode in English consists of an initiating event, an internal response, a plan, an attempt, a consequence and a reaction (Stein & Glenn, 1979). Each component is described in Table 11.2. While only 50 percent of kindergarten children can retell narratives with well-formed episodes, this percentage increases to 78 percent by sixth grade. Episodes may be linked additively, temporally, causally, or in a mixed fashion. A story may consist of one or more interrelated episodes.

There appears to be a sequence of stages in the development of English story grammars (Glenn & Stein, 1980). Certain structural patterns appear early and persist, while others are rather late in developing. The resultant narratives can be described as *descriptive sequences, action sequences, reaction sequences, abbreviated episodes, complete episodes, complex*

TABLE 11.2 Story Grammar Components

COMPONENT	DESCRIPTION	EXAMPLE
Setting statement	Introduce the characters; describe their habitual actions and the social, physical and/or temporal contexts; introduce the protagonist.	There was this boy and
Initiating event	Event that induces the character(s) to act through some natural act, such as an earthquake; a notion to seek something, such as treasure; or the action of one of the characters, such as arresting someone.	. . . he got kidnapped by these pirates.
Internal response	Characters' reactions, such as emotional responses, thoughts, or intentions, to the initiating events. Internal responses provide some motivation for the characters.	He missed his dog.
Internal plan	Indicates the characters' strategies for attaining their goal(s). Young children rarely include this element.	So he decided to escape.
Attempt	Overt action(s) of the characters to bring about some consequence, such as to attain their goal(s).	When they were all eating, he cut the ropes and
Direct consequence	Characters' success or failure at attaining their goal(s) as a result of the attempt.	. . . he got away.
Reaction his	Characters' emotional response, thought, or actions to the outcome or preceding chain of events.	And he lived on an island with dog. And they played in the sand every day.

episodes, and *interactive episodes*. The structural qualities of each type of story grammar are listed in Table 11.3.

Descriptive sequences consist of descriptions of characters, surroundings, and habitual actions. There are no causal or temporal links. The entire story consists of setting statements:

> There was this magician. He had a big hat like this. He turned elephants into mice. And he had birds in his coat. The end.

This type of structure is characteristic of the initial narratives of preschool children, described as *heaps*.

Action sequences have a chronological order for actions but no causal relations. The story consists of a setting statement and various action attempts:

> We got up early on Christmas morning. We lighted the tree. We opened gifts. Mommy made cinnamon buns. Then we played with the toys.

TABLE 11.3   Structural Properties of Narratives

STRUCTURAL PATTERN	STRUCTURAL PROPERTIES
Descriptive sequence	Setting statements (S) (S) (S)
Action sequence	Setting statement (S) Attempts (A) (A) (A)
Reaction sequence	Setting statement (S) Initiating event (IE) Attempts (A) (A) (A)
Abbreviated episode	Setting statement (S) Initiating event (IE) or Internal response (IR) Direct consequence (DC)
Complete episode	Setting statement (S) Two of the following: 　　Initiating event (IE) 　　Internal response (IR) 　　Attempt (A) Direct consequence (DC)
Complex episode	Multiple episodes 　Setting statement (S) 　Two of the following: 　　Initiating event (IE_1) 　　Internal response (IR_1) 　　Attempt (A_1) 　Direct consequence (DC_1) 　Two of the following: 　　Initiating event (IE_2) 　　Internal response (IR_2) 　　Attempt (A_2) 　Direct consequence (DC_2) Expanded complete episode 　Setting statement (S) 　Initiating event (IE) 　Internal response (IR) 　Internal plan (IP) 　Attempt (A) 　Direct consequence (DC) 　Reaction (R)
Interactive episode	Two separate but parallel episodes that influence each other

This type of story grammar is the type seen in early sequential and temporal chain narratives of preschool children.

Reaction sequences consist of a series of events in which changes cause other changes with no goal-directed behaviors. The sequence consists of a setting, an initiating event, and action attempts:

> There was a little puppy. He smelled a kittie. The kittie scratched the puppy. The puppy ran away. He smelled a girl. The girl took the puppy home and gave the pu . . . him milk. And that's the end.

In contrast, *abbreviated episodes* contain an implicit or explicit goal. At this level, the story may contain either an event statement and a consequence or an internal response and a consequence:

> This girl hated spinach. And she had a big plate of it. And she fed the spinach to the dog under the table. After her plate was all clean, she got a big dessert. That's all.

Although the character's behavior is purposeful, it is usually not premeditated or planned. Reaction sequences and abbreviated episodes are characteristic of the narratives of school-age children until approximately age nine (Westby, 1984).

Complete episodes contain an entire goal-oriented behavioral sequence consisting of a consequence statement and two of the following: initiating event, internal response, and attempt:

> Once this man went hunting. He woke up a big bear. The bear chased him up a tree and climbed up. To get away, the man waved at a helicopter. The helicopter gave the man a rope. He climbed up and got away from the bear. The end.

Complex episodes are expansions of the complete episode or contain multiple episodes:

> Spiderman saw a bank robber. He jumped down and captured one of them with a punch. And he called the police. One bank robber got away in his truck. Spiderman ran after the truck. He threw his net over the truck and got the bank robber. And that was the end of the bank robbers.

Finally, *interactive episodes* contain two characters who have separate goals and actions that influence the behavior of each other:

> Mary decided to build a doghouse. She bought all the wood she needed. Her cat got jealous. Mary cut all the wood and hammered it. The cat rubbed her leg and meowed. Mary was too busy to stop and she painted it. The cat meowed more. When Mary was all done, she let the dog go to sleep. And then she hugged the kitty too.

Complete, complex, and interactive story grammars are seen in the narratives of mid- and late-elementary school children, adolescents, and adults. Most children produce all the elements of story grammar by age nine or ten.

Narrative Differences

As might be expected, not all children of a given age exhibit the same levels of narrative competence. The narratives of underachieving children may be shorter, have less internal organization and cohesion, and contain fewer story grammar components and less sentence complexity (Hayes, Norris, & Flaitz, 1998).

Narration varies with the context or situation and with the culture of the speaker. Situational variables may influence the type of storytelling as much as the developmental level of the narrator. Contextual constraints include the type and size of the audience, the goal, time allotment, and competition for the floor (Scott et al., 1992). The more familiar the audience, the longer the clauses and the more use of embedded clauses. Across languages, the number of characters varies with the style and purpose of the narrative (Clancy, 1980; Guttierrez-Clellan & Heinrichs-Ramos, 1993;).

The narratives of some African American children, especially girls, have a distinct structure that differs from the story grammar model presented previously. Characterized as *topic-associating*, these narratives consist of thematically related incidents that make an implicit point, such as the need to help your baby brother or to avoid someone. These narratives often lack clear indicators of characters, place, or shifts in time (Gee, 1989; Michaels, 1981, 1991).

Narratives are culturally based and development will differ by culture and language. Linguistic differences will account for differing methods of introducing new elements, referring to old information, and providing cohesion. Still, we find that narratives become increasingly more complex and more coherent. More characters and dialogue are used and multiple and complex episodes.

As Spanish-speaking children mature, their narratives become more detailed and contain more embedding, although overall length increases little (Guttierrez-Clellan & McGrath, 1991). These narratives exhibit an increase in cohesion, ellipsis, and more accurate reference and a decrease in ambiguities and redundancies with age (Guttierrez-Clellan & Heinrichs-Ramos, 1993). Cohesion is achieved through the use of articles and nouns (*un nene/a boy*), pronouns (*ella/she*), ellipsis (*El fue a la tienda, cogio un poco de comida/he went to the store, got some food*) and demonstratives (*este/this*). In fact, ellipsis may be even more pronounced because Spanish verb endings indicate person, eliminating the need for pronouns. The increasing use of ellipsis with locations is consistent with that noted in the narratives of English-speaking children (Black, 1985). Props in Spanish narratives are usually referenced by name. Similarly, in English narratives props not primary to the narrative are also referenced by name (Clancy, 1980; Karmiloff-Smith, 1981).

As in English, Italian-speaking children use nouns to introduce new information. Pronouns and inflected verbs are also used. School-aged Italian-speaking children rely more on nouns, thus reducing ambiguity on the part of the listener. In addition, school-aged children are more adept at integrating the content of the narrative (Orsolini, Rossi, & Pontecorvo, 1996).

Across languages such as English, German, French, and Mandarin, clear marking of new information in the form of a noun does not emerge until age seven (Hickman, Hendriks, Roland, & Liang, 1996). Because languages differ in form, it might be expected that the development of sentence structure to indicate newness would also differ. For example, in English, new information is often placed at the end of the sentence and does not emerge fully until adulthood. In contrast, use of sentence structure to introduce newness is used more frequently by French-speaking children. An interplay exists between discourse factors governing information flow, cognition relative to narrative complexity, and language-specific forms.

Dialogue is increasingly used within narratives as they mature. As in English, children developing other languages, such as Turkish, gain increasing ability to relate conversations by adopting different roles within their narratives, switching from character to narrator and back again (Ozyurek, 1996).

Conversational Abilities

Successful communication rests on the participants' *social cognition*, their knowledge of people, relationships, and events (Shantz, 1983). Participants must be actively involved, asking and answering questions, making voluntary replies and statements, and being sensitive to the contributions of others. They collaborate to ensure mutual understanding. Great individual variability exists, and some seven-year-olds are more effective than the least effective forty-three-year-olds (Anderson, Clark, & Mullin, 1994).

The most successful communicators use questions to probe before introducing a possibly unfamiliar topic. Although the number of questions does not increase with age, more successful communicators use more questions and have more answered than do the least successful. In addition, regardless of age, more successful school-age communicators are quick to recognize communication breakdown and to offer further explanation or to repair (Anderson et al., 1994).

Adults still exercise control over much of the conversation of the young school-age child by asking questions. Role, power, and control relationships are evident in children's responses. In general, responses to adult queries by first-graders are brief, simple, and appropriate, with little elaboration. In contrast, responses to peer questions are more complex and more varied.

In peer interaction among young school-age children, approximately 60 percent of the utterances are effective, measured by the clarity and structural completeness of the utterance sent, the clarity of reference and relevance to the situation, the form of the utterance, the requirement for and maintenance of attention, and approximately four feet of communication distance. The style-switching behavior reported for four-year-olds is even more pronounced by age eight. When speaking with peers, the child makes more nonlinguistic noises and exact repetitions and engages in more ritualized play. With adults, the child uses different codes for his parents and for those outside the family. In general, parents are the recipients of more demands and whining, and of shorter, less conversational narratives.

Language Uses

Almost from the time the child begins to speak, he or she is able to provide information and to discuss topics briefly. Language functions increase greatly with the demands of the classroom. Children are required to explain, express, describe, direct, report, reason, imagine, hypothesize, persuade, infer cause, and predict outcomes. New vocabulary and syntactic forms accompany these functions. For example, hypothesizing uses *how about . . .*, *what if . . .*, and so on, while persuading uses *yes but, on the other hand, because if . . . then . . .*, and the like. By age thirteen, the adolescent is able to synthesize information rather than parrot what he or she has heard or read.

Mastery of these functions comes gradually and varies with the function. Even some seventeen-year-olds have difficulty offering and supporting their opinions in a well-formed, logical fashion (Stephens, 1988).

By late adolescence, the child is aware that a communication partner's perspective and knowledge may differ from his own and that it is important to consider these differences. Social perspective-taking, the ability to understand and adopt varying points of view, is necessary for successful communication and is used to persuade, comfort, and to be polite (Bliss, 1992). The largest gains in social perspective-taking and subsequent tailoring of individualized messages occur in middle childhood (ages seven to nine).

The high-schooler uses language creatively in sarcasm, jokes, and double meanings. These begin to develop in the early school years. It can be a memorable event when a child devises his first joke. I remember my daughter's first one very well. We were discussing groupings of animals, such as *herds* of cattle, *flocks* of chickens, *packs* of wolves, and so on when someone asked about bees. One son ventured *hive*, another *school*. At this point Jessica, age seven, chimed in with "If bees went to school, they'd have to ride the school *buzz*!" Even if she heard it elsewhere, she gets some credit for good timing.

High-schoolers also make deliberate use of metaphor and can explain complex behavior and natural phenomena. These changes reflect overall development within all five aspects of language.

Because of cultural difference, the expectations of the classroom teacher may differ from that of the child. For example, majority English-speaking teachers may prefer individual recitation, while children from populations such as the native Canadian Inuit participate best within cooperative group interactions, the cultural norm (Crago, Eriks-Brophy, Pesco, & McAlpine, 1997). The reluctance of Inuit children to respond individually may be misinterpreted by the teacher as being uncooperative. Similarly, Algonquin narration is a cooperative group effort that may not be appreciated by the teacher demanding individual storytelling. In addition, the teacher's stopping of a narrative to correct grammar may violate the function of narratives in Algonquin culture, which is to amuse or tell a troubling experience.

The communication experiences and needs of adults result in a language system characterized by many special *registers*, or styles of speech, not found in childhood. For example, most adults have jobs that require specific language skills—talking on the phone, writing, giving directives—or terminology, called *jargon*. Also, special communication rules reflect the power structure of the workplace. Special styles exist for those with whom the adult is intimate, such as pet names (*poobear*, *wissycat*, *mertz*) or terms of endearment (*honey*, *dear*), that are distinct from those reserved for strangers or business associates.

Focus.

Many adults also belong to ethnic, racial, or sexual-orientation minorities or to social groups that require still other styles. These act as a bond for these groups, whether they are African American teenage males, Jewish elders, lesbians, avid CB or shortwave radio enthusiasts, or art patrons. Adults also engage in diverse social functions, such as funerals, public speaking, sports, or even card playing, that require special lexicons and manners of speaking. It is even possible to detect political orientation from the adult's choice of terms. For example, in the present political climate, the contrasts between *women's lib–women's movement*, *Negroes–African Americans*, and *pro-life–antiabortion* signal conservatism by the first term, liberalism by the second. Most adults use several different registers. Exposure and need are the determining factors in acquisition, and registers disappear from a person's repertoire because of infrequent use.

The conversational abilities of adults continue to diversify and to become more elaborate with age if health is maintained (Obler, 1985). Except for the small percentage of older adults who have suffered some brain injury or disease, most continue to be effective communicators throughout their lives.

Topic Introduction and Maintenance

The school-age child is able to introduce a topic into the conversation, sustain it through several turns, and close or switch the topic. These skills develop only gradually throughout elementary school and contrast sharply to preschool performance. The three-year-old, for example, sustains the topic only 20 percent of the time if the partner's preceding utterance was a topic-sharing response to one of the child's prior utterances. In other words, topics change rapidly. Four-year-olds can remain on topic when explaining how a toy works but still cannot sustain dialog.

In general, the proportion of introduced topics maintained in subsequent turns increases with age, with the most change occurring from late elementary school to adulthood (Brinton & Fujiki, 1984). A related decrease in the number of different topics introduced or reintroduced occurs during this same period. Thus, there is a growing adherence to the concept of relevance in a conversation. The eight-year-old's topics tend to be concrete. Sustained abstract discussions emerge around age eleven.

Adults effectively use *shading*, or modifying the focus of the topic, as a means of gradually moving from one topic to another while maintaining some continuity in the conversation. The topic-shading utterance includes some aspect of the preceding utterance but shifts the central focus of concern.

Conjuncts and Disjuncts

In conversation, the child is slowly learning to link sentences with devices that are peripheral to the clause (Scott, 1984a). By bridging utterances, these devices provide continuity within discourse. The devices consist of *adverbial disjuncts*, which comment on or convey the speaker's attitude toward the content of the connected sentence, such as *frankly, to be honest, perhaps, however, yet*, and *to my surprise*, and *adverbial conjuncts*, which signal a logical relation between sentences, such as *still, as a result of*, and *to conclude*. The following are examples of adverbial disjuncts used in conversation:

> *Honestly*, I don't know why you bought that car.
> *In my opinion*, it was a bargain.
> *Well, to be honest*, I think it's a lemon.

Adverbial conjuncts are cohesive and connective devices and may be concordant (*similarly, moreover, consequently*) or discordant (*in contrast, rather, but, nevertheless*). Conjuncts express a logical intersential relationship and are more common in literature than in conversation. In the following example, the conjunct *as a result of* signals the relationship of the two sentences:

> We were up all night. As a result of our effort, our group won the
> competition.

Development of conjuncts occurs gradually from school age into adulthood. Both production and understanding increase with age, although comprehension exceeds production even in young adults (Nippold, Schwarz, & Undlin, 1992). By age six, the child uses the adverbial conjuncts *now, then, so,* and *though*, although disjuncts are rare. By age twelve, the youth has added *otherwise, anyway, therefore,* and *however*, plus the disjuncts *really* and *probably*. This development continues well into the adult years, with adults using twelve conjuncts per 100 utterances compared to the twelve-year-old's four (Scott, 1988).

Indirect Requests

One verbal strategy adults use widely is the indirect request that does not refer directly to what the speaker wants. For example, "The sun sure is a scorcher today" may be an indirect, nonconventional request for a drink. Development of indirect requests is particularly noteworthy because such requests represent a growing awareness of the importance of both socially appropriate requests and the communication context.

Indirect requests are first produced in the preschool years. The proportion of indirect to direct requests increases between ages three and five. This proportion does not change markedly between ages five and six, although the internal structure of requests develops (Levin & Rubin, 1982). In general, the five-year-old is successful at directly asking, commanding, and forbidding. By age seven, he or she has acquired greater facility with indirect forms. Flexibility in indirect request forms increases with age. For example, the proportion of hints—"That's a beautiful jacket, and it would go so well with my tan"—increases from childhood through adulthood (Ervin-Tripp, 1980).

The school-age child seems to be following two rules: be brief and be devious (or avoid being demanding) (Ervin-Tripp & Gordon, 1986). The school-age child is more creative and more aware of social roles than the preschooler. He or she is also aware that overpoliteness is inappropriate. As with preschoolers, however, the eight-year-old can be more polite to adults and to those perceived as uncooperative than he is to his peers (Parsons, 1980).

After age eight, a change occurs in the child's awareness of others, and he or she increasingly takes their intentions into consideration (Ervin-Tripp & Gordon, 1986). While the younger child acts as if expecting compliance, the eight-year-old may signify the possibility of something else. In general, the eight-year-old is more polite when not from the listener's peer group, when interrupting the listener's activities, and when the task requested is difficult. Although the child's use of requests is similar to that of adults, he or she still has some difficulty with indirect requests and may interpret them literally. It's not until adolescence that the child approaches adult proficiency.

The preschool child has difficulty understanding many forms of indirect request Although six-year-olds generally respond to literal meanings, eight-year-olds and adults recognize most nonliteral requests for action as well (Ackerman, 1978). For example, the six-year-old who is asked "Can you pass the cup?" may respond "Yes" but not follow through.

More mature language users consider the context more fully and deduce that these questions are indirect requests for action. Decisions about the nature of a request—for information or compliance—can be difficult. By age eleven, children are able to use the utterance and context to infer the speaker's intent accurately (Abbeduto, Nuccio, Al-Mabuk, Rotto, & Maas, 1992).

There seems to be a general developmental pattern to the comprehension of indirect requests (Carrell, 1981). As a child matures, comprehension of most types of indirect request increases. Interrogative forms, such as *shouldn't you?* and *should you?*, are more difficult than declarative forms, such as *you shouldn't* and *you should*. Negative forms, such as *please don't* and *you shouldn't*, are more difficult for four- to seven-year-olds than positive forms, such as *please do* and *you should*. Polarity is a strong factor, especially when it differs from the literal meaning. *Shouldn't you?*, for example, is in a negative form but is a prod for positive action, as in "Shouldn't you leave?" In contrast, *Must you?*, although positive in form, conveys caution or cessation, as in "Must you stop now?" These levels of relative difficulty change little from childhood to adulthood and reflect the same comprehension difficulties experienced by adults.

In part, development of comprehension also reflects the words used. Four- and five-year-olds understand most simple indirect requests containing *can* and *will* but have difficulty with others, such as *must* and *should* .

Conversational Repair

More mindful of the listener's needs, the school-age child attempts to clarify the conversation through a variety of strategies (Konefal & Fokes, 1984). Rather than merely repeating, as most three- to five-year-olds do, the six-year-old may elaborate some elements in the repetition, thus providing more information. Until age nine, however, the predominant repair strategy is repetition. The nine-year-old clearly provides additional input for the listener. Although not as proficient as adults, nine-year-olds are capable of addressing the perceived source of a breakdown in communication by defining their terms, providing more background context, and talking about the process of conversational repair (Brinton et al., 1986).

The ability to detect communication breakdown also improves with age. By adulthood, linguistic anomalies are detected almost instantaneously (Fodor, Ni, Crain, & Shankweiler, 1996).

Deictic Terms

By school age, most children can produce deictic terms (*here*, *there*) correctly. By about age seven, a child should be able to produce and comprehend both singular and plural *demonstratives* (*this*, *that*, *these*, *those*) or words that indicate to which object or event the speaker is referring. Children under age seven do not incorporate all semantic features of demonstratives. First, the child must understand that *this* and *that* are pronouns when used alone, as in "See *that*," and articles when followed by a noun, as in "*That* one's big." Second, the child must comprehend the feature of more or less far, that is, of distance. Third, the child must realize that the speaker is the referent, the deictic aspect of demonstratives. The last two features overlap with those of *here* and *there*.

An initial strategy for the production of deictic verbs, such as *bring* and *take*, is to use them with locational terms for directionality, as in *bring it here* or *bring it there*. The causal meaning of the verb—it causes something to happen—is acquired first. Later, the child learns the deictic meaning (Abkarian, 1988).

Gender Differences

In the early elementary school years, the language of boys and girls begins to reflect the gender differences of older children and adults (Haas, 1979). These differences can be noted in vocabulary use and conversational style. Although the changing status of women in our society may lessen these differences, they nonetheless exist currently.

It is important to remind ourselves that males and females have more similarities than differences in their language use (Pillon, Degauquier, & Duquesne, 1992). In addition, other factors such as the context and topic have a greater influence on conversational style than gender (McMullen & Pasloski, 1992).

Finally, any communicative act must be interpreted in light of context, the conversational style of the participants, the interaction of these styles, and the cultural background of the participants (Tannen, 1994). Interrupting may be interpreted by some speakers as rudeness or pushiness and by others as enthusiastic participation.

Vocabulary Use

The lexical differences between men and women are generally quantitative rather than qualitative (B. Thorne, Kramerae, & Henley, 1983). In general, women avoid swearing and coarse language in conversation and tend to use more polite words, such as *please*, *thank you*, and *good-bye* (Greif & Berko Gleason, 1980). Other descriptive words, such as *adorable*, *charming*, *sweet*, *lovely*, and *divine*, are also associated with women. In addition, women use a fuller range of color terms.

Considerable differences can be found in emphatic or emotional expressions. Women tend to use expressions, such as *oh dear*, *goodness*, and *gracious me*, while men tend to use expletives like *damn it*. Even first-graders are reasonably accurate at selecting the gender of a speaker who says, "Damn it, you broke the TV" or "My goodness, you broke the TV." In emergency situations in which an active, assertive response is needed, interjections, such as *oh dear*, are rare even for women.

Conversational Style

Although American English-speaking men and women may possess the same language, they use and understand it in very different ways (Tannen, 1990). While women tend to be more indirect, to seek consensus, and to listen carefully, men tend to lecture and may seem inattentive to women. Women see their role as conversation facilitators, while men see theirs as information providers. Thus, women face their conversational partners, giving vocal or verbal feedback and often finishing the listener's thought. Men often do not face their partners, looking around the room and making only fleeting eye contact. Body posture differences can be observed in young teens with males more distant and not facing each other. In contrast, girls sit closer and may touch during the conversation (Tannen, 1994).

The cartoon of the wife and husband at the breakfast table, she talking while he reads the newspaper, has its basis in adult conversational styles. In short, men talk more in public and less at home. The most frequent reason for divorce given by women in the United States is lack of communication. Much of this difference stems from the different expectations of men and women in conversation. Men see conversations as an opportunity for debate or competition, and thus act combative. When listening, they are silent, giving little vocal feedback, which they may consider to be interruptive. For men, conversations are events in which talk maintains status and independence. The goal, therefore, becomes "scoring" on one's opponent and protecting oneself. To score, a man may dismiss the topic and, by association, the conversational partner as trivial or unimportant.

Among American men, topics are changed often and rarely involve personal issues or feelings. One unfortunate result is the lack of intimacy experienced by many men throughout adulthood. It is difficult to build intimate relationships based on talk of sports, work, and politics.

In contrast, women see conversations as a way to create intimacy. For women, intimacy is built through talking. The topics discussed are not as important as closeness and the sharing of feelings and emotions. Topics are often shared at length and explored thoroughly. Girls' and women's topics are more focused, less diffuse than those of boys and men (Tannen, 1994). At all ages, females have less difficulty finding something to talk about and topics are changed less frequently.

As good conversationalists, women see their role as an agreeable and supportive one. They try to avoid anger and disagreement (Tannen, 1994). Women and girls tend to face each other directly and to look into each others' faces. Women also make more "listener noise" to let the speaker know that they are attending. These responses consist of *uh-huh* and *yeah*. Men usually use these responses to signal agreement (Maltz & Borker, 1982).

It is not surprising, therefore, to find that men and women differ in the amount of talking, in nonlinguistic devices, and in turn-taking behaviors. In general, men tend to be more verbose than women. In a conversational context, the longest speaking time occurs when men speak with other men. Contrary to contemporary "wisdom," women's conversations with men or with other women are shorter. Women maintain more eye contact and smile more often than men.

Within a conversation, men and women use different turn-taking styles. In general, adult listeners of either sex are more likely to interrupt a female speaker than a male. Men typically interrupt to suggest alternative views, to argue, to introduce new topics, or to

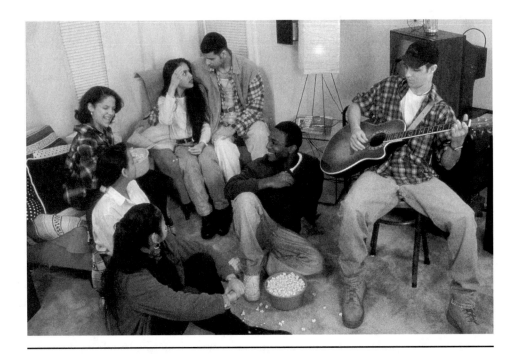

Gender differences in the speech and language of males and females become evident in early elementary school and increase with age.

complete the speaker's sentence (P. Smith, 1985). In contrast, women interrupt to clarify and support the speaker. In general, however, interrupting is more related to the context than to the gender of the interrupter (Nohara, 1992).

Women relinquish their conversational turns more readily than men. A frequently used device is a question, compliment, or request. Women ask more questions, thus indirectly introducing topics into the conversation. Only about 36 percent of these topics become the focus of conversation. In contrast, 96 percent of male-introduced topics are sustained (Ehrenreich, 1981).

Given these characteristics and the societal roles of men and women, men may feel no need to talk at home because there are no other men to whom they must prove themselves. In contrast, women may feel secure within the home and feel that they are free to talk without offending or being seen as combative.

Development

Parental speech to children of different sexes varies. As early as two years of age, daughters are imitated more by their mothers and talked to longer than are sons. Fathers use more imperatives and more insulting terms, such as *ding-a-ling* and *butthead*, with their sons (Berko Gleason & Greif, 1983) and address their daughters as *honey* and *sweetie*. These terms may reflect the nature of adult male conversations. Fathers use the diminutive form (adding a suffix to denote smallness or affection) more frequently and interrupt daughters more often than sons (Warren-Leubecker, 1982). The overall effects of these parental behaviors are not yet known.

Preschool boys seem more aware of the differences between male and female adults than girls do. As early as kindergarten, boys' topics tend to be space, quantity, physical movement, self, and value judgments. In contrast, kindergarten girls talk more about "traditional" female roles. Boys begin to talk about sports and girls about school possibly as early as age four (Haas, 1979; Staley, 1982).

From early childhood, boys' relationships are based less on talking and more on doing. Boys' groups tend to be larger and more hierarchical than those of girls. Actions and talking are used in the struggle to avoid subordination. The listener role is seen as one of passivity and submissiveness, while the talker role is assertive. In this competitive environment, preadolescent boys posture and counterposture, using verbal aggression such as practical jokes, put-downs, and insults (Maltz & Borker, 1982). Speech is used to assert dominance and to hold attention.

In contrast to boys, girls usually play in pairs, sharing the play, talking, and telling "secrets." Personal problems and concerns are shared, with agreement and understanding by the participants. In this cooperative environment, preadolescent girls spend considerable time talking, reflecting, and sharing. Their language is more inclusive than that of boys with frequent use of words such as *let's* and *we* (Goodwin, 1980).

Genderlect, as the collective stylistic characteristics of men and women is called, is well-established by mid-adolescence. Communicative competence is valued by adolescents as a way of presenting themselves to peers and great pressure exists to conform.

Conclusion

The communication behaviors of men and women may reflect the traditional status of women within our society. As in other cultures, words associated with masculinity are judged to be better or more positive than those associated with femininity (Konishi, 1993).

Women demonstrate nonlinguistic behaviors, such as increased eye contact, which suggest that they hold a less dominant position within conversations. The freedom to interrupt and the sustaining of male-introduced topics reflect a higher relative status for males. In addition, women's use of "feminine" exclamations, such as *oh dear*, suggests a lack of power or a lack of conviction in the importance of the message.

As one might imagine, these conditions make it difficult for adolescent girls to acquire adult self-confidence. The behaviors to which they are expected to conform deny women interactional control and send a devaluing message.

The actual basis for these gender differences has not been determined. It will be interesting to see the effects of more women in the workplace on the communicative behavior of both sexes.

It is impossible to separate conversational behaviors from culture. Men and women around the world interact in very different manners. For example, in Greece, both men and women use indirect styles of address at about the same rate as American women (Tannen, 1994). Nor is the interrupting behavior of American men universal among males. In Africa, the Caribbean, the Mediterranean, South America, Jewish and Arab cultures, and Eastern Europe, women interrupt men far more frequently than in the majority American culture.

Finally, many cultures, such as Thai, Japanese, Hawaiian, and Antiguan, exhibit a cultural style of overlapping speech that is cooperative rather than interruptive (Hayashi, 1988; Moerman, 1988).

Summary

As the child gains greater facility with the form and content aspects of language, he or she is able to concentrate more on language use in narratives and in conversational give-and-take. As he or she develops, the child requires less and less of his or her limited-capacity system for planning and encoding the message. More capacity is therefore available for adapting messages to specific audiences and situations. Gradually, the child is able to reallocate these limited resources and so to increase the effectiveness of the system. Contrast the sample of the speech and language of a seven-year-old child presented on track eleven of the CD that accompanies this text with that of a twelve-year-old child presented on track twelve.

SEMANTIC DEVELOPMENT

During the school-age period and the adult years, the individual increases the size of his or her vocabulary and the specificity of definition. Gradually, the child acquires an abstract knowledge of meaning that is independent of particular contexts or individual interpretations. In the process, the individual reorganizes the semantic aspects of language (Table 11.1). The new organization is reflected in the way the child uses words. One outgrowth is the creative or figurative use of language for effect. This entire process of semantic growth, beginning in the early school years, may be related to an overall change in cognitive processing.

Throughout life, the average healthy person will continue to add new words to his or her lexicon. Other than for reasons of poor health, language growth should continue, albeit at a slower rate. Although the ability to access or recall words rapidly may decline some after age seventy, lexical items are not lost (Obler, 1985). Older adults are as able as younger language users to define words appropriately. In some ways, the language performance of older adults may seem to others to be deteriorating. For example, seniors generally do not hear as well as the young. They may therefore miss critical pieces of information. Senior citizens also tend to use older terminology, which makes them appear to be less adept at using language. Newer terms may be more difficult for them to recall. Thus, the older adult might use the terms *dungarees* and *tennis shoes* in place of *jeans* and *sneakers*. The popular image of the incoherent, rambling older adult with poor word memory is untrue and unfair to most seniors.

Vocabulary Growth

School-age and adult years are a period of continued growth in the understanding of words and relationships. It is estimated that, by graduation from high school, a young adult has meanings for some 80,000 words (G. Miller & Gildea, 1987). Actually, this number of words is increased with the addition of morphological prefixes and suffixes that change word meanings (Anglin, 1995b). Morphemes are added throughout the school years. Many words are added from context, often while reading, especially after fourth grade.

Added lexical items are only a portion of the change. Vocabulary growth is not the same as semantic sophistication or depth of understanding—the overall development of the child's semantic system (Pease & Berko Gleason, 1985). While new words may increase the size of the child's lexicon, they may not cause any changes in interrelated semantic concepts, semantic classes, synonyms, homonyms, and antonyms. These are all part of a child's understanding of a word. In fact, even adults have incomplete mastery of some words.

More than other areas of language, development of semantics varies widely with educational level, socioeconomic status, gender, age, and cultural background. Definitional skill is highly correlated with involvement in an academic culture. As a result, some working class fourth graders outperform their parents in providing oral definitions (Kurland & Snow, 1997).

During school-age and adult years, there are two types of increases in word meanings: horizontal and vertical. In horizontal increases, the child adds features to the definition that are common to the adult definition. Vertical increases involve bringing together all the definitions that can fit a single word. The multiple meanings of school-age children and the less flexible semantic systems of younger children are illustrated in the following closing retort of an argument between my two nieces, Michelle and Katie, her younger sister:

| *Michelle:* | Well, when I have children, I hope they don't get any of your genes. |
| *Katie* (after a short pause): | No, and they won't get any of my sneakers, either. |

Between the ages of seven and eleven, there are significant increases in comprehension of spatial, temporal, familial, disjunctive, and logical relationships. The child acquires many dictionary-like and multiple meanings during this period. In non-English languages, children also continue to acquire more informative and complete definitions (Benelli, Arcuri, & Marchesini, 1988). The rate of growth slows and stabilizes during the teen years.

New words may reflect the cognitive and linguistic activities of education, such as *remember*, *doubt*, *conclude*, *assert*, *interpret*, and *predict* (Astington & Olson, 1987). Others, such as connectives—*but*, *although*, *however*—are used for narratives and in reading and writing. Full understanding of most connectives occurs gradually, and some are still not mastered by eighth grade. Finally, as the child attempts to be more precise, he or she adds adverbs of magnitude, such as *slightly*, *somewhat*, and *unusually*. Acquisition of these terms continues into adulthood.

Semantic constraints may delay full mature use of even seemingly simple words such as *in*, *on*, and *at* (Arlin, 1983). Many prepositions can mark both locative and temporal relationships. For example, prepositions such as *in* and *on* represent periodicity of duration, whereas *at* represents a moment in time. In general, *in* and *on* are used for periods of time, such as days (*on Monday*) or parts of days (*in the morning*), or for months (*in May*). In contrast, *at* is used for specific moments (*at midnight*, *at 9:15*). The temporal concept of periodicity develops much later than the locative—not until about age ten. A child is into teenage years before he or she can explain the periodicity/moment distinction.

In the early years of elementary school, a change occurs in the use of spatial relational terms. There is a decrease in the use of nonspecific and general terms and a corresponding increase in the use of specific spatial terms from ages four to seven (Cox, 1985). Usage shifts gradually from nonspecific deictic terms, based on the speaker's perspective (*here*, *there*), through environmental-based terms (*away from the window*, *toward the door*), to correct spatial terms (*top*, *up*, *left*) (Cox & Richardson, 1985). From age three on, the child gains increasing knowledge of horizontal-frontal (*front/back*) and horizontal-lateral (*left/right*) relationships. Increasing precision of use continues into adulthood.

These new relations also require new, more complex syntactic structures. Although *first* and *last* can be applied to single words, newly acquired *before* and *after* are clausal or phrasal connectives requiring a more complex structure.

As discussed in Chapter 8, words refer to categories that are defined by prototypes or best exemplars. As he or she matures, the child acquires more features of the exemplar. Some instances are more typical than others and are easier for children to learn. In general, the child has a less definitive exemplar than the adult and relies more on perceptual knowledge (M. Bernstein, 1983). In contrast, adult definitions reflect both perceptual attributes and functions.

The child's ability to define words may progress in two ways during the early school years. First, the child progresses conceptually from definitions based on individual experience to more socially shared meaning. Second, he or she moves syntactically from single-word action definitions to sentences expressing complex relationships. This shift in form occurs at around second grade (Wehren, DeLisi, & Arnold, 1981). Similar shifts in definition content occur throughout grade school.

Supplying precise semantic content seems to develop prior to using correct syntactic form to provide a definition (Johnson & Anglin, 1995). In addition, high-quality definitions develop for root words prior to inflected or derived words.

Supplying word definitions is a metalinguistic skill. In general, both quantitative and qualitative improvement in definitions occurs in adolescence. Synonym-type definitions increase. A greater tendency exists to include categorical membership (*an apple is fruit*), function, description, and degree (*almost*, *nearly*).

In general, adult definitions are abstract. They tend to be descriptive, with concrete terms or references to specific instances used to modify the concept. In addition, adult definitions include synonyms, explanations, and categorizations of the word defined. During adolescence, a number of changes occur in definitions with the inclusion of category membership, the sharpening of core features of a word, and the addition of subtle aspects of meaning (Nippold, Hegel, Sohlberg, & Schwarz, 1999).

Unlike child meanings, adult definitions are exclusionary and also specify what an entity is not (Wehren et al., 1981). Adult definitions reflect an individual's personal biases and experiences, in addition to the constraints of the situation (D. Johnson, Toms-Bronowski, & Pittelman, 1982)

Vocabulary knowledge is highly correlated with general linguistic competence. A relationship may exist between stored word knowledge and comprehension of discourse. Throughout the school years, the child becomes better at deducing word meaning from context. While the five-year-old defines a word narrowly in terms of sentence meaning, the eleven-year-old abstracts and synthesizes meaning to form a definition.

Syntagmatic-Paradigmatic Shift

Around age seven, the child begins to associate words in a different way than previously. Young children's word associations are primarily heterogeneous, in contrast to the homogeneous associations of adults. This change from one system of association to the other is called the **syntagmatic-paradigmatic shift**. A syntagmatic association is based on a syntactic relationship. For example, the stimulus word *girl* might elicit a child response *run*. In contrast, a paradigmatic association is based on semantic class, resulting from semantic attributes. In this case, the word *girl* might elicit *boy* or *woman*. The shift may represent either a refinement and organization of semantic features or a change in general cognitive-processing strategies.

The shift is gradual, beginning in preschool and continuing into adulthood. The period of most rapid change occurs between five and nine years. It is not until the adult years, however, that paradigmatic associations become consistent and fully integrated. Adults also use conceptual categorization, especially with abstract relations. For example, words from the sensory domain, such as *hot* and *cold*, may be associated with psychological states in order to form sentences such as "She is a *cold* person."

Some of this shift in cognitive organization is reflected in children's definitions. In addition to becoming more elaborate, the school-age child's definitions contain more superordinate categories, such as *furniture* and *clothing*. Some superordinate categories—*animal*, for example—are established as early as age three.

As the school-age child's definitions gradually become more literate or dictionarylike, they share certain characteristics. The definitions become more explicit, conventional representations of the implicit word meanings found in conversation. The linguistic form becomes more constrained with age until around age eleven, when the child has acquired all the elements of the conventional adult definition. The developmental sequence of required elements for definitions is presented in Table 11.4. The preschooler's individual, experientially based definition thus shifts to a more conventional, socially shared one.

Related Cognitive Processing

During the school years, there appears to be a change in cognitive processing, storage, and retrieval that reflects a shift from a nonlinguistic visual-perceptual mode to linguistic categorization. The initial change occurs in elementary school, with a shift from concrete to abstract during adolescence. The increasing reliance on linguistic categorization allows the child to process greater amounts of linguistic information.

TABLE 11.4 Developmental Sequence of Definitions

ELEMENTS REQUIRED	EXAMPLE
Noun phrase$_1$ . . .	*Dogs* have yukky breath.
NP$_1$ is . . .	*Dogs are* always barking and breathing.
NP$_1$ is NP$_2$ . . .	*Dogs are things* with four legs, a tail, bad breath, and barking.
NP$_1$ is NP$_2$ (superordinate category)	*Dogs are animals* that usually live in people's houses.

Several factors affect vocabulary acquisition (D. Johnson et al., 1982). First, both children and adults use a strategy of "chunking" semantically related information into categories for remembering. Seventh-graders rely more on chunking for recall than do first-graders. Second, the use of semantic relations resolves word ambiguities. For example, *there*, *their*, and *they're* sound very similar and could be confused, except for the very different semantic relations they represent. Third, categorical structures are stored hierarchically. Fourth, facilitative neural networks connect related word-concept structures. Thus new vocabulary acquisitions are associated with previous knowledge.

Individuals may use several levels of linguistic processing simultaneously:

Surface—syntactic rules and phonetic strings
Deep—semantic categories and relations
Contextual—situation or image

The mode or modes of processing relied on reflect the properties of the sentence and the maturation of the processor.

Children show a shift in linguistic processing from reliance on surface to deep structure strategies during early school years. This shift may reflect decreasing cognitive reliance on visual input for memory and recall, a gradual change from visual encoding by preschoolers to overt naming as the dominant memory process of school-age children. Kindergarteners also employ a naming strategy to enhance recall. Dependence on visual input for recall does not appear to lessen greatly until approximately age nine.

The processing shift may also reflect the child's increasing ability to integrate situational nonlinguistic information with linguistic information. These abilities are needed for effective daily communication. An example is the use of stress or emphasis in sentence decoding. There is a progression in the ability to use stress cues throughout elementary school and into the teenage years (F. Myers & R. Myers, 1983). Adults may use the following sequence of processing strategies:

1. Segment the message into the underlying sentences.
2. Mark the relations between the underlying sentences.
3. Determine the semantic relations of the lexical items.
4. Determine the semantic probabilities of co-occurrence.
5. Label the functions and properties of specific lexical items.

Children may begin to employ these strategies as early as age five.

The evolution of processing strategies may be reflected in the shifting recall patterns that occur with adult changes. The free recall of linguistic material with increased complexity decreases with age. These changes in cognitive operations may be more quantitative than qualitative (Spilich, 1983). The elderly have more difficulty with linguistic processing that requires greater organization in order to recall. In general, the elderly are more sensitive to theme or underlying meaning but are less able than young adults to recall syntax.

Figurative Language

The school-age child also develops figurative language, which enables use of language in a truly creative way. Figurative language is words used in an imaginative sense, rather than a literal one, to create an imaginative or emotional impression. Conversation, classroom teaching, and reading use figurative expressions frequently (Lazar, Warr-Leeper, Nicholson, & Johnson, 1989; Nippold, 1991).

The primary types of figurative language include idioms, metaphors, similes, and proverbs. Idioms are short expressions that cannot be analyzed grammatically. These colorful terms are not learned as part of a rule system and cannot be interpreted literally. They are acquired through continual use, and their meanings are inferred from context. For example, *hit the road* does not mean to strike a sharp blow to the asphalt but, rather, to leave. Table 11.5 presents some American English idioms.

Metaphors and similes are figures of speech that compare actual entities with a descriptive image. In a metaphor, a comparison is implied, such as "She kept a *hawk-eyed* surveillance." In contrast, a simile is an explicit comparison, usually introduced by *like* or *as*, such as "He ran *like a frightened rabbit*." To form a metaphor or a simile, the speaker must perceive a resemblance between two separate elements. The basis of the similarity is not literally true.

Preschool children produce many inventive figures of speech, such as the following examples (H. Gardner & Winner, 1979):

> A bald man is described as having a "barefoot" head.
> A stop sign is described as a "candy cane."
> A folded potato chip is described as a "cowboy hat."

I recall my daughter Jessica's description of the Lincoln Memorial, with its many columns, as "Lincoln's crib." My son Jason referred to his bruise as a "rotten spot." One of my students reported her daughter crying because she had hurt her "foot thumb" or big toe. The same child requested "ear gloves" or earmuffs for her cold ears. Heather Leary, upon seeing snow for the first time, described it as "white rain like bubbles." a rather poetic image. These early figures of speech are usually based on physical resemblance or on similarities of use or function. They appear to be an extension of, or an accompaniment to, symbolic play. Children as young as age three can produce intentional, appropriate, descriptive metaphors

TABLE 11.5 Common American English Idioms

strike a bargain	jump the gun	superior *to* (better *than*)
hit the road	break a date	in search *of* (search *for*)
take a cab	hop a plane	throw a party
robbed blind	do lunch	off the wall
in the pink	on a lark	

(Gottfried, 1997). There is significant development of metaphorical expressions in later preschool years.

The young child's creative descriptions do not imply that he or she can use figurative language (Hakes, 1982). This linguistic creativity often results from not knowing the correct word to use.

Metaphors become less frequent in spontaneous speech after age six. Two possible reasons for this decline are, first, that the child now has a basic vocabulary and is less pressured to stretch his or her vocabulary to express new meanings and, second, that the rule-guided linguistic training of school leaves little room for creativity. The remaining figures of speech, although less numerous, are more adultlike. Usually, the quantity of metaphors in creative writing increases in later elementary school.

The decline in what children produce spontaneously, however, does not reflect a decline in what they are capable of producing (Hakes, 1982). Rather, the decline is evidence of the young elementary school child's orientation toward the real and the literal.

While the spontaneous generation of figures of speech declines with age, comprehension improves. Some idioms are comprehended during late preschool (Abkarian, Jones, & West, 1992). Even by age seven, however, comprehension seems to be context-dependent, and production by the child lags well behind (Levorato & Cacciari, 1992). The five- to seven-year-old avoids crossing from physical into psychological domains and prefers to associate two terms rather than equating them. Child interpretation thus alters the relationship. For example, "She is a cold person" may be interpreted as "She lives at the North Pole." In contrast, the eight- to nine-year-old is beginning to appreciate the psychological process. The child still misinterprets the metaphor, however, because he or she does not fully understand the psychological dimension.

The older school-age child is able to make metaphoric matches across several sensory domains. For example, colors can be used to describe psychological states, as in "I feel *blue*." Child explanations for the matches change markedly with age.

Proverbs, the last type of figurative speech, are short, popular sayings that embody a generally accepted truth, useful thought, or advice. Often quite picturesque, proverbs are very difficult for young school-age children to comprehend. Examples of proverbs are:

> Don't put the cart before the horse.
> A new broom sweeps clean.
> You can't have your cake and eat it, too.
> Look before you leap.

The six-, seven-, or eight-year-old child interprets proverbs quite literally. Development of comprehension continues throughout adolescence and adulthood.

The ability to comprehend proverbs is strongly correlated with perceptual analogical reasoning ability (Nippold, Martin, & Erskine, 1988). Analogical reasoning problems follow the format "——— is to ——— as ——— is to ———." In similar fashion, the child attempting to comprehend a proverb must understand the underlying relationships between the proverb and the context. Both figurative language comprehension and analogical reasoning are strongly related to receptive vocabulary development, underscoring the semantic link between these skills (Nippold & Sullivan, 1987).

Accuracy in interpreting idioms and proverbs slowly increases throughout late childhood and adolescence (Gibbs, 1987; Nippold & Martin, 1989; Nippold et al., 1988). Although five-year-olds interpret most figurative expressions literally, even they can interpret some idioms in context. Figurative understanding begins gradually and continues into adulthood (Gibbs, 1987; Nippold & Martin, 1989; Prinz, 1983; Thorum, 1980). Of course, development of individual figurative expressions varies widely and depends, among other things, on world knowledge, learning context, and metaphoric transparency (Gibbs, 1987).

A general ability to interpret figurative expressions is related to world knowledge . For example, *smooth sailing* and *fishing for a compliment* have more meaning if you've sailed or fished.

Figurative expressions are easier for adolescents to comprehend in context than in isolation, possibly because figurative language is learned in context. Frequency of exposure, in contrast, has only a minor effect (Cacciari & Levorato, 1989; Levorato & Cacciari, 1992)

A figurative expression may be learned and stored as a large single lexical item—just as a word is learned and stored—rather than as individual words within the expression. As with single words, the meanings of figurative expressions are inferred from repeated exposure to these expressions in different contexts. For example, after the election, Grandpa says of the side with the poor showing, "They better *throw in the towel*." After working hard at her job, Mom sighs exhaustedly and says, "I'm *throwing in the towel*." Soon the child infers that the expression means something akin to *admitting defeat*. This task is an analytical one in which the child must actively think about the meaning of the expression in context and perceive the metaphoric comparisons.

Metaphorically transparent idioms are easier for children and adults to interpret than metaphorically opaque ones (Gibbs, 1987). **Metaphoric transparency**, or the extent of the literal–figurative relationship, directly affects ease of interpretation. Idioms, such as *hold your tongue,* have closely related literal and figurative meanings or are metaphorically transparent, because the meanings relate to speaking and to the tongue. In contrast, *beat around the bush* and *kick the bucket* do not have closely related meanings and are therefore metaphorically opaque. Even adults find less literal idioms difficult to interpret (Cronk, Lima, & Schweigert, 1993).

For preteens and adolescents, idioms that are more familiar, supported by context, and more transparent are easier to understand than those that are less familiar, isolated or out of context, and more opaque (Nippold & Taylor, 1995; Nippold, Taylor, & Baker, 1995; Spector, 1996). These factors are also important in the interpretation of proverbs (Nippold & Haq, 1996). Language experience and the development of metalinguistic abilities (see Chapter 12) are important determiners of individual skill. For adults in their twenties, concrete proverbs are easier to interpret than abstract. This difference is not seen in older adults where the ease of interpreting is related to overall level of education (Nippold, Uhden, Schwarz, 1997).

Although high-use idioms, such as *to put their heads together*, are easy for all American English-speaking children, low-use idioms, such as *to paper over the cracks*, are more easily understood by children who represented the majority culture (Qualls & Harris, 1999). In other words, regional and cultural differences affect idiom understanding.

The figurative and literal interpretations of figurative language may be retrieved in simultaneous but separate processes (Cacciari & Tabossi, 1988; Cronk & Schweigert, 1992;

Glass, 1983). The figurative meaning is stored in the child's lexicon as a single unit. The less frequently the expression is accessed, the more difficult it is to locate.

With interpreting, the literal process occurs as it would with any incoming signal. Meanwhile, lexical figurative analysis of the entire expression occurs. If the context supports the figurative interpretation, literal interpretation is interrupted and does not precede (Gibbs, 1985, 1986; Needham, 1992).

CONCLUSION

By adulthood, each individual is a truly versatile speaker who can tailor his or her message to the context and the participants. Adults are able to move flexibly from work to the gym to a cocktail party and home to tuck in the kids and alter their language effortlessly as needed. Within these contexts and many more, the mature communicator can change style and topic rapidly or remain in both almost indefinitely.

With increased age, the individual sharpens word definitions and relationships, resulting in more accurate communication. At the same time, he or she learns to use language figuratively to create nonliteral relationships. As a result of both processes, communication is both more precise and more creative. Again, the language user has gained increased flexibility.

DISCUSSION

Go back to the school-age and adult section of Chapter 3 for a quick review of the highlights of this chapter. All the major parts are outlined there. What can you add to each one?

Vocabulary expands rapidly, thus requiring increasingly better organization. The result is a shift from a word order type of organization to a categorical, semantic-based organization. The result is flexibility and easy access. New items in the vocabulary are multiple definitions and figurative language.

Pragmatics continues with the development of conversational and narrative skills. Narratives focus on internal narrative development called story grammars. A new element is the development of distinctive male and female styles of talking. If nothing else, that part of the chapter usually leads to lively discussion in class.

These changes—both pragmatic and semantic—can be subtle and some deficits may go unnoticed, yet it is just these very deficits that may make some otherwise high-functioning individuals seem odd or inappropriate. Not being able to vary one's style of talking for given contexts, being slightly off in the timing of turns, and even poor eye contact will make a teenager the target of derision by other adolescents. Likewise, not knowing the meaning of slang terms can lead to isolation. It is these differences and more that separate the preschool speaker from the adult. It may seem odd, but there are situations in which it may be appropriate to teach slang to some adolescents with language impairments.

REFLECTIONS

1. The conversational abilities of the school age child increase dramatically. Describe these pragmatic abilities.

2. Describe the differences between the speech of men and women and suggest possible related factors.

3. Between the ages of five and nine, the child undergoes the syntagmatic paradigmatic shift in his concept formation. What is this shift? What is its effect on the child's definitions?

4. Figurative language cannot be taken literally; the child must use other cues to interpret. What are the major types of figurative language? Explain the development of this form of language.

12

School-Age and Adult Language Form and Mode Development

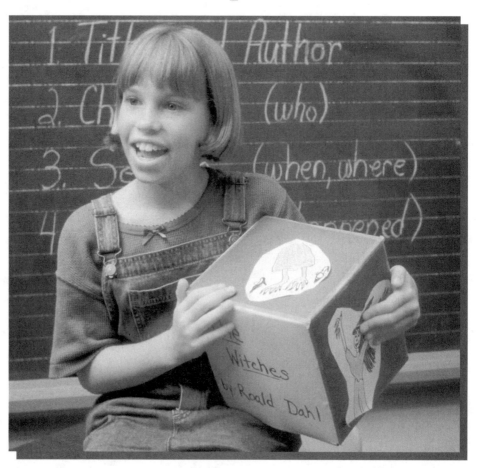

CHAPTER OBJECTIVES

Much of language form is refined during school-age and adult development. Along with increased vocabulary and use, the child and adult master the fine points of American English form. In addition, a new mode of communication—reading and writing—increases the possibilities for interacting with many conversational partners, even those who are no longer living. When you have completed this chapter, you should understand

- the different types of passive sentences and their development.
- the continued development of embedding and conjoining and possible reasons for the sequence of conjunction development.
- morphophonemic changes.
- metalinguistic abilities.
- the bottom-up and top-down theories of reading processing.
- the development of reading and writing.
- the following terms:

        metalinguistic   morphophonemic
                                                       phonological awareness

Much of the syntactic development in the school years is intrasentential, at the noun- and verb-phrase level. Other development involves the refinement of features learned earlier, such as determiners, pronouns, and embedding. The child continues to operate from his or her own mini-theories about language, which are correct for some situations but not all (Karmiloff-Smith, 1986). These theories become broadened and more flexible as they blend with the language-use skills that the child continues to acquire.

The primary manner of joining clauses shifts gradually from conjoining to embedding. While many rules are learned during the preschool years, many exceptions are discovered during the school years. Finally, with a more flexible language system at hand, the child learns to be more economical in its use and to avoid redundancy such as the double negative.

Metalinguistic ability, the awareness that enables a language user to think about and reflect on language, also becomes well-developed during the school-age period. The ability to think about language in the abstract is reflected in the development of writing and reading skills.

Reading and writing, plus the demands of the classroom, require major changes in the way a child uses language. Very different rules for talking apply between the classroom and conversation. The child must negotiate a turn by seeking recognition from the teacher and responding in a highly specific manner to questions, which may represent over half the teacher's utterances. "Text-related" or ideational language becomes relatively more important than social, interpersonal language. The child is held highly accountable for responses and is required to use precise word meanings. The child who comes to school with different language skills and expectations may suffer as a consequence.

SYNTACTIC AND MORPHOLOGIC DEVELOPMENT

Language development in the school-age period consists of simultaneous expansion of existing syntactic forms and acquisition of new forms (Table 12.1). The child continues with internal sentence expansion by elaborating the noun and verb phrases. Conjoining and embedding functions also expand. Additional structures include the passive form.

TABLE 12.1   Summary of School-Age Child's Development of Language Form

AGE IN YEARS	SYNTAX/MORPHOLOGY	PHONOLOGY
5	• Produces short passives with *lost*, *left*, and *broken*	
6	• Comprehends parallel embedding, imperative commands, *-man* and *-er* suffix • Uses many plural nouns	• Identifies syllables • Masters rule for /s/, /z/, and /əz/ pluralization • Is able to manipulate sound units to rhyme and produce stems
7	• Comprehends *because* • Follows adult ordering of adjectives	• Recognizes unacceptable sound sequences
8	• Uses full passives (80% of children • Uses *-er* suffix to mark initiator of an action (*teacher*) • Is able to judge grammatical correctness separate from semantics	• Is able to produce all American English sounds and blends
9	• Comprehends and uses *tell* and *promise*	
10	• Comprehends and uses *ask* • Comprehends *because* consistently • Uses pronouns to refer to elements outside immediate sentence • Understands difference between *definitely*, *probably*, and *possibly*	
11	• Comprehends *if* and *though* • Creates *much* with mass nouns • Uses *-er* for instrument (*eraser*)	
12		• Uses stress contrasts
13–15	• Comprehends *unless* • Comprehends all types of embedding	
16–18		• Uses vowel-shifting rules (*divine–divinity*)

Although the child has achieved basic sentence competence by age five, fewer than 50 percent of first-graders can produce correct pronouns, "cause" clauses, and gerunds. Fewer than 20 percent can produce *if* and *so* clauses and participles. You will recall that gerunds are verbs to which *-ing* has been added to produce a form that fulfills a noun function. For example,

He enjoys *fishing*.
Running is his favorite exercise.

In participles, the same form fills an adjectival role, as in

We bought *fishing* equipment.
Do you like your new *running* shoes?

Morphologic Development

Learning to use a morphological rule begins with the hypothesis that a small set of words are treated in a certain way grammatically. The first uses of a morphological marker are probably the result of rote memorization. This is followed by morphological generalizations about phonological marking (/d, t/) and meaning (past tense) (Bybee & Slobin, 1982). Gradually, the child forms a rule.

While some inflectional suffixes are refined during the school-age years, the main developments occur in the addition of inflectional prefixes (*un-*, *dis-*, *non-*, *ir-*) and derivational suffixes (Nagy, Diakidoy, & Anderson, 1991). The development of inflectional prefixes is very gradual and protracted, continuing into adulthood. I, for one, know that *flammable* written on a truck means *keep your distance*, but I'm easily confused by *inflammable*.

Derivational suffixes—those that change word classes—are a much larger set of word parts than inflectional suffixes and are usually used to change the part of speech of the base word. As a group, they have a smaller range of use and have many irregularities. Often, use is very restricted, as in the use of *-hood* or *-ment*. For example, *-ment* changes the verb *attach* to the noun *attachment* but cannot be used with common verbs, such as *talk*, *eat*, *drink*, and *sit*. Over 80 percent of words with derivational suffixes do not even mean what the parts suggest (Nagy & Anderson, 1984; White, Power, & White, 1989). Despite this fact, knowledge of derivational suffix meaning is a significant factor in interpreting novel words (Lewis & Windsor, 1996).

Derivational suffixes are first learned orally, although reading strengthens learning, especially for more complex forms (Carlisle, 1987). A very limited general order of acquisition is *-er*, *-y*, noun compounds, and *-ly*. Mastery continues into late adolescence (Carlisle, 1987, 1988). The *-y* marker used to form adjectives such as *sticky* and *fluffy* is not acquired until age eleven, and the *-ly* marker used to form adverbs such as *quickly* is learned in adolescence.

Difficulty in learning is related to **morphophonemic** *processes*, discussed later in the chapter, and to semantic distinctions. For example, the *-er* suffix is initially acquired to mark the initiator of some action, such as paint*er* for the person who paints and teach*er* for the

TABLE 12.2   School-Age Development of Irregular Verbs

AGE	VERBS
5-0 to 5-5	*took, fell, broke, found*
5-6 to 5-11	*came, made, threw, sat*
6-0 to 6-5	*ran, flew, wore, wrote, cut, fed, drove, bit*
6-6 to 6-11	*blew, read, shot, rode*
7-0 to 7-5	*drank*
7-6 to 7-11	*hid, rang, slept, drew, dug, swam*
8-0 to 8-5	*left, caught, slid, hung*
8-6 to 8-11	*sent, shook, built*

Note: Nine words did not reach criterion by 8-5 through 8-11 years. These were *bent, chose, fought, held, sang, sank, stood, swang,* and *swept.*

Source: Adapted from Shipley, K., Maddox, M., & Driver, J. (1991). Children's development of irregular past tense verb forms. *Language, Speech and Hearing Services in Schools, 22,* 115–122.

person who teaches. Although this suffix may appear in late preschool with some specific words, children are not able to use it generatively until age eight (Derwing & Baker, 1986).

The *-er* used to mark the instrument for accomplishing some action is acquired even later, around age eleven (Clark & Hecht, 1982). Examples of the instrumental *-er* include lighting a cigarette with a light*er* or erasing with an eras*er.* In part, the late development of the instrumental *-er* can be explained by the child's use of other more common words in place of the "verb + er" form, such as the more appropriate *stove* for *cooker* and *shovel* for *digger.* Other words have no non-*er* equivalent.

Although only a few hundred word definitions are taught directly, children use their morphologic knowledge generalized to new words for semantic decoding (Tyler & Nagy, 1987; Wysocki & Jenkins, 1987). This process becomes increasingly important with maturity as less frequently used words are encountered more.

Noun- and Verb-Phrase Development

Children of five to seven years use most elements of noun and verb phrases but frequently omit these elements, even when they are required. Even at age seven, they omit some elements but expand others redundantly. The rhythm of a sentence seems to be more salient, and children often miss small, unstressed functor words. In addition, school-age children still have difficulty with some prepositions, verb tensing and modality, and plurals. Unique instances or rule exceptions, such as irregular past and plural, are particularly difficult.

Noun Phrases

Within the noun phrase, pronoun and adjective development continues. The child learns to differentiate better between subject pronouns, such as *I, he, she, we,* and *they,* and object pronouns, such as *me, him, her, us,* and *them,* and to use reflexives, such as *myself, himself, herself*, and *ourselves*. In addition, he or she learns to carry pronouns across sentences and to analyze a sentence to determine to which noun a pronoun refers. For example, the child must perform some complex analysis in order to interpret the following sentences:

> Mary's mother was very sick. Mary knew that *she* must obtain a doctor for *her*.

The child must be able to hold more than one dimension of the noun phrase or of an entire clause and to comprehend or use a pronoun in its place. This procedure is demonstrated in the following sentences:

> The earth began to tremble shortly before rush hour, reaching full force forty minutes later. *It* was devastating.

By age ten, the child is able to use pronouns to make this type of reference outside the immediate sentence (Karmiloff-Smith, 1986).

Adjective ordering also becomes evident within the noun phrase. In English, multiple properties are generally described by a string of sequentially ordered adjectives. As noted in Table 10.6, different semantic classes of adjectives have definite positions based on a complex rule system. During school age, the most evident change comes in the addition of post-noun modifiers in the form of embedded phrases and clauses.

Three-year-olds display the same ordering preference as adults for the first adjective in a sequence (Richards, 1980). The child does not show positional preferences that approximate adult ordering for the other adjectives until school age. Earlier ordering preferences may reflect an imitative strategy rather than an analytical approach to the separate adjectives. The period from age five to seven marks a phase of improved cognitive ability to discriminate perceptual attributes and their relationships.

The distinction between mass and count nouns and their quantifiers is acquired only slowly throughout the school years (Gathercole, 1985; P. Gordon, 1988). Mass nouns refer to homogeneous, nonindividual substances, such as *water*, *sand*, and *sugar*. Count nouns refer to heterogeneous, individual objects, such as *cup*, *bicycle*, and *house*. Mass nouns take quantifying modifiers, such as *much* and *little*, while count nouns take quantifiers, such as *many* and *few*.

Although children as young as age two can make a distinction between count and mass nouns, it is not until much later that they learn to use the determiner (*this, that*) with count nouns and not with mass nouns (P. Gordon, 1988). By early elementary school, the child has learned most of the correct noun forms so that words like *monies* and *mens* are rare. *Many* then appears with plural count nouns, as in "many houses." *Much* is usually learned by late elementary school, although the adolescent still makes errors. Early on, the child discovers a way around the quantifier question by using *lots of* with both types of nouns.

Verb Phrases

Verbs appear to offer greater difficulty for school-age children than nouns. These difficulties may be related to varied syntactic marking (Gentner, 1982). For example, verb action can be reversed in three ways:

1. Use of the prefix *un-*: "She is tying her shoe. She is *untying* her shoe."
2. Use of a particle following the verb: "Pull *on* your boots. Pull *off* your boots."
3. Use of separate lexical items: "She *opened* the door. She *closed* the door."

Certain forms may be used only with specific verbs. The child's resultant confusion produces sentences such as these (Bowerman, 1981):

> I had to untake the sewing. (take out the stitches)
> I'll get it after it's plugged out. (unplugged)

The difficulty of learning how to state underlying verb relationships may account for the greater amount of time needed for acquisition of verbs compared to common nouns.

During the school years, the child adds verb tenses, such as the perfect [*have* + *be* + *verb(en/ed)* as in *has been eaten*, or *have* + *verb(en/ed)* as in *has finished*], additional irregular past-tense verbs (see Table 12.2), and modal auxiliary verbs.

Modality is a semantic notion of possibility, obligation, permission, intention, validity, truth, and functionality expressed in modal auxiliary verbs and in different sentence types. School-age children and adults also express modality in adverbs (*possibly*, *maybe*), adjectives (*possible*, *likely*), nouns (*possibility*, *likelihood*), verbs (*believe*, *doubt*), and suffixes (*-able*). Obviously, all forms of modality do not develop simultaneously. In general, the possibility, obligation, permission, and intention forms develop before the validity, truth, and functionality forms (Stephany, 1986). Even twelve-year-olds do not have an adult sense of modality (Coates, 1988).

Adverbs of likelihood, such as *definitely*, *probably*, and *possibly*, can pose a problem even for school-age children. In general, preschoolers don't understand the distinction between the terms. By fourth grade, however, most children know the difference. The terms are not learned at the same time, but *definitely* is learned first and understood best by most children (Hoffner, Cantor, & Badzinski, 1990).

Even within a form, such as *will*, different functions develop at different rates. Cognitively, *will-do* (I will go) seems to develop before *will-happen* ("It will take some effort.") (Pea & Mawby, 1981). This is true in languages as different as English, Greek, and Turkish (Goossens, 1981; Slobin & Aksu, 1982; Stephany, 1986).

Sentence Types

In general, comprehension of linguistic relationships expressed in sentences improves throughout the school years (Table 12.1). The comparative relationship, as in *as big as*, *smaller than*, and *more fun than*, is the easiest one for first- to third-graders to interpret. The cognitive skills needed for comparative relationships develop during the preschool years but must await linguistic development. Other sentential relations, such as passive, are more difficult for school-age children to interpret.

Linguists are only now beginning to explore the effect of prosody—rate and pausing—on the sentence comprehension of older children and adults. Syntax does not fully represent the organization of a spoken sentence. Prosody seems to aid mature listeners by segmenting linguistic units, just as it helps language-learning children and is one of the characteristics of motherese (Gerken, 1996). When speakers pause at inappropriate boundaries, they interfere with their listeners' syntactic processing (Speer, Kjelgaard, & Dobroth, 1996). It is possible that the rhythmic outline of a sentence forms a frame in auditory working memory into which the syntactic elements are placed for analysis. Prosodic information can aid older children and adults in identifying sentence elements, even when these elements are jumbled or misplaced (Nagel, Shapiro, Tuller, & Nawy, 1996).

Sentence production continues to expand during the school-age through adult years across individuals at all socioeconomic levels and of all racial/ethnic groups (Craig, Washington, & Thompson-Porter, 1998). In both English and Spanish, sentences become longer with the addition of more words, embedded phrases and embedded clauses. As in English, Spanish-speaking children with low school achievement have less complex syntax (Gutierrez-Clellen, 1998).

Passive Sentences

Passive sentences are troublesome, both receptively and expressively, for English-speaking children. The passive form is acquired earlier in non-Indo-European languages, such as Inuktitut (S. Allen & Crago, 1996); Sesotho (Demuth, 1989, 1990), a West African language; Zulu (Suzman, 1987); and Quiche Mayan (Pye, 1988), a native Mexican language. The English passive varies from the predominant *agent + action + object* arrangement, requiring a change in sentence-processing strategy. American English-speaking adults use the passive form infrequently. As you might imagine, then, five-year-old children rarely produce full passive sentences.

Children do not truly comprehend passive sentences until about age five-and-a-half. Prior to this age, children use extralinguistic strategies, such as contextual support, to interpret sentences (Bridges, 1980). Children may also rely on action verbs for interpretation. True comprehension skill is related to the ability to view an event from another person's perspective and to alternate or shift perspective.

An additional clue for passive interpretation may be the presence of a preposition (Shorr & Dale, 1981). In general, young school-age children interpret a sentence as passive when *from* or *by* is present and as active when *to* is used. Thus, "The picture was painted *by* Mary" is passive, and "The picture was given *to* John" is active.

Production of passives begins in the late preschool years with short sentences containing noun + *be/get* + verb(-*en/-ed*), such as "It got broken" or "It was crushed." In these early passives, the noun is almost always inanimate. These forms may be based on the predicate adjective form seen with the copula, such as "He was sad" (Bowey, 1982). Verbs of state, such as *lost*, *left*, and *broken*, tend to predominate in these short passives. Later, the child uses action verbs, such as *killed*, *hit*, and *crashed*, in both short and full passives.

Approximately 80 percent of seven-and-a-half- to eight-year-olds produce full passive sentences. In general, a full passive contains some form of *be* or *got*, a past-tense marker, and a preposition followed by a noun phrase that is agentive or instrumentive, as in "The window was broken by Diego." Some passive forms do not appear until eleven years of age.

Passives may be of three general types: *reversible*, *instrumental nonreversible*, and *agentive nonreversible*. In the reversible type, either noun could be the actor or the object: "The dog was chased by the cat" could be reversed to read "The cat was chased by the dog." In the nonreversible type, the nouns cannot be reversed. The two nonreversible passives include one in which the subject is an instrument, such as *ball*, and another in which the subject is an agent, such as *boy*. An example of the instrumental type is "The window was broken by the ball." In the agentive type, "The window was broken by the boy." Both are nonreversible since we could not say "The ball/boy was broken by the window." These semantic distinctions appear to be important for development of the passive form.

As a group, children use about an equal number of reversible and nonreversible passives. Prior to age four, children produce more reversible passives with considerable word-order confusion. Children say "The boy is chased by the girl" when in fact the boy is in pursuit. This confusion is reflected in sentence interpretation as well. Only about 50 percent of five-year-olds can correctly interpret reversible passives (Bridges, 1980).

A marked increase in nonreversible passive production occurs just prior to age eight. The type of nonreversible passive that is most prominent changes with age. Agentive non-reversibles appear at age nine. Instrumental nonreversible passives are the most frequent nonreversibles for eleven- to thirteen-year-olds. For this age group, semantic distinctions are also signaled by preposition use. Reversible passives use *by*, whereas nonreversibles use *with*. Adults may use either *by* or *with* in the instrumental nonreversible type. Both children and adults use *by* with the agentive nonreversible passive. Children's passives thus seem to be semantically different from those of adults.

Conjoining and Embedding

The child's repertoire of embedded and conjoined forms increases throughout the school years. Syntactic rules for both forms are observed more frequently. Clausal conjoining expands with the use of the following conjunctions:

Type	Examples
Causal	*because, so, therefore*
Conditional	*if*
Disjunctive	*but, or, although*
Temporal	*when, before, after, then*

The conjunction of choice for narration, however, remains *and*. Between 50 and 80 percent of the narrative sentences of school-age children begin with *and* (Scott, 1987). This percentage decreases as the children mature. By eleven to fourteen years of age, only approximately 20 percent of narrative sentences begin with *and*. This percentage decreases to 5 percent under the somewhat more formal constraints of writing (Scott, 1987).

Other conjunctions are more frequently used for clausal conjoining. Up to age twelve, *because* and *when* predominate, with *if* and *in order to* also used frequently (Scott, 1987).

Even though *if*, *so*, and *because* are produced relatively early in the school years, full understanding does not develop until much later. Semantic concepts of time and pragmatic aspects of propositional truth may affect comprehension.

Learning to understand and use *because* is not an easy task. To understand a sentence with *because*, the child must comprehend not only the relationship between two events, but also their temporal sequence. This sequence is not necessarily the same as the order presented in the sentence. In "I went because I was asked," the speaker was invited before he or she actually left, although the linguistic ordering is the reverse. At first, the child tends to confuse *because* with *and* and *then*, using them all in a similar fashion. In both comprehension and production, the preschool child appears to follow an order-of-mention strategy. Although the causal relationship appears to be understood prior to age seven, knowledge of the ordering role of *because* seems to be weak.

Comprehension of *because* does not seem to develop until age seven. Consistently correct comprehension may not occur until around age ten or eleven.

Pragmatic factors may also affect the development of conjunctions. Children are more accurate at judging the speaker's meaning if the speaker expresses belief in the truthfulness of the utterance and if the two clauses are related positively. The conjunction *because* expresses both strong belief and a positive relationship. Other conjunctions express different relations. For example, both *because* and *although* presuppose that the speaker believes the two expressed propositions to be true:

It is a block because it is cubical.
It is a block, although it is made of metal.

In contrast, *unless* and *if* presuppose speaker uncertainty about at least one of the propositions:

It is a block unless it is round.
It is a block if it is wooden.

Similarly, *because* and *if* express a positive relationship between the two clauses, while *although* and *unless* express a negative relationship. *Although* expresses an exception or an illogical relationship. *Unless* requires that the truth of one proposition be denied in order for the relationship to be logical. Figure 12.1 expresses these concepts. In general, the more positive the relationship, the easier it is to comprehend the conjunction. Thus *because* is learned before *if* and *although*, which in turn are followed by *unless*. Even fifth-graders may have difficulty understanding *unless* (Wing & Scholnick, 1981). Younger children do not understand the appropriate pragmatic cues for disbelief and uncertainty. Therefore, they rely on syntactic cues.

FIGURE 12.1 Concepts Expressed by Conjunctions

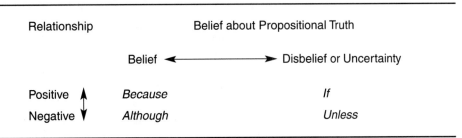

Relationship	Belief about Propositional Truth	
	Belief ←————————→ Disbelief or Uncertainty	
Positive ↑	*Because*	*If*
Negative ↓	*Although*	*Unless*

Source: Adapted from Wing, C., & Scholnick, E. Children's comprehension of pragmatic concepts expressed in "because," "although," "if," and "unless." *Journal of Child Language*, 1981, *8*, 347–365.

Syntactic strategies are also important in the production and interpretation of embedding. The percentage of embedded sentences increases steadily to 20 to 30 percent in children's narratives throughout the school years (Scott, 1984b). Relative pronoun use is expanded with the addition of *whose*, *whom*, and *in which* (Scott, 1988). Multiple embeddings also increase with maturity and are one of the most significant differences between the narrative syntactic structure of six- to eight-year-olds and ten- to twelve-year-olds.

Although school-age clausal embeddings include relative pronoun deletions and center or subject-relative clause embedding, these forms are rarely produced prior to age seven. Examples of each of these forms include the following:

> I'm engaged to someone (*whom*) you know. (Relative pronoun deletion)
> The book *that Reggie read* was exciting. (Center or subject-relative clause
> embedding)

Center embedding is particularly difficult.

For children, semantic role is also an important factor in interpretation . If the object of a center embedding is inanimate, it is less likely to be misinterpreted than an animate object is. In the following, *window* cannot *run*, so there is no confusion in the first sentence, but the second may be misinterpreted:

> The boy, who broke the window, ran away. (Interpreted correctly)
> The boy, who hit the girl, ran away. (Could be interpreted to mean that the
> girl ran away)

Faced with confusion, the child resorts to a *subject + verb + object* interpretation strategy.

Comprehension of embedded sentences also seems to be based on the place and manner of the embedding. Embeddings may occur at the end of a sentence or in the center. The two clauses may be parallel, in which both share the same subject or object, or nonparallel, in which they do not:

> The *boy who* lives next door gave me a present. (parallel central embedding:
> the same subject—*boy*—serves both clauses)
> He gave me a *present that* I didn't like. (parallel ending embedding: the same
> object—*present*—serves both clauses)
> He gave me the *present that* is on the table. (nonparallel ending embedding:
> the object of one—*present*—is the subject of the other)
> The *dog that* was chased by the boy is angry. (nonparallel central embedding:
> the subject of the main clause—*dog*—is the object of the embedded clause)

This order is the general developmental sequence from easiest to most difficult (Abrahamsen & Rigrodsky, 1984). The relative difficulty of center embedded clauses may be due to limitation in auditory working memory (R. Lewis, 1996). As the child matures, auditory working memory is able to hold more items for longer periods of time.

First-graders rely heavily on word order for interpretation and are confused by semantic class reversals between subject and object class. By seventh grade, the child has little difficulty interpreting these sentences and relies primarily on grammatical cues (Abrahamsen & Rigrodsky, 1984). This change probably reflects the child's underlying cognitive development.

Summary

During the school-age years, the child adds new morphological and syntactic structures and expands and refines existing forms. These developments enable expression of increasingly complex relationships and use of more creative language. Underlying semantic concepts are often the key to this complex learning.

PHONOLOGICAL DEVELOPMENT

During the early school years, the child completes the phonetic inventory (Table 12.1). By age eight he or she can produce all English speech sounds competently. Sounds in longer words or blends may still be difficult. The acquisition of sounds, however, is only one aspect of a child's phonological competence.

By age six, the child can identify syllables (Hakes, 1980). Very few four-year-olds are able to identify these units. Not until later in the school years does the child recognize that spoken language is composed of phoneme-sized units.

Phonemic competence is evident in the child's rhyming ability. Children become sensitive to phonetic patterns in the preschool years and often rhyme words by substituting one sound or syllable for another, producing *cat, bat, rat, fat, hat,* and so on. This process is spontaneous, automatic word play; a more deliberate, controlled process evolves later. It is not until the school years that the child understands the basis of the sound similarity. From kindergarten to third grade, the child is increasingly able to discriminate words that rhyme from those with other similarities. For example, *hug* and *rug* rhyme, but *rug* and *rig,* although similar, do not.

By age seven, the child is able to produce a resultant word after one sound is removed from a word. For example, removing /s/ from *sink* produces *ink.* Younger children can repeat a stem (*ink* in *sink*) better if the stem forms a meaningful word. Removing /s/ from *soap,* for example, produces *oap,* a meaningless word, and hence a more difficult stem to repeat. Thus, the child may rely more on semantic than on structural rules.

The four-year-old child is able to decide if a sound sequence conforms to the phonological rules of English. He or she will repeat words that contain possible sequences, even when the words are not real, but will modify impermissible sequences when repeating them in order to produce sequences more like English. A seven-year-old tends to replace the meaningless words with actual words. These changes most likely reflect the child's increasing metalinguistic skills, which will be discussed later.

Morphophonemic Development

Morphophonemic changes are phonological or sound modifications that result when morphemes are placed together. For example, the final /k/ in *electric* changes to a /s/ in *electricity.* Several rules for morphophonemic change are learned gradually throughout elementary school.

One rule, usually learned by first grade, pertains to the regular plural -s mentioned in Chapter 10. The five- to six-year-old has learned the rule for /s/ and /z/ but not for /əz/. Nouns ending in -sk and -st clusters may be difficult for some students to pluralize, even in third grade. Is the plural of *desk* /desks/ or /deskəz/?

During the school years, the child also learns the rules for vowel shifting. For example, the /aI/ sound in *divine* changes to an /I/ in *divinity*. Other examples are as follows:

/aI/—/I/	/eI/—/æ/	/i/—/ɛ/
divine—divinity	explain—explanation	serene—serenity
collide—collision	sane—sanity	obscene—obscenity

Knowledge of vowel shifting is gained only gradually. The five-year-old child does not understand the rules, and it is not until age seventeen that most individuals learn to apply all the rules.

Stress, or emphasis, is also learned during the school years. The stress placed on certain syllables or words reflects the grammatical function of that unit. In English, stress varies with the relationship between two words and with the word's use as a noun or verb. For example, two words may form a phrase, such as *green house*, or a compound word, such as *greenhouse*. If you repeat the two, you will find that you stress *house* in the phrase and *green* in the compound word. Here are some other examples:

Phrase	Compound Word
red *head*	*red*head
black *board*	*black*board
high *chair*	*high*chair

Noun–verb pairs also differ. In the noun *record*, emphasis is on the first syllable, whereas the verb *record* is pronounced with stress on the last. Other examples are:

Noun	Verb
*pre*sent	pre*sent*
*con*duct	con*duct*

Initially acquired on isolated words, pitch contours are gradually integrated into larger units. The period from age three to five seems to be particularly important in several languages for the acquisition of stress patterns (Allen, 1983). It is not until age twelve, however, that the full adult stress and accent system is acquired (Ingram, 1986).

Summary

It is not enough for the child to acquire the sounds of the native language. These are only the building blocks. Throughout the school years, the child learns rules for permissible combinations and for the use of stress, which is related to syntactic and semantic growth as well. Thus, the child is again forming rule systems that bring order to the linguistic world. The child is not just mirroring the speech heard around him or her.

METALINGUISTIC ABILITIES

Metalinguistic abilities enable the language user to think about language independently of comprehension and production abilities. As such, the child focuses on and reflects on language as a decontextualized object (van Kleeck, 1982). It is these "linguistic intuitions" that let us make decisions about the grammatical acceptability of an utterance. Thus, the child treats language as an object of analysis and observation, using language to describe language. This ability develops only gradually throughout the school years.

In adults, comprehension and production are almost automatic, and processing occurs at the rate of communication. There is no inordinate burden. Even children's comprehension strategies seem to be unconscious. Controlled, conscious processes tend to be minimal, because comprehension includes the total linguistic and nonlinguistic contexts.

Although metalinguistic abilities appear in the preschool years, full awareness is not found until age seven to eight years (Saywitz & Cherry-Wilkinson, 1982). Prior to this age, children view language primarily as a means of communication, rather than focusing on the manner in which it is conveyed (van Kleeck, 1982). After age seven or eight, the development of decentration enables the child to concentrate on and process simultaneously two aspects of language: message meaning and linguistic correctness. Thus, the child is able to judge grammatical correctness without being influenced by semantics.

Preschool children tend to make judgments of utterance acceptability based on the content rather than on the grammatical structure. Thus, a four-year-old might judge "Daddy painted the fence" as unacceptable since, in the child's realm of experience, "Daddies don't paint fences, they paint walls" (Hakes, 1980). By kindergarten, the child is just beginning to separate what is said from how it is said, to separate referents from words, and to notice structure. Even so, school-age children may still judge correctness more on semantic intent or meaning than on grammatical form (Sutter & Johnson, 1990).

The ability to detect syntactic errors develops first. The school-age child demonstrates an increasing ability to judge grammatical acceptability and to correct unacceptable sentences (Bowey, 1986). The metalinguistic skills to correct regular and irregular nouns and verbs appear at about age six (Cox, 1989). This change reflects a growing knowledge of language structure.

Metalinguistic abilities usually emerge after the child has mastered a linguistic form. Therefore, it is possible that the young school-age child becomes aware at a metalinguistic level of language forms and content unconsciously used in the preschool years. Some metalinguistic abilities are an almost unconscious or implicit aspect of feedback, whereas others are extremely explicit and conscious. An order of development based on this continuum is presented in Table 12.3.

Metalinguistic awareness may be essential to the changes in semantic organization discussed in Chapter 11. Morphological awareness of root words, such as *like*, and derived forms, such as *likable, unlike, likely,* and *unlikely,* is necessary for the formation of associational

TABLE 12.3   Development of Metalinguistic Skills and Awareness

APPROXIMATE AGE	ABILITIES

1½–2 yrs.	1. Monitor one's own on-going utterances
	  a. Repair spontaneously
	  b. Practice sounds, words, and sentences
	  c. Adjust one's speech to different listeners

3–4 yrs.	2. Check the result of one's utterance
	  a. Check whether the listener has understood; if not, repair or try again
	  b. Comment explicitly on own utterances and those of others
	  c. Correct others
	3. Test for reality
	  a. Decide whether a word or sentence "works" in furthering listener understanding
	4. Attempt to learn language deliberately
	  a. Practice new sounds, words, and sentences
	  b. Practice speech styles of different roles

School age	5. Predict the consequences of using particular forms (inflections, words, phrases, sentences)
	  a. Apply appropriate inflections to "new" words
	  b. Judge utterances as appropriate for a specific listener or setting
	  c. Correct word order and wording in sentences judged as "wrong"
	6. Reflect on the product of an utterance (structure independent of use)
	  a. Identify specific linguistic units (sounds, syllables, words, sentences)
	  b. Provide definitions of words
	  c. Construct puns, riddles, or other forms of humor
	  d. Explain why some sentences are possible and how to interpret them

Source: Adapted from E. Clark, "Awareness of Language: Some Evidence from What Children Say and Do." In A. Sinclair, R. Jarvella, and W. Levelt (Eds.), *The Child's Conception of Language.* New York: Springer-Verlag, 1978.

networks (Nagy, Anderson, Schommer, Scott, & Stallman, 1989). These networks are constructed of highly similar words, and activation of one opens access to others.

    Like emerging pragmatic skills, metalinguistic abilities depend on development of all aspects of language. With increased structural and semantic skills, the child is freed from the immediate linguistic context and can attend to how a message is communicated. In addition, metalinguistic skill development is related to language use, cognitive development, reading ability, academic achievement, IQ, environmental stimulation, and play (Kemper & Vernooy, 1993; Saywitz & Cherry-Wilkinson, 1982).

READING AND WRITING: A NEW MODE

With entry into school, the child is required to learn a new mode of communication through the visual channel. Although there is only moderate overlap between the processes of oral and visual communication, among the best indicators of a child's potential for success with reading and writing are oral language and metalinguistic skills (R. Katz, Shankweiler, & Liberman, 1981; R. Kemper, 1985; Mann, Shankweiler, & Smith, 1984).

Metalinguistic skills enable the child to decontextualize and segment linguistic material. A strong relationship exists between early segmentation skills and reading and spelling. About half of kindergartners and 90 percent of first-graders are able to segment words into syllables. By the end of first grade, with some formal instruction, approximately 70 percent of children can segment by phoneme. Awareness of the sound system is also very important. The abilities to recognize and create rhymes and to create words that begin with certain sounds in kindergarten correlate highly with reading success later on.

Children with a history of preschool speech and language problems frequently have difficulty with reading (Maxwell & Wallach, 1984; P. Weiner, 1985). There are strong indications that speech/audition and writing/reading share, at least in part, a common linguistic base, although they differ in other ways.

Both reading and writing are complex processes that are not totally understood by development and education professionals. It is understood, though, that reading is the synthesis of a complex network of perceptual and cognitive acts along a continuum from word recognition and decoding skills to comprehension and integration. Beyond the printed page, the skilled reader draws conclusions and inferences from what he or she reads. Of all the factors involved in early reading success, early exposure to reading by parents and a literate atmosphere at home seem to be most important (Goldfield & Snow, 1985; C. Snow, 1983).

The Process of Reading

Reading is a language-based skill. As such, it requires the processing of language that is decontextualized from any ongoing event. Decontextualized language is characterized by the fact that the speaker and listener do not directly share the experience being communicated. The speaker must create the context through language, as in narration. It is not surprising, therefore, that poor readers also exhibit poor narrative skills, especially with linguistic cohesion (Norris & Bruning, 1988). The narratives of poor readers tend to be shorter and less well developed than those of better readers.

Familiarity with nursery rhymes is also correlated with better reading skills (Bryant, Bradley, MacLean & Crossland, 1989). In addition to helping the child become sensitive to rhyming and to phonemes, nursery rhymes provide experience with language play, a building block for metalinguistic skills.

Two major theoretical positions attempt to explain the processes involved in reading. Dubbed the *bottom-up* and *top-down* approaches, they describe the extremes of a theoretical continuum. An interactive processing model somewhere between the two is more likely.

According to the bottom-up theory, reading is translating written elements (Perfetti, 1984). Hence, bottom-up theories emphasize lower-level perceptual and phonemic processes and their influence on higher cognitive functioning. Knowledge of both perceptual features in letters and grapheme–phoneme correspondence, as well as lexical retrieval, aid word recognition and decoding. Evidence exists that for the mature reader, the basic units of analysis are not individual letters or graphemes but groupings of letters that form recognizable segments of words (Bowey, 1996).

In contrast, the top-down, or problem-solving, theory emphasizes the cognitive task of deriving meaning. Higher cognitive functions, such as concepts, inferences, and levels of meaning, influence the processing of lower-order information. The reader generates hypotheses about the written material based on his or her knowledge, the content, and the syntactic structures used. Sampling of the reading confirms or does not confirm these hypotheses. The relationship between these two theories is illustrated in Figure 12.2.

The bottom-up theory assumes that the child must learn to decode print. In English, the input for the child is *orthography*, or a written alphabetic system containing twenty-six letters. The child must be able to segment, or divide, each word into phonemic elements and learn the alphabetic code that corresponds (Juel, 1984). Only when this process is automatic can the child give sufficient attention to the meaning. The progression may be one in which the child gains increasing automaticity at each stage as he or she develops and as the

FIGURE 12.2   Theories of Reading Processing

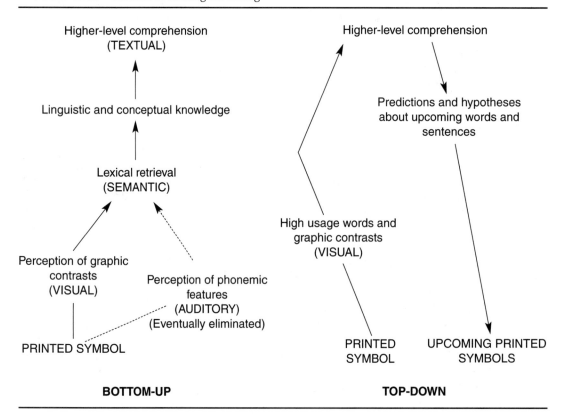

process becomes less conscious. Thus, the child first gains automatic processing at the visual and auditory levels; the other stages are still processed consciously (Figure 12.2).

Information processing theory (Chapters 4 and 5) may help to explain how automaticity develops. Each word has a switchboard that activates the visual, auditory, and semantic features of that word. If the reader has enough information from these features, the information is automatically presented to the other parts of the system for processing. It takes a child approximately 0.5 second to recognize a familiar short word; adults average 0.25 second. If processing facilities are limited, poor or early readers, who spend relatively more capacity on lower-level decoding, have less available for higher-level, comprehension-type tasks (Wolf, Bally, & Morris, 1984).

The most basic difference between oral and visual language is the input. At the level of word recognition, the two inputs share the same cognitive processes. Auditory and visual features from perceptual analysis are used to enter the reader's mental dictionary, or lexicon. Initially, a child performs oral reading; therefore, both inputs are available. Eventually, the more indirect auditory route is deleted. The child goes directly from visual analysis to word recognition. The route used depends on the sophistication of the reader (Barron, 1981; Frith, 1985). Higher processing involves linguistic and conceptual knowledge. Reading information is stored temporarily in a speech-sound code for processing, regardless of the input mode.

Initial slow learning of reading in English, according to the bottom-up theory, is caused by the lack of correspondence between English speech sounds and letters. The twenty-six letters of the English alphabet are used to form approximately twenty-four consonants and twenty-one vowels or diphthongs, plus consonant clusters (*str*, *cl*) and vowel doubling. Most of you have probably seen the example of *ghoti*, which for the uninitiated is pronounced "fish." The analysis is as follows:

$$\underset{/f/}{(enou)gh} + \underset{/\text{I}/}{(w)o(men)} + \underset{/\text{ʃ}/}{(na)ti(on)} = \underset{/\text{fIʃ}/}{ghoti}$$

The letters used in English writing and reading are abstractions that can only be mastered by continual exposure to phonemic patterns.

The bottom-up theory may explain some of the initial difficulties children have with reading, but it cannot account for the entire reading process, such as sentence comprehension, the effects of context on comprehension, or the use of hypothesis testing with unfamiliar or upcoming words in the text. The top-down, or problem-solving, model of reading addresses these inadequacies by viewing reading as a "psycholinguistic guessing game" (K. Goodman, 1976) in which the reader uses language and conceptual knowledge to aid in recognizing words sequentially. As he or she reads, the child makes predictions from syntactic and semantic cues about upcoming words and sentences. The text acts as confirmation. At first, a child will learn high-usage words, such as *the* and *is*, on sight and then use them plus the overall text to form hypotheses regarding unknown words. In other words, the child uses his or her knowledge of language to help figure out the word.

The mature silent reader doesn't even read whole words. Rather, the child samples enough of a word to confirm the hypothesis and recognizes others quickly by sight. In this manner, he or she can read rapidly for overall meaning.

Most likely, reading consists of parallel processes, both top-down and bottom-up, that provide information simultaneously at various levels of analysis (Stanovich, 1980). This information is then synthesized. The processes are interactive, and relative reliance on each varies with the material being read and the skill of the reader. By third or fourth grade, children employ both a bottom-up strategy when reading isolated words and a top-down strategy when reading text. Thus, faster top-down processes are used with textual material and slower, bottom-up processes when such support is lacking.

The complex process of reading is closely related to linguistic processing. In addition to the initial use of two input modes, the reader processes material on at least two levels: bit-by-bit and holistically. The relative reliance of the reader on each level varies with reading competence.

Reading Development

Like speech and language, prereading in our culture is acquired through social interaction rather than formal instruction (Ferreiro, 1984; Pflaum, 1986; C. Snow, 1983). Reading together is a highly social activity in which both parents and children participate. The adult uses many of the conversational techniques described in Chapter 7 for oral language development, including focusing attention, asking questions, and reinforcing the child's attempts at reading (Teale, 1984).

Many parents introduce books to their children prior to age one, using a naming activity in which the child identifies pictures (C. Snow & Ninio, 1986). Parents sometimes provide a narrative, thus indirectly teaching the child about story structure. Actual text reading by parents usually begins late in the second year or in the third year. A relationship exists between the age of onset of home reading routines and the child's oral language skills, especially oral comprehension (Debaryshe, 1993).

Parent–child reading is not the only way of developing a concept of literacy (Teale, 1984). Television shows, such as "Sesame Street," and parental activities, such as the use of cookbooks and TV schedules or bill paying, are also important (Anderson & Stokes, 1984; Brice Heath, 1983). The child learns that books and writing or print convey information.

There are several phases of reading development (Chall, 1983). In the prereading phase, which occurs prior to age six, the child learns letter and number discrimination, recognition, and scanning. As children mature, parents gradually require more active participation by the child during reading. More cognitively demanding input is introduced.

Most four-year-olds are "consumers" of print and are able to recognize their names in print and a few memorized words (Dickinson, Wolf, & Stotsky, 1993). Usually learned within an environmental context, such as signs and package labels, these words gradually become decontextualized until they are recognized in print alone. Approximately 60 percent of three-year-olds and 80 percent of four- and five-year-olds recognize the word *stop* (Y. Goodman, 1986), and they all probably know McDonald's golden "M." In addition, they gain some general concept that print is distinct from the pictures and that books are used in certain ways.

Young children often will pretend to read, using the vocabulary and syntax associated with books. This different style of language gradually evolves from language about the text to language that recreates the text (Sulzby & Zecker, 1991).

In the first phase of reading development, the alphabetic phase, up to approximately second grade, the child concentrates on decoding single words in simple stories. In order to read, the child needs to know what reading is, what it does, and the principles of the writing system; he or she also needs to exploit this knowledge to achieve an increasingly automatic, fluent, error-free performance (P. Smith, 1986). Undoubtedly, the most difficult part of this learning involves the metalinguistic skills needed in order to integrate the sound and writing systems. In English, the phoneme, as represented by a grapheme or letter, is the basis for the orthographic system. Among such systems, only Korean (I. Taylor, 1980) has phonemic features such as place and manner of sound production included in the written symbols. Other languages, such as Japanese, use an orthography system based on the syllable or word as the basic unit. Alphabetic systems, such as English or German, are easier for recovering the phonological form, although such recovery is unnecessary for mature silent reading (Hardin, O'Connell, & Kowal, 1998).

Prereading activities, such as joint book reading, facilitate the learning of letter names, shapes, and sounds. Individuals who have difficulty recognizing letters will have decoding problems. It is quite another problem, however, to know that individual letters stand for individual sounds. Not only must the child know about letters, but he or she must be aware that words consist of discrete bits of sound, something called **phonological awareness**. More than just awareness and auditory discrimination, phonological awareness includes the ability to manipulate these components of spoken words (Snowling, Hulme, Smith, & Thomas, 1994). At a conscious level, the child must be able to consider the form of speech as a separate entity (Yopp, 1992).

It is unclear exactly which aspects of phonological awareness a child must possess in order to read effectively. A list of phonological awareness skills would include rhyming, segmentation of sentences and words, alliteration (big bright bundles bounced by blithely), blending and breakdown skills, and manipulation of sounds to create new words.

As early as age two some children show awareness of sounds in their speech repairs, in rhyming, and in sound play (Kamhi & Catts, 1999). Rhyming activities may also increase awareness of syllables and smaller units. Although some three-year-olds demonstrate alliterative skills, many preschoolers are unable to segment words into smaller units (MacLean, Bryant & Bradley, 1987; van Kleeck & Schuele, 1987). While children are aware of sounds, most will require some formal instruction in order to break words down into individual phonemes.

Phonological awareness progresses gradually from an awareness of larger segments to smaller ones (Gombert, 1992). Many four-year-olds are able to detect syllables and rhyme but are unable to detect phonemes until age five or six. Children with language impairment often lack knowledge of rhyme, letter names, and concepts related to print (Boudreau & Hedberg, 1999).

The child's cognitive and linguistic abilities are also important for early reading development. Especially important are memory and the access to the lexicon or language word storage.

Unfortunately, knowing that a phoneme roughly corresponds to a grapheme is not enough. As discussed previously, the correspondence is not one to one. In addition, English orthography sometimes favors morphological stability over phonemic difference, as in using *-ed* for the past-tense marker, even though it may be pronounced as /t/, /d/, or /əd/.

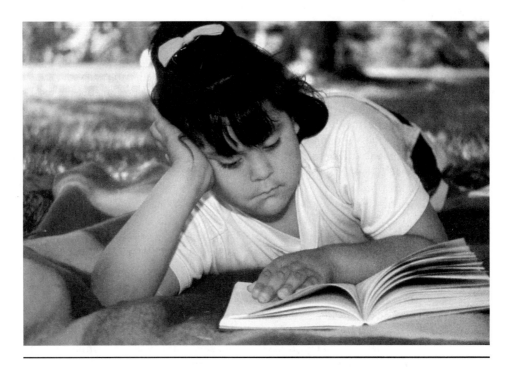

By fourth grade, it is expected that children will be able to read alone and silently for comprehension.

Syllable knowledge is needed in order to decode and pronounce written words. Along with syllable knowledge is a knowledge of syllable stress. The noun *"entrance"* differs from the verb *"entrance"* only in the stress placed on each syllable. By age seven, the child has a rigid stress rule that is the same for all words. This is gradually modified into a more flexible system as the child matures.

The child also must be aware of word boundaries. The child must begin to realize that *jumping rope* is two words and that forms such as *jump-roping* are incorrect.

By age seven or eight, most children have acquired the graphemic (sound-symbol), syllabic, and word knowledge they need to become competent readers. This knowledge is acquired in school in most countries. Among the Vai, a Liberian population, however, knowledge of written syllabic symbols is learned informally within the family (Scribner & Cole, 1981).

Once the child gains some control over letter discrimination and syllable and word boundaries, he or she becomes a more efficient attender, and some higher comprehension skills become evident. Meaningful words in context are read faster than random words. At this stage, the child begins by relying heavily on visual configuration for word recognition by paying particular attention to the first letter and to word length, ignoring letter order and other features (Marsh, Friedman, Welch, & Desberg, 1981). The child is aware of the importance of the letters but is unable to use them in analyzing the word (Allington, 1984).

Next, the child learns sound–spelling correspondence rules and is able, using this phonetic approach, to sound out novel words (Frith, 1985). Thus, segmental detail, or the arrangement of sound and letter sequences, becomes more important (Barron, 1981). In addition, the child learns that the text, not the reader, is the bearer of the message and that the text does more than just describe the pictures (Ferreiro & Teberosky, 1982). Successful first-grade oral readers are able to use the text to analyze unknown words. Along with phonological and orthographics or spelling, semantics is an important factor in word decoding (Swank, 1997). Poor readers tend to guess wildly.

By the second or orthographic stage, roughly third and fourth grades, the child is able to analyze unknown words using orthographic patterns and contextual references. Phase 3, from grades four to eight, seems to be a major watershed in which the emphasis in reading shifts from decoding skills to comprehension. Thus, the scanning rate continues to increase steadily. By secondary school, firmly within phase 4, the adolescent uses higher-level skills such as inference and recognition of viewpoint to aid comprehension. Lower-level skills are already firmly established. Finally, at phase 5, the college level and beyond, the adult is able to integrate what reads into his or her current knowledge base and make critical judgments about the material.

From age seven or eight through adulthood, reading becomes more automatic, with direct access to both phonological-orthographic and semantic coding. Adjustments in reading strategy that depend on one more than the other are based on text difficulty. The differences between the seven-year-old and the adult reader are primarily quantitative, not qualitative, although there are some obvious differences (P. Smith, 1986). Adults have a larger, more diverse vocabulary and a more flexible pronunciation system, and they are able to comprehend larger units than elementary school children (P. Harris, Kruithof, Terwogt, & Visser, 1981).

Comprehension is also aided by cohesion within the text. In general, the more cohesive ties in the text, the more understandable (Irwin, 1980). More explicit texts are more readable. As in oral development, more mature readers interpret ties more readily and have less difficulty with complex, intersential cohesion (Chapman, 1983; Monson, 1982).

Not all children follow the same progression. Children have different cognitive styles that influence the manner in which they approach tasks. In addition, which language is being read and whether it is the reader's first or second language will influence the processes emphasized (Hakes, 1980).

The Process of Writing

Written language is not just transcription of oral language. Therefore, children must learn to use constructions other than those they use in speech. Initially, the structures in both are very close, but they display less maturity in the written form. This is probably because the physical process is so laborious. Once writing becomes automatic, however, the grammar in writing becomes more advanced than that in speech.

Children with language impairments often experience difficulty learning to write. The most significant factor in writing problems seems to be the presence of phonological disorders (Lewis, O'Donnell, Freebairn, & Taylor, 1998).

Some structures are common to speech but occur rarely, if at all, in writing. Other structures are more typical of writing than of speech. Structures found almost exclusively in speech include dysfluencies, fillers (*well, you know*), vague expletives (. . . *and all*, . . . *and everything*), *this* and *these* used for old information (*And there was this man* . . .), and pronoun apposition (*My dog, he got a bath*) (Perera, 1986). Dysfluencies, such as false starts, reformulations, redundant repetitions, and ungrammatical strings of words, are nine times as frequent in the speech of ten-year-olds as in their writing. No doubt this reflects the additional time that writers have to plan, reflect upon, and modify their message.

Studies of older elementary children who speak standard dialects indicate that dialectal structures also do not occur in written communication. These studies have not included younger or nonstandard dialectal speakers.

In general, writing is more formal and more complex, and the structures found more frequently in writing reflect this quality. By ages twelve to thirteen, the syntax used in writing far exceeds that used in speech (Gillam & Johnston, 1992). This is a gradual process. For example, post-noun modifiers become more common in writing at about age eight and embedded clauses at about age ten.

While complex subjects are rare in speech, they are found more frequently in the writing of nine-year-olds than in the speech of adults (Crystal, 1980). This reflects the use of embedded phrases and clauses, some of which, such as *whose, whom, on which*, and *in which*, occur almost exclusively in writing. In addition, written sentences include more prepositional and adverbial phrases (*opposite the drug counter* . . . , *about 5 miles down the beach* . . .).

In general, by age nine or ten, writing is free of many of the features of speech. At about this time, writing becomes more mature than speech, reflecting linguistic performance that is closer to linguistic knowledge.

For most of childhood and adolescence, writing ability lags behind reading comprehension. This asymmetry cannot be totally explained by English orthography. The sound–letter correspondence is not found in kanji, a Japanese writing system using Chinese characters for words and concepts, but the reading-writing asymmetry persists in children (Yamada, 1992).

Writing Development

There is only a moderate amount of overlap between writing and reading. In general, better writers are better readers, and vice versa. The process of writing is close to drawing in that both represent an underlying symbolization (Dyson, 1983; Gourley, Bennett, Gundersheim, & McClellan, 1983). The two systems are different, however, and become differentiated around age three.

Development of spelling can be described as a five-stage process (Henderson & Beers, 1980). From preliterate scribbling, drawing, and some letters, the child progresses to a letter–name stage in which letters represent sounds and the child uses invented spelling. In the next or within-word patterns stage the child uses orthographic patterns to govern short and long vowel use. These patterns often take precedence over sound, as in using *-ed* for regular past tense despite the varying phonological patterns. In the last two stages, syllable juncture and derivational constancy, the child pays attention to patterns in stressed and unstressed syllables and uses roots and their derivations for spelling. Of course, learning to write is much more than just spelling.

Most preschoolers have been exposed to print in such forms as letters to Santa, grocery lists, and party invitations. Their "writing" goes through a hierarchy from drawing through scribbling to creating forms that resemble letters. Figure 12.3 is an example of the drawing of a four-year-old. Initially, play, drawing, writing, and speaking are intertwined (Baghban, 1984; Dyson, 1989; Harste, Woodward, & Burke, 1984). Well-learned words appear next, followed by inventive spelling and, finally, conventional spelling (Sulzby, 1986). At first, the child may pretend to write, even though he or she doesn't know letter names or that print represents words (Sulzby, 1981). Well-learned words, such as *stop* or the child's name, help the child learn that different letters represent different sounds.

With inventive spelling, the child tries to impose some regularity on his or her writing system by matching sounds and letters (Read, 1981). The sounds in the letter name are matched to the sounds the child hears. Initially, the first letter represents the entire word, with little attention given to the other letters. For example, *MBRS* might represent *Mommy*. This is similar to the initial stage of reading, in which the child pays attention to the first letter only. Next, the child represents syllables, without some vowels and some spacing. For example, *grass* might be written as *GRS* or *game* as *GM*. Several of the following characteristics of inventive spelling are important because they let us know the salient features of words for children (Pflaum, 1986):

FIGURE 12.3 With drawings such as this (entitled *Me*), children begin to communicate information graphically prior to the development of writing.

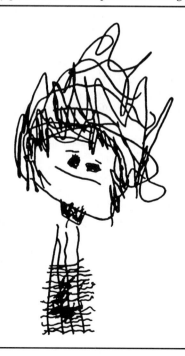

Use vowel names if the vowel is long:

DA = day   *LIK = like*

But do not use vowel names if the vowel is short:

FES = fish   *LAFFT = left*

Spell the word the way it's pronounced:

BEDR = better   *WOODR = water*   *PREDE = pretty*

Spell according to placement of the tongue (Temple, Nathan, & Burris, 1982). (Note that different vowels are used for *a* and that medial *n* is often omitted.):

PLAT = plant   *WOTED = wanted*

Do not use vowels with medial and final nasals (/m/, /n/) or liquids (/r/, /l/):

GRDN = garden   *LITL = little*

Write past and plural endings generally as they are heard. (*T* is used first, then both *T* and *D*.):

STOPT = stopped   *DAZ = days*   *FESEZ = fishes*   *PLATS = plants*

In the final phase of inventive spelling, called *phonemic spelling*, the child is aware of the alphabet and the correspondence of sound and symbol. The following is a short story (Temple, Nathan, & Burris, 1982):

HE HAD A BLUE CLTH. IT TRD IN TO A BRD.
(He had a blue cloth. It turned into a bird.)

With school instruction, the child develops a more conventional system.

Initially, spelling seems to be very phonologically based, although word recognition seems to be more visually based (Bryant & Bradley, 1980). Many spelling errors resemble phonological processes in preschool children, such as weak syllable deletion, cluster reduction, and sound substitution based on phonological similarity rather than visual resemblance (Hoffman & Norris, 1989). If this is true, then simplification strategies for words in spelling and in early pronunciation are similar.

Writing, of course, involves more than spelling. Young writers, like preschool speakers, are often oblivious of the needs of the reader. (See the discussion of presuppositional skills in Chapter 9.) The six-year-old pays very little attention to format, spacing, spelling, and punctuation.

Often, other aspects of writing will deteriorate when one aspect is stressed. For example, spelling and sentence structure deteriorate when the child changes from printing to script. Writing on a difficult topic may also result in spelling, handwriting, or text deterioration. Despite these deficiencies, the stories of young children are often direct and beautiful in their simplicity, as evidenced by the short story that follows. Created especially for this book by my friend Christina, aged six, the story concerns two frogs (*tow forg*).

Tow forg

Tow forg on a TV. Where anr tow forgs? I will go to The TV. This is My Tow forgs. My forgs are fun. I Love forgs. I Love forgs To.

by Christina

Another six-year-old friend, Lauren, had written a story about people she loved and liked, two very distinct groups. When challenged by her mother, she replied, "I might change it; this is my first draft."

By the middle school years, the length and diversity of children's productions increase. Along with the longer writing required in school come increasing cognitive demands on the child for coherence of ideas. First using drawings to highlight important portions and to help organize the text, the child moves on to order of recall, usually the order of occurrence. Text forms, such as letter format, are used later to help organize material.

Around third or fourth grade, there is a shift in the child's writing from an egocentric focus to a concern for reader reaction. Writers begin to revise and to proofread their work (Bartlett, 1982). This is influenced by the writer's syntactic knowledge. In general, the school years bring a decrease in incomplete oral and written sentences and in dependence on the *subject + verb + object* format and an accompanying increase in complex clauses and phrases and in sentence format variety. Near the end of elementary school, the complexity of written language surpasses that of spoken language (Gillam & Johnston, 1992; Gundloch, 1981). Organizational changes continue also, and in high school adolescents are able to organize arguments logically and to produce persuasive writing (Nold, 1981).

Four phases in the development of writing are probable (Kroll, 1981): preparation, consolidation, differentiation, and integration. In the preparation phase, the child learns the physical aspects of handwriting by copying words written by adults.

At around age seven, the child enters the consolidation phase. In this phase, the child can write independently using structures from speech in the same proportion as they appear in speech.

In the differentiation phase, the child's writing begins to take on its own grammatical characteristics. Speech and writing become differentiated. This occurs at about age ten.

Finally, a minority of mature writers enter the integration phase. In this phase, writing has become sufficiently differentiated and integrated that the personality of the writer can come through when desired and appropriate. Change is not smooth but appears to occur in a series of spurts at ages nine, thirteen, and seventeen, followed by periods of consolidation.

The last writing style to develop is expository writing. Essays contain a logical, very condensed organization with complex syntactic structures. Each sentence is linked to the topic, and the overall organization is coherent and unambiguous.

Grammatical development can be described for writing, as we have done for speech (Perera, 1986). For example, the types of sentences change. There is a threefold increase in the number of written passive sentences between ages eight and thirteen.

At the sentence level, clause length increases in writing, as it does in speech. The mean length of the written clause is 6.5 words for the eight-year-old writer, 7.7 for the thirteen-year-old, 8.6 for the seventeen-year-old, and 11.5 for the adult. As in speech, there is also an increase in embedded subordinate clauses and a decrease in coordination or compound sentences. Relative clauses double in frequency between ages seven and seventeen and continue to increase into adulthood. Adverbial clauses, especially those signifying time (*when . . .*), also increase and diversify.

At the phrase level, there is an increase in pre- and post-noun modifiers. By adolescence, writers are modifying nouns with adverbs as well as adjectives and are often using four or more modifiers with a noun. Verb phrases are expanded by increasing use of modality, tense, and aspect.

Summary

Once children have gained a working knowledge of spoken language, most adapt to the new mode of written language with relative ease. Initial difficulties with symbol relationships slow the first stages. The underlying linguistic relationships between spoken and written language, however, make eventual success possible and help explain the process. In addition to the child's linguistic knowledge, emerging metalinguistic skills enable him or her to decontextualize language and thus use that knowledge to understand language in another form or mode.

CONCLUSION

By kindergarten age, the child has acquired much of the structure of the mature oral language user. Development continues, however, as the child adds new forms and gains new skills in transmitting messages. The process continues throughout life, especially in the semantic aspects of language.

Through formal instruction, the child learns a new mode of language transmission. Reading and writing open new avenues of exploration and learning for the child and are essential skills in the modern literate society.

Older children and adults have the linguistic skills to enable them to select, from among several available communication strategies, the one best suited to a specific situation. Mature language is efficient and appropriate. It is efficient because words are more specifically defined and because forms do not need repetition or paraphrasing in order to be understood. It is appropriate because utterances are selected for the psychosocial dynamics of the communication situation. Less mature language users are less able to select the appropriate code because they have a limited repertoire of language forms.

DISCUSSION

Syntax has slowed and many forms, such as conjunctions take a long time to develop fully. The development of language form has become very complicated as sentence complexity increases and as morphophonemic changes occur in the child's expanding vocabulary.

At about the time the child begins school, he or she gains an increased ability to manipulate language out of the physical context. Thus, the language of narratives can be used to create the context of the narrative, and the child can begin to read with understanding. This ability is called metalinguistics; it lets us consider language in the abstract and make judgments of correctness or appropriateness. Most importantly for our purposes, it enables us to develop a new mode of communication: reading and writing.

Just as SLPs and teachers are concerned with oral language, so they are also concerned with written language. Many SLPs include a portfolio of a child's writing in an assessment of a child's language skills. Remember that the single best indicator of a child's potential in written language is oral language skills. It would seem essential, then, that this mode of communication be assessed and that necessary training be attempted, usually in conjunction with the classroom teacher and reading specialist.

REFLECTIONS

1. Explain the different types of passive sentences and briefly sketch their developmental sequence.

2. Embedding and conjoining, begun in preschool, continue to develop during the school years. Explain this development briefly and give possible reasons for the sequence of conjunction development.

3. Morphophonemic development is the major phonological change present in the school years. Describe the morphophonemic changes and provide an example.

4. Explain metalinguistic abilities.

5. Reading may be either symbol generated or the result of predictive hypotheses. Describe briefly the bottom-up and top-down theories of reading processing.

6. As in oral language, the child goes through a developmental sequence in written language. Describe the development of reading and writing.

13

Language Differences: Bidialectism and Bilingualism

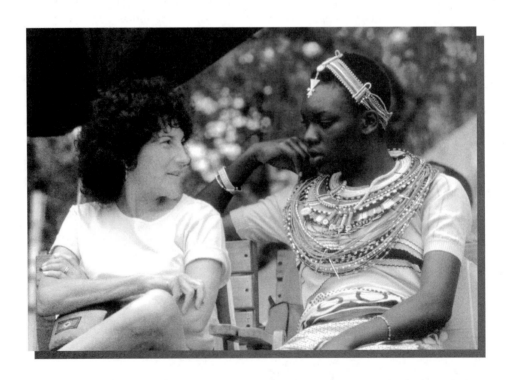

CHAPTER OBJECTIVES

In actual usage, a language is a collection of dialects, or rule-governed variations, of a nonexistent standard. Dialects represent a difference, not a disorder. Some dialects are the result of learning English as a second language. Differences in the way children learn two languages depend on which languages are being learned and the age of the child. When you have completed this chapter, you should understand

- a definition of a dialect and its relation to its parent language.
- the major factors that cause dialects to develop.
- the major characteristics of African American English.
- the major characteristics of Latino English.
- the major characteristics of Asian English.
- the differences between simultaneous and successive second-language acquisition.
- the educational problems encountered by dialectal and second-language children.
- the following terms:

archiform	free alternation
bilingual	interlanguage
code-switch	pidgin
creole	register
deficit approach	style shifting
dialect	vernacular

The United States is becoming an increasingly pluralistic society. The notion of the melting pot is giving way to one of a *stew* in which cultural and ethno-racial groups contribute to the whole but retain their essential character. One characteristic of these groups may be either language or dialect. Most minority groups continue to embrace their culture and, when non-English, their language.

It is conservatively projected that the minority population in the United States will increase to forty-five million by the year 2000 and to sixty-three million by 2030 (Spencer, 1984). At the same time, the majority white population will increase at a slower rate and will thus become a smaller proportion of the entire U.S. population. If current trends continue, white non-Hispanics will be the largest *minority* by the year 2080 (Bouvier & Gardner, 1986).

At present, in the United States approximately one in four Americans identifies as other than white non-Hispanic. In the state of California, a score of cities, and several counties, minorities represent more than 50 percent of the population. This situation reflects traditional demographics and a population shift that is the result of recent immigration, internal migration, and natural increase.

Within the last twenty years, 80 percent of the legal immigrants to the United States have come from Asia and Latin America (Robey, 1985; Russell, 1983). Approximately 40 percent of all recent legal immigrants are Asian. As a result, there are over five million Asians and Asian Americans residing in the United States. Although this number represents only about 2 percent of the total U.S. population, it does not indicate the impact of Asians and Asian Americans on the country. Asians and Asian Americans tend to settle in coastal states, especially in the West, where they form large segments of the population. In addition, Asians and Asian Americans represent the fastest-growing segment of the U.S. population. Approximately three-fourths of the legal Asian immigrants come from the five countries of Vietnam, the Philippines, Korea, China, and India. They represent several languages and dialects of those countries.

There are approximately nineteen million Hispanics in the United States. In addition, there are several million more Spanish-surnamed individuals who identify with Hispanic culture to a lesser degree. Approximately 40 percent of all recent legal immigrants are Hispanic. These immigrants come primarily from Mexico and Central America, Puerto Rico and Cuba, and South America and speak various dialects of Spanish.

In addition, there are approximately 80,000 legal black immigrants per year from the Caribbean, South and Central America, and Africa. It is estimated that this group will represent slightly less than 1 percent of the U.S. population by the year 2000. This minority represents a number of languages, as is evident from the many geographic areas of origin.

The exact number of illegal immigrants is unknown. Estimates range from five to ten million, with a growth of approximately 500,000 per year (Bouvier & Gardner, 1986; Robey, 1987). These immigrants also add to the numbers of various minorities.

The largest internal migration is and has been that of African Americans who number thirty million, or 12 percent of the U.S. population. Reversing the trend of the early-to-mid twentieth century, African Americans began returning to the South in the early 1970s (Robinson, 1986; Russell, 1982). Many of these individuals speak regional and/or ethno-racial dialects, such as African American English.

To a smaller extent, Native Americans, totaling 1.6 million, or 0.7 percent of the population, have also experienced internal migration. At present, just over 20 percent of Native Americans live on reservations or historic trust properties, compared to 90 percent in 1940 (U.S Department of Health and Human Services, 1985, 1986). Their language may reflect their native language or the specific dialect of American English they learned.

Currently, the 1.2 million Native Americans who are affiliated with some native community are divided among approximately 450 "tribes" or nations varying in size from the Cherokee nation of over 300,000 to groups of just a handful (Robinson-Zanatu, 1996). In addition to representing a variety of cultures, Native Americans speak over 200 different languages (Leap, 1993). Seventy-eight percent of Native Americans live in urban areas, creating an invisibility that is treated by those in the majority culture as an insignificance.

Birth rates differ across groups and also contribute to the changing demographics of the U.S. population. The majority white birth rate is 1.7, inadequate to maintain the relative proportion of whites in the United States (Hodgkinson, 1986). Birth rates for minority populations are higher, for example, 2.4 for African Americans, 2.5 for Hispanic Americans, and 1.8 for Vietnamese Americans (R. Gardner, Robey, & Smith, 1985; National Center for Health Statistics, 1983, 1985).

Linguists have terms for the changes languages undergo when they come into contact with another language. Speakers of a nondominant language will often obtain limited vocabulary in the dominant language. This vocabulary, with little or no grammar, is the basis for a **pidgin**. What grammar is present usually reflects the less dominant language. Pidgins are the languages of New Guinea, the Solomon Islands, parts of northeast Australia, rural Hawaii, and West Africa. When Britain's Prince Charles visited New Guinea, he was introduced as *nambawan pikinini bilong misis kwin* [number one (*first*) pikininni (*son*) belonging to (*of*) Mrs. Queen (*Queen Elizabeth*)].

Pidgins develop from a need to communicate. For example, sixty-five African slaves on a plantation in French Guinea in 1695 spoke twelve different languages (Berreby, 1992). A pidgin developed.

Over many years, pidgins evolve, develop grammars, and become **creoles** that borrow words and grammar from both languages, but mostly from the dominant language. An example is the language of Jamaica's population.

We cannot discuss language development adequately without considering dialectal variations, such as African American English and what we shall call Latino English and Asian English and their effect on the learning of American English and on the learner. In addition, recent immigrations raise issues of bilingualism, second-language learning, and language use within the majority language. Many of the issues discussed will also apply to dialectal differences in British and Canadian English and to bilingual countries such as Canada.

DIALECTS

In the musical comedy *My Fair Lady* (Lerner & Loewe, 1956), Professor Higgins laments that the English can't teach their children how to speak. His anxiety relates to the various dialects of British English. His contention, and that of George Bernard Shaw, the author of *Pygmalion* (1916), upon which *My Fair Lady* is based, is that language is related to the way others view us and make judgments about us. Inherent in his argument is the notion that there is one correct English language and that all variations are substandard. This **deficit approach** seems unfounded in light of recent research on dialectal differences.

Although we have been discussing the English language and others throughout this text, it is important to realize that to some extent the languages we have been discussing are theoretical entities. The view of a monolithic, unchanging, immutable language does not fit reality. Languages are fluid and changing. Different individuals use the same language differently. Most of us have met or will meet someone speaking English who might as well be speaking Farsi or Urdu for all the sense it makes to us.

Languages are especially changeable "around the edges, where they interact with other languages" (Backus, 1999). For example, in many bilingual communities, speakers develop new varieties of communication incorporating both languages and these varieties function as the basic vernacular or everyday speech of the community.

Not all speakers of a language use the same language rules. Variations that characterize the language of a particular group are collectively called a dialect. A dialect is a language–rule system used by an identifiable group of people that varies in some way from an ideal language standard. Dialects usually differ in the frequency of use of certain structures rather than in the presence or absence of these structures. The ideal standard is rarely used except in formal writing, and the concept of a standard spoken language is practically a myth. Each dialect shares a common set of grammatical rules with the standard language. Thus, dialects of a language are theoretically mutually intelligible to all speakers of that language. No dialect is better than any other, nor should a dialect be considered a deviant or inferior form of a language. "To devalue his language or to presume Standard English is a 'better system' is to devalue the child and his culture and to reveal a naïveté concerning language" (Baratz, 1968, p. 145). Each dialect is a systematic rule system that should be viewed within its social context. Sociolinguists assume that a dialect is adequate to meet the demands of the speech community in which it is found. Like languages, dialects evolve over time to meet the needs of the communities in which they are used.

Despite the validity of all dialects, society places relative values on each one. The standard dialect becomes the "official" criterion. Speakers of the language determine what is acceptable, often assuming that their own dialect is the most appropriate. In a stratified society, such as that of the United States, some dialects are accorded higher status than others. But, in fact, the relative value of a dialect is not intrinsic; it represents only the listener's bias. Dialects are merely differences within a language.

The two ways of classifying dialects—the deficit approach and the sociolinguistic approach—are illustrated in Figure 13.1. In the diagram, dialects that are closer to each other in the frequency of rule use are separated by less distance. Under the deficit approach, each dialect has a different relative status. Those closer to the idealized standard are considered to be better. Status is determined relative to the standard. The sociolinguistic approach views each dialect as an equally valid rule system. Each dialect is related to the others and to the ideal standard. No value is placed on a dialect.

FIGURE 13.1   The Relationship of the Idealized Standard Language and Its Dialects

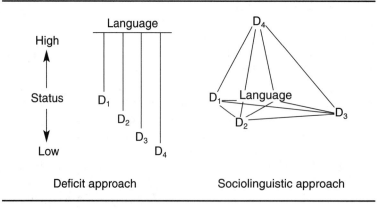

Related Factors

Several factors are related to dialectal differences. These include (a) geography, (b) socio-economic level, (c) race and ethnicity, (d) situation or context, (e) peer-group influences, and (f) first- or second-language learning. A child born and raised in Boston will not sound like a child from Charleston, South Carolina. In turn, a poor child and a wealthy preparatory school child from Charleston will not speak the same way. These differences are called *dialectal differences*. In general, the language of these children reflects the environmental influences of the language spoken around them. No children learn dialect-free English. From birth, each child hears English spoken with some dialectal variation. The study of these dialectal influences is an integral part of sociolinguistics. Before you continue, it might be helpful to listen again to track one of the accompanying audio CD. Several speakers represent different geographic locations within the United States. Two speakers demonstrate dialects that result when a first language interacts with American English. Do you think you sound like any of these speakers or is your dialect different?

The United States was established by settlers who spoke many different languages and several dialects of British English. Members of various ethnic groups chose to settle in specific geographic areas. Other individuals remained isolated by choice or by natural boundaries. In an age of less mobility, before there were national media, American English was free to evolve in several separate ways. A New York City dialect is very different from an Ozark dialect, yet both are close enough to Standard American English (SAE) to be identified as variants of SAE. As a child matures, he or she learns the dialect of the region and learns to distinguish it from other dialects. Each region has lexical items and grammatical structures that differ slightly. What are *sack* and *pop* to the Midwestern American are *bag* and *soda* to the Middle Atlantic speaker. The Italian sandwich changes to *submarine*, *torpedo*, *hero*, *wedge*, *hoagie* and *poo'boy* as it moves about the United States. Within each region there is no confusion. Order a milkshake in Massachusetts and that's what you get—flavored milk that's been shaken. If you want ice cream in it, you need to ask for a *frappe*.

Some regions of the United States seem to be more prone to word invention or to novel use than others. In the southern Appalachian region, for example, you might encounter the following (J. Miller, 1985):

> A man might raise enough corn to *bread* his family over the winter.
> To do something without considering the consequences is to do it
> *unthoughtedly*.
> Something totally destroyed would be torn to *flinderation*.
> Long-lasting things are *lasty*.

Note that the form of each word follows generally accepted morphological marking rules, such as the *-ly* in *unthoughtedly*.

One of my sons was given a vivid example of regional dialectal differences while conversing with a child from the Southern United States. Although she was white, the child's older half-brother was the product of a racially mixed marriage. Trying to figure out this situation, my son ventured the opinion, "Your brother is really *tan*." He was corrected quickly with, "No he ain't; he's *eleven*."

A second factor in dialectal differences is socioeconomic level. This factor relates to social class, educational and occupational level, home environment, and family interactional styles, including maternal teaching and child-rearing patterns. In general, people from lower socioeconomic groups use more restricted linguistic systems. Their word definitions often relate to one particular aspect of the underlying concept. Those from higher socioeconomic levels generally have more education and are more mobile. These factors generally contribute to the use of a more standard dialect. For example, among African American children, boys from lower-income homes are more likely than middle-class boys or girls to use features of a dialect called African American English (AAE) (Washington & Craig, 1998).

Racial and ethnic differences are a third factor that contributes to dialect development. By choice or as a result of de facto segregation, racial and ethnic minorities may become isolated and a particular dialectal variation may evolve. It has been argued that the distinctive Brooklyn dialect reflects the strong influence of Irish upon American English. Yiddish influences have also affected the New York City dialect. The largest racial group in the United States with a characteristic dialect is African American. This dialect, called *African American English*, is spoken by working-class African Americans, primarily in large industrial areas and in the rural South. Not all African Americans speak African American English.

Fourth, dialect is influenced by situational and contextual factors. These variations may be structural, stylistic, or pragmatic. With a single speaker, the particular situation may result in the use of different dialects. All speakers alter their language in response to situational variables. These situationally influenced language variations are called **registers**. Motherese, the special form of adult language addressed to language-learning children, is an example of a register. The selection of a register depends on the speaker's perception of the situation and the participants, attitude toward or knowledge of the topic, and intention or purpose. A casual, informal, or intimate register is called a **vernacular** variation. For example, informal American English uses more contractions and particles than formal American English. Thus, there is greater reliance on *can't* and *don't* and on phrases such as *get up* instead of *rise* and *go away* instead of *leave*. The variation from formal to informal styles or the reverse is called **style shifting** and is practiced by all speakers. Regardless of the socioeconomic status of the speaker, style shifts seem to be in the same direction for similar situations. For example, in formal reading there is greater use of *-ing* (/h/), while informal conversation is characterized by an increase in the use of *-in* (/n/). Most shifts are made unconsciously. Thus, we might read aloud "I am writing" but say in conversation "I'm writin'."

A fifth influence on language is peer group. In the United States, groups such as teens or lesbians and gay men have their own lexicons and idioms that are not understood by the society as a whole. Peer influence is particularly important during adolescence. Generally, the adolescent dialect is used only with peers. Linguists have labeled two strains of the current teen dialect as "mallspeak" and "pagerspeak." Minimalist and repetitive, the rather imprecise mallspeak is a spoken dialect that overuses the words such as *like, y'know,* and *whatever*. In contrast, pagerspeak is a written language of numbers and asterisks used to leave messages on friends' pagers. For example, 50538 when rotated upside down resembles *besos* or kisses. In yet another form, 90*401773 is *go home* with 9 representing a "g," 4 a legless "h," 177 the outline of an "m," and 3 an "e." Other signals are codes memorized by users.

Much of youth slang can be traced back to earlier roots. The current word *phat* actually began in the 1960s with the same meaning (Dalzell, 1996). Many rap words have their roots in 1940s jive talk used among jazz musicians.

Finally, a dialect may reflect the primacy of another language. Speakers with a different native language often retain vestiges of that language. These people typically **code-switch** from one language to the other. In this process, one language may interfere with the other. The area where the two languages conflict is called an *interference point*. The speaker's age and education and the social situation influence the efficacy of code-switching.

American English Dialects

Standard American English (SAE) is an idealized version of American English that occurs rarely in conversation, although many Americans can be classified as users. It is the form of American English that is used in textbooks and on network newscasts.

There are at least ten regional dialects in the United States (presented in Figure 13.2): Eastern New England, New York City, Western Pennsylvania, Middle Atlantic, Appalachian, Southern, Central Midland, North Central, Southwest, and Northwest. In general, the variations are greatest on the East Coast and decrease to the West. Each geographic region has

FIGURE 13.2   Major American Geographic Dialects

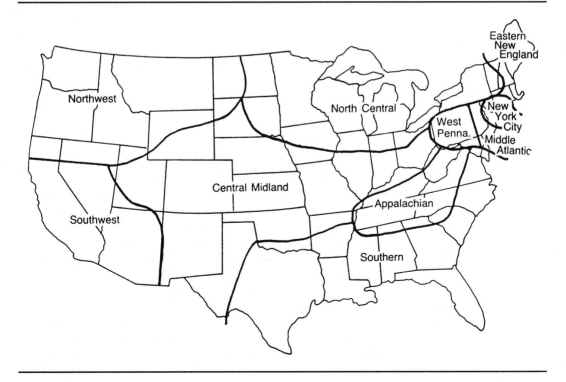

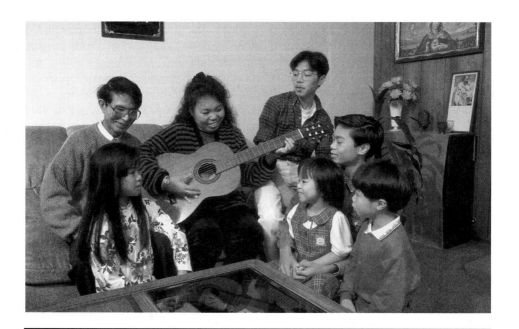

Attitudes toward the culture and language of the parents, the size of the immigrant community, and the language spoken at home are some of the factors that affect bilingualism.

a dialect marked by distinct sound patterns, words and idioms, and syntactic and prosodic systems.

The major racial and ethnic dialects in the United States are African American English, Spanish-influenced or Latino English, and Asian English. In part, these dialects are influenced by geographic region and by socioeconomic factors. Spanish influences also differ depending on the country or area of origin. Colombian Spanish is very different from Puerto Rican Spanish. Asian English differs with the country of origin and the native language.

African American English

For the purposes of description, we shall consider African American English (AAE) to be the relatively uniform dialect used by African Americans in the inner cities of most large urban areas and in the rural South, when speaking casually. In short, it is the linguistic system used by working-class African American people within their speech community. As such, AAE shares many of the characteristics of Southern and working-class dialects. Obviously, not all African Americans speak the dialect. Even among speakers of AAE, a difference exists in the amount of dialectal features used by different individuals. Conversely, white speakers who live or work with speakers of AAE may use some of its features. It is also important to remember that there are variations of AAE that its speakers use for certain situations. As with other dialects, there is a formal–informal continuum. Individual differences may be related to age, geographic location, income, occupation, and education (Terrell & Terrell, 1993).

AAE is a systematic language rule system, not a deviant or improper form of English. Its linguistic variations from SAE are not errors. The linguistic differences between AAE and SAE are minimal. Most of the grammatical rules and underlying concepts are similar. Variations are the result of a different and equally complex rule system. Many aspects of AAE are shared with other dialects. There is considerable overlap between AAE and both Southern English and Southern white nonstandard English. Some aspects, however—such as the use of *be* in the habitual sense, as in "She *be* working there since 1985," and the triple negative, as in "Nobody don't got none"—are primarily characteristic of AAE. Much of the sense of the dialect can also be found in its intonational patterns, speaking rate, and distinctive lexicon.

The major characteristics of AAE are listed in Tables 13.1 and 13.2. It is unlikely that any given individual who speaks AAE will exhibit all of these characteristics. The frequency of appearance of each feature will change with situational variations and over time. There is decreasing use of some features of AAE in favor of more SAE as children advance through elementary school.

We shall discuss some of the more outstanding differences between SAE and AAE. The phonemic differences, especially the weakening of final consonants, relate to some of the more evident structural contrasts. Many morphological endings are omitted or not pronounced. Other words tend to sound similar because of omission, weakening, or substitution. The following are a few examples:

SAE	↔	AAE	SAE	↔	AAE	SAE	↔	AAE
guard		god	Carol		Cal	past		pass
sore		saw	fault		fought	boot		boo
court		caught	toll		toe	death		deaf
called		caught	hits		hit	feed		feet

Sociolinguists have yet to determine if the *called–call* contrast reflects consonant cluster simplification or a syntactic rule relating to the fact that the regular past-tense marker is nonobligatory, since past tense can be inferred from the context.

The speech of young African American children does not reflect many of the phonological contrasts presented in Table 13.1 (Seymour & Seymour, 1981). Four- and five-year-old African American children have not mastered the adult AAE phonological system. Their phonological rules reflect their developmental level (Seymour & Seymour, 1981). The most consistent syntactic features found in the speech of many African American preschoolers are deletion of the copula and lack of the third-person marker (Washington & Craig, 1994).

Many AAE structural rules reflect a recognition of the redundant nature of many SAE constructions. For example, the possessive *'s* is unnecessary when the relationship is expressed by word order. Similar arguments can be made for certain cases of the plural *-s*, the third-person *-s*, and verb-tense markers. If a numerical quantifier such as *five* or *dozen* appears before a noun, the listener knows that the noun is plural and that the plural *-s* is thus redundant. Likewise, the use of *he*, *she*, or a singular noun subject marks the third person, negating the need for the third-person *-s*. In addition, context often signals the verb tense. Similar arguments about redundancy have been advanced by linguists to explain the

TABLE 13.1   Phonemic Contrasts Between AAE and SAE

	POSITION IN WORD		
SAE PHONEMES	**INITIAL**	**MEDIAL**	**FINAL***
/p/		Unaspirated /p/	Unaspirated /p/
/n/			Reliance on preceding nasalized vowel
/w/	Omitted in specific words (*I'as, too!*)		
/b/		Unreleased /b/	Unreleased /b/
/g/		Unreleased /g/	Unreleased /g/
/k/		Unaspirated /k/	Unaspirated /k/
/d/	Omitted in specific words (*I'on't know*)	Unreleased /d/	Unreleased /d/
/ŋ/		/n/	/n/
/t/		Unaspirated /t/	Unaspirated /t/
/l/		Omitted before labial consonants (*help–hep*)	"uh" following a vowel (*Bill–Biuh*)
/ɹ/		Omitted or /ə/	Omitted or prolonged vowel or glide
/θ/	Unaspirated /t/ or /f/	Unaspirated /t/ or /f/ between vowels	Unaspirated /t/ or /f/ (*bath–baf*)
/v/	Sometimes /b/	/b/ before /m/ and /n/	Sometimes /b/
/ð/	/d/	/d/ or /v/ between vowels	/d/, /v/, /f/
/z/		Omitted or replaced by /d/ before nasal sound (*wasn't–wud'n*)	

Blends

/stɹ/ becomes /skɹ/
/ʃɹ/ becomes /stɹ/
/θɹ/ becomes /θ/
/pɹ/ becomes /p/
/bɹ/ becomes /b/
/kɹ/ becomes /k/
/gɹ/ becomes /g/

Final Consonant Clusters (second consonant omitted when these clusters occur at the end of a word)

/sk/	/nd/	/sp/
/ft/	/ld/	/dʒ d/
/st/	/ɹd/	/nt/

---

*Note weakening of final consonants.

TABLE 13.2   Grammatical Contrasts Between AAE and SAE

AAE GRAMMATICAL STRUCTURE	SAE GRAMMATICAL STRUCTURE

Possessive -'s
Nonobligatory where word position expresses possession
   Get *mother* coat.
   It *be* mother's.
	Obligatory regardless of position
	
	   Get *mother's* coat.
	   It's *mother's*.

Plural -s
Nonobligatory with numerical quantifier
   He got ten *dollar*.
   Look at the *cats*.
	Obligatory regardless of numerical quantifier
	   He has ten *dollars*.
	   Look at the *cats*.

Regular past -ed
Nonobligatory, reduced as consonant cluster
   Yesterday, I *walk* to school.
	Obligatory
	   Yesterday, I *walked* to school.

Irregular past
Case by case, some verbs inflected, others not
   I *see* him last week.
	All irregular verbs inflected
	   I *saw* him last week.

Regular present-tense third-person singular -s
   Nonobligatory
      She *eat* too much.
	Obligatory
	   She *eats* too much.

Irregular present-tense third-person singular -s
   Nonobligatory
      He *do* my job.
	Obligatory
	   He *does* my job.

Indefinite an
Use of indefinite *a*.
   He ride in *a* airplane.
	Use of *an* before nouns beginning with a vowel.
	   He rode in *an* airplane.

Pronouns
Pronominal apposition: pronoun immediately follows noun
   Momma *she* mad. She . . .
	Pronoun used elsewhere in sentence or in other sentence; not in apposition
	   Momma *is* mad. She . . .

Future tense
More frequent use of *be going to* (*gonna*)
   I *be going to* dance tonight.
   I *gonna* dance tonight.
Omit *will* preceding *be*
   I *be* home later.
	More frequent use of *will*
	   I *will* dance tonight.
	   I *am going* to dance tonight.
	Obligatory use of *will*
	   I *will* (I'll) *be* home later.

Negation
Triple negative
   Nobody don't never like me.
Use of *ain't*
   I *ain't* going.
	Absence of triple negative
	   No one ever likes me.
	Ain't is unacceptable form
	   I'm *not* going.

(continued)

TABLE 13.2   Continued

AAE GRAMMATICAL STRUCTURE	SAE GRAMMATICAL STRUCTURE
Modals	
Double modals for such forms as *might*, *could*, and *should*	Single modal use
I *might could* go.	I *might be able to* go.
Questions	
Same form for direct and indirect	Different forms for direct and indirect
What *it is*?	What *is it*?
Do you know what *it is*?	Do you know what *it is*?
Relative pronouns	
Nonobligatory in most cases	Nonobligatory with *that* only
He the one stole it.	He's the one *who* stole it.
It the one you like.	It's the one (*that*) you like.
Conditional *if*	
Use of *do* for conditional *if*	Use of *if*
I ask *did* she go.	I asked *if* she went.
Perfect construction	
Been used for action in the distant past	*Been* not used
He *been* gone.	He left a long time ago.
Copula	
Nonobligatory when contractible	Obligatory in contractible and uncontractible forms
He sick.	He's sick.
Habitual or general state	
Marked with uninflected *be*	Nonuse of *be*; verb inflected
She *be* workin'.	She's *working* now.

Sources: Data drawn from Baratz (1969); Fasold & Wolfram, (1970); Williams & Wolfram (1977).

development of some syntactic structures. Other AAE forms introduce redundancy. These include double and triple negatives, pronominal apposition, and certain double modal forms.

The verb *to be* offers a special case. The verb may be nonobligatory in AAE as a contractible copula or as a contractible auxiliary in the present progressive. Some linguists have used these omissions as evidence that the verb *to be* does not exist at a deep structural or conceptual level. On the other hand, the verb *to be* is used to mark the future, a habitual state, or the distant past. The verb *to be* is also present in all uncontractible positions. Thus, it appears that the SAE rule for contractibility is similar to the AAE rule for nonobligatory use. The rules of the verb *to be* represent not the presence or absence of a structure, but differences in use. Question inversion rules offer a similar example when compared to indirect questions and to the use of the conditional *if* (Table 13.2).

In addition to the phonological and structural differences between SAE and AAE, there are also vocabulary differences. In any dialect, words may take on broadened definitions or, conversely, either more restricted meanings or new definitions. AAE words and phrases often influence and change SAE. Many slang expressions used in SAE originated in AAE. These include *rock 'n' roll, cool, rap,* and *jivin'.* Other terms, such as *chitlins* or *crackers,* a derisive term for whites, are used almost exclusively in AAE. A sample of idioms is presented in Table 13.3 (Smitherman, 1994). No one speaker uses all of these idioms, and they represent speakers of different ages and geographic locations.

Language use also differs. There is a strong oral tradition in some African American communities, and superior verbal skills are highly regarded. In inner-city groups, youths with good verbal skills are usually in high positions within the group power structure. *Raps,* now popularized in modern music, are used to boast, put down, or humiliate an opponent.

Other nonlinguistic differences may be found between some speakers of AAE and other dialects. For example, touching someone's hair may be considered an offense to some AAE speakers but a sign of affection by users of dialects closer to SAE. Similarly, indirect eye contact, the use of personal questions, and interrupting are acceptable conversational conduct in some African American communities but would be considered rude in those closer to SAE. Conversational silence may signal opposite messages: refutation for AAE speakers and acceptance or agreement for SAE speakers. Finally, emotional or demonstrative, even abusive, outbursts may be tolerated in AAE but not in SAE.

AAE and the Wider Society. For an individual child, the main effects of using AAE are social and educational. To the extent that AAE is stigmatized within our multidialectal society, the child may also be stigmatized. Unfortunately, many people attach relative values to certain dialects and to the speakers of those dialects. Individuals tend to respond to dialects in terms of stereotypes. This generalized or stereotypic response may, in turn, affect other

TABLE 13.3   Selected AAE Idioms

IDIOM	DEFINITION AND EXAMPLE
All that	Excellent, fantastic, superb, all that it seems to be, as in "She bad, she definitely *all that.*"
Amen corner	Place where older individuals usually sit in traditional African American church.
Barefoot as a river duck	Not wearing shoes, as in "It too cold for you be runnin' around *barefoot as a river duck.*"
Crack on	To insult seriously or in fun, as in "He jus' *crackin on* you."
Eagle-flyin' day	Pay day.
Old head	Older and wiser person.
On it	In control of the situation, as in "Don't worry, I *on it.*"
That how you livin'?	Why are you acting like that?
Word	Affirmative response to an action or statement. "Right on, *word up!*"

Source: From Smitherman (1994).

judgments. Employment and educational opportunities may be denied because of dialectal differences. In general, AAE speakers are granted shorter employment interviews, offered fewer positions, and offered lower-paying positions (Terrell & Terrell, 1983) than speakers of more standard English dialects. Apparently, this discrimination does not significantly affect the self-concept of AAE speakers. Research has indicated that African American children who speak AAE seem to have a higher self-concept than those who do not.

It has been found that some educators exhibit a bias in favor of SAE or a regional dialect. Teachers may use any of the following reasons for assuming that minority students are inferior to white children speaking dialects closer to SAE:

1. Minority students demonstrate a lack of verbal capacity in formal or threatening situations.
2. Poor school performance is a result of this verbal deficit.
3. Middle-class speech habits are necessary for learning, as evidenced by the better school achievement of middle-class children.
4. Dialectal differences reflect differences in the capacity for logical analysis.
5. Logical thinking can be fostered by teaching children to mimic the formal speech patterns of their teachers.
6. Children who adopt these formal patterns think logically and thus do better in reading and arithmetic.

Unfortunately, scores on norm-referenced tests, usually based on standard language skill usage, can be, and often are, used to bolster this position.

Throughout this book we have concentrated on the "generic" child, most typically white and middle class. Some studies have shown, however, that lower-class African American children do not acquire language within a similar social context. Urban African American children may pass through three stages of language acquisition. First, they learn the basics of language at home; then, from ages five to fifteen, they learn a local vernacular dialect from their peers; and, finally, they develop the more standard AAE dialect. Southern, rural, lower-class African American children are not encouraged to communicate conversationally or to ask questions. In a southeastern Appalachian working-class town, dubbed "Trackton," children are addressed indirectly and are not expected to provide information (Brice Heath, 1983). Children are exposed to a wide variety of language through extended families and neighbors who tease and verbally challenge toddlers. The children often begin to speak by imitating the ending phrases of these speakers. Children who try to interrupt adult conversation may be scolded for their speech inaccuracies or for their less mature language. Within other regions, language stimulation may appear in other forms, such as rhymes, songs, or stories. In general, the mothers of these children do not feel obligated to teach language. Development differs in the demands for communication placed on the child. Therefore, children differ in their expectations of appropriate communication behavior.

Although preschool African American children from homes using AAE do not develop all forms of the dialect, there is a marked increase in use during school age, especially from grades three to five (Isaacs, 1996). As mentioned earlier, prepubescent boys are especially likely to use AAE (Washington & Craig, 1998).

Classroom teachers, faced with dialectal differences, may assume that the differences signify inferior abilities. Language-based testing encourages such thinking. Teachers may assume that students who speak AAE do not understand SAE. But this does not appear to be the case. African American children's comprehension seems to be as good for SAE as for AAE. In fact, African American students perform better at sentence completion when cued in SAE. Finally, there is no difference between African American lower-class and white middle-class children in imitation of SAE sentences The ability of African American children to comprehend AAE and SAE continues into adulthood. African American adults find child speakers of both dialects equally intelligible, whereas adult SAE speakers find child SAE speakers significantly more intelligible than AAE speakers.

Speakers of AAE may have difficulty with reading and spelling in SAE. In general, children read orally in accordance with their dialects. The resultant differences are not errors in word recognition (Burke, Pflaum, & Knafle, 1982). Phonemic differences may make it difficult, however, for the teacher to interpret the child's oral reading. Surface phonemic differences may also account for the child's spelling errors. In addition, AAE speakers may not recognize the significance of the grammatical markers that they omit. This suggests that the AAE-speaking child may not hear a difference or may not understand its significance. It is easy to see how this difficulty could be transferred to other academic areas.

Latino English

Within the United States, the largest ethnic population is Hispanic. Not all people with Spanish surnames speak Spanish; some do exclusively; and still others are **bilingual**, speaking both Spanish and English. The form of English spoken depends on the amount and type of Spanish spoken. The two largest Hispanic groups in the United States are of Puerto Rican–Caribbean and Mexican–Central American origin. Although both groups speak Spanish, their Spanish dialectal differences influence their comprehension and production of American English. The dialect of American English spoken in the surrounding community also has an effect. As a result, the interference points may be very different for individual speakers. We will discuss the general characteristics of these speakers and refer to their dialect as *Latino English* (LE). Tables 13.4 and 13.5 summarize the major differences found between LE and SAE.

As expected, there are phonological differences between Spanish and English. Some English speech sounds, such as /θ/, /ð/, /z/, /ʃ/, /ʒ/, /I/, /æ/, and /ʌ/, do not exist in Spanish. As a result, these sounds are frequently distorted, or replaced with other sounds, by speakers of LE. In addition, all final plosives are voiceless in Spanish, and initial voiceless plosives are not aspirated. In LE, sounds may be altered from their English articulation. Finally, Spanish does not distinguish between /b/ and /v/, and the Spanish /ɪ/ and /l/ are produced differently from their English equivalents. As expected, speakers of LE use /b/ and /v/ interchangeably, while they use Spanish /ɪ/ and /l/ in place of their English equivalents.

Spanish vowels are a special consideration. There are five vowels and four diphthongs in Spanish. In contrast, English has many more. In addition, Spanish vowels have the same quality or length, whether in a stressed or an unstressed syllable. English vowels vary with stressing. As a result, English vowels can present a special problem in perception and production.

TABLE 13.4 Phonemic Contrasts Between LE and SAE

	POSITION IN WORD		
SAE PHONEMES	**INITIAL**	**MEDIAL**	**FINAL***
/p/	Unaspirated /p/		Omitted or weakened
/m/			Omitted
/w/	/hu/		Omitted
/b/			Omitted, distorted, or /p/
/g/			Omitted, distorted, or /k/
/k/	Unaspirated or /g/		Omitted, distorted, or /g/
/f/			Omitted
/d/		Dentalized	Omitted, distorted, or /t/
/ŋ/	/n/	/d/	/n/ (sing–sin)
/j/	/dʒ/		
/t/			Omitted
/ʃ/	/tʃ/	/s/, /tʃ/	/tʃ/ (wish–which)
/tʃ/	/ʃ/ (chair–share)	/ʃ/	/ʃ/ (watch–wash)
/ɪ/	Distorted	Distorted	Distorted
/dʒ/	/d/	/j/	/ʃ/
/θ/	/t/, /s/ (thin–tin, sin)	Omitted	/ʃ/, /t/, /s/
/v/	/b/ (vat–bat)	/b/	Distorted
/z/	/s/ (zip–sip)	/s/ (razor–racer)	/s/
/ð/	/d/ (then–den)	/d/, /θ/, /v/ (lather–ladder)	/d/

Blends

/skw/ becomes /eskw/*
/sl/ becomes /esl/*
/st/ becomes /est/*

Vowels

/ɪ/ becomes /i/ (bit–beet)

*Separates cluster into two syllables.

Structural contrasts between LE and SAE also reflect interference points between Spanish and English. Many redundant SAE markers are nonobligatory, as they are in AAE. Other markers, such as the postnoun possessive, reflect Spanish constructions. A similar example can be found in the placement of adjectives following the noun in Spanish and in LE. In addition, the speaker of LE may scatter his or her speech with many vocabulary words of Spanish origin.

Nonlinguistic differences also persist between LE and SAE. In general, a closer or smaller relative distance is tolerated among many LE speakers, as is a greater incidence of touching between conversational partners. Other differences, such as avoidance of direct

TABLE 13.5   Grammatical Contrasts Between LE and SAE

LE GRAMMATICAL STRUCTURE	SAE GRAMMATICAL STRUCTURE
Possessive -'s	
Use postnoun modifier	Postnoun modifier used rarely
This is the homework of *my brother*.	This is *my brother's* homework.
Article used with body parts	Possessive pronoun used with body parts
I cut *the finger*.	I cut *my* finger.
Plural -s	
Nonobligatory	Obligatory, excluding exceptions
The *girl* are playing.	The *girls* are playing.
The *sheep* are playing.	The *sheep* are playing.
Regular past -ed	
Nonobligatory, especially when understood	Obligatory
I *talk* to her yesterday.	I *talked* to her yesterday.
Regular third-person singular present-tense -s	
Nonobligatory	Obligatory
She *eat* too much.	She *eats* too much.
Articles	
Often omitted	Usually obligatory
I am going to store.	I am going to *the* store.
I am going to school.	I am going to school.
Subject pronouns	
Omitted when subject has been identified in the previous sentence	Obligatory
Father is happy. Bought a new car.	Father is happy. *He* bought a new car.
Future tense	
Use *go + to*	Use *be + going to*
I *go to* dance.	I *am going to* the dance.
Negation	
Use *no* before the verb	Use *not* (preceded by auxiliary verb where appropriate)
She *no* eat candy.	She does *not* eat candy.
Question	
Intonation; no noun–verb inversion	Noun–verb inversion usually
Maria is going?	*Is Maria* going?
Copula	
Occasional use of *have*	Use of *be*
I *have* ten years.	I *am* ten years old.
Negative imperatives	
No used for *don't*	*Don't* used
No throw stones.	*Don't* throw stones.

(continued)

TABLE 13.5   Continued

LE GRAMMATICAL STRUCTURE	SAE GRAMMATICAL STRUCTURE

***Do* insertion**
Nonobligatory in questions
  You like ice cream?
	Obligatory when no auxiliary verb
	  Do you like ice cream?

Comparatives
More frequent use of longer form (*more*)
  He is *more* tall.
	More frequent use of shorter -*er*.
	  He is tall*er*.

eye contact, may signal attentiveness and respect for LE speakers while signaling the opposite for speakers of more standard American English dialects.

Asian English

Although we shall use the term *Asian English* (AE), it is clearly a misnomer because no such entity exists. It is merely a term that enables us to discuss the various dialects of Asian Americans as a group.

The most widely used languages in Asia are Mandarin Chinese, Cantonese Chinese, Filipino, Japanese, Khmer, Korean, Laotian, and Vietnamese. Of these, Mandarin Chinese has had the most pervasive influence on the evolution of the others. Indian and colonial European cultures, as well as others, have also influenced these languages. Each language has various dialects and features that distinguish it from the others. Thus, there is, in reality, no Asian English as a cohesive unit.

Nonetheless, the English of Asian language speakers has certain characteristics in common. These are listed in Tables 13.6 and 13.7. The omission of final consonants, for example, is prevalent in AE. In contrast to English, most Asian languages have open or vowel-final syllables.

BILINGUALISM

We cannot really discuss LE or AE without addressing the issue of bilingualism. Spanish, the various Asian languages, and English are separate languages with their own lexicons and rule systems; children from other than English-speaking families are encouraged to become speakers of English in the public schools. LE and AE reflect the effects of Spanish and the various Asian languages on English. Neither LE nor Spanish is spoken by all Hispanic Americans. Similarly, not all Asian Americans speak some variety of AE or an Asian language. Those individuals who speak both Spanish and English are said to be bilingual as are speakers of both Korean and English.

The prevalence of bilingualism reflects the cultural mixing within a nation. In an isolated country, such as Iceland, the rather homogeneous nature of the culture is reflected in

TABLE 13.6   Phonemic Contrasts Between AE and SAE

SAE PHONEMES	POSITION IN WORD		
	INITIAL	MEDIAL	FINAL
/p/	/b/§	/b/§	Omission
/s/	Distortion*	Distortion*	Omission
/z/	/s/†	/s/†	Omission
/t/	Distortion*	Distortion*	Omission
/tʃ/	/ʃ/§	/ʃ/§	Omission
/ʃ/	/s/†	/s/†	Omission
/ɹ/, /l/	Confusion‡	Confusion‡	Omission
/θ/	/s/	/s/	Omission
/dz/	/d/ or /z/§	/d/ or /z/§	Omission
/v/	/f/Ê	/f/‡	Omission
	/w/†	/w/†	Omission
/ð/	/z/*	/z/*	Omission
	/d/§	/d/§	Omission

Blends

Addition of /ə/ between consonants‡
Omission of final consonant clusters§

Vowels

Shortening or lengthening of vowels (*seat–sit, it–eat**)
Difficulty with /ɪ/, /ɔ/, and /æ/, and substitution of /ə/ for /æ/†
Difficulty with /ɪ/, /æ/, /ʊ/, and /ə/§

Source: Adapted from Cheng, L. (June, 1987). Cross-cultural and linguistic considerations in working with Asian populations. *Asha, 29*(6), 33–38.

*Mandarin Chinese only.
†Cantonese Chinese only.
‡Mandarin, Cantonese, and Japanese.
§Vietnamese only.

the scarcity of bilingualism. In the United States, approximately 17 percent of the population is bilingual, mostly speaking Spanish and English. Canada, which fosters more cultural diversity than its neighbor to the south and has two official languages, has a 24 percent bilingual population (deVries & Vallee, 1980). Other countries may have large bilingual populations because of a large, influential neighbor with a different language, because the official language differs from the indigenous one, or because of a large immigrant population.

True balanced bilingualism, or equal proficiency in two languages, is rare. Nonbalanced bilingualism, in which an individual has obtained a higher level of proficiency in one of the languages, is more common. The language in which the individual is more proficient may not be the native language, which can recede if devalued or used infrequently (Hakuta, 1987).

TABLE 13.7   Grammatical Contrasts Between AE and SAE

AE GRAMMATICAL STRUCTURE	SAE GRAMMATICAL STRUCTURE
Plural -s	
Not used with numerical adjective: *three* cat	Used regardless of numerical adjective: *three cats*
Used with irregular plural: *three sheeps*	Not used with irregular plural: *three sheep*
Auxiliaries *to be* and *to do*	
Omission: *I going home. She not want eat.*	Obligatory and inflected in the present progressive form: *I am going home. She does not want to eat.*
Uninflected: *I is going. She do not want eat.*	
Verb *have*	
Omission *You been here.*	Obligatory and inflected: *You have been here. He has one.*
Uninflected *He have one.*	
Past-tense -ed	
Omission: *He talk yesterday.*	Obligatory, nonovergeneralization, and single marking: *He talked yesterday. I ate yesterday. She didn't eat.*
Overgeneralization: *I eated yesterday.*	
Double marking: *She didn't ate.*	
Interrogative	
Nonreversal: *You are late?*	Reversal and obligatory auxiliary: *Are you late? Do you like ice cream?*
Omitted auxiliary: *You like ice cream?*	
Perfect marker	
Omission: *I have write letter.*	Obligatory: *I have written a letter.*
Verb–noun agreement	
Nonagreement: *He go to school. You goes to school.*	Agreement: *He goes to school. You go to school.*
Article	
Omission: *Please give gift.*	Obligatory with certain nouns: *Please give the gift. She went to school.*
Overgeneralization: *She go the school.*	
Preposition	
Misuse: *I am in home.*	Obligatory specific use: *I am at home. He goes by bus.*
Omission: *He go bus.*	
Pronoun	
Subjective/objective confusion: *Him go quickly.*	Subjective/objective distinction: *He gave it to her.*
Possessive confusion: *It him book.*	Possessive distinction: *It's his book.*

TABLE 13.7 Continued

AE GRAMMATICAL STRUCTURE	SAE GRAMMATICAL STRUCTURE
Demonstrative	
Confusion: *I like those horse.*	Singular/distinction: *I like that horse.*
Conjunction	
Omission: *You I go together.*	Obligatory use between last two items a series: *You and I are going together. Mary, John, and Carol went.*
Negation	
Double marking: *I didn't see nobody.*	Single obligatory marking: *I didn't see anybody. He didn't come.*
Simplified form: *He no come.*	
Word order	
Adjective following noun (Vietnamese): *clothes new.* Possessive following noun (Vietnamese): *dress her.*	Most noun modifiers precede noun: *new clothes.* Possessive precedes noun: *her dress.*
Omission of object with transitive verb: *I want.*	Use of direct object with most transitive verbs: *I want it.*

Source: Adapted from Cheng, L. (June, 1987). Cross-cultural and linguistic considerations in working with Asian populations. *ASHA*, 29(6), 33–38.

It is also possible for a person to be semiproficient or semilingual in both languages. This situation may occur for any number of reasons explained later in the chapter.

Decreased proficiency may also reflect mixed input. Children who hear "Spanglish" (Spanish + English) in south Florida and in the southwestern United States or "Franglais" (French + English) in parts of Quebec province can be expected to have more mixing in their own language (Redlinger & Park, 1980). Examples of Spanglish among Miami adolescents include *chileado* (chilling out), *coolismo* (ultra-cool or way cool), *eskipeando* (skipping class), *friquado* (freak out), and *Que wow!* More detrimental to the learning of either language is the mixing of syntax as in *Como puedo ayudarlo?*—literally *How can I help you*, following English word order—in place of the Spanish *Que desea?*

There is a not-so-subtle prejudice against other languages in the general American culture. Again, the users of dialects closer to the standard tend to respond to these languages or to AE or LE stereotypically. Unfortunately, this prejudice can even be seen in the speech of bilingual adults. For example, when speaking Spanish with an Anglo, Hispanic adults tend to Americanize Spanish words, but they do not do so with an Hispanic audience.

The non-English-speaking or bilingual child faces some danger in the schools, including educational placement. In at least one case in my experience, a non-English-speaking child was classified as mentally retarded based on an English-receptive vocabulary test. It can only be hoped that this case is a rarity.

Effects of Bilingualism on Language Learning

It has long been assumed that bilingual children are at a disadvantage when learning language and that their progress in one or both languages is delayed. The effects of bilingualism differ with the age of the individual and the manner of language acquisition. It is important to make a distinction between simultaneous and successive acquisition.

Simultaneous Acquisition

Simultaneous acquisition is the development of two languages prior to age three. Simultaneous bilingual acquisition can be characterized as follows (Grosjean, 1982):

1. Initial language mixing, followed by a slow separation and increasing awareness of the differences.
2. Influence of one on the other when one is favored by the environment.
3. Avoidance of difficult words and constructions in the weaker language.
4. Rapid shifts in the dominance of either language with environmental shifts.
5. Final separation of the phonological and grammatical systems but enduring influence of the dominant system in vocabulary and idioms.

The rate and manner of development appear to be the same whether the child is monolingual or bilingual (Oller, Eilers, Urbano, & Cobo-Lewis, 1997). In spite of the bilingual linguistic load, the child acquires both languages at a rate comparable to that of monolingual children. The degree of dissimilarity between the two languages does not appear to affect the rate of acquisition. The key to development is the consistent use of the two languages within their primary-use environments.

There seem to be three stages in the simultaneous acquisition of two languages in young children. During the first stage, the child has two separate lexical systems (Pearson, Fernandez, & Oller, 1995). Vocabulary words rarely overlap (Genesee, Nicoladis, & Paradis, 1995). The child learns one word from either language for each referent. When there is an overlap, the child does not treat the words as equals. Some words are treated as corresponding, although they are not considered so by adults. This is similar to the early meaning differences found between adult words and words of the monolingual child. Initially, words from both languages are combined indiscriminately (Vihman, 1985).

In the initial stage of simultaneous bilingual development, children may actually have two different language systems that they are able to use in different contexts or in functionally different ways (Genesee, 1989). Thus, the child may use one system with adults of one language and one with adults of the other. Rather than signifying a mixing of the two languages, such things as the use of words from both languages may be an example of overextension. The child uses whatever vocabulary he or she has available. Mixing of grammatical elements may reflect lack of development of structures in one of the languages, possibly because these structures are too difficult at present.

Phonological differentiation is also occurring. The earliest phonology is usually a combination of the two different inputs into a single system, although the least interference seems to occur in this aspect of language. Differentiation of the phonological systems begins between twenty-four to thirty months. "By age 2, children have acquired a conception of their native phonology that specifies certain contrasts as relevant and others . . . as irrelevant to the language's meaning system" (Oller & Eilers, 1983, p. 53). Thus, in tasks involving identification of meaning, the child may ignore contrasts that do not pertain.

In the second stage, the child has two distinct lexicons but applies the same syntactic rules to both. This lexical generalization process is difficult and occurs slowly. The child must separate a word from its specific context and identify it with the corresponding word in the other language. Each word tends to remain tied to the particular context in which it was learned, and corresponding words are not usually learned simultaneously. The child is able to move between the two lexicons and to translate words freely. Unfortunately, this flexibility is not found at the syntactic level. The nonparallel sequence of syntactic learning reflects the difference in linguistic difficulty of particular syntactic structures within the two languages. In general, the child learns structures common to both languages first, the simpler constructions before the more complex. Thus, if a construction is more complex in one language, it will be learned first in the other language in its simpler form.

Finally, in the third stage, the child correctly produces lexical and syntactic structures from each language. Although there is still a great deal of interference, it is mostly confined to the syntactic level. As few as 2 percent of bilingual preschoolers' utterances may contain some mixing . In general, mixes are used when the child lacks an appropriate word in one language or when the mixed entry is a more salient word to the child. The child's mixing seems to result from a mixed adult input. For Spanish-speaking children in the United States, mixing consists primarily of inserting English nouns into Spanish utterances. The structural consistency of the utterance is maintained.

To decrease interference, the child may try to keep the two languages as separate as possible, associating each with a particular person (Redlinger & Park, 1980). As the child becomes more familiar with the syntactic differences, the tendency to label people with a certain language decreases. The child becomes truly bilingual and can manage two separate languages at about age seven.

The truly bilingual person possesses a dual system simultaneously available during processing. In addition, semantic input may be processed in each language regardless of the language of input. Most information is processed at the semantic level, because the interpretation of surface syntax requires much greater proficiency.

Successive Acquisition

Most bilingual children develop one language (L_1), such as Spanish, at home and a second (L_2), such as American English, with peers or in school, usually after age three. Although humans are capable of acquiring a second language at any age, by the late teens it is difficult for a speaker to acquire native-speaker pronunciation characteristics in a second language. In part, this difficulty may reflect the tendency of adult speakers to use the discourse-processing strategies of their native language to interpret the second language (Tao & Healy, 1996).

Although young children do not necessarily acquire L_2 faster or more easily than adults, they eventually outperform adults in L_2. In addition, children are less susceptible than adults to interference from L_1.

Early exposure to L_2 may result in a delay in L_1 before it is mature. In turn, competence in L_2 may be a function of relative maturity in L_1 (Cummins, 1980, 1984). The result may be *semilingualism*, a failure to reach proficiency in either language. Children learning language at school age have acquired some metalinguistic skills that may facilitate L_2 learning (Schiff-Meyers, 1992).

Success in nonsimultaneous language acquisition is more closely related to the learner's attitude toward, and identity with, the users of the language being acquired, and his or her positive attitude toward the first language and culture. Need is another strong motivating factor, although intelligence seems to have little effect (Pinsleur, 1980). Most children acquire a second language rapidly, although the strategies used differ with age, the child's linguistic knowledge, and the nature of the two languages. The more the child's learning style matches the teaching style the better the development of L_2. Children tend to learn in immediate contexts through sensory activity, while adults prefer explicit rule training. Such home factors as literacy and a positive attitude toward both languages are also very important (Hamayan & Damico, 1991; Weinstein, 1984).

Successive acquisition of L_2 outside the classroom may occur in three stages. In the first stage, the child establishes social relations with speakers of the second language. The interaction is more important than information exchange, and the child relies on "fixed verbal formulas." These fixed formulas are learned as single units, such as *lookit, okay, ya know*, and *wait a minute*. During this stage, the child assumes that what is being said is relevant to the situation or to what the speaker is experiencing. The child scans the formulas for recurring linguistic patterns. The social strategy is to join the group and act as if he or she knows what is being communicated. The child tries to use the few phrases and words that give the impression of being able to speak the second language.

Speakers seem to adopt one of two strategies: other-directed or inner-directed. Those choosing the other-directed strategy approach the language-learning task as an interpersonal one. The goal is to get the message across in any way possible. In contrast, those who choose an inner-directed strategy approach the task as an intrapersonal one. Focus is less on communication and more on breaking the language code. Inner-directed individuals may appear to be rather quiet and withdrawn (Kessler, 1984). Actually, they are engaging in "private" speech in which they repeat the utterances of others, recall and practice phrases, create new utterances, modify and expand existing utterances, and rehearse for future social performance (Saville-Troike, 1988).

In the second stage, communication becomes the goal. The child's strategies include using to the utmost the linguistic units he or she understands and working on overall communication, while saving the details for later. The child begins talking with whatever units he or she can produce and comprehend.

At this point, a child may develop a hybrid form called **interlanguage**, a jumble of L_1 and L_2 rules plus the child's creative ones. As a transitional system, the child's individualistic interlanguage is constantly changing (Tarone, 1988).

Finally, in the third stage, the child concentrates on correct language forms. He or she is more mature than the typical simultaneous bilingual learner and can apply general knowledge of language to an analysis of this particular language (Keller-Cohen, 1987). From previous learning, the child recognizes that language is organized sequentially and that order is important. In addition, he or she recognizes that, although language units may have multiple meanings or functions, meaning is often related to the immediate context. The child scans the speech of others, paying attention to order and sequences. In production, the child attempts not to interrupt or rearrange these sequences and to present his or her message as simply as possible.

L_1 can form the foundation for L_2. Certain language processes are basic, and knowledge in L_1 can be transferred to L_2. Although interference can occur, fewer than 5 percent of the errors in the second language are traceable to this source.

Since the child already has one linguistic system, he or she has an acoustic-perceptual system, an articulatory repertoire, and a cognitive-semantic base from which to begin acquiring a second language. Therefore, errors, although similar, are more limited than in first language acquisition. Errors cannot be predicted based on the linguistic form of the two languages. The effects of either language upon the other vary with each child, and interference appears to be minimal. Children do not use their knowledge of L_1 to formulate utterances in L_2. Instead, they treat the new language as an independent system and gradually construct it from the speech they hear.

Usually, the first language continues to develop to adult norms, while the second achieves a somewhat lower level. This isn't always the case, however, and L_1 may be forgotten unless it is maintained at home. In actual practice, use determines which language will become dominant.

In general, second-language learning by young children mirrors first-language learning. At first, the child begins with single words or common short phrases and then moves to short sentences and morphological markers. Semantic relations are expressed first by order and then with morphological markers. Sentence alterations, such as negation and interrogation, follow acquisition patterns similar to those found in first-language learning. The errors made by the child learning English as a second language are also similar to those made by those learning English first.

Common differences noted in L_2 learning include omission and overextension of morphological inflections, double marking, misordering of sentence constituents, and the use of archiforms and free alternation. An **archiform** is one member of a word class used exclusively, such as *that* for all demonstratives. As more members of a class are acquired, perhaps *this*, *these*, and *those*, the child may vary usage among the members without concern for the different meanings; this is called **free alternation**.

Phonological development also follows a similar pattern in first and second languages. The phonological system from the first language forms a foundation for the second. Gradually the two phonological systems become differentiated.

Although the school-age child may have no conversational difficulties, he or she may experience problems with the decontextualized language of the classroom. It may take six to seven years to obtain cognitive-academic proficiency (Cummins, 1980).

Code Switching and Development

Bilingual speakers often exhibit code-switching, or shifting from one language to another, especially when both languages are used in the environment, as in the southwestern United States, in Quebec, or in sections of many major U.S. cities. The behavior is not random, nor does it reflect an underlying language deficit. Rather, code switching is the result of functional and grammatical principles and is a complex, rule-governed phenomenon that is system-atically influenced by the context and the situation (Auer, 1984; Genesee, 1984; McClure, 1981; Penalosa, 1981; Poplack, 1981; Sanchez, 1983; Sprott & Kemper, 1987). Code switching is confined almost exclusively to free morphemes, most frequently nouns, and tends to occur where the surface structures are similar (Poplack, 1981). Children begin by code switching single words from one language to another (Lanza, 1992). In contrast, adults tend to substitute whole sentences (Huerta-Macias, 1981). Certain words and phrases tend to be switched predictably across different conversations by the same speaker.

Rather than representing the integration of both grammars into a third, new grammar, code-switching rules demonstrate the continuing separation of the two languages (Leder-berg & Morales, 1985). Two of these rules are as follows:

1. Code switching occurs only when code-switched words are positioned in accordance with the rules for the language from which the word is selected.
2. Code switching cannot occur within word boundaries.

A corollary of the first rule is that code switching occurs at natural word and phrase bound-aries that correspond to monolinguals' processing units (Azuma, 1996). Although the first rule is observed by bilinguals of all ages, the second is frequently violated by children under ten.

For children, systematic code switching appears to be a function of the participants in a conversation (McClure, 1981). Three characteristics of the participants are important: their perceived language proficiency, their language preference, and their social identity. In general, children under age five combine proficiency and preference decisions. A listener either knows a language or does not. Older children make finer distinctions and may, there-fore, consider their speaker more often. Their behavior reflects the developing presupposi-tional skills seen in school-age children. Children also identify certain people with certain languages. If unsure, they try to use physical characteristics as a guide. For example, in the Southwestern United States, Anglo teachers may be addressed in English even though they are proficient in Spanish (McClure, 1981).

Other functional variables also influence code switching (McClure, 1981). Although physical setting alone has little influence, the type of discourse is a factor. Interviews and narratives contain few switches, instead remaining in one language or the other. Conversa-tions, in contrast, are characterized by frequent switches. In addition, code switching can be a stylistic device used for direct quotes, emphasis, clarification or repetition, elaboration, focus on a particular portion of a message, attention getting and maintenance, and personal interjections or asides. Although topics alone do not usually influence switching, the lan-guage of a specific group may be used when discussing that group, and code switching may signal topic changes. In the southwestern United States, for example, Spanish-speaking families may use English when discussing the Anglos (Huerta-Macias, 1981).

The exact developmental function of code switching is unknown. The function may be twofold (Huerta-Macias, 1981). First, it may be an aid for retention of the first language while a second is learned. Once the two languages are learned, code switching may ensure that both are used.

Bilingualism and Cognition

Learning a second language may result in modified brain organization. The resultant pattern depends on a number of factors, including the age at second-language acquisition, the manner of learning, the patterns of usage, and the similarity of characteristics of the languages. Second-language learning may involve right-hemisphere mechanisms not involved in single-language learning. If a second language is learned before puberty, there may be symmetrical representation within the two hemispheres. Later language learning may result in more complex, less symmetrical lateralization.

Not all researchers agree. In contrast to what was just stated, there may be more right-hemisphere involvement the later the second language is acquired relative to the first and the more informal the exposure to the second (Vaid, 1983), especially if the second language was learned after age six (Sussman, Franklin, & Simon, 1982). In addition, the right hemisphere is more likely to be involved if the languages differ greatly. The more advanced the second language, however, the greater the left-hemisphere involvement. Obviously, the resultant hemispheric pattern will reflect an interaction of these variables. Overall, the reported differences between monolinguals and bilinguals may reflect different processing strategies rather than distinctive organizational and functional differences (Vaid, 1983).

There is a very strong relationship between bilingualism and cognitive development. Bilinguals are superior in classifying objects, creativity, concept formation, memory, metalinguistic awareness, perceptual disembedding, problem solving, role taking, science concepts social sensitivity, and understanding complex instructions (Eckstein, 1986; Fang, 1985; Kessler & Quinn, 1987; Powers & Lopez, 1985; Sperling, 1990; Whitaker, Rueda, & Prieto, 1985). Bilinguals must achieve high levels of proficiency, however, before the effects are evident in cognitive development. Even high functioning five- to six-year-olds exhibit higher divergent thinking, imagination, grammatical awareness, perceptual organization, and reading achievement (Ricciardelli, 1992).

Language may also affect memory of personal events (Javier, Barroso, & Munoz, 1993). Both L_1 and L_2 can serve as the reference or coding language depending on the linguistic context. Recall is considerably better if the reference language is used in the recall process. Likewise, word identification also depends on past experience with and actual use of the words in question (Frenck-Mestre, 1993).

Cultural Diversity

It is easy for many middle-class, English-speaking, white Americans to assume that the manner in which they function is the only way or the right way. Just as there are dialectal differences within American English, there are child-nurturing and language-teaching differences as well. Not all cultures within the United States place the same emphasis on verbal communication. Among some Latinos, silence is associated with aloofness and self-restraint, certainly admirable qualities. Children are expected to be silent and thoughtful, to listen, and to hesitate before speaking. Apache Native Americans value silence. Individuals developing within these cultures will have different communication standards.

Neither the model of mother-as-communication-partner nor the use of motherese is universal. For example, among Mexican Americans, mothers may act as a language assistant or coach, helping the child imitate, and thus maintain an interaction with, a third party (A. Eisenberg, 1982). By the later preschool years, the child is very adept in conversations involving multiple participants and is able to perform before an audience. Inner-city Puerto Rican and African American children, on the other hand, are generally raised in an environment in which much of the socialization is accomplished through peers (Iglesias, 1986).

The prospective teacher or speech-language pathologist should be aware that his or her expectations and the communication abilities of minority children may differ. For example, middle-class children come to school with the basics of the literary strategy. Their narratives are topic-oriented and sequentially organized. Children from Hispanic and some Native American cultures may be more visually oriented. Stories may be descriptive rather than narrative or may deviate from the middle-class story pattern (Iglesias, 1986). In general, the stories the child encounters in reading texts and those he or she is expected to write follow the literary pattern of the narrative.

In each of the cases discussed, the minority culture or individual is not wrong, just different. Even if the methods of middle-class American mothers and their children had been proven to be the most efficient way to learn language—which they haven't—these methods would not necessarily be so in cultures in which other conditions exist.

CONCLUSION

Dialectal differences and bilingualism can pose special problems for the language-learning child, especially when the child enters school. Yet children who speak with a dialect of American English seem to understand SAE. These young children, if motivated, follow a developmental sequence and learn a second language or dialect relatively easily. They already have a language rule system that enables them to understand other dialects and learn other languages. Although different from SAE, other dialectal systems are not deviant. The U.S. district court for eastern Michigan, in a ruling known as the *Ann Arbor decision* (Joiner, 1979), has ruled that AAE is a rule-governed linguistic system. Furthermore, educators must develop methods for teaching SAE to dialectal speakers.

Bilingual children appear to learn two languages with a minimum of delay. The key to development seems to be the pattern of use within the language community. Even young monolingual children can learn a second language easily. This second-language development seems to mirror the sequence found in the initial language.

Poor performance of minority children in school is often related to a lack of genuine respect for linguistic and cultural differences and an expectation of inferiority by the teacher and/or the child. Teachers' failure to understand the nature of the child's language in his or her culture may result in a situation in which classroom experiences are incompatible with the child's cultural background.

DISCUSSION

I sound fine, but everyone else has an accent! Not so fast. If nothing else, please take from this chapter that a standard American English really doesn't exist in your and my daily use of language. You speak a dialect while I use the standard. I'm having fun with you. We all speak a dialect. The important thing to recognize is that no one dialect is better than any other. They are all rule-based variations.

In the real world, however, some dialects are rewarded, while others are punished by the culture as a whole. Still, within a community, a dialect that is punished by the larger society may be rewarded and may give status to its user. It is very difficult to separate a dialect from its culture.

As you know, languages are also closely related to culture. Bilingualism may represent biculturalism. To suggest that bilingualism is a disorder is to insult the speaker.

The SLP, teacher, or school psychologist will be confronted by children who use non-standard dialects or who are bilingual. These children may or may not have language and speech impairments, too. Can you imagine the difficulty a monolingual SLP would have in determining the type and extend of an impairment in this situation? It happens daily for some SLPs. For those SLPs who are bilingual, the situation is somewhat easier.

REFLECTIONS

1. How do dialects relate to each other and to the parent language?

2. What factors contribute to the development of dialects? Relate these to the dialects found in the United States.

3. List the major differences between AAE and SAE.

4. List the major differences between LE and SAE.

5. List the major differences between AE and SAE.

6. Explain the differences between simultaneous and successive second-language acquisition.

7. What are some of the special problems encountered in the educational system by children who speak AAE or LE or who are bilingual?

14

Language Research
and Analysis

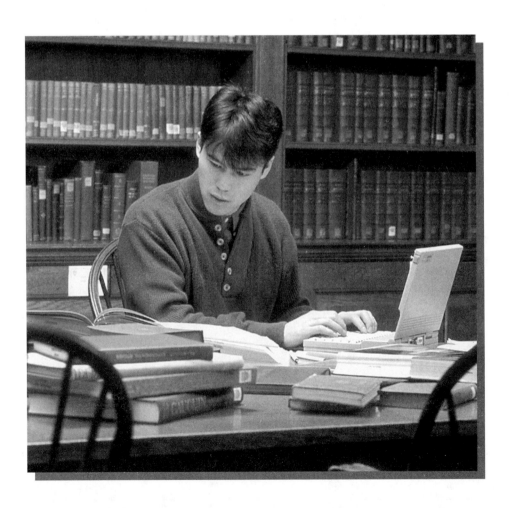

CHAPTER OBJECTIVES

Our knowledge of child language development is only as good as the research data that we possess. In turn, these data reflect the questions that researchers ask and the studies they design to answer these questions. This chapter explores these questions and presents actual language samples and a description of each. When you have completed this chapter, you should understand

- the effect of the method of data collection on the resultant data.
- the effect of the sample size and variability on the resultant data.
- the issues of naturalness and representativeness.
- collection and analysis procedures.
- the value of cross-language studies.

Throughout this text, we have been discussing child language development information that has been gathered from studies of child language. These data are difficult to collect and often require extraordinary procedures in order to ensure valid, reliable, and objective reporting.

In general, there are four goals of child language research (Bennett-Kaster, 1988):

1. To confirm general linguistic principles.
2. To discover principles of language development.
3. To clarify the relationship of language to developments in other areas, such as cognition.
4. To provide a more or less theoretical description of language development.

The purpose and the researcher's theoretical predisposition will influence the type of data-collection procedure used. The researcher's behavioral, linguistic, cognitive, or eclectic theories will influence the specific language features studied and the overall study design. Research is usually based on a model of language or language development that may not reflect the actual language hypotheses of the child. Thus, the results might describe the child's fit or lack of fit to a model rather than the child's actual operating principles, hypotheses, or linguistic performance.

Just as there are different methods of collection, there are many considerations that influence the data gathered by these procedures. In this chapter, we will briefly explore issues related to child language study, such as the method of study, the population and language sample size and variability, the naturalness and representativeness of the language sample, data collection, and data analysis. I shall refer frequently to two studies that we have discussed previously, those of R. Brown (1973) and Wells (1985). Other studies will be mentioned, as appropriate, without burdening the discussion with specific details of each. Cross-linguistic studies and data will also be discussed. Finally, we shall examine portions of actual language samples and note differences and similarities between children.

ISSUES IN THE STUDY OF CHILD LANGUAGE

While the notion of collecting and analyzing child language data may seem simple, in fact it is very complex. Several decisions must be made prior to data collection. The methods and procedures used can influence the resultant data and may unintentionally color the conclusions drawn from these data.

Method of Data Collection

Language-development data are usually collected in two ways: spontaneous conversational sampling or natural observation and structured testing or experimental manipulation. Each method raises issues of appropriateness for the language feature being studied. Either one alone may be insufficient to describe the child's linguistic competence, that is, what he or she knows about language. Data yielded in one context may not appear in another. For example, in a study of pronouns in which I participated, children produced a wider variety in conversation and produced more advanced forms in more formal testing (Haas & Owens, 1985). Other researchers have also found that formal elicitation tasks, such as testing procedures, produce more advanced child language than conversational sampling (Eisenberg, 1997). Ideally, the linguist would employ both approaches, using the structured procedures to obtain more in-depth information on the data collected by the more broad-based naturalistic procedures (Wells, 1985).

Some researchers prefer testing or experimental manipulation in order to control for some of the variables inherent in more naturalistic collection. Within a test or experimental procedure, various linguistic elements may be elicited using verbal and nonverbal stimuli in a structured presentation. Such control of the context, however, may result in rather narrow sampling.

Formal procedures also enable researchers to gather data that may not be readily available using conversational or observational techniques. For example, it is difficult to assess children's comprehension or their metalinguistic skills without direct testing. Many hypotheses cannot be tested directly for ethical reasons, however, so researchers must test indirectly or observe some features of language development.

Language and experimental factors must be manipulated with caution. One aspect of language can affect others, even though the researcher does not intend for this to happen. For example, among both children and adults, new information introduced into a conversation is consistently more phonologically accurate than older, shared information.

Likewise, experimental factors can have unintended consequences. For example, a researcher may highlight an item in a picture upon which the child is to comment. Although the accuracy of the message is not increased when one item is marked, the amount of redundancy or inclusion of irrelevant information does increase (Lloyd & Banham, 1997).

Unfortunately, testing and experimental tasks do not necessarily reflect the child's performance in everyday use. For example, in an experimental task, the child may rely on on-the-spot problem-solving techniques rather than on his or her own everyday operating theories and hypotheses (Karmiloff-Smith, 1986). In addition, noncompliance with testing or experimental procedures may not mean noncomprehension or lack of knowledge. Especially with preschoolers, incorrect responding may indicate a lack of attention or interest.

The results of testing can be especially suspect unless they are analyzed thoroughly. Test scores alone tell researchers nothing about performance on individual items. Two children may have the same score and very different responses. Scoring of individual items may be limited to a wrong-or-right dichotomy, with little analysis of the types of incorrect responses and the underlying processes that these answers may reflect. Testing contexts may provide more or fewer stimuli than are found in the real world, thus modifying the difficulty of the task for the child.

Language processing is not a single unitary operation as is often assumed in test construction, but consists of component operations, such as lexical access, syntactic decoding, and discourse processing, that are engaged at different times and with varying degrees depending on the linguistic task. So-called *off-line test tasks*, as in fill-ins, measure only the endpoints of several linguistic processes, such as providing the missing word.

During off-line testing, components of the overall process are overlooked. For example, the process of guessing the missing word may be the reverse of what happens in rapid-fire conversational processing. Conscious guessing is too slow in conversation. Rather than context aiding in predicting the next word or phrase of the speaker, contextual information seems to provide a check that correct items have been uttered. Although off-line techniques may tell us what children know, they tell us little about how children process or access language.

Various techniques, called *on-line tasks*, attempt to measure operations at various temporal points during processing and describe individual and integrative components (Shapiro, Swinney, & Borsky, 1998). For example, at what point in the cue "Mary has a blue dress and a red dress; she has two _____" does the child access the word *dresses*? We might be able to determine this information by the on-line technique of asking the child to paraphrase or answer yes/no questions after only limited information is presented. Techniques can be much more elaborate than this simple example suggests. Although still in their infancy, on-line techniques are beginning to provide valuable linguistic processing data.

In short, testing and experimental data may be very accurate but very limited. The results must be examined within the context of the specific tasks designed to elicit certain behaviors. A better measure is the consistency of use of a language feature across tasks (Bennett-Kaster, 1988; Derwing & Baker, 1986).

Sampling spontaneous conversation is more naturalistic and, ideally, ensures analysis of real-life behaviors. Such collection is not without its problems. For example, the data collected may be affected by several variables, such as the amount of language, the intelligibility of the child, and the context. To date, linguists have not identified all the possible variables that can affect performance or the extent of their influence. As a result, certain linguistic elements may not be exhibited even when they are present in the child's repertoire. Some linguistic elements occur infrequently, such as passive-voice sentences, and others are optional, such as the use of pronouns. Usually, a single conversational sample is inadequate to demonstrate the full range of a child's communication abilities. It is difficult to estimate the child's competence or ability based on actual behavior. In addition, information on the child's production provides only a general estimate of comprehension.

Sampling techniques exist along a continuum from very unstructured, open-ended situations to more structured, restrictive ones in which the researcher attempts to control or manipulate one or more variables. For example, the researcher interested in narratives may want to elicit a particular variety, such as recounts, and directs the child to provide a story about something that happened to him or her. Pictures also might be used to elicit narratives. All such manipulations affect the child's language. For example, pretend play involving routine events facilitates communication with more topic maintenance and less miscommunication among children than less familiar interactive situations (Short-Meyerson & Abbeduto, 1997).

Child language data may also be obtained from the CHILDES system of database transcripts. The system also includes programs for computer analysis, methods of linguistic coding, and systems for linking these transcripts to digitized audio and video. A corpus of language samples is available along with studies from English and other languages. The internet address for CHILDES is given at the end of the chapter.

Any given naturalistic situation may be insufficient for eliciting the child's systematic knowledge of language. Nor is there certainty that a given test situation will represent the child's naturally occurring communication. Thus, it is best to have data from a combination of collection procedures. In either case, the linguist is sampling the child's performance. The child's linguistic competence—what he or she knows about language—must be inferred from this performance.

Sample Size and Variability

The researcher must be concerned about two samples: the sample or group of children from whom data are collected and the sample of language data. In both samples, the researcher must be concerned with size and variability. Too small a sample will restrict the conclusions that can be drawn about all children, and two large a sample may be unwieldy. The two samples, subjects and language, also interact, one influencing the other.

The number of children or subjects should be large enough to allow for individual differences and to enable group conclusions to be drawn. The overall design of the study will influence the number of subjects considered adequate. For example, it may be appropriate to follow a few children for a period of time, called a *longitudinal study*, but inappropriate to administer a one-time-only test to the same limited number of children. Other considerations will also influence the number of children studied. In a longitudinal study, for example, as many as 30 percent of the children may be lost because of family mobility, illness, or unwillingness to continue over a four- or five-year period. It might be better, therefore, to adopt an overlapping longitudinal design with two different age samples, each being observed for half the length of time that would have been needed in a longitudinal study (Wells, 1985).

Wells (1985) sampled 128 children for two years each, using such an overlapping longitudinal model. R. Brown (1973) studied three children intensively for ten to sixteen months. Wells recorded each child for analysis for twenty-seven minutes at three-month intervals throughout the study, collecting an average of 120 utterances on each occasion. In contrast, Brown averaged two hours of sampling each month.

The sample of children should accurately reflect the diversity of the larger population from which they were drawn. In other words, the children sampled should represent all socioeconomic, racial and ethnic, and dialectal variations found in the total population, and in the same proportions found there. Other variables that may be important include size of family, birth order, presence of one or both parents in the home, presence of natural parents in the home, and amount of schooling. Some variables, such as socioeconomic status, may be difficult to determine, although parental education and employment seem to be important contributing factors. Mixed-race children may force the researcher to make decisions about racial self-identity that are not appropriate. Other variables, such as birth order, may be more important than more traditional variables, such as gender (Bennett-Kaster, 1988).

Characteristics of the tester, experimenter, or conversational partner are also important. In general, preschool children will perform better with a familiar adult. There is also some indication that minority children may perform better with adults from the same minority group.

Some children found in the general population may be excluded when the study attempts to determine normal development. These may include children with known handicaps; bilingual children; twins, triplets, and other multiple births; and children in institutional care or full-time nursery school. Children may also be excluded who are likely to move during the course of the study or whose parents were deemed uncooperative or unreliable (Wells, 1985). For example, children with parents in the military are likely to move frequently, possibly prior to the completion of a longitudinal study. With each exclusion, the "normal" group becomes more restricted and, thus, less representative.

In order to draw group conclusions, subjects must be matched in some way. Although the most common way to group children is by age, such matching of subjects in language-development studies may be "fundamentally inappropriate" (Pine & Lieven, 1990). Many language differences reflect developmental changes in other areas. Therefore, reliable age-independent measures of development, such as level of cognitive development, may be a better gauge of real developmental differences and may allow more appropriate comparisons of children's language development.

The problem of the appropriate amount of the child's language to sample becomes especially critical with low-incidence elements. Usually at least 100 utterances are needed in order to have an adequate sample, although the sample size depends on the purpose for which it is collected. High reliability on measures such as number of different words, MLU, and mean sentence length in morphemes may require at least 175 complete and intelligible utterances (Gavin & Giles, 1996). Elements that occur less than once in 100 utterances may not occur within the typical sample of that length. In addition, a single occurrence is very weak evidence upon which to base an assumption that the child has this linguistic element within his or her repertoire. This assumption is strengthened, however, if a large proportion of the individuals being studied exhibit this linguistic element (Wells, 1985).

As mentioned, the amount of language collected will vary with the language feature being studied. Pragmatic aspects of language, which vary with the context, may require the inclusion of several contexts to provide an adequately varied sample. Such language uses as conversational openings, which occur only once in each conversation, would require varied contexts in order to allow the researcher to reach even tentative conclusions.

In general, the larger the sample of children and/or speech, the fewer data it is possible to analyze. Conversely, the more detailed the analysis, the fewer children or the smaller the amount of speech it is possible to sample. Resources such as personnel, time, and money are always limited. The linguist must decide on an appropriate sample size and an adequate level of analysis.

Naturalness and Representativeness of the Data

Any sample should fulfill the twin requirements of naturalness and representativeness. Even testing should attempt to use familiar situations with the child. The conversational sample will be more natural if the participants are free to move about and are uninhibited by the process of sample collection. A representative sample should include as many of the child's everyday experiences as possible. Unfortunately, little is known about the range and frequency of children's activities. To address this issue, Wells (1985) sampled randomly throughout the day for short periods.

Each day, Wells collected twenty-four randomly scheduled samples of ninety seconds' duration each. Samples were scheduled so that four occurred within each of six equal time periods throughout the day. Eighteen of the twenty-four samples, totaling twenty-seven minutes of recording, were needed for analysis. This allowed a possible 25 percent of the samples to be blank as a result of having been recorded while the child was beyond the range of the microphone's transmission. Two samples from each of the six time blocks were randomly chosen for transcription. After these had been transcribed, the process continued randomly with the remaining six samples until 120 intelligible utterances had been amassed. The remaining utterances were not transcribed for analysis. This procedure was followed once every three months for two years for each child.

As you can see, it is not always easy to obtain natural and representative language data. At least three potential factors may be problems (Wells, 1985). One problem is that of the "observer paradox" (Labov, 1972). Stated briefly, it is that the absence of an observer may result in uninterpretable data, but the presence of an observer may influence the language obtained, so that it lacks spontaneity and naturalness.

The presence of an observer can also affect the sample being collected. The behavior of the child and the conversational partner may be influenced by the presence of another person. For this reason, Wells (1985) collected samples on a tape recorder, with no observer present. The recorder was programmed to begin taping at randomly assigned times throughout the day. In contrast, R. Brown (1973) included two observers: one to keep a written transcript of the linguistic and nonlinguistic behaviors of the parent and child and the other to tend the tape recorder and to be a playmate for the child.

The absence of an observer may also complicate the process of determining the exact context of the language sample. At the end of each recording day, parents might be asked to identify contexts by the activity and participants present, although the reliability of such recalled information is doubtful (Wells, 1985). In addition, the immediate nonlinguistic context of each utterance cannot be reconstructed from audiotape alone.

A second problem is the child's physical and emotional state at the time the information is collected. Usually, the child's caregiver is asked to comment on the typicalness of the child's performance.

A third problem relates to the context in which the sample is collected. Occasionally, information is collected in experimental or test-type situations. The rationale for collecting this type of data is that through manipulation of the context, the linguist can obtain language features from the child that may not be elicited in conversation. Unfortunately, the language obtained is likely to be divorced from meaningful contexts in the child's experience and thus does not represent the child's use of language to communicate with familiar conversational partners in everyday contexts. Theoretically, the most representative sample should be elicited in the home for preschoolers and in the home or classroom for older children, with a parent, sibling, or teacher as the conversational partner.

Language samples should be representative in the two ways discussed previously. First, the population sample from which the language is collected should be representative of all aspects of the total population. Second, each child's language sample should be representative of his or her typical language performance. This is best ensured if the sample is collected in a variety of typical settings in which the child is engaged in everyday activities with his or her usual conversational partners.

Collection Procedures

Questions relative to collection of the language sample must of necessity concern the presence or absence of a researcher and the actual recording method. Wells (1985) attempted to minimize observer influences by having the child wear a microphone that transmitted to a tape recorder preprogrammed to record at frequent but irregular intervals throughout the day. Of course, there are problems with this process, such as the compactness and sensitivity of the microphone transmitter. In contrast, R. Brown (1973) used two researchers in the setting, while data were recorded on a tape recorder.

Several collection techniques exist, such as diary accounts, checklists, and parental report, as well as direct and taped observation. The first three are alternatives to researcher observation and have been used effectively in the study of early semantic and morphologic growth (Marchman & Bates, 1994; Reznick & Goldfield, 1994). Such methods enable researchers to collect from more children because they are less time-consuming and have been pronounced reliable and valid while remaining highly representative (Marchman & Bates, 1994).

Electronic means of collection seem essential for microanalysis. Videotaping, while more intrusive, is better than audiotaping alone, because it enables the researcher to observe the nonlinguistic elements of the situation in addition to the linguistic elements. Written transcription within the collection setting is the least desirable method for several reasons. First, it is easy to miss short utterances. Second, it is nearly impossible to transcribe the language of both the child and the conversational partner because of the large number of utterances within a short period of time. Third, transcription within the conversational setting does not enable the researcher to return to the child's speech for missed or misinterpreted utterances.

The language sample should be transcribed as soon after it is collected as possible. Caregivers familiar with the child's language should be consulted to determine if the sample is typical of the child's performance.

Analysis Procedures

Transcription may also be difficult. The result will vary with the playback unit used. Transcribers can check each other's work, but they must be careful not to be influenced by the initial transcript. It is best if two independent transcriptions are prepared and compared for discrepancies. The life experiences of each transcriber will affect expectations for various conversational samples and, thus, modify what each believes he or she hears.

Because transcription offers many opportunities for error, studies should ensure intratranscriber reliability. This is not always easy to accomplish. Many published studies either do not establish intratranscriber reliability or do not report it. Several factors contribute to transcription errors, including the type of speech sampled, the intelligibility of the child, the number of transcribers, the level of transcription comparison, and the experience of the transcriber(s) (Pye, Wilcox, & Siren, 1988). In general, the more defined the speech sampled, the better the intelligibility; the greater the number of transcribers, the larger the unit of comparison; and the more experienced the transcriber, the better the chance of having an accurate transcript. The type of speech sample may range from individual words to whole conversations. Larger units are more difficult to transcribe accurately. The use of more than one transcriber reduces the possibility of errors if the transcribers compare their transcriptions and resolve their differences in a consistent manner. Finally, lower levels of comparison, such as phonemes, increase the likelihood of error because of the precise nature of such units.

Actual analysis may be even more ticklish, especially when trying to determine the bases for that analysis. For example, MLU is still the most common measure of language growth, although its value is questionable. Numerical scores and measures, such as MLU, are inadequate for describing language development in detail. Other values might include total number of words or number of words per clause. Such values collapse data to a single figure. Breadth of behavior might be obtained by the number of different forms used by a child, such as number of different words and number of unique syntactic types (Hadley, 1999).

It is also difficult to determine when a child or group of children actually knows or has mastered a language feature. The criteria for establishing that a child knows a word or a feature have not been preestablished. For example, with word knowledge, the researcher must have clear evidence that a child comprehends the word. In contrast, production criteria would probably be based on spontaneous use and consistent semantic intent. With young children, the researcher would also note consistent phonetic form and semantic intent, with decisions of knowledge not necessarily based on whether the form and meaning are related to an adult word.

Usually, mastery can be based on children using a feature in 90 percent of the obligatory locations or on 90 percent of the children using the feature consistently, but these percentages vary with the researcher. Some researchers consider the average age for acquisition

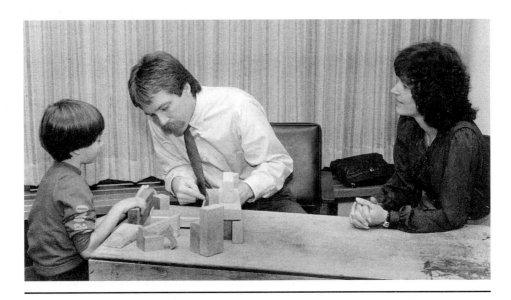

Child language studies attempt to describe the process of language development and to note linguistic differences and their effect on the process.

to be that at which 50 percent of children use a language feature consistently. Of course, such measures are complicated by the complex nature of most language features and the extended period of time often needed for mastery. As we have seen, forms such as passive voice may take several years from first appearance to full, mature use.

An example of one real-life analysis difficulty may be illustrative. In a study of preschool pronoun development (Haas & Owens, 1985), a colleague and I were very surprised to find no errors in pronoun use in conversations among children even as young as two. The children had adopted the rule *when in doubt, use a noun*. Thus, analysis that focused on pronouns yielded no errors. When analysis expanded beyond pronouns, however, we found overuse of nouns.

CROSS-LANGUAGE STUDIES

Cross-language studies are usually undertaken in order to investigate universality, linguistic specificity, relative difficulty, or acquisitional principles (Berman, 1986). Studies of universality attempt to determine which aspects of language, such as nouns and verbs, appear in all languages. One underlying question is the innateness and universality of linguistic processes.

Yes/no questions, for example, are treated differently in different languages. Positive questions, such as "Are you a dog?", are answered *yes* for a right or true proposition to express agreement and *no* for the opposite. In contrast, negative questions, such as "Aren't you a dog?", are answered in language-specific ways: as if positive in English and Spanish, on the truthfulness or falseness in French and German, and on agreement or disagreement in Japanese, Chinese, Korean, and Navajo (Akiyama, 1992). In all of these languages, however, children begin as in English and Spanish, suggesting an underlying process.

Studies of linguistic specificity attempt to determine whether development is the result of universal cognitive development or unique linguistic knowledge. The development of spatial and temporal terms, for example, seems to be based on cognitive temporal knowledge as well as on specific linguistic forms used to mark that knowledge. English uses *in* for containment and *on* for support. In contrast, Spanish uses *en* for both and German uses *auf, an,* and *um* just for *on*. In Chalcatongo Mixtec, an Otomanguecan language of Mexico, speakers use body parts for spatial terms, such as "The man is *animal-back* the house" for "The man is *on* the roof" and "The cat rug's *face*" for "The cat is *on* the rug" (Bowerman, 1993). While the English concepts *in* and *on* seem very straightforward, linguistic expression differs greatly.

Relative difficulty studies look for language-development differences that may be explained by the relative difficulty of learning structures and forms in different languages. For example, the passive sentence form is very difficult in English and is mastered much later than the relatively easier form in Egyptian Arabic, Turkish, Sesotho, and Zulu (Demuth, 1990; Perera, 1994). These languages are very different from each other, a situation that raises many other questions. Unlike Turkish, Sesotho, an African language, has a complex tonal grammatical system applied at the morphologic level (Demuth, 1993).

Finally, studies that investigate acquisitional principles try to find underlying language-learning strategies that children apply regardless of the language being acquired. The learning principles described in Chapter 7 are the result of this type of study.

There are two basic methods of collecting cross-linguistic data. The first is to gather a range of studies completed in different languages, although these studies may differ in their aims and methods (MacWhinney, 1978; Peters, 1983; Slobin, 1985). While this method may be quicker, because the studies have already been completed, it may not be easy to draw conclusions from such a diverse collection. The second method is to use a similar design across subjects from different language groups (Bates et al., 1984; Clark & Berman, 1984; Clark & Hecht, 1982; Mulford, 1983; Slobin, 1982). This method yields much more definitive data, with fewer complicating variables, but takes much more time and effort to organize, coordinate, and collect. This type of cross-linguistic study can be extremely difficult.

EXAMPLES OF CHILD LANGUAGE DATA

It might be helpful to examine a few child language samples and to comment on the language demonstrated in each. In this section, we shall examine the language of three children from monolingual, English-speaking homes. I have not included the entire sample, but rather one contiguous segment that is somewhat illustrative. Surface differences will be obvious.

The first segment (Table 14.1) was collected in the home and is a conversation between a twenty-two-month-old child and her mother. The overall MLU of the child, T.,

TABLE 14.1   Toddler Language Sample

What do you see?
1. Birthday cake Kelly house.
    A birthday cake at Kelly's house? What else was at Kelly's house?
2. Birthday cake mommy.
    Mommy had a birthday cake. What else did you have?
3. Kelly house.
    Kelly's house. Oh, look.
4. Color on the table.
    The man colored on the table. Well, that's all right. What are you making?
5. Doggie.
    Are you making a doggie?
6. Okay.
    All right. Oh, that's nice, T.
7. Where more doggie there?
    Is there another doggie underneath?
8. Yeah.
    Where can you find the picture? Is that what you're looking for, the picture of
    the doggie? Where's the doggie?
9. A doggie.
10. Color a doggie.
    Okay, you color the doggie.
11. Mommy color crayon.
    Mommy has crayons. Mommy's coloring. What's mommy making?
12. Doggie.
    A doggie?
13. Okay.
    All right, I'll make a doggie. Is this the doggie's tail?
14. The doggie's tail.
    Doggie's tail.
15. More.
    More doggie?
16. Okay.
    Can T. color? Hum?
17. More doggie there.
18. More doggie daddy.
    More doggie daddy?
19. Wants a more doggie.
20. More doggie.
21. Put more doggie there.
    Okay, you color doggie on this.

is approximately 1.9, placing her in the upper end of Brown's stage I. It should be noted that this MLU was calculated from two different situations. Although it has not been calculated, the mother's MLU is also low. The mother makes extensive use of imitation, expansion, and extension.

At first reading, it is obvious that the conversation is very concrete and concerned with the task of coloring. There is no great variety in the words used, and the child repeats these words frequently. The child engages in turn-taking and is very responsive. Many of the child's utterances, such as 9 and 14, are whole or partial imitations. The child has a wide range of illocutionary functions in the entire sample. Within this segment, she answers (1, 2, 3, 5, 8, 12) and asks questions (7), replies to her mother's utterances (4, 6, 13, 16), makes declarations (10, 18), gives directions to her mother (11, 17, 21), and makes demands (15, 19, 20).

The second segment (Table 14.2) was also collected in the home and is also a conversation between a child and her mother. The two are engaged in role play with a child's sink, table, and dishes. The mother's speech is complicated by her taking two roles: that of

TABLE 14.2   Early Preschool Language Sample

1. She wants some coffee.
    Oh, well, do you have a cup? Where's it at?
2. I don't know where in here.
    Well, just find a cup for her. This is her cereal.
3. Don't know where is it.
    Well, she can't have coffee.
4. Can't have coffee.
5. What's that?
    Coffee.
6. She have coffee?
    Okay. Do you want to feed her and I'll finish ironing?
7. Yeah.
    Okay. Boy, this iron gets hot.
8. What do you do?
    I burned myself.
9. Oh.
    I got burned.
10. Oh, let me . . .
11. No, it's not hot.
    Pshew.
12. It's coldy.
13. I touch it.
    Oh, I think it's hot. Feel it.
14. It's coldy.
    I think it's hot. Okay, the ironing's finished. What are you feeding her?

TABLE 14.2   Continued

15. The apple.
16. Michelle eat cereal.
    Gee, okay.
17. She wants some, some, some coffee.
    Oops.
18. That's her coffee.
    Okay, I'll pour some more. Oh, my goodness.
19. It's hot.
    I better put this back on the stove, don't you think?
20. Yeah, don't think.
    Where's the milk?
21. In the refrigerator.
    Okay, let me get some milk. There, got her bottle ready for you.
22. All right.
    Okay.
23. She eated it alldone.
24. She has to go sleep.
    She has to go to sleep. Well well, you better wipe her face.
25. Oh.
    Gee, J., you don't know what you're doing, do you?
26. Yeah.
    Oh, come here, Michelle. Oh, she's still hungry. Can you feed her some more?
27. She wants one that's good.
    Oh.
28. I fix.
    What are you fixing now?
29. I fixing her cereal.
    Oh, the poor little baby's so hungry. Don't you ever feed her?
30. Yeah.
    I think you need to buy her . . .
31. She want some bottle.

the baby, Michelle, and that of another person in the situation. The child, J., plays herself as the mother of Michelle. The adult uses turnabouts to a greater extent than the mother in the first segment. Expansion is very limited and occurs only after child utterance 24. The child is thirty-two months old, and her MLU from the larger sample is approximately 3.3. In general, the child is very responsive. As might be expected, her greater output of language compared to T. (Table 14.1) also demonstrates many more language features. Like T., J. has much variety in her language, and she initiates and responds to conversation.

Noun and verb phrases are present or understood in many utterances and have expanded with the use of articles, adjectives, and pronouns and auxiliary verbs, respectively. When expanded, noun phrases usually contain only one additional element, such as an article or adjective (*some*), but not both. The child demonstrates some of her own rule application in utterances 12 and 14, in which she uses the rule of adding *-y* to a noun to produce an adjective (*coldy*), and in 23, in which she places *-ed* on an irregular verb (*eated*). She also has some difficulty with the irregular verb *have* in 6, but not in 24. Auxiliary verbs are omitted in 13, 16, and 29. In addition, the third-person singular *-s* is used inconsistently (1, 17, 27, 31). As might be expected at this level of development, the child demonstrates some embedding of infinitive phrases in 24 (*to go*) but has not mastered this form, as noted in the same utterance [*(to) sleep*]. Her only embedded clauses are of the early object noun-phrase complement type seen in 3 (*where is it*) and a relative clause attached to the object in 27 (*that's good*). Number 3 demonstrates confusion with the *wh-* question form and the *wh-* embedded clause form. The child has some difficulty with the interrogative form (6, 18) and with the comprehension of tag questions (20).

The third segment (Table 14.3) is a conversation between two preschool children, M. and E., both forty-eight months of age. They are role-playing in an area of a preschool in which there is a child's kitchen. We shall concentrate on M.—the numbered utterances— whose MLU is approximately 5.1. The longer utterances, the imaginative use of language, and the frequent interruption of speakers are very evident. It's an enjoyable sample to read. The conversational behaviors of two preschool partners are not as organized as those of a preschooler and an adult.

M.'s noun phrases have been expanded to include a noun and an adjective in utterances 1 (*the other*) and 25 (*a real*), and M. has a much better command of auxiliary verbs than J., although she omits the auxiliary in 18 [*(are) just kidding*]. Most singular and plural nouns are used correctly, although an irregular, such as *leaf, leaves*, still offers some difficulty (25). Conjunctions appear, alone (19), at the beginning of utterances (9, 31), and in

TABLE 14.3 Late Preschool Language Sample

---

1. Oh, this almost looks like the other one.
2. See?
    But it has the same hat.
3. Hey, I'm gonna put the sticker right here, okay?
4. Put your stickers right here.
    So we can pretend these are the TV's.
5. Okay.
    I'm making dinner.
6. Oh, onions.
    Oh.
7. Oh, let me toast it.
    No way.
8. I'm gonna cook, okay?

TABLE 14.3   Continued

9. While you do your stuff, okay?
   > I'm toasting. I'm making a piece of bread.

10. I'm eating this bread.

11. Good bread.

12. I think I'm gonna go to work soon.

13. Get this orange out of here.
   > Honey . . .

14. What?

15. Let's get married now.

16. Just a place to get married . . . under the table.
   > We have to have our toast under. . . . You be married too. Don't touch me.

17. Mine.
   > No, you can touch me, you can touch me. I just kidding. . . .

18. I know you just kidding.
   > Why'd you say "bye"?

19. Because.

20. I said "bye." . . .
   > Here have a piece of bread.

21. I said "bye" just because . . . I said "bye" 'cause I had to go to work and you won't let me.

22. That's why.
   > Go to work, honey.

23. Mmmm.

24. It got real leaves.

25. This is a real leaves.

26. They're real leaves, you know?

27. See?
   > What? 'Cause they come off?

28. Uh-huh.

29. Wanna see?
   > Don't do it. You'll break their toys.

30. Mmmm, bye, I'm going to work.
   > Bye-bye. Pretend you came back with that hat on from work and I made you a piece of bread and put a piece of bread.

31. And I won't eat it.
   > Okay. When you came back from work, I'll give you a piece of bread.

32. Okay, then I won't eat it.

33. Bye.
   > Bye-bye, hon.

joining clauses (21). Several infinitive phrases are present, usually of the *gonna X* variety (3, 8, 12), but there are other forms as well (21). Prepositional phrase embedding is also evident in 16 (*under the table*), as well as clausal embedding, again of the object noun-phrase complement type, in 18 [*(that) you (are) just kidding*] and 26 [*(that) they're real leaves*]. This last utterance is very complex in that the statement would be *You know that they're real leaves* and must be changed considerably to form the question seen in 26.

These three samples offer great variety and demonstrate the differences in child language as children develop. It is much easier to comment on the behaviors demonstrated by a few children than it is to collect samples from a number of children in the hope of analyzing them definitively and extrapolating data about the language development of all children.

CONCLUSION

Complex topics such as language and language development require a great amount of study and research. If the data that result from such research are to be of value beyond the children from whom they were collected, researchers must consider a great variety of questions relative to the language features studied, the children selected, the amount of data, and the collection and analysis procedures. Describing child language development accurately is a difficult and time-consuming job.

DISCUSSION

Without linguistic research, this book could not exist. Look at the bibliography and you will get some idea of the range of this research. I have given you some of the issues in collection and analysis of linguistic data. Some of you may be interested in such research. We can always use new data, especially in other languages.

You may be interested in the research data collected by linguists and others who study child language. The Child Language Data Exchange System or CHILDES database contains information on child language, actual child language transcripts, and software tools for analysis. You can access this database at http://childes.psy.cmu.edu/.

REFLECTIONS

1. Explain the two primary methods of data collection and the types of data generated by each.

2. Explain the way in which language sample and population sample size and variability affect the data collected.

3. Why are natural and representative language samples desired, and what are the potential problems that can interfere with collecting these types of samples?

4. How can the method of collection affect the language sample collected?

5. Discuss the issues related to analysis that may affect the results of language studies.

6. Discuss the primary areas of investigation undertaken in cross-language studies.

15

Disorders and Development

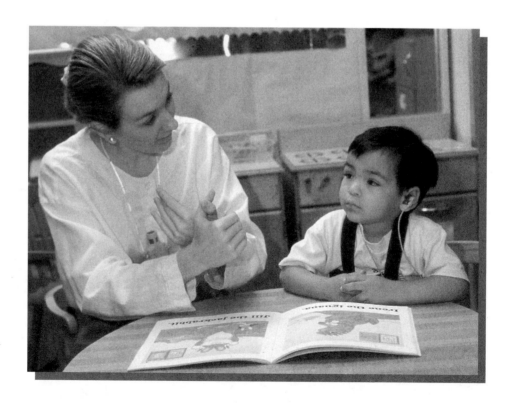

CHAPTER OBJECTIVES

When you have completed this chapter, you should be able to discuss the applicability of your knowledge of speech and language development to language disorders.

Not all children develop speech and language as outlined in the preceding chapters. Approximately 5 percent of the total population, including about 10 percent of the children in elementary school, have communication disorders of various types and severity. These range from the common /w/-for-/r/ articulation substitution—as in *wun* (/wʌn/) for *run*—to the lack of language use of children with severe autism.

> In addition to their disorder, affected individuals must also bear the stigma of difference. Even speech disorders considered minor and easily remediable . . . are apparently viewed as stigmatizing by large groups of listeners in the general public. . . . Speech, language, and hearing disorders which greatly reduce intelligibility of conversation and therefore limit the communicative exchange of thoughts and feelings are often met with outright public rejection and result in obvious social isolation. (Love, 1981, p. 486)

Communication disorders have traditionally been classified as organic, nonorganic, or combined in origin. Organic disorders have some physical origin, such as brain damage or hearing loss. Nonorganic causes include such things as faulty learning or environmental deprivation. In actual practice, most communication disorders have both organic and nonorganic origins. For example, cerebral palsy results from brain injury, an organic etiology, but may have nonorganic correlates. Suppose that a child with cerebral palsy has been allowed to communicate with grunts and gestures even though capable of short, spoken (albeit difficult-to-understand) phrases. His or her use of grunts and gestures reflects a combined origin.

Even seemingly obvious causes, such as various syndromes that result in mental retardation, usually do not produce strictly organic language disorders. Several factors, such as residence at home or in an institution and the type of language intervention, usually influence the rate and form of language development.

Some children may be language-delayed for various nonspecific or unknown reasons. Language-delayed children often show severe, broad impairments in all aspects of language. As these children mature, their deficits may become milder and more narrow. By sixty months, most of these children may seem to have overcome their earlier delay; however, lingering problems may be seen when these children begin to read (Scarborough & Dobrich, 1990). Other children, such as those with retardation or learning disabilities, may have serious language problems that persist in both breadth and severity. At present, the speech and language of many individuals with autism remains extremely impaired throughout their lives. Finally, adults with deafness, even those with a good education, may have language skills in English well below those expected for their chronological age.

Similar behaviors may also result from very different origins. For example, hypernasal or overly nasal speech may result from cleft palate or poor learning, to name just two of the many possible causes. Immature or delayed language acquisition may also result from causes as diverse as mental retardation and environmental deprivation. This situation is further complicated when we consider the higher incidence of mild mental retardation among lower socioeconomic groups than among the general population. The poor are also more likely to experience environmental deprivation, so the two causes may become combined.

Children with speech and language disorders are the special charge of the speech-language pathologist and, to a lesser extent, of the special education and resource teacher. These professionals often employ a developmental approach in remediation.

THE DEVELOPMENTAL APPROACH

Although not all communication disorders lend themselves to a developmental intervention strategy, a developmental approach seems most justifiable in the area of language disorder or delay. The speech-language pathologist should base intervention decisions, in part, on knowledge of language development. For individuals who are severely delayed or low-functioning, training may begin at a prelinguistic level, targeting the early social, communicative, cognitive, and perceptual skills outlined in Chapters 5 and 6 (Owens, 1982, 1995). It seems especially important to establish an early communication base for the delayed or disordered child (Reichle, 1990). With a knowledge of language development and its prerequisites, professionals do not need to wait until a child starts to speak before beginning intervention. Intervention should begin as soon as there is any indication of possible language delay or disorder. Infants with syndromes associated with delay or disorder, such as Down syndrome, should begin training shortly after birth in infant stimulation programs in order to achieve their potential in language skill development.

Early intervention is especially important for children with deafness and should emphasize language input. The hearing infant is exposed to thousands of brief verbal interactions before he or she produces the first meaningful word. In contrast, the child with deafness misses much of this prelinguistic interaction that is so important for later language development. Early use of signs, gestures, and speech could help establish a communication base for this child.

For children with autism or retardation, an environmental approach to communication training that includes the child's conversational partners and contexts seems justified (Nietupski, Scheutz, & Ockwood, 1980; Owens, 1982, 1995). An isolated therapy model is not sufficient. All those who interact with the child are potential language trainers. In addition, conversational approaches may result in avoidance of the stereotypic responsive behavior observed in many children with autism. Unfortunately, many language training programs seem to assume that spontaneous communication will naturally emerge from receptive and expressive training that is primarily responsive. Language training should occur within a communication framework.

Once a child begins to use language expressively, the knowledgeable clinician can select training targets based on normal language development. In addition to first words, semantic and illocutionary functions of early language may be targeted (Owens, 1982,

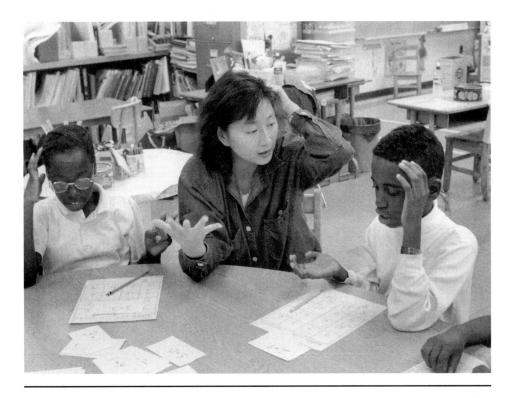

Language development knowledge can act as a guide for speech-language pathologists and others concerned with children's development.

1995). Prutting (1979) has suggested a stage approach to training that follows the guidelines of normal development. The child progresses from one developmental stage to the next.

Not all professionals support a developmental intervention strategy, especially stage proposals such as Prutting's. While pronouncing the developmental intervention model "basically sound," Winitz (1983) contended that it is "generally used incorrectly" (p. 26). According to Winitz, the basic premises of the developmental approach are that intervention should begin at the lowest level of functioning and should continue within that level and succeeding ones until the client demonstrates expertise in all aspects of language associated with that level. He contended that testing measures achievement rather than underlying rule systems. Therefore, programming reflects "age points at which mastery has been achieved, but does not indicate successive points in a learning sequence" (p. 32). Language learning is not a linear process. Winitz concluded: "Developmental language profiles should . . . serve as a guide for the 'emphasis' of certain structures and, perhaps, the avoidance of others. However, these profiles should not be used as a fixed set of sequences from which the clinician cannot deviate" (p. 33).

It would be a gross misuse of the developmental model to assume that children will all follow in the same lockstep sequence. Language intervention should be individualized. Each child with language impairment must be considered in terms of his or her own communicative context and needs.

Age-related developmental data, such as those supplied within this text, can supplement the intervention data from the child with language impairment (Chapman & Miller, 1980). Behavioral descriptions from different stages can be used to aid intervention planning. This information can provide a rationale for individual programming decisions.

In short, normal development is a guide for language remediation and assessment. Language benchmarks can alert parents and professionals to expected behaviors and to the approximate point in development when a behavior usually appears. In addition, normal development can provide direction for training those children who are not developing normally.

Normal development is not the only intervention guide, but it is one of the most useful. A teacher or speech-language pathologist must rely on many sources of information and "should be a behaviorist, a pragmatist, a cognitivist, a linguist, a developmentalist, and an optimist in order to put together an effective means of teaching language to children" (Schiefelbusch, 1978, p. 461). I hope this text has provided a basis for your own development of some of these skills.

Appendix

American English Speech Sounds

The smallest unit of speech is the phoneme. It consists of a family of sounds that are close enough in perceptual qualities to be distinguished from other phonemes. Thus, although phonemes are meaningless, they make semantic difference in actual use. For example, the final sounds in *kiss* and *kick* are perceptually different enough to alert the listener to differences in meaning. Recognition of this distinction could be crucial, especially on a first date. Phonemes are written between slashes (as in /s/) to distinguish them from the alphabet. The International Phonetic Alphabet (IPA) is used rather than the English alphabet for two reasons. First, a sound may be spelled several ways, as in g*o*, r*ow*, h*oe*, and th*ough*. In contrast, some letters, such as *c*, can be pronounced more than one way (as *s* or *k*). Similarly, the *o* in *comb* differs from the one in *come*. Second, the pronunciation of the English alphabet cannot be applied to other languages. Although French uses an identical alphabet, the pronunciation of the individual letters is quite different.

The actual sound produced by a speaker at a given time is called a **phone**, and no two phones are alike. Phones may be grouped perceptually as **allophones**, but even allophones may differ slightly. For example, the /p/ in *stop* may or may not be accompanied by a puff of air, or aspiration. The /p/ sound in *spot* is not aspirated. These two allophones are similar enough, however, to be classified as the phoneme /p/. A phoneme is thus made up of a group of allophones. As speakers of English, we have no difficulty recognizing the phonemic variations in *pop*, *pot*, *top*, and *tot*. Many English words differ by only one consonant or vowel. Consider *bet*, *get*, *let*, *met*, *net*, *pet*, *set*, *vet*, and *wet* or *bat*, *bet*, *bit*, and *but*. Perception of the different phonemes is extremely important for interpretation.

Each spoken language employs particular phonemes. In English, these sounds are classified as vowels or consonants. The distinction is based mainly on sound production characteristics. Vowels are produced with a relatively unrestricted air flow in the vocal tract. Consonants require a closed or narrowly constricted passage that results in friction and air turbulence. The number of phonemes attributed to American English differs with the classification system used and the dialect of the speaker. In this text we discuss forty-five phonemes—twenty-one vowels and twenty-four consonants.

Phonemes can be described as being voiced or voiceless. **Voiced phonemes** are produced by phonation, or vibration, at the vocal folds of the larynx; **voiceless phonemes** are produced without vibration. All vowels in English are voiced; consonants may be either voiced or voiceless.

Two classification systems are currently used for English phonemes. The more traditional approach emphasizes the phoneme and classifies each according to place or manner of articulation. In contrast, the second, called the *distinctive feature approach*, emphasizes the characteristics or constituents of each phoneme.

TRADITIONAL PHONEMIC CLASSIFICATION

Traditional classification of English phonemes is based on the locus or place of articulation, usually the position of the tongue; and additionally, for consonants, on the manner of articulation, usually the type of release of air. Vowels are classified by the highest arched portion of the tongue and by the presence or absence of lip rounding. Consonants can be described by the site of articulation, by the manner of articulation, and by the presence or absence of voicing.

Vowels

Vowels can be described in terms of tongue height and front-to-back positioning (Schane, 1973). Heights can be characterized as close, close-mid, open-mid, or open, depending on the position of the highest portion of the tongue and on lip closure. The location of this high point within the mouth can be described as front, central, or back. For example, a vowel can be described as close front, or open back, or any position in between. The English vowels are displayed graphically by position in Figure A.1. Words using each sound are printed next to each phoneme.

Lip rounding is an additional descriptive term used in vowel classification. During lip rounding, the lips protrude slightly, forming an O shape. Rounding is characteristic of some, but not all, back vowels, such as the last sound in *construe*. In contrast, there is no lip rounding in *construct*.

One group of vowel-like sounds is more complex than the single-vowel phonemes. These sounds are called *diphthongs*. A **diphthong** is a blend of two vowels within the same syllable. In other words, the sound begins with one vowel and glides smoothly toward another position. When the word *my* is repeated slowly, the speaker can feel and hear the shift from one vowel to another.

Consonants

Consonant sounds are somewhat more complex than vowel sounds. They are described by their manner of articulation, place of articulation, and voicing (Table A.1). *Manner* refers to the type of production, generally with respect to the release of air. The six generally recognized categories of manner are:

FIGURE A.1   Classification of English Vowels by Tongue Position

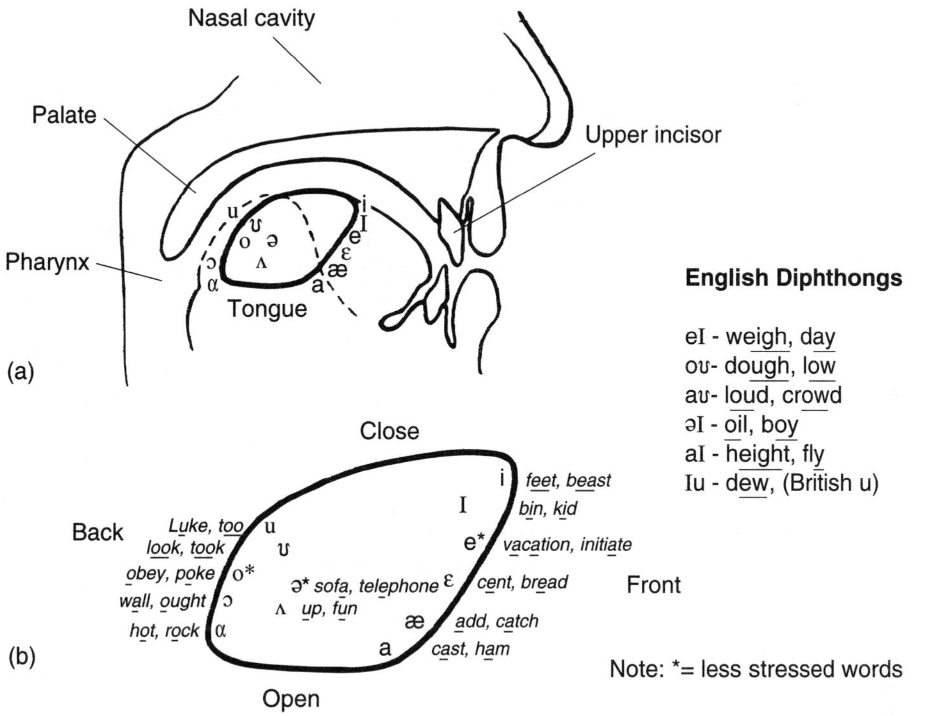

English Diphthongs

eI - we<u>igh</u>, d<u>ay</u>
oʊ- d<u>ough</u>, l<u>ow</u>
aʊ- l<u>oud</u>, cr<u>ow</u>d
ɔI - <u>oil</u>, b<u>oy</u>
aI - h<u>eight</u>, fl<u>y</u>
Iu - d<u>ew</u>, (British u)

Note: *= less stressed words

- Plosive (/p/, /b/, /t/, /d/, /k/, /g/)—Complete obstruction of the airstream, with quick release accompanied by an audible escape of air; similar to an explosion.
- Fricative (/f/, /v/, /θ/, /ð/, /s/, /z/, /ʃ/, /ʒ/, /h/)—Narrow constriction through which the air must pass, creating a hissing noise.
- Affricative (/tʃ/, /dʒ/)—A combination that begins with a plosive followed by a fricative, as the IPA symbols suggest.
- Approximant (/w/, /j/, /ɹ/)—Produced by the proximity of two articulators without turbulence.
- Lateral approximant (/l/)—Produced is similar manner to an approximant with the addition of the lateral flow of the airstream.
- Nasal (/m/, /n/, /ŋ/)—Oral cavity closed to exiting air but velum lowered to allow breath to exit via the nasal cavity. Variations result from constriction within the oral cavity.

The *locus* or place of articulation varies across the six manner categories and describes the position where the maximum constriction occurs. Constriction may be partial or complete. The seven locations are:

- Bilabial (/p/, /b/, /m/)—Lips together.
- Labiodental (/f/, /v/)—Lower lip touches upper incisors.
- Dental (/θ/, /ð/)—Tongue tip protruding slightly between the lower and upper incisors.
- Alveolar (/t/, /d/, /s/, /z/, /l/, /ɹ/, /n/)—Front of tongue to upper alveolar (gum) ridge.
- Postalveolar (/ʃ/, /ʒ/, /j/)—Tongue blade gently approximates postalveolar ridge area.
- Palatal (/tʃ/, /dʒ/)—Tongue blade raised to hard palate.
- Velar (/k/, /g/, /ŋ/)—Back of tongue raised to soft palate or velum.
- Glottal (/h/)—Restriction at glottis or opening to larynx.

Three sounds are considered combinations because of their location or movement during production. These are /tʃ/, /dʒ/, and /w/.

Many pairs of English consonant sounds differ only in voicing. When two phonemes have the same manner and place of articulation but differ in voicing, they are called **cognates**. For examples, the /f/ and /v/ phonemes are cognates. If you repeat the words *face* and

TABLE A.1   Traditional Classification of English Consonants

	MANNER OF PRODUCTION						
PLACE OF CONSTRICTION	**PLOSIVE** U	V	**FRICATE** U	V	**APPROXIMANT**[†] V	**LATERAL APPROXIMANT**	**NASAL**[†] V
Bilabial	p (pig)	b (big)			w (watt)		m (sum)
Labiodental			f (face)	v (vase)			
Dental			θ (thigh, thin)	ð (thy, this)			
Alveolar	t (tot)	d (dot)	s (seal)	z (zeal)	ɹ (rot)	l (lot)	n (sun)
Postalveolar			ʃ (shoe, mission)	ʒ (visual, measure)	j (yacht)		
Palatal			tʃ (choke, nature)	dʒ (joke, gentle)			
Velar	k (coat)	g (goat)					ŋ (sung)
Glottal			h (happy)				

U = unvoiced; V = voiced.

[†]All voiced.

vase, you can feel the difference at the level of the larynx. The place and manner of articulation do not differ. All English plosives, and fricatives, except /h/, are organized in voiced and voiceless pairs.

You should be aware that the voicing distinction is indefinite. This problem can be explained by **voice onset time** (VOT), which is the interval between the burst of a plosive and the commencement of phonation. In other words, no English plosives are truly voiceless; rather, they have a delayed VOT. The VOT is usually less than thirty milliseconds for voiceless plosives. The mean delay is 58 milliseconds for /p/ and 70 milliseconds for /t/ (Lisker & Abramson, 1965).

Theoretically, speech sounds could be produced in almost any tongue position and in all configurations of manner, placing, and voicing. Other languages use some of the phonemes of English, plus additional speech sounds, even some with other production characteristics. Some English distinctions are not present in other languages. In Spanish there is no distinction between /s/ and /z/; they are not separate phonemes. Other languages make finer distinctions. In Zulu, meaning is often differentiated by the degree of aspiration, or breathiness, of a sound. Thus, there are different varieties of /t/, /k/, and /p/ that are not relevant to speakers of English (and are difficult for those speakers to distinguish).

DISTINCTIVE FEATURE CLASSIFICATION

The distinctive feature approach to the study of speech sounds is an attempt to break phonemes into smaller analytic units. A phoneme's **distinctive features** are the significant acoustic or articulatory characteristics that distinguish it from other phonemes. There are several theoretical classification systems based on acoustic (Jakobson, Fant, & Halle, 1951), articulatory (N. Chomsky & Halle, 1968), and perceptual characteristics (Singh, Woods, & Becker, 1972). Some systems are binary, noting merely the presence or absence of a feature, while others are scaled, noting the strength of the feature on a continuum.

In general, the greater the agreement on distinctive features between two phonemes, the more alike the phonemes. Thus, common features describe the relationship between two phonemes. Table A.2 displays the Chomsky and Halle (1968) classification system. Note the similarity between sounds such as /t/ and /d/ and between /s/ and /z/. In contrast, /n/ and /l/ are very dissimilar.

Although helpful in analysis, distinctive-feature classification systems are abstractions. There is little indication that the features noted have any psychological reality for children, nor do these features tend to spread rapidly to all affected phonemes.

SOUNDS IN SPEECH

Although we can describe English speech sounds in isolation, they rarely occur alone in actual use. Plosives cannot be produced in isolation but must be combined with some other phoneme. Speech is a dynamic process in which individual sounds are seldom treated as discrete units. Movement patterns for more than one sound may occur simultaneously, their features overlapping (MacNeilage, 1970). This co-occurrence of production characteristics

TABLE A.2 English Consonants Including the Glottal Stop by Chomsky-Halle Extended Features

CONSONANTS

FEATURES	k	q	t	d	p	b	f	v	θ	ð	s	z	ʃ	ʒ	tʃ	dʒ	m	n	ŋ	l	ɹ	h	w	j	?
Vocalic	–	–	–	–	–	–	–	–	–	–	–	–	–	–	–	–	–	–	–	+	+	–	–	–	–
Consonantal	+	+	+	+	+	+	+	+	+	+	+	+	+	+	+	+	+	+	+	+	+	–	–	–	–
High	+	+	–	–	–	–	–	–	–	–	–	–	+	+	+	+	–	–	+	–	–	–	+	+	–
Back	+	+	–	–	–	–	–	–	–	–	–	–	–	–	–	–	–	–	+	–	–	–	+	–	–
Low	–	–	–	–	–	–	–	–	–	–	–	–	–	–	–	–	–	–	–	–	–	+	–	–	+
Anterior	–	–	+	+	+	+	+	+	+	+	+	+	–	–	–	–	+	+	–	+	–	–	–	–	–
Coronal	–	–	+	+	–	–	–	–	+	+	+	+	+	+	+	+	–	+	+	+	+	–	–	–	–
Round																							+	–	–
Tense																							–	–	
Voice	–	+	–	+	–	+	–	+	–	+	–	+	–	+	–	+	+	+	+	+	+	–	+	+	–
Continuant	–	–	–	–	–	–	+	+	+	+	+	+	+	+	–	–	–	–	–	+	+	+	+	+	+
Nasal	–	–	–	–	–	–	–	–	–	–	–	–	–	–	–	–	+	+	+	–	–	–	–	–	–
Strident	–	–	–	–	–	–	+	+	–	–	+	+	+	+	+	+	–	–	–	–	–	–	–	–	–

Blank   =   not relevant.
  –   =   binary feature not present.
  +   =   binary feature present.

- *Vocalic*—Constriction in the oral cavity is not greater than required for the high vowels /i, u/.
- *Consonantal*—The sound is made with a radical constriction in the midsagittal region of the oral cavity.
- *High*—The body of the tongue is elevated above the neutral position.
- *Back*—The body of the tongue retracts from the neutral position.
- *Low*—The body of the tongue is lowered below the neutral position.
- *Anterior*—The sound is produced further forward in the mouth than /ʃ/.
- *Coronal*—The sound is produced with the blade of the tongue raised from the neutral position.
- *Round*—The lip orifice is narrowed.
- *Tense*—The sound is produced deliberately, accurately, and distinctly.
- *Voice*—During the production of the sound, the larynx vibrates periodically.
- *Continuant*—The vocal tract is partially constricted during the production of the sound.
- *Nasal*—The velopharyngeal valve is sufficiently open during the production of the sound to permit the air-sound stream to be directed through the nose.
- *Strident*—The air stream is directed over a rough surface in such a way as to produce an audible noise.

Source: R. Owens, Jr., "Communication, Language, and Speech," in G. Shames & E. Wiig, *Human Communication Disorders: An Introduction*, Columbus, Ohio: Merrill Publishing Co., 1986, p. 41. Reprinted with permission. 2nd ed.

of two or more phonemes is called *coarticulation*. **Coarticulation** is the result of the motor commands from the brain and the mechanical response of the speech muscles. As a good organizer, the brain sends movement and position commands in advance of the actual occurrence in an utterance. Through high speed X-ray studies, we can demonstrate that movement may occur several phonemes prior to the appearance of the phoneme associated with this movement (Daniloff & Moll, 1968). For example, in the word *construe*, lip rounding begins well before the /u/ sound. You can see this movement with the aid of a mirror. These anticipatory movements are a clear indication that the brain is not functioning on a phoneme level but rather with larger organizational units. The type of coarticulation demonstrated by anticipatory movements is called *anticipatory*, or *forward*, *coarticulation*.

In any mechanical system, including the speech mechanism, there is also some built-in inertia, or drag. Muscle movements lag behind brain commands and continue after the commands have ceased. The result is that the production characteristics of one phoneme may persist during production of a following phoneme. The nasalization of the /z/ in *runs* (/rʌnz/) is caused by the insufficient time available for the velum to return to its upward position after /n/. This type of coarticulation is called *carryover*, or *backward*, *coarticulation*.

Glossary

Accommodation   Process of reorganizing cognitive structures or schemes or creating new schemes in response to external stimuli that do not fit into any available scheme. Piagetian concept.

Account   A type of narrative in which the speaker relates a past experience in which the listener did not share.

Action relational words   Words that define the manner in which objects are related through movement; semantic category.

Adaptation   Process by which an organism adapts to the environment; occurs as a result of two complementary processes, assimilation and accommodation. Piagetian concept.

Adjective   A syntactic unit used to modify a noun, including possessive nouns (*mom's*), ordinals (*first*), adjectives (*blue, old*), and descriptors (*shopping center*).

Adverb   A syntactic unit used to modify a word or phrase other than a noun or pronoun, such as a verb (ran *quickly*), an adjective (*extremely* old man), another adverb (*very* quickly), or a whole clause (*Obviously* you do not understand). Adverbs may indicate the time (*later, today, previously*), place (*here*), manner (*quietly, slowly*), or degree (*overly, last*).

Agent   Semantic class of words that labels entities that cause or are the source of action.

Allophone   Perceptual grouping of phones of similar speech sounds. Together form a phoneme.

Anaphoric reference   Grammatical mechanism that notifies the listener that the speaker is referring to a previous reference. Pronouns are one type of word used in anaphoric reference.

Angular gyrus   Association area of the brain, located in the posterior portion of the temporal lobe, responsible for linguistic processing, especially word recall.

Antonyms   A word that differs only in the opposite value of a single important feature.

Archiform   One member of a word class used to the exclusion of all others. For example, *a* may be used for all articles or *he* for all third-person pronouns.

Arcuate fasciculus   White, fibrous tract of axons and dendrites underlying the angular gyrus in the brain. Language is organized in Wernicke's area and transmitted through the arcuate fasciculus to Broca's area.

Article   A syntactic unit that precedes a noun or noun equivalent, marking definite (*the*) or indefinite (*a, an*) references or new (*a, an*) or old (*the*) information.

Articulation   Dynamic process of producing speech sounds by movement of speech organs and the resultant modification of the laryngeal tone.

Aspect   The dynamics of an event, noted by the verb, relative to the event's completion, repetition, or continuing duration.

Assimilation   Process by which external stimuli are incorporated into existing cognitive structures or schemes. Piagetian concept.

Associative complex hypothesis   Theory that each example of a meaning category shares something with a core concept. In other words, there are common elements in the meanings of *pants, shirt, shoes,* and *hat* that classify each as clothing. Vygotskyan concept.

Attribution relational words   Words that mark the attributes, characteristics, or differences between two objects; semantic category.

Auxiliary verb   A "helping" or nonprimary verb used to form tenses (*do* want, *did* read, *am* going, *was* eating, *have been* running) and to express mood or intention (*can, could, may, might, must, shall, should*). The latter type are called **modals** or modal auxiliary verbs.

Babbling   Long strings of sounds that children begin to produce at about four months of age.

Bilingual   Fluent in two languages; uses two languages on a daily basis.

Bootstrapping   Process of learning language in which the child uses what he or she knows to decode more mature language. For example, the child may use semantic knowledge to aid in decoding and learning syntax.

Bound morpheme   Meaning unit that cannot occur alone but must be joined to a free morpheme; generally includes grammatical tags or markers that are derivational, such as *-ly*, *-er*, or *-ment*, or inflectional, such as *-ed* or *-s*.

Bracketing   Process of breaking a speech stream into analyzable units by detecting end points or divisions through the use of intonational cues.

Broca's area   Cortical area of the left frontal lobe of the brain responsible for detailing and coordinating the programming of speech movements.

Case   A distinct semantic role such as *agent* or *location*.

Centering   The linking of entities in a narrative to form a story nucleus. Links may be based on similarity or complementarity of features, sequence, or causality.

Central nervous system (CNS)   Portion of the nervous system consisting of the brain and spinal cord.

Cephalocaudal   Head-to-foot developmental progression.

Cerebrum   Upper brain, consisting of the cortex and the subcortical structures.

Chaining   Narrative form consisting of a sequence of events that share attributes and lead directly from one to another.

Clause   Group of words containing a subject and the accompanying verb; used as a sentence (independent clause) or attached to an independent clause (dependent clause).

Clustering   Process of breaking speech stream into analyzable units based on predictability of syllables and phoneme structures.

Coarticulation   Co-occurrence of the characteristics of two or more phonemes as one phoneme influences another in perception or in production; may be forward (anticipatory) or backward (carryover).

Code switching   Process of varying between two or more languages.

Cognates   Phoneme pairs that differ only in voicing; manner and place of articulation are similar. For example, /f/ and /v/ are cognates, as are /s/ and /z/.

Cognitive determinism   Theoretical construct that considers linguistic content to reflect the developmental order of cognitive structures.

Cognitive stimulation   Process of providing stimuli for comparison to stored referents, thus requiring evaluation and comparison.

Communication   Process of encoding, transmitting, and decoding signals in order to exchange information and ideas between the participants.

Communication competence   Degree of success in communicating, measured by the appropriateness and effectiveness of the message.

Communication functions   Uses or purposes of communication, such as requesting information or replying.

Complex sentence   Sentence consisting of a main clause and at least one subordinate clause.

Compound sentence   Sentence consisting of two or more main clauses.

Conjoining   Joining two or more main clauses with a conjunction.

Conjunction   A syntactic unit used to connect words, phrases, or clauses, such as *and, but, or, if, so, since, because, therefore, though, although*, and so on.

Consonant cluster reduction   Phonological process seen in preschool children in which one or more consonants are deleted from a cluster of two or more (/tɹ, stɹ, sl, kɹ/) in order to simplify production.

Constituent   Unit, or component, of a sentence.

Contingent query   Request for clarification, such as "What?" or "Huh?"

Convergent semantic production   Process of recalling or producing a unique semantic unit, such as a word, phrase, or sentence, to fit a given linguistic restriction, such as the meaning of a stimulus. For example, convergent abilities are needed in completing crossword puzzles.

Copula   Form of the verb *to be* as a main verb. Signifies a relationship between the subject and a predicate adjective (*fat, tired, young*) or another noun (*teacher, farmer, pianist*).

Corpus callosum   Main transverse tract of neurons running between the two hemispheres of the brain.

Cortex   Outermost gray layer of the brain, made up of neuron cell bodies.

Count noun   A noun that can be singular (*cat*) or plural (*cats*), regular (*dog–dogs*) or irregular (*woman–women*) and can be preceded by a numerical term (two *rabbits*) or by *many* (many *cars*).

Creole   Grammar and structure from two or more languages used as a single language system. Usually follows development of a pidgin.

Critical period   Hypothesized period, prior to age five, in which language learning must occur.

Decentration   Process of moving from one-dimensional descriptions of entities and events to coordinated multiattributional ones.

Deep structure   Basic structure or meaning that underlies a sentence; generated through the use of phrase-structure rules. Chomskyan concept.

Deficit approach   Notion that only one dialect of a language is inherently correct or standard and that others are substandard or exhibit some deficit.

Deictic gaze   Gaze directed at a referent rather than a communication partner.

Deixis   Process of using the speaker's perspective as a reference. For example, deixis can be seen in words such as *this, that, here, there, me,* and *you.*

Demonstratives   Articles that indicate, from the speaker's perspective, to which entity the speaker is referring. Examples include *this, that, these,* and *those.*

Dialect   Language rule system of an identifiable group that varies from the rule system of an ideal standard.

Diminutive   Form of the noun used to denote that it refers to something small, as in *dog–doggie,* and *cat–kittie.*

Diphthong   Vowel-like speech sound produced by blending two vowels within a syllable.

Direct object   A noun or noun equivalent, such as a phrase or clause, that answers the question What? or Whom? following a transitive verb [He threw the *ball* (noun). She likes *to fish* (infinitive phrase). I know *where you went* (clause).]. Direct objects receive or are affected by the action of the verb.

Distancing   Gradual increase in the perceptual distance of infants and the accompanying shift from the senses of touch, taste, and smell to vision and hearing.

Distinctive features   Significant acoustic or articulatory characteristics of a phoneme that distinguish it from other phonemes.

Divergent semantic production   Process of recalling or producing a variety of words, phrases, or sentences on a topic. Divergent semantic abilities give language its originality, flexibility, and creativity.

Echolalia   Immediate, whole or partial vocal imitation of another speaker; characterizes the child's speech beginning at about eight months.

Ellipsis   Conversational device of omitting redundant information. For example, when asked "Who saw the movie?" we reply "I did," not "I saw the movie."

Embedded *wh-* question   Object noun-phrase complement using a *wh-* word as a connector for the dependent clause.

Embedding   Placing a phrase or dependent clause within a phrase or clause.

Epenthesis   Process of inserting a vowel sound where none is required.

Equilibrium   State of cognitive balance or harmony between incoming stimuli and cognitive structures. Piagetian concept.

Event structure   Set of event sequences including the events, relationships and relative significance.

Eventcast   A type of narrative that explains some current or anticipated event. Eventcasts often accompany the play of young children.

Evocative utterance   Toddler language-learning strategy in which the child names an entity and awaits adult evaluative feedback as to the correctness of the name or label.

Expansion   Adult's more mature version of a child utterance that preserves the word order of the original child utterance. For example, when a child says "Doggie eat," an adult might reply, "The doggie is eating."

Extension   Adult's semantically related comment on a topic established by a child. For example, when a child says "Doggie eat," an adult might reply, "Yes, doggie hungry."

Extinction   Behavioral concept of removing all reinforcement until a behavior decreases or ceases.

Fast mapping   Word-learning strategy in which the child infers a connection between a word and its referent after only one exposure.

Figurative language   Expressions that use words or phrases in an impression or represent an abstract concept; cannot be interpreted literally. For example, "My father *hit the roof*" cannot be explained at a syntactic level. Types of figurative language include idioms, metaphors, similes, and proverbs.

Fissure   A valley, or depression (also called a *sulcus*), between two gyri on the surface, or cortex, of the brain.

Formula   Memorized verbal routine or unanalyzed chunk of language often used in everyday conversation.

Free alternation   Variable use of members of a word class without consideration of different meanings. For example, *the* and *a* may be used randomly.

Free morpheme   Meaning unit that can occur alone, such as *dog, chair, run,* and *fast.*

Fully resonant nuclei (FRN)   Vowel-like sounds that are fully resonated laryngeal tones.

Functional-core hypothesis   Theory that word meanings represent dynamic relationships, such as actions or functional uses, rather than static perceptual traits. Concept usually associated with Nelson.

Genderlect   The style of talking used by men and women.

Gerund   A verb (*swim*) plus *-ing* that functions as a noun in the subject (*Swimming* is great exercise) or object (I like *swimming*) position of a sentence or as the object of a preposition (By *swimming* for shore, he saved himself). Gerunds can be modified by adjectives (graceful *swimming*) or adverbs (*swimming* gracefully).

Government-binding theory   Linguistic theory that attempts to describe the way in which the human mind represents an autonomous system of language that is diverse and flexible and yet learned from limited input.

Grammars   Systems of rules or underlying principles that describe the five aspects of language.

Gyrus (Plural **gyri**)   Hill between two fissures, or sulci, on the surface, or cortex, of the brain.

Habituation   Expectation of occurrence formed for frequently occurring stimuli. Habituation is one method of testing infants' perceptions of changing stimuli.

Heschl's gyrus   Area located in the auditory cortex of each hemisphere of the brain that receives incoming auditory signals from the inner ear.

Hypothesis-testing utterance   Toddler language-learning strategy in which the child seeks confirmation of the name of an entity by naming it with rising intonation, thus posing a yes/no question.

Idiom   Short, figurative expression, such as *blow your mind, hit the roof,* or *split my sides.*

Illocutionary force   Speaker's intention or attitude toward his or her utterance.

Index   Shared property of a motor act that indicates recognition by an infant.

Indicating   Following a line of regard by commenting. Mothers follow their infant's line of regard and comment on the object or event that is the focus of the child's attention.

Indirect object   A noun or noun equivalent that is indirectly affected by the verb in that the action is performed for the indirect object (Give the notes to *her.* She gave *me* a gift.). Indirect objects usually are preceded by or can be rewritten to be preceded by *for* or *to.*

Infinitive   A verb (*swim*) preceded by *to* that functions as a noun (I love *to swim. To swim* is such a joy.) and occasionally as an adjective (I have a project *to finish.*) or adverb (She worked *to become* a teacher.). The *to* may be omitted following certain words, such as *help, dare,* and *let* (He helped *fix* my bike. We dared not *tell* our secret. Let's *go* now.).

Information processing   Theoretical model of brain function that stresses methods employed in dealing with information.

Integrative rehearsal   Use of repetition or rehearsal to transfer information to long-term memory. Information-processing concept.

Interlanguage   Transitional system in which a person uses rules from two or more languages simultaneously.

Interrogative utterance   Toddler language-learning strategy in which the child attempts to learn the name of an entity by asking *What?, That?,* or *Wassat?.* Not to be confused with adultlike interrogative sentences, which are more varied (*what, where, who, why, how, when*).

Intransitive verb   A verb that does not take a direct object (I *waited* quietly for hours) and is not able to be made passive.

Irregular past-tense verb   A verb that takes a marker other than the *-ed* past-tense marker (*eat–ate, stand–stood, throw–threw*).

Jargon   Strings of unintelligible speech sounds with the intonational pattern of adult speech.

Joint action   Shared action sequences of mother and child, often routines. Provide basis for many scripts.

Joint (shared) reference   Process of differentiating or noting a particular object, action, or event for the purpose of communication.

Language   Socially shared code or conventional system for representing concepts through the use of arbitrary symbols and rule-governed combinations of those symbols.

Larynx   Anatomical structure that surmounts the trachea and houses the vocal folds. Made of several separate cartilaginous elements, the larynx's primary function is to protect the lungs from the entrance of foreign material.

Lexicon Individual dictionary of each person containing words and the underlying concepts of each. The lexicon is dynamic, changing with experience.

Linguistic competence Native speaker's underlying knowledge of the rules for generating and understanding conventional linguistic forms.

Linguistic determinism Theory that language determines thought; all higher thought is dependent upon language. Whorf hypothesis.

Linguistic performance Actual language use, reflecting linguistic competence and the communication constraints.

Linguistic relativism Theory that the experiences of speakers of different languages vary; that groups with the same language think in the same manner. Whorf hypothesis.

Location relational words Words that define the geographic, physical, directional, or spatial relationship of two objects; semantic category.

Main clause Clause within a multiclause sentence that can occur alone.

Mass noun Noun referring to homogeneous, nonindividual substances (*water, sand, sugar, salt, milk*) that cannot take a numerical term (*one, 300*). Unlike count nouns, mass nouns take *much* (*much sand*) rather than *many*.

Mean length of utterance (MLU) Average number of morphemes per utterance.

Metalinguistic cues Linguistic intuitions on the acceptability of communication.

Metalinguistics The use of language knowledge to make decisions about and to discuss processes of language.

Metaphor Figure of speech in which a comparison or resemblance is implied between two entities. Meaning is extended on the basis of some natural relationship, such as *mouth of a bottle*.

Metaphoric transparency Amount of literal-figurative relationship. High or strong relationships result in easy interpretation.

Modal auxiliary Auxiliary or helping verb used to express mood or attitude, such as ability (*can*), permission (*may*), intention (*will*), possibility (*might*), and obligation (*must*).

Morpheme Smallest unit of meaning; indivisible (*dog*) without violating the meaning or producing

meaningless units (*do, g*). There are two types of morphemes, free and bound.

Morphology Aspect of language concerned with rules governing change in meaning at the intraword level.

Morphophonemic Term used to refer to changes in sound production related to meaning changes.

Motherese Style of talking used most often by white middle-class American mothers when addressing their eighteen- to twenty-four-month-old toddlers.

Mutual gaze Eye contact with a communication partner; used to signal intensified attention.

Myelination Process of maturation of the nervous system in which the nerves develop a protective myelin sheath, or sleeve.

Narrative Consists of self-generated story; familiar tale; retelling of a movie, television show, or previously heard or seen story; and personal experience recounting.

Narrative level Overall organization of a narrative.

Nasal cavity Nose; cavity between the pharynx and the nares, separated from the oral cavity by the palate.

Neonate Newborn.

Neurolinguistics Study of the anatomy, physiology, and biochemistry of the brain responsible for language processing and formulation.

Neuron Nerve cell; basic unit of the nervous system.

Nonegocentrism Ability to take another person's perspective.

Nonlinguistic cues Coding devices that contribute to communication but are not a part of speech. Examples include gestures, body posture, eye contact, head and body movement, facial expression, and physical distance or proxemics.

Noun A syntactic unit noting a person, place, thing, quality, or activity (*Juan, New York, automobile, courage, departure*) that can usually be made possessive (*woman's*) and plural (*women*). Nouns can serve as the subject, object, or indirect object of a sentence [*Mary* (subject) gave the *ball* (object) to *John* (indirect object)] or as the object of a preposition (to *school*, at the old *mill*). The noun is the only element required in a noun phrase.

Noun phrase A noun element consisting of a noun, pronoun, or phrasal noun substitute, such as an infinitive or gerund, and the associated words that describe or modify that element. The noun element is the only obligatory portion.

Object   A sentence element filled by a noun or noun substitute upon which the action is performed, as in "She threw the *ball*" (direct object), or for whom the action is performed, as in "She bought the flowers for *him*" (indirect object).

Object noun-phrase complement   Subordinate clause that serves as the object of the main clause, as in "I remember *what you did to me*."

Open syllable   Syllable, usually CV, ending in a vowel.

Operant conditioning   Behavioral training as a result of reinforcement and punishment.

Oral cavity   Mouth; cavity between the pharynx and the lips, bounded below by the tongue, and above by the palate.

Organization   Tendency for all living things to systemize or organize behaviors. Piagetian concept.

Overextension   Process in which a child applies a word's meaning to more exemplars than an adult would. The child's definition is too broad and is thus beyond acceptable adult usage.

Paralinguistic codes   Vocal and nonvocal codes that are superimposed on a linguistic code to signal the speaker's attitude or emotion or to clarify or provide additional meaning.

Participle   A verb (*swim*) plus *-ing*, *-ed*, *-t*, or *-en* used as an adjective (Let's go to the *swimming* pool. He had a *concealed* weapon. It was a *lost* cause. He was a *broken* man.).

Perceptual (or sensory) stimulation   Reception of stimuli and recognition of their parameters.

Peripheral nervous system   All elements of the nervous system outside of the skull and spinal cord.

Pharynx   Cavity extending from the larynx to the nasal cavity.

Phonation   Process of producing a low-pitched hum or buzz from the vibration of the vocal folds.

Phone   Actual produced speech sound.

Phoneme   Smallest linguistic unit of sound, each with distinctive features, that can signal a difference in meaning when modified.

Phonetically consistent forms (PCFs)   Consistent vocal patterns that accompany gestures prior to the appearance of words.

Phonological awareness   Consideration of phonology at a conscious level, including syllabification; sound identification, manipulation, segmentation, and blending; rhyming; and illiteration. A metalingistic skills, phonological awareness is necessary for the development of reading.

Phonology   Aspect of language concerned with the rules governing the structure, distribution, and sequencing of speech-sound patterns.

Phrasal coordination   Process of conjoining clauses and deleting common elements.

Phrase   Group of words that does not contain a subject or predicate and is used as a noun substitute or as a noun or verb modifier.

Phrase-structure rules   Rules that delineate basic relationships underlying sentence organization. Chomskyan concept. Chomsky found the phrase-structure rules to be universal and thus concluded that they were innate.

Pidgin   Vocabulary of a dominant language used by speakers of a nondominant one with little or no grammatical structure.

Possession relational words   Words that recognize an association between an object and a particular person; semantic category.

Pragmatics   Aspect of language concerned with language use within a communication context.

Preposition   A syntactic unit noting the relation—usually in space or time—of a noun or its equivalent to some other word in the sentence (*on* the dresser, *in* my heart, *at* five o'clock). Common prepositions include *after*, *at*, *before*, *between*, *by*, *for*, *from*, *in*, *of*, *on*, *over*, *to*, *under*, and *with*.

Present progressive   A verb tense consisting of *be* + *Verb-ing* and used to express a continuous action occurring at the present time (*am eating*, *are running*).

Presupposition   Process of assuming which information a listener possesses or may need.

Primitive speech act (PSA)   Act, prosodic pattern, or word that conveys the early intentions of children. Term coined by Dore.

Pronominal   Adjective form of the word pronoun, as in "This sentence uses a *pronominal* form."

Pronoun   A syntactic unit that can take the place of a noun. Pronouns may fulfill syntactic functions such as subject (*I*, *you*, *he*, *she*, *it*, *we*, *they*), object (*me*, *you*, *him*, *her*, *it*, *us*, *them*), possessive (*my*, *your*, *his*, *her*, *its*, *our*, *their*), and reflexive (*myself*, *yourself*, *himself*, *herself*, *itself*, *ourselves*, *yourselves*, *themselves*). In addition, pronouns may be classified as interrogative (*Who* is she?), relative (The girl *who* sits behind me never does her homework), and indefinite (*all*, *any*, *anyone*, *each*, *either*, *everyone*, *few*, *no one*, *one*, *some*, *someone*).

Propositional force   Conceptual content or meaning of speech acts.

Protoconversation   Vocal interactions between mothers and infants that resemble the verbal exchanges of more mature conversations.

Prototypic complex hypothesis   Theory that word meanings represent an underlying concept exemplified by a central referent, or prototype, that is a best exemplar or a composite of the concept.

Proverb   Figure of speech that often gives advice or states some folk wisdom, such as "Don't put all your eggs in one basket."

Psycholinguistics   Study of the psychological aspects of language, especially as they apply to the psychological processes involved in learning, processing, and using language.

Punisher   Response that follows a behavior and decreases the probability of recurrence of that behavior.

Quasi-resonant nuclei (QRN)   Partial resonance of speech sounds found in neonates.

Recount   A type of narrative that relates past experiences of which the child and the listener partook, observed, or read.

Reduplicated babbling   Long strings of consonant-vowel syllable repetitions, such as *ba-ba-ba-ba-ba*, which appear in the vocal play of six- to seven-month-old infants.

Reduplication   Phonological process in which child repeats one syllable in a multisyllabic word, as in producing *wawa* for *water*.

Referencing   Differentiation of one entity from many; noting the presence of a single object, action, or event for one's communication partner.

Reflexes   Automatic, involuntary motor patterns. Although many neonatal behaviors are reflexive, this condition changes quickly with maturity.

Reflexive relational words   Words that relate objects to themselves in such ways as existence, nonexistence, disappearance, and recurrence; semantic category.

Register   Situationally influenced language variations, such as motherese.

Regular past-tense verb   A verb that takes the *-ed* marker for the past tense (*walked*, *jumped*, *typed*).

Rehearsal   Process of maintaining information within long-term memory; repetition, drill, or practice.

Reinforcement   Response that follows a behavior and increases the probability of recurrence of that behavior.

Relational words   Words that refer across entities, including action, location, appearance, disappearance, and possession; semantic category.

Relative clause   Subordinate clause that follows and modifies a noun, as in "I really like the car *that we test-drove last night.*"

Request for clarification   Request from the listener for restatement of or additional information on some unclear utterance of the speaker.

Resonation   Process of modifying the laryngeal tone by altering the shape of the pharyngeal, oral, and nasal cavities.

Respiration   Process of inhalation and exhalation, plus the resultant gas exchange.

Reticular formation   Unit of neurons within the brain stem responsible for sensory integration and for inhibition or facilitation of sensory information.

Rich interpretation   Process of interpreting child language by considering both the linguistic and nonlinguistic contexts.

Schemes   Cognitive structure or concept that an individual uses to process incoming sensory information; manifested as an organized pattern or reaction to stimuli. Piagetian concept.

Script   Scaffolding or predictable structure of an event which provides "slots" for participation and aids comprehension.

Segmentation   Process of dividing conversation so that utterances encode the relevant dynamic elements of a situation; accompaniment to joint action.

Selection restrictions   Constraints of specific word meanings that govern possible word combinations.

Selective imitation   Toddler language-learning strategy in which the child imitates those language features that he or she is in the process of learning. Toddlers do not imitate randomly.

Semantic features   Perceptual or functional aspects of meaning that characterize a word.

Semantic-feature hypothesis   Theory that word meanings represent universal semantic features or attributes, such as animate/inanimate and male/female. For young children, meanings represent perceptual attributes. Hypothesis usually associated with Clark.

Semantics   Aspect of language concerned with rules governing the meaning or content of words or grammatical units.

Semantic-syntactic rules   Word-order rules that describe the early multiword utterances of young children. Examples include *agent + action* and *negative + X*.

Sensorimotor   Stage of cognitive development (approximately from birth to two years) in which a child acquires knowledge of actions and objects through sensory and motor input. Piagetian concept.

Sentence   An independent clause (*subject + verb* that can stand alone) that may be classified as simple (independent clause alone), compound (two or more independent clauses joined together), complex (an independent clause plus one or more dependent clauses), or compound-complex (two or more independent clauses plus one or more dependent clauses).

Sentential coordination   Conjoining of full clauses.

Sibilants   Sounds produced by forcing air through a narrow constriction formed by the tongue and palate. The turbulence produced results in a hissing sound. Examples include /s/, /z/, /ʃ/, and /ʒ/.

Sign   Symbol that represents a cognitive structure; denotes thought about some entity or event. A word is an example.

Signal   Indicator that elicits an action schema and in which there is no differentiation between the form of the action (signifier) and the content (significant). An example is maternal posturing for "I'm going to get you."

Simile   Figure of speech that states an explicit comparison, such as *eats like a pig* or *lovely as a flower*.

Simple sentence   Linguistic structure that contains one full clause.

Social smile   Infant's smile in response to an external social stimulus.

Sociolinguistics   Study of the sociological influence on language learning and use, especially cultural and situational variables, including dialects, bilingualism, and parent–child interactions.

Speech   Dynamic neuromuscular process of producing speech sounds for communication; a verbal means of transmission.

Speech act   Basic unit of communication; an intentional, verbally encoded message that includes the speaker's intentions, the speaker's meaning, the message's meaning, and the listener's interpretation. Concept specified by Searle.

Story   Type of narrative, fictionalized.

Story grammar   Narrative framework that specifies the underlying relationship of the story components.

Style shifting   The process of varying the style of talking used, such as shifting between formal and informal styles.

Subordinate clause   Clause that cannot occur alone but functions in support of the main clause.

Substantive words   Words that refer to specific entities or classes of entities that have certain shared features.

Sulcus (Plural **Sulci**)   See *Fissure*.

Supramarginal gyrus   Association area of the brain, located in the posterior portion of the temporal lobe, responsible for linguistic processing, especially of longer syntactic units such as sentences.

Suprasegmental devices   Paralinguistic mechanisms superimposed on the verbal signal to change the form and meaning of the sentence by acting across the elements or segments of that sentence. Examples include intonation, stress, and inflection.

Surface structure   Structural characteristics of the actual spoken message; result of application of the phrase structure and transformational rules to the deep structure.

Symbol   Entity that represents another entity containing similar features. For example, a word is a symbol for the entity it represents.

Synapse   Miniscule space between the axon of one neuron and the dendrites of another.

Synonym   Word that shares the same or a similar meaning with another word.

Syntagmatic-paradigmatic shift   Change in word associational behavior from a syntactic to a semantic basis; occurs during the school-age years.

Syntax   Organizational rules specifying word order, sentence organization, and word relationships.

Tense   A marking of the verb, such as past or future, that relates the speech time in the present to the event time or time when the event occurs.

Thalamus   Organ located in the higher brain stem that receives incoming sensory information, except smell, and relays this information to the appropriate portion of the brain for analysis.

Topic   Content or subject about which conversational partners speak.

Topic-comment Process by which a topic is established and then elaborated upon. The infant may establish a topic by a look, gesture, or word; the infant or mother may then elaborate.

Transactional model Communication-first model of language development, evidenced in the give and take of early child–parent dialogs.

Transformational rules Rules that operate on strings of symbols, rearranging phrase-structure elements to form an acceptable sentence for output. There are rules for negatives, passive voice, interrogatives, and so on. Chomskyan concept.

Transitive verb A verb that must take a direct object to complete its meaning (The woman *sold* his books). Transitive verbs can be made into passive voice (The books *were sold* by the woman).

Turnabout Conversational device used by a mother with a preschooler to maintain the conversation and aid the child in making on-topic comments. In its usual form, the turnabout consists of a comment on or reply to the child's utterance followed by a cue, such as a question, for the child to reply.

Underextension Process in which a child applies a word meaning to fewer exemplars than an adult would. The child's definition is too restrictive and more limited than in adult usage.

Uninflected verb Verb containing no marking for person (*runs*, *eats*, *jumps*) or for tense (**will** run, **has been** eating, jump**ed**), as in *run*, *eat*, and *jump*.

Variegated babbling Long strings of nonidentical syllables that appear in the vocal play of some eight- to ten-month-old infants.

Verb A syntactic unit noting action (*run*, *jump*, *eat*) or being/state (*be*, *want*, *feel*) that changes form to indicate time or tense (*go*, *went*, *will go*, *is going*), person (*am–is*, *run–runs*), number (*is–are*), mood (*could*, *might*), and aspect. Verbs can be classified as transitive, intransitive, or equative.

Verb phrase Verb and the words or phrases, such as prepositional phrases, that accompany it.

Vernacular Casual, informal, or intimate language register or style.

Vocal folds Laryngeal vibrators responsible for phonation.

Voice Change made in the verb to indicate whether the subject of the sentence acts (active voice), e.g., *The cat chases the dog*, or is acted upon (passive voice), e.g., *The dog is chased by the cat*.

Voiced phonemes Phonemes that are produced with vibration at the level of the larynx.

Voiceless phonemes Phonemes that are produced without vibration at the level of the larynx.

Voice onset time (VOT) Interval between the burst of a voiced plosive and the commencement of phonation.

Wernicke's area Language-processing area of the brain, located in the left temporal lobe; responsible for organizing the underlying structure of outgoing messages and analyzing incoming linguistic information.

Word knowledge Verbal word and symbol definitions.

World knowledge Autobiographical and experiential understanding and memory of events reflecting personal and cultural interpretations.

References

Abbeduto, L., Nuccio, J. B., Al-Mabuk, R., Rotto, P., & Maas, F. (1992). Interpreting and responding to spoken language: Children's recognition and use of a speaker's goal. *Journal of Child Language, 19*, 677–693.

Abbeduto, L., & Rosenberg, S. (1985). Children's knowledge of the presuppositions of *know* and other cognitive verbs. *Journal of Child Language, 12*, 621–641.

Abkarian, G. (1988). Acquiring lexical contrast: The case of *bring-take* learning. *Journal of Speech and Hearing Research, 31*, 317–326.

Abkarian, G., Jones, A., & West, G. (1992). Young children's idiom comprehension: Trying to get the picture. *Journal of Speech and Hearing Research, 35*, 580–587.

Abrahamsen, E., & Rigrodsky, S. (1984). Comprehension of complex sentences in children at three levels of cognitive development. *Journal of Psycholinguistic Research, 13*, 333–350.

Ackerman, B. (1978). Children's understanding of speech acts in unconventional directive frames. *Child Development, 49*, 311–318.

Acredolo, L., & Goodwyn, S. (1988). Symbolic gesturing in normal infants. *Human Development, 28*, 40–49.

Acredolo, L., & Goodwyn, S. (1990). Sign language in babies: The significance of symbolic gesturing for understanding language development. In R. Vasta (Ed.), *Annals of Child Development* (pp. 1–42). London: Jessica Kingsley Publishers Ltd.

Adams, A., & Gathercole, S. E. (1995). Phonological working memory and speech production in preschool children. *Journal of Speech, Language, and Hearing Research, 38*, 403–414.

Adamson, L., & Bakeman, R. (1985). Affect and attention: Infants observed with mothers and peers. *Child Development, 56*, 582–593.

Adler, S. A., Gerhardstein, P., & Rovee-Collier, C. (1998). Levels-of-processing effects in infant memory? *Child Development, 69*, 280–294.

Akhtar, N., Dunham, F., & Dunham, P. J. (1991). Directive interactions and early vocabulary development: The role of joint attentional focus. *Journal of Child Language, 18*, 41–49.

Akiyama, M. M. (1992). Cross-linguistic contrasts of verification and answering among children. *Journal of Psycholinguistic Research, 21*, 67–85.

Aksu, A., & Slobin, D. (1985). Acquisition of Turkish. In D. Slobin (Ed.), *The crosslinguistic study of language acquisition*. Hillsdale, NJ: Erlbaum.

Allen, G. (1983). Linguistic experience modifies lexical stress perception. *Journal of Child Language, 10*, 535–549.

Allen, R., & Shatz, M. (1983). "What says meow?" The role of context and linguistic experience in very young children's responses to what questions. *Journal of Child Language, 10*, 321–335.

Allen, S. E. M., & Crago, M. B. (1996). Early passive acquisition in Inuktitut. *Journal of Child Language, 23*, 129–155.

Allington, R. (1984). Oral reading. In P. Pearson, R. Barr, M. Kamil, & P. Mosenthal (Eds.), *Handbook of reading research*. New York: Longman.

Altman, G., & Steedman, M. (1988). Interaction with context during human sentence processing. *Cognition, 30*, 191–238.

Amayreh, M. M., & Dyson, A. T. (1998). The acquisition of Arabic consonants. *Journal of Speech, Language, and Hearing Research, 41*, 642–653.

Andersen, E., & Kekelis, L. (1983). *The role of children in determining the nature of their linguistic input.* Paper presented at the Eighth Annual Conference on Language Development, Boston University.

Anderson, A., & Stokes, S. (1984). Social and institutional influences on the development and practice of literacy. In H. Goelman, A. Oberg, & F. Smith (Eds.), *Awakening to literacy*. Exeter, NH: Heinemann.

Anderson, A. H., Clark, A., & Mullin, J. (1994). Interactive communication between children: Learning how to make language work in dialogue. *Journal of Child Language, 21*, 439–463.

Anderson, E. (1992). *Speaking with style: The sociolinguistic skills of children.* London: Routledge.

Anderson, R., & Smith, B. (1987). Phonological development of two-year-old monolingual Puerto Rican Spanish-speaking children. *Journal of Child Language, 14,* 57–78.

Anderson, R. T. (1998). The development of grammatical case distinctions in the use of personal pronouns by Spanish-speaking preschoolers. *Journal of Speech, Language, Hearing Research, 41,* 394–406.

Anglin, J. M. (1985). The child's expressible knowledge of word concepts: What preschoolers can say about the meanings of some nouns and verbs. In K. E. Nelson (Ed.), *Children's language, Volume 5* (pp. 77–127). Hillsdale, NJ: Erlbaum.

Anglin, J. M. (1993). Vocabulary development: A morphological analysis. *Monographs of the Society for Research in Child Development, 58* (10).

Anglin, J. M. (1995a). Classifying the world through language: Functional relevance, cultural significance, and category name learning. *International Journal of Intercultural Relations, 19,* 161–181.

Anglin, J. M. (1995b, April). *Word knowledge and the growth of potentially knowable vocabulary.* Paper presented at the biennial meeting of the Society for Research in Child Development, Indianapolis, IN.

Arlin, M. (1983). Children's comprehension of semantic constraints on temporal prepositions. *Journal of Psycholinguistic Research, 12,* 1–15.

Arnold, P., & Murray, C. (1998). Memory for faces and objects by deaf and hearing signers and hearing nonsigners. *Journal of Psycholinguistic Research, 27,* 481–491.

Aslin, R. N. (1992). Segmentation of fluent speech into words: Learning models and the role of maternal input. In B. deBoysson-Bardies, S. DeSchonen, P. Jusczyk, P. MacNeilage, & J. Morton (Eds.), *Developmental neurocognition: Speech and face processing in the first year of life.* Dordrecht: Kluwer.

Aslin, R. N., & Pisoni, D. (1980). Some developmental processes in speech perception. In G. Yeni-Komshian, J. Kavanaugh, & C. Ferguson (Eds.), *Child phonology: Vol. 2, Perception.* New York: Academic Press.

Aslin, R. N., & Smith, L. (1988). Perceptual development. *Annual Review of Psychology, 39,* 435–473.

Astington, J. W., & Olson, D. R. (1987, April). *Literacy and schooling: Learning to talk about thought.* Paper presented at the annual meeting of the American Educational Research Association, Washington, DC.

Au, K. (1990). Children's use of information in word learning. *Journal of Child Language, 17,* 393–416.

Auer, J. C. P. (1984). *Bilingual conversation.* Amsterdam: Benjamins.

Austin, J. (1962). *How to do things with words.* London: Oxford University Press.

Axtell, R. E. (1991). *Gestures: The do's and taboos of body language around the world.* Baltimore, MD: Wiley & Sons.

Azuma, S. (1996). Speech production units among bilinguals. *Journal of Psycholinguistic Research, 25,* 397–416.

Backus, A. (1999). Mixed native language: A challenge to the monolithic view of language. *Topics in Language Disorders, 19*(4), 11–22.

Baddeley, A. D. (1986). *Working memory.* Oxford: Oxford University Press.

Baghban, M. (1984). *Our daughter learns to read and write.* Newark, DE: International Reading Association.

Baldwin, D. A. (1993). Infants' ability to consult the speaker for clues to word reference. *Journal of Child Language, 20,* 395–418.

Banigan, R., & Mervis, C. (1988). Role of adult input in young children's category evolution: II. An experimental study. *Journal of Child Language, 15,* 493–504.

Baratz, J. (1968). Language in the economically disadvantaged child: A perspective. *Asha, 10,* 145–146.

Barnes, S., Gutfreund, M., Satterly, D., & Wells, G. (1983). Characteristics of adult speech which predict children's language development. *Journal of Child Language, 10,* 65–84.

Barrett, M. D. (1982). Distinguishing between prototypes: The early acquisition of meaning of object names. In S. Kuczaj (Ed.), *Language development:* Vol. 1. *Syntax and semantics.* Hillsdale, NJ: Erlbaum.

Barrett, M. D. (1983). *Scripts, prototypes, and the early acquisition of word meaning.* Paper presented at the annual conference of the British Psychological Society.

Barrett, M. D. (1986). Early semantic representations and early word usage. In S. A. Kuczaj & M. D. Barrett (Eds.), *The development of word meaning.* New York: Springer-Verlag.

Barrett, M. D., Harris, M., & Chasin, J. (1991). Early lexical development and maternal speech: A comparison of children's initial and subsequent uses of words. *Journal of Child Language, 18*, 21–40.

Barron, R. (1981). Development of visual word recognition: A review. In G. Mackinnon & T. Waller (Eds.), *Reading research: Advances in theory and practice*. New York: Academic Press.

Bartlett, C. (1982). Learning to write: Some cognitive and linguistic components. In R. Shuy (Ed.), *Linguistic and literacy series, No. 2*. Washington, DC: Center of Applied Linguistics.

Barton, M. E., & Strosberg, R. (1997). Conversational patterns of two-year-old twins in mother-twin-twin triads. *Journal of Child Language, 24*, 257–269.

Bates, E. (1976). *Language and context: The acquisition of pragmatics*. New York: Academic Press.

Bates, E., Benigni, L., Bretherton, I., Camaioni, L., & Volterra, V. (1979). *The emergence of symbols: Cognition and communication in infancy*. New York: Academic Press.

Bates, E., Bretherton, I., Shore, C., & McNew, S. (1983). Names, gestures and objects: The role of context in the emergence of symbols. In K. Nelson (Ed.), *Children's language* (Vol. 4). Hillsdale, NJ: Erlbaum.

Bates, E., Bretherton, I., & Snyder, L. (1988). *From first words to grammar: Individual differences and dissociable mechanisms*. New York: Cambridge University Press.

Bates, E., Bretherton, I., Snyder, L., Shore, C., & Volterra, V. (1980). Vocal and gestural symbols at 13 months. *Merrill-Palmer Quarterly, 26*, 407–423.

Bates, E., Camaioni, L., & Volterra, V. (1975). The acquisition of performatives prior to speech. *Merrill-Palmer Quarterly, 21*, 205–216.

Bates, E., MacWhinney, B., Caselli, C., Devescove, S., Natale, F., & Vanza, V. (1984). Cross-linguistic study of the development of sentence interpretation strategies. *Child Development, 55*, 341–354.

Bates, E., Marchman, V., Thal, D., Fenson, L., Dale, P., Reznick, J., Reilly, J., & Hartung, J. (1994). Developmental and stylistic variation in the composition of early vocabulary. *Journal of Child Language, 21*, 85–123.

Bates, E., & Snyder, L. (1987). The cognitive hypothesis in language development. In I. Uzgiris & J. Hunt (Eds.), *Infant performance and experience: New findings with the ordinal scales*. Urbana: University of Illinois Press.

Bateson, M. (1979). The epigenesis of conversational interaction: A personal account of research development. In M. Bullow (Ed.), *Before speech*. New York: Cambridge University Press.

Bayles, K., Tomoeda, C., & Boone, D. (1985). A view of age-related changes in language function. *Developmental Neuropsychology, 1*, 231–264.

Bedrosian, J., Wanska, S., Sykes, K., Smith, A., & Dalton, B. (1988). Conversational turn-taking violations in mother–child interactions. *Journal of Speech and Hearing Research, 31*, 81–86.

Behrend, D. (1988). Overextensions in early language comprehension: Evidence from a signal detection approach. *Journal of Child Language, 15*, 63–75.

Behrend, D. A., Harris, L. L., & Cartwright, K. B. (1995). Morphological cues to verb meaning: Verb inflections and the initial mapping of verb meanings. *Journal of Child Language, 22*, 89–106.

Bellinger, D. (1980). Consistency in the pattern of change in mothers' speech: Some discriminant analyses. *Journal of Child Language, 7*, 469–487.

Bellugi, U. (1967). *The acquisition of negation*. Unpublished doctoral dissertation. Harvard University.

Bellugi, U., & Brown, R. (1964). The acquisition of language. *Monographs of the Society for Research in Child Development, 29* (No. 92).

Benedict, H. (1979). Early lexical development: Comprehension and production. *Journal of Child Language, 6*, 183–200.

Benelli, B., Arcuri, L., & Marchesini, G. (1988). Cognitive and linguistic factors in the development of word definitions. *Journal of Child Language, 15*, 619–635.

Bennett-Kaster, T. (1983). Noun phrases and coherence in child narratives. *Journal of Child Language, 10*, 135–149.

Bennett-Kaster, T. (1986). Cohesion and predication in child narrative. *Journal of Child Language, 13*, 353–370.

Bennett-Kaster, T. (1988). *Analyzing children's language*. Oxford: Blackwell.

Benson, N. J., & Anglin, J. M. (1987). The child's knowledge of English kin terms. *First Language, 7*, 41–66.

Berko Gleason, J., & Greif, E. (1983). Men's speech to young children. In B. Thorne, C. Kramerae, & N.

Henley (Eds.), *Language, gender, and society*. Rowley, MA: Newbury House.

Berman., R. (1985). Acquisition of Hebrew. In D. Slobin (Ed.), *The crosslinguistic study of language acquisition*. Hillsdale, NJ: Erlbaum.

Berman, R. (1986). A crosslinguistic perspective: Morphology and syntax. In P. Fletcher & M. Garman (Eds.), *Language acquisition* (2nd ed.). New York: Cambridge University Press.

Berninger, G., & Garvey, C. (1982). Tag constructions: Structure and function in child discourse. *Journal of Child Language, 9*, 151–168.

Bernstein, M. (1983). Formation of internal structure in a lexical category. *Journal of Child Language, 10*, 381–399.

Bernstein Ratner, N., & Pye, C. (1984). Higher pitch in BT is not universal: Acoustic evidence from Quiche Mayan. *Journal of Child Language, 11*, 515–522.

Bertoncini, J., Bijeljac-Babic, R. V., Blumstein, S. E., & Mehler, J. (1987). Discrimination in neonates of very short CVs. *Journal of the Acoustic Society of America, 82*, 31–37.

Black, J. B. (1985). An exposition on understanding expository text. In B. K. Britton & J. B. Black (Eds.), *Understanding expository text*. Hillsdale, NJ: Erlbaum Associates.

Blake, J., & deBoysson-Bardies, B. (1992). Patterns of babbling: A cross-linguistic study. *Journal of Child Language, 19*, 51–74.

Blake, J., Quartaro, G., & Onorati, S. (1993). Evaluating quantitative measures of grammatical complexity in spontaneous speech samples. *Journal of Child Language, 20*, 139–152.

Blanck, G. (1990). Vygotsky: The man and his cause. In L.C. Moll (Ed.), *Vygotsky and education* (pp. 31–58). New York: Cambridge University Press.

Bliss, L. S. (1992). A comparison of tactful messages by children with and without language impairment. *Language, Speech, and Hearing Services in Schools, 23*, 343–347.

Bloom, K. (1988). Quality of adult vocalizations affects the quality of infant vocalizations. *Journal of Child Language, 15*, 469–480.

Bloom, K., & Lo, E. (1990). Adult perceptions of vocalizing infants. *Infant Behavior and Development, 13*, 209–213.

Bloom, K., Russell, A., & Wassenberg, K. (1987). Turn-taking affects the quality of infant vocalizations. *Journal of Child Language, 14*, 221–227.

Bloom, L. (1970). *Language development: Form and function of emerging grammars*. Cambridge: MIT Press.

Bloom, L. (1973). *One word at a time: The use of single-word utterances before syntax*. The Hague: Mouton.

Bloom, L. (1983). Of continuity, nature, and magic. In R. Golinkoff (Ed.), *The transition from preverbal to verbal communication*. Hillsdale, NJ: Erlbaum.

Bloom, L., & Lahey, M. (1978). *Language development and language disorders*. New York: Wiley.

Bloom, L., Lahey, P., Hood, L., Lifter, K., & Fiess, K. (1980). Complex sentences: Acquisition of syntactic connectors and the semantic relations they encode. *Journal of Child Language, 7*, 235–262.

Bloom, L., Lifter, K., & Hafitz, J. (1980). Semantics of verbs and the development of verb inflection in child language. *Language, 56*, 386–412.

Bloom, L., Tackeff, J., & Lahey, M. (1984). Learning to speak in complement constructions. *Journal of Child Language, 11*, 391–406.

Bloom, P. (1990). Syntactic distinctions in child language. *Journal of Child Language, 17*, 343–355.

Bohannon, J., & Marquis, A. (1977). Children's control of adult speech. *Child Development, 48*, 1002–1008.

Bohannon, J., & Stanowicz, L. (1988). The issue of negative evidence: Adult responses to children's language errors. *Developmental Psychology, 24*, 684–689.

Boswell, M. (1988). *Gesture and speech in the one-word stage*. Unpublished doctoral dissertation, University of Chicago.

Boudreau, D. M., & Hedberg, N. L. (1999). A comparison of early literacy skills in children with specific language impairment and their typically developing peers. *American Journal of Speech-Language Pathology, 8*, 249–260.

Bouvier, L., & Gardner, R. (1986). *Immigration to the U.S.: The unfinished story*. Washington, DC: Population Reference Bureau.

Bower, T. (1977). *The perceptual world of the child*. Cambridge: Harvard University Press.

Bowerman, M. (1974). Discussion summary—Development of concepts underlying language. In R. Schiefelbusch & L. Lloyd (Eds.), *Language perspectives—Acquisition, retardation, and intervention*. Baltimore: University Park Press.

Bowerman, M. (1978). Systematizing semantic knowledge: Changes over time in the child's organization of word meaning. *Child Development, 49*, 977–987.

Bowerman, M. (1981). *The child's expression of meaning: Expanding relationships among lexicon, syntax and morphology*. Paper presented at the New York Academy of Science Conference on Native Language and Foreign Language Acquisition.

Bowerman, M. (1993). Learning a semantic system: What role do cognitive predispositions play? In P. Bloom (Ed.), *Language acquisition: Core readings*. Cambridge, MA: MIT Press.

Bowey, J. (1982). The structural processing of the truncated passive in children and adults. *Journal of Psycholinguistic Research, 11*, 417–436.

Bowey, J. (1986). Syntactic awareness and verbal performance from preschool to fifth grade. *Journal of Psycholinguistic Research, 15*, 285–308.

Bowey, J. A. (1996). Orthographic onset as functional units in adult word recognition. *Journal of Psycholinguistic Research, 25*, 571–595.

Bowles, N., & Poon, L. (1985). Aging and retrieval of words in semantic memory. *Journal of Gerontology, 40*, 71–77.

Braine, M. (1976). Children's first word combinations. *Monographs of the Society for Research in Child Development, 41* (Serial No. 164).

Brener, R. (1983). Learning the deictic meaning of third person pronouns. *Journal of Psycholinguistics Research, 12*, 235–262.

Bretherton, I. (1984). Representing the social world in symbolic play: Reality and fantasy. In I. Bretherton (Ed.), *Symbolic play: The development of social understanding*. New York: Academic Press.

Bretherton, I., & Beeghly, M. (1982). Talking about internal states: The acquisition of an explicit theory of mind. *Developmental Psychology, 18*, 906–921.

Brice Heath, S. (1983). *Ways with words: Language, life, and work in communities and classrooms*. Cambridge: Cambridge University Press.

Bridges, A. (1980). SVD comprehension strategies reconsidered: The evidence of individual patterns of response. *Journal of Child Language, 7*, 89–104.

Briggs, C. L. (1984). Learning how to ask: Native metacommunicative competence and incompetence of fieldworkers. *Language in Society, 13*, 1–28.

Brinton, B., & Fujiki, M. (1984). Development of topic manipulation skills in discourse. *Journal of Speech and Hearing Research, 27*, 350–358.

Brinton, B., Fujiki, M., Loeb, D., & Winkler, E. (1986). Development of conversational repair strategies in response to requests for clarification. *Journal of Speech and Hearing Research, 29*, 75–81.

Brockman, L. M., Morgan, G. A., & Harmon, R. J. (1988). Mastery motivation and developmental delay. In T. D. Wachs & R. Sheehan (Eds.), *Assessment of young developmentally disabled children*. New York: Plenum.

Brown, B., & Leonard, L. (1986). Lexical influences on children's early positional patterns. *Journal of Child Language, 13*, 219–229.

Brown, R. (1956). Language and categories. Appendix in J. Bruner, J. Goodner, & G. Austin, *A study of thinking*. New York: Wiley.

Brown, R. (1958). *Words and things*. New York: Free Press.

Brown, R. (1965). *Social psychology*. New York: Free Press.

Brown. R. (1973). *A first language: The early stages*. Cambridge: Harvard University Press.

Brown, R. (1977). Preface. In C. Snow & C. Ferguson (Eds.), *Talking to children: Language input and acquisition*. New York: Cambridge University Press.

Brown, R., & Bellugi, U. (1964). Three processes in the child's acquisition of syntax. *Harvard Educational Review, 34*, 133–151.

Brownell, C. (1988). Combinatorial skills: Converging developments over the second year. *Child Development, 59*, 675–685.

Bruner, J. (1975). The ontogenesis of speech acts. *Journal of Child Language, 2*, 1–19.

Bruner, J. (1976). *On prelinguistic prerequisites of speech*. Paper presented to the Stirling Conference on Psychology of Language.

Bruner, J. (1977a). Early social interaction and language acquisition. In R. Schaffer (Ed.), *Studies in mother-infant interaction*. New York: Academic Press.

Bruner, J. (1978b). Learning how to do things with words. In J. Bruner & A. Gurton (Eds.), *Wolfson College Lectures 1976: Human Growth and Development*. Oxford: Oxford University Press.

Bruner, J. (1983). *Child's talk*. New York: W.W. Norton.

Bryant, P., & Bradley, L. (1980). Why children sometimes write words which they do not read. In U. Firth (Ed.), *Cognitive processes in spelling*. New York: Academic Press.

Bryant, P., Bradley, L., MacLean, M., & Crossland, J. (1989). Nursery rhymes, phonological skills, and reading. *Journal of Child Language, 16*, 407–428.

Buhr, R. (1980). The emergence of vowels in an infant. *Journal of Speech and Hearing Research, 23*, 73–94.

Burke, S., Pflaum, S., & Knafle, J. (1982, January). The influence of black English on diagnosis of reading in learning disabled and normal readers. *Journal of Learning Disabilities, 15,* 19–22.

Bybee, J., & Slobin, D. (1982). Rules and schemas in the development and use of the English past. *Language, 58,* 265–289.

Cacciari, C., & Levorato, M. C. (1989). How children understand idioms in discourse. *Journal of Child Language, 16,* 387–405.

Cacciari, C., & Tabossi, P. (1988). The comprehension of idioms. *Journal of Memory and Language, 27,* 669–683.

Capirci, O., Iverson, J. M., Pizzuto, E., & Volterra, V. (1996). Gestures and words during the transition to two-word speech. *Journal of Child Language, 23,* 645–673.

Carey, S. (1981). The child as word learner. In M. Halle, J. Bresnan, & G. Miller (Eds.), *Linguistic theory and psychological reality.* Cambridge, MA: MIT Press.

Carlisle, J. F. (1987). The use of morphological knowledge in spelling derived forms by learning disabled and normal students. *Annals of Dyslesia, 37,* 90–108.

Carlisle, J. F. (1988). Knowledge of derivational morphology and spelling ability in fourth, sixth, and eighth graders. *Applied Psycholinguistics, 9,* 247–266.

Carpenter, K. (1991). Later rather than sooner: Extralinguistic categories in the acquisition of Thai classifiers. *Journal of Child Language, 18,* 93–113.

Carrell, P. (1981). Children's understanding of indirect requests: Comparing child and adult comprehension. *Journal of Child Language, 8,* 329–345.

Casby, M. W. (1986). A pragmatic perspective of repitition in child language. *Journal of Psycholinguistic Research, 15,* 127–140.

Case, R. (1985). *Intellectual development: A systematic reinterpretation.* New York: Academic Press.

Case, R. (1992). *The mind's staircase.* Hillsdale, NJ: Erlbaum.

Caselli, M. (1990). Communicative gestures and first words. In V. Bolterra & C. Erting (Eds.), *From gesture to sign in hearing and deaf children* (pp. 56–67). New York: Springer-Verlag.

Chafe, W. (1970). *Meaning and the structure of language.* Chicago: University of Chicago Press.

Chalkley, M. (1982). The emergence of language as a social skill. In S. Kuczaj (Ed.), *Language development: Vol. 2, Language, thought and culture.* Hillsdale, NJ: Erlbaum.

Chall, J. (1983). *Stages of reading development.* New York: McGraw-Hill.

Chapman, L. J. (1983). *Reading development and cohesion.* London: Heineman Educational Books.

Chapman, R., & Miller, J. (1980). Analyzing language and communication in the child. In R. Schiefelbusch (Ed.), *Nonspeech language and communication.* Baltimore: University Park Press.

Charney, R. (1980). Speech roles and the development of personal pronouns. *Journal of Child Language, 7,* 509–528.

Cheng, L. (1987, June). Cross-cultural and linguistic considerations in working with Asian populations. *Asha, 29* (6), 33–38.

Chi, M. (1985). Changing conception of sources or memory development. *Human Development, 28,* 50–56.

Chiat, S. (1986). Personal pronouns. In P. Fletcher & M. Garman (Eds.), *Language acquisition* (2nd ed.). New York: Cambridge University Press.

Choi, S. (1988). The semantic development of negation: A cross-linguistic longitudinal study. *Journal of Child Language, 15,* 517–531.

Choi, S., & Gopnik, A. (1995) Early acquisition of verbs in Korean: A cross-linguistic study. *Journal of Child Language, 22,* 497–529.

Chomsky, N. (1957). *Syntactic structures.* The Hague: Mouton.

Chomsky, N. (1959). A review of Skinner's Verbal Behavior. *Language, 35,* 26–58.

Chomsky, N. (1965). *Aspects of the theory of syntax.* Cambridge: MIT Press.

Chomsky, N. (1968). *Language and mind.* New York: Harcourt, Brace & World.

Chomsky, N. (1981). *Lectures on government and binding.* Dordrecht, Holland: Foris.

Chomsky, N. (1986). *Knowledge of language.* New York: Praeger.

Chomsky, N. (1992). A mimimalist program for linguistic theory. *MIT Occasional Papers in Linguistics, 1.* Cambridge: Massachusetts Institute of Technology.

Chomsky, N. (1995). *A mimimalist program.* Cambridge: MIT Press.

Chomsky, N., & Halle, M. (1968). *The sound pattern of English.* New York: Harper & Row.

Cicchetti, D. (1989). How research on child maltreatment has informed the study of child development: Perspectives from developmental psychopathology.

In D. Cicchetti & V. Carlson (Eds.), *Child maltreatment: Theory and research on causes and consequences of child abuse and neglect*. New York: Cambridge University Press.

Clancy, P. M. (1980). Referential choice in English and Japanese narrative discourse. In W. Chafe (Ed.), *The pear stories: Cognitive, cultural, and linguistic aspects of narrative production* (pp. 127–199). Norwood, NJ: Ablex.

Clancy, P. M. (1985). Acquisition of Japanese. In D. Slobin (Ed.), *The cross-linguistic study of language acquisition*. Hillsdale, NJ: Erlbaum.

Clancy, P. M. (1989). Form and function in the acquisition of Korean *wh-* questions. *Journal of Child Language, 16*, 323–347.

Clark, E. V. (1971). On the acquisition of the meaning of "before" and "after." *Journal of Verbal Learning and Verbal Behavior, 10*, 266–275.

Clark, E. V. (1973a). Non-linguistic strategies and the acquisition of word meanings. *Cognition, 2*, 161–182.

Clark, E. V. (1973b). What's in a word? On the child's acquisition of semantics in his first language. In T. Moore (Ed.), *Cognitive development and the acquisition of language*. New York: Academic Press.

Clark, E. V. (1975). Knowledge, context and strategy in the acquisition of meaning. In D. Dato (Ed.), *Developmental psycholinguistics: Theory and application*. Washington, DC: Georgetown University Press.

Clark, E. V. (1978). Awareness of language: Some evidence from what children say and do. In A. Sinclair, R. Jarvella, & W. Levelt (Eds.), *The child's conception of language*. New York: Springer-Verlag.

Clark, E. V. (1981) Lexical innovations: How children learn to create new words. In W. Deutsch (Ed.), *The child's construction of language*. New York: Academic Press.

Clark, E. V. (1983). Meaning and concepts. In P. Mussen (Ed.), *Handbook of child psychology* (Vol. 3). New York: Wiley.

Clark, E. V. (1985). Acquisition of Romance, with special reference to French. In D. Slobin (Ed.), *The crosslinguistic study of language acquisition*. Hillsdale, NJ: Erlbaum.

Clark, E. V. (1990). On the pragmatics of contrast. *Journal of Child Language, 17*, 417–431.

Clark, E. V., & Berman, R. (1984). Structure and use in the acquisition of word formation. *Language, 60*, 542–594.

Clark, E. V., Gelman, S., & Lane, N. (1985). Compound nouns and category structure in young children. *Child Development, 56*, 84–94.

Clark, E. V., & Hecht, B. (1982). Learning to coin agent and instrument nouns. *Cognition, 12*, 1–24.

Clark, E. V., & Sengul, C. (1978). Strategies in the acquisition of deixis. *Journal of Child Language, 5*, 457–475.

Clark, H., & Chase, W. (1972). On the process of comparing sentences against pictures. *Cognitive Psychology, 3*, 472–517.

Coates, J. (1988). The acquisition of the meaning of modality in children aged eight and twelve. *Journal of Child Language, 15*, 425–434.

Cohen, S., & Beckwith, L. (1975). *Maternal language input in infancy*. Paper presented to the American Pscyhological Association.

Committee on Language, American Speech-Language-Hearing Association. (1983). Definition of language, *Asha, 25*, 44.

Constable, C. M. (1986). The application of scripts in the organization of language intervention contexts. *Event knowledge, 10*, 205–230.

Cooper, R. P., & Aslin, R. N. (1990). Preference for infant-directed speech in the first month after birth. *Child Development, 61*, 1584–1595.

Coulson, A. (1999, August 20). Language is more than words and sentences. Rochester, NY *Democrat & Chronicle*, 8A.

Cox, M. (1985). *The child's point of view: Cognitive and linguistic development*. Brighton, Eng.: Harvester Press.

Cox, M. (1989). Children's over-regularization of nouns and verbs. *Journal of Child Language, 16*, 203–206.

Cox, M., & Richardson, J. (1985). How do children describe spatial relationships? *Journal of Child Language, 12*, 611–620.

Crago, M. B., Eriks-Brophy, A., Pesco, D., & McAlpine, L. (1997). Culturally based miscommunication in classroom interaction. *Language, Speech, and Hearing Services in Schools, 28*, 245–254.

Craig, H. K., Washington, J. A., & Thompson-Porter, C. (1998). Average c-unit lengths in the discourse of African American children from low-income, urban homes. *Journal of Speech, Language and Hearing Research, 41*, 433–444.

Crais, E. (1987). Fast mapping of novel words in oral story content. *Dissertation Abstracts International, 48*, Part 3b, 724.

Crais, E. R. & Chapman. R. (1987). Story recall and inferencing skills in language-learning disable and nondisabled children. *Journal of Speech and Hearing Disorders, 52*, 50–55.

Cronk, B. C., Lima, S. D., & Schweigert, W. A. (1993). Idioms in sentences: Effects of frequency, literalness, and familiarity. *Journal of Psycholinguistic Research, 22*, 59–82.

Cronk, B. C., & Schweigert, W. A. (1992). The comprehension of idioms: The effects of familiarity, literalness, and usage. *Applied Psycholinguistics, 13*, 131–146.

Crystal, D. (1980). Neglected grammatical factors in conversational English. In S. Greenbaum, G. Leech, & J. Svartvik (Eds.), *Studies in English linguistics for Randolph Quirk*. London: Longman.

Cummins, J. (1980). Psychological assessment of immigrant children: Logic or intuition. *Journal of Multicultural Multilingual Development, 1*, 97–111.

Cummins, J. (1984). *Bilingualism and special education: Issues in assessment and pedogogy*. Austin, TX: Pro-Ed.

Dale, P. S., & Crain-Thoreson, C. (1993). Pronoun reversals: Who, when, & why? *Journal of Child Language, 20*, 573–589.

Dalzell, T. (1996). *Flappers 2 rappers: American youth slang*. New York: Merriam Webster.

Daniloff, R., & Moll, K. (1968). Coarticulation of lip rounding. *Journal of Speech and Hearing Research, 11*, 707–721.

Davis, F. A., & DeCasper, A. J. (1989). *Intrauterine heartbeat sounds are reinforcing for newborns because of active right-lateralized processes*. Paper presented at the Society for Research in Child Development, Kansas City, MO.

Debaryshe, B. D. (1993). Joint picture-book reading correlates of early language skill. *Journal of Child Language, 20*, 455–461.

deBoysson-Bardies, B. (1989). *Material evidence of infant selection from the target language: A cross-linguistic phonetic study*. Paper presented at the conference on Phonological Development, Stanford University.

deBoysson-Bardies, B., Halle, P., Sagart, L., & Durand, C. (1989). A crosslinguistic investigation of vowel formants in babbling. *Journal of Child Language, 16*, 1–17.

deBoysson-Bardies, B., Sagart, L., & Durand, C. (1984). Discernible differences in the babbling of infants according to target language. *Journal of Child Language, 11*, 1–15.

DeCasper, A. J., & Fifer, W. P. (1980). Of human bondage: Newborns prefer their mothers' voices. *Science, 208*, 1174–1176.

DeCasper, A. J., & Spence, M. (1986). Prenatal maternal speech influences newborns' perceptions of speech sounds. *Infant Behavior and Infant Development, 9*, 133–150.

DeHart, G., & Maratsos, M. (1984). Children's acquisition of presuppositional usages. In R. Schiefelbusch & J. Pickar (Eds.), *The acquisition of communicative competence*. Baltimore: University Park Press.

DeLemos, C. (1981). Internal processes in the child's construction of language. In W. Deutsch (Ed.), *The child's construction of language*. New York: Academic Press.

Della Corte, M., Benedict, H., & Klein, D. (1983). The relationship of pragmatic dimensions of mothers' speech to the referential-expressive distinction. *Journal of Child Language, 10*, 35–43.

Demetras, M., Post, K., & Snow, C. (1986). Feedback to first language learners: The role of repetitions and clarification questions. *Journal of Child Language, 13*, 275–292.

Demuth, K. (1989). Maturation, continuity and the acquisition of Sesotho passive. *Language, 65*, 56–80.

Demuth, K. (1990). Subject, topic and Sesotho passive. *Journal of Child Language, 17*, 67–84.

Demuth, K. (1993). Issues in the acquisition of the Sesotho tonal system. *Journal of Child Language, 20*, 275–301.

Dennis, M., Sugar, J., & Whitaker, H. (1982). The acquisition of tag questions. *Child Development, 53*, 1254–1257.

Derwing, B., & Baker, W. (1986). Assessing morphological development. In P. Fletcher & M. Garman (Eds.), *Language acquisition* (2nd ed.). New York: Cambridge University Press.

de Villiers, J. (1984). Form and force interactions: The development of negatives and questions. In R. Schiefelbusch & J. Pickar (Eds.), *The acquisition of communicative competence*. Baltimore: University Park Press.

de Villiers, J. (1985). Learning how to use verbs: Lexical coding and the influence of the input. *Journal of Child Language, 12*, 587–595.

de Villiers, P. (1982). *Later syntactic development: The contribution of semantics and pragmatics*. Paper presented at the convention of the New York State Speech-Language-Hearing Association.

deVries, J., & Vallee, F. (1980). *Language use in Canada.* Ottawa: Statistics Canada.

Diamond, J. (1993, February). Speaking with a single tongue. *Discover,* 78–85.

Dickinson, D. (1984). First impressions: Children's knowledge of words gained from a single exposure. *Applied Psycholinguistics, 5,* 359–373.

Dickinson, D. Wolf, M., & Stotsky, S. (1993). Words move: The interwoven development of oral and written language. In J. B. Gleason (Ed.), *The development of language.* Boston: Allyn and Bacon

Diesendruck, G., & Shatz, M. (1997). The effect of perceptual similarity and linguistic input on children's acquisition of object labels. *Journal of Child Language, 24,* 695–717.

Dobrich, W., & Scarborough, H. S. (1992). Phonological characteristics of words young children try to say. *Journal of Child Language, 19,* 597–616.

Dodd, B., & McEvoy, S. (1994). Twin language or phonological disorder. *Journal of Child Language, 21,* 273–289.

D'Odorico, L., Cassibba, R., & Salerni, N. (1997). Temporal relatiohships between gaze and vocal behavior in prelinguistic and linguistic communication. *Journal of Psycholinguistic Research, 26,* 539–556.

D'Odorico, L., & Franco, F. (1985). The determinants of baby talk: Relationship to context. *Journal of Child Language, 12,* 567–586.

Dollaghan, C. (1985). Child meets word: "Fast mapping" in preschool children. *Journal of Speech and Hearing Research, 28,* 449–454.

Dollaghan, C. (1994). Children's phonological neighborhoods: Half empty or half full. *Journal of Child Language, 21,* 257–271.

Donahue, M. L., & Pearl, R. (1995). Conversational interactions of mothers and their preschool children who had been born preterm. *Journal of Speech and Hearing Research, 38,* 1117–1125.

Dore, J. (1974). A pragmatic description of early language development. *Journal of Psycholinguistic Research, 3,* 343–350.

Dore, J. (1986). The development of conversational competence. In R. Schiefelbusch (Ed.), *Language competence: Assessment and intervention.* San Diego: College-Hill Press.

Dore, J., Franklin, M., Miller, R., & Ramer, A. (1976). Transitional phenomena in early language acquisition. *Journal of Child Language, 3,* 13–28.

Dromi, E. (1987). *Early lexical development.* New York: Cambridge University Press.

Dromi, E., & Berman, R. (1982). A morphemic measure of early language development from Modern Hebrew. *Journal of Child Language, 9,* 403–424.

Duchan, J. (1986). Learning to describe events. *Topics in Language Disorders, 6(4),* 27–36.

Dunst, C., & Lowe, L. (1986). From reflex to symbol: Describing, explaining, & fostering communicative competence. *Augmentative & Alternative Communication, 2,* 11–18.

Dyson, A. H. (1983). *Early writing as drawing: The developmental gap between speaking and writing.* Paper presented at the convention of the American Educational Research Association.

Dyson, A. H. (1989). *Multiple worlds of child writers: Friends learning to write.* New York: Teachers College Press.

Eckstein, A. (1986). Effect of the bilingual program on English language and cognitive development. In M. Clyne (Ed.), *An early start: Second language at primary school* (pp. 82–98). Melbourne: River Seine Publications.

Ehrenreich, B. (1981). The politics of talking in couples. *Ms., 5,* 43–45, 86–89.

Eisen, J. M., & Fernald, A. (in preparation). *Prosodic modifications in the infant-directed speech of rural Xhosa-speaking mothers.*

Eisenberg, A. (1982). *Language acquisition in cultural perspective: Talk in three Mexicano homes.* Unpublished doctoral dissertation, University of California, Berkeley.

Eisenberg, A. (1985). Learning to describe past experiences in conversation. *Discourse Processes, 8,* 177–204.

Eisenberg, R. (1976). *Auditory competence in early life: The roots of communicative behavior.* Baltimore: University Park Press.

Eisenberg, S. (1997). Investigating children's language: A comparison of conversational sampling and elicited production. *Journal of Psycholinguistic Research, 26,* 519–538.

Elbers, M. (1990). Language acquisition: Blends, overgeneralization and self-produced input. In P. Coopman, B., Shouten, & W. Lonneveld (Eds.), *OTS Yearbook 1990.* Dordrecht: ICG.

Elias, G., & Broerse, J. (1996). Developmental changes in the incidence and likelihood of simultaneous talk during the first two years: A question of function. *Journal of Child Language, 23*, 201–217.

Elliot, A. (1981). *Child language.* New York: Cambridge University Press.

Emmorey, K. (1993). Processing a dynamic visual-spatial language: Psycholinguistic studies of American Sign Language. *Journal of Psycholinguistic Research, 22*, 153–187.

Emslie, H., & Stevenson, R. (1981). Preschool children's use of the articles in definite and indefinite referring expressions. *Journal of Child Language, 8*, 313–328.

Erbaugh, M. (1980, December). *Acquisition of Mandarin syntax: 'Less' grammar isn't easier.* Paper presented at the meeting of the Linguistic Society of America, San Antonio, TX.

Erbaugh, M. (1982). *Coming to order: Natural selection and the origin of syntax in the Mandarin-speaking child.* Unpublished doctoral dissertation, University of California, Berkeley.

Erreich, A. (1984). Learning how to ask: Patterns of inversion in yes/no and wh- questions. *Journal of Child Language, 11*, 579–592.

Ervin-Tripp, S. (1980). Lecture. University of Minnesota. May 14, 1980.

Ervin-Tripp, S., & Gordon, D. (1986). The development of requests. In R. Schiefelbusch (Ed.), *Language competence: Assessment and intervention.* San Diego: College-Hill Press.

Ervin-Tripp, S., O'Connor, M., Rosenberg, J., & O'Barr, A. W. (1984). Language and power in the family. In C. Kramerae & M. Schulz (Eds.), *Language and power* (4th ed.). Beverly Hills, CA: Sage.

Fang, F. (1985). An experiment on the use of classifiers by 4- to 6-year olds. *Acta Psycholgica Sinica, 17*, 384–392.

Farrar, M. J. (1990). Discourse and the acquisition of grammatical morphemes. *Journal of Child Language, 17*, 607–624.

Farrar, M. J., Friend, M. J., & Forbes, J. N. (1993). Event knowledge and early language acquisition. *Journal of Child Language, 20*, 591–606.

Feagans, L. (1980). Children's understanding of some temporal terms denoting order, duration, and simultaneity. *Journal of Psycholinguistic Research, 9*, 41–57.

Fenson, L., & Ramsey, D. (1980). Decentration and integration of the child's play in the second year. *Child Development, 51*, 171–178.

Ferguson, C. (1978). Learning to pronounce: The earliest stages of phonological development in the child. In F. Minifie & L. Lloyd (Eds.), *Communicative and cognitive abilities—Early behavioral assessment.* Baltimore: University Park Press.

Fernald, A. (1981). *Four-month-olds prefer to listen to "motherese."* Paper presented at a meeting of the Society for Research in Child Development.

Fernald, A. (1985). Four-month-old infants prefer to listen to motherese. *Infant Behavior and Development, 8*, 181–195.

Fernald, A. (1994). Human maternal vocalizations to infants as biologically relevant signals: An evolutionary perspective. In P. Bloom (Ed.), *Language acquisition: Core readings.* Cambridge, MA: MIT Press.

Fernald, A., & Kuhl, P. (1987). *Fundamental frequency as an acoustic determinant of infant preference for motherese.* Paper presented at a meeting of the Society for Research in Child Development.

Fernald, A., & Morikawa, H. (1993). Common themes and cultural differences in Japanese and American mothers' speech to infants. *Child Development, 64*, 637–656.

Fernald, A., & Simon, T. (1984). Expanded intonation contours in mothers' speech to newborns. *Developmental Psychology, 20*, 104–113.

Fernald, A., Taeschner, T., Dunn, J., Papousek, M., deBoysson-Bardies, B., & Fukui, I. (1989). A cross-language study of prosody modifications in mothers' and fathers' speech to preverbal infants. *Journal of Child Language, 16*, 477–501.

Ferreiro, E. (1984). The underlying logic of literacy development. In H. Goelman, A. Oberg, & F. Smith (Eds.), *Awakening to literacy.* Exeter, NH: Heinemann.

Ferreiro, E., & Teberosky, A. (1982). Literacy before schooling. Exeter, NH: Heinemann.

Fillmore, C. (1968). The case for case. In E. Bach & R. Harmas (Eds.), *Universals in linguistic theory.* New York: Holt, Rinehart & Winston.

Fischer, K. (1980). A theory of cognitive development: The control and construction of hierarchies of skill. *Psychological Review, 87*, 477–526.

Fischer, K. W., & Bidell, T. (1991). Constraining nativist inferences about cognitive capacities. In S. Carey & R. Gelmans (Eds.), *The epigenesis of mind: Essays on biology and cognition* (pp. 199–235). Holmsdale, NJ: Erlbaum.

Fischer, K. W., & Farrar, M. J. (1987). Generalizations about generalizations: How a theory of skill development explains both generality and specificity. *International Journal of Psychology, 22,* 643–677.

Fivush, R. (1984). Learning about school: The development of kindergarteners' school scripts. *Child Development, 55,* 1697–1709.

Flavell, J. (1977). *Cognitive development.* Englewood Cliffs, NJ: Prentice Hall.

Flavell, J. (1982). On cognitive development. *Child Development, 53,* 1–10.

Flavell, J., & Wellman, H. (1977). Metamemory. In R. Kail & J. Hagen (Eds.), *Perspectives on the development of memory and cognition.* Hillsdale, NJ: Erlbaum.

Fodor, J. D., Ni, W., Crain, S., & Shankweiler, D. (1996). Tasks and timing in the perception of linguistic anomaly. *Journal of Psycholinguistic Research, 25,* 25–57.

Fogel, A., Toda, S., & Kawai, M. (1988). Mother–infant face-to-face interaction in Japan and the United States: A laboratory comparison using 3-month-old infants. *Developmental Psychology, 24,* 398–406.

Forbes, J. N., & Poulin-DuBois, D. (1997). Representational change in young children's understanding of familiar verb meaning. *Journal of Child Language, 24,* 389–406.

Foster, S. (1981). The emergence of topic type in children under 2; 6: A chicken-and-egg problem. *Proceedings and Reports in Child Language Development, 20,* 52–60.

Foster, S. (1986). Learning topic management in the preschool years. *Journal of Child Language, 13,* 231–250.

Franco, F., & Butterworth, G. (1996). Pointing and social awareness: Declaring and requesting in the second year. *Journal of Child Language, 23,* 307–336.

Frazier, L. (1987). Theories of sentence processing. In J. L. Garfield (Ed.), *Modularity in knowledge representation and natural language understanding.* Cambridge, MA: MIT Press.

Frazier, L. (1993). Processing Dutch sentence structures. *Journal of Psycholinguistic Research, 22,* 85–108.

Frazier, L., & Clifton, C. (1995). *Construal.* Cambridge, MA: MIT Press.

Fremgen, A., & Fay, D. (1980). Overextensions in production and comprehension: A methodological clarification. *Journal of Child Language, 7,* 205–211.

French, A. (1989). The systematic acquisition of word forms by a child during the first-fifty-word-stage. *Journal of Child Language, 16,* 69–90.

French, L., & Brown, A. (1977). Comprehension of "before" and "after" in logical and arbitrary sequences. *Journal of Child Language, 4,* 247–256.

French, L., & Nelson, K. (1985). *Young children's knowledge of relational terms: Some ifs, ors, and buts.* New York: Springer-Verlag.

Frenck-Mestre, C. (1993). Use of orthographic redundancies and word identification speed in bilinguals. *Journal of Psycholinguistic Research, 22,* 397–409.

Frith, V. (1985). Beneath the surface of developmental dyslexia. In K. Patterson, J. Marshall, & M. Coltheart (Eds.), *Surface dyslexia: Neuropsychological and cognitive studies of phonological reading.* London: Erlbaum.

Furman, L. N., & Walden, T. A. (1989, April). *The effect of script knowledge on children's communicative interactions.* Paper presented at the meeting of the Society for Research in Child Development, Kansas City, MO.

Furrow, D. (1984). Young children's use of prosody. *Journal of Child Language, 11,* 203–213.

Furrow, D., Baillie, C., McLaren, J., & Moore, C. (1993). Differential responding to two- and three-year-olds utterances: The role of grammaticality and ambiguity. *Journal of Child Language, 20,* 363–375.

Furrow, D., Moore, C., Davidge, J., & Chiasson, L. (1992). Mental terms in mothers' and children's speech: Similarities and relationships. *Journal of Child Language, 19,* 617–631.

Furrow, D., & Nelson, K. (1984). Enviromental correlates of indivual differences in language acquisition. *Journal of Child Language, 11,* 523–534.

Furth, H. (1966). *Thinking without language.* New York: Free Press.

Furth, H. (1971). Linguistic deficiency and thinking: Research with deaf subjects, 1964–1969 *Psychological Bulletin, 75,* 58–72.

Gainotti, G., Caltagirone, C., Miceli, G., & Masullo, C. (1981). Selective semantic-lexical impairment to language comprehension in right brain-damaged patients. *Brain and Language, 13,* 201–211.

Galda, L. (1984). Narrative competence: Play, storytelling and comprehension. In A. Pellegrini & T. Yawkey (Eds.), *The development of oral and written language in social context.* Norwood, NJ: Ablex.

Gale, D., Liebergott, J., & Griffin, S. (1981). *Getting it: Children's requests for clarification.* Paper presented at the convention of the American Speech-Language-Hearing Association.

Gallagher, T. (1981). Contingent query sequences within adult-child discourse. *Journal of Child Language, 8,* 51–62.

Galligan, R. (1987). Intonation with single words: Purposive and grammatical use. *Journal of Child Language, 14,* 1–21.

Gardner, H., & Winner, E. (1979, May). The child is father to the metaphor. *Psychology Today,* 81–91.

Gardner, R., Robey, B., & Smith, P. (1985). Asian Americans: Growth, change, and diversity. *Population Bulletin, 40(4).*

Gathercole, V. (1985). "Me has too much hard questions": The acquisition of the linguistic mass-count distinction in much and many. *Journal of Child Language, 12,* 395–415.

Gathercole, V. (1989). Contrast: A semantic constraint? *Journal of Child Language, 16,* 685–702.

Gavin, W. J., & Giles, L. (1996). Sample size effects on temporal reliability of language sample measures of preschool children. *Journal of Speech and Hearing Research, 39,* 1258–1262.

Gee, J.P. (1989). Two styles of narrative construction and their linguistic and educational implications. *Discourse Processes, 12,* 287–307.

Genesee, F. (1989). Early bilingual development: One language or two? *Journal of Child Language, 16,* 161–179.

Genesee, F., Nicoladis, E. & Paradis, J. (1995). Language differentiation in early bilingual development. *Journal of Child Language, 22,* 611–631.

Gentner, D. (1982). Why nouns are learned before verbs: Linguistic relativity versus natural partitioning. In S. Kuczaj (Ed.), *Language development: Vol 2. Language, thought, and culture.* Hillsdale, NJ: Erlbaum.

George, S. W., & Krantz, M. (1981). The effects of preferred partnerships on communication adequacy. *Journal of Psychology, 109,* 245–253.

Gerken, L. (1996). Prosody's role in language acquisition and adult parsing. *Journal of Psycholinguistic Research, 25,* 345–356.

Gertner, B. L., Rice, M. L., & Hadley, P. A. (1994). Influence of communicative competence on peer preferences in a preschool classroom. *Journal of Speech and Hearing Research, 37,* 913–923.

Geschwind, N., & Galaburda, A. (1985). Cerebral lateralization, biological mechanisms, associations and pathology: I. A hypothesis and a program for research. *Archives of Neurology, 42,* 428–459.

Gibbs, R. W. (1985). On the process of understanding idioms. *Journal of Psycholinguistic Research, 14,* 465–472.

Gibbs, R. W. (1986). Skating on thin ice: Literal meaning and understanding idioms in conversation. *Discourse Processes, 9,* 17–30.

Gibbs, R. W. (1987). Linguistic factors in children's understanding of idioms. *Journal of Child Language, 14,* 569–586.

Gibson, E. (1991). A computational theory of human linguistic processing: Memory limitations and processing breakdown. Unpublished doctoral dissertation, Carnegie Mellon University, Pittsburgh, PA.

Gibson, E., & Levin, H. (1975). *The psychology of reading.* Cambridge: MIT Press.

Gillam, R. B., & Johnston, J. R. (1992). Spoken and written language relationships in language/learning-impaired and normal achieving school-age children. *Journal of Speech and Hearing Research, 35,* 1303–1315.

Ginsberg, G., & Kilbourne, B. (1988). Emergence of vocal alternation in mother–infant interchanges. *Journal of Child Language, 15,* 221–235.

Girbau, D. (1996). Private and social speech in communication: Terminology and distinctive traits. *Journal of Psycholinguistic Research, 25,* 507–513.

Girouard, P. C., Ricard, M., & DeCarie, T. G. (1997). The acquisition of personal pronouns in French-speaking children. *Journal of Child Language, 24,* 311–326.

Glass, A. (1983). The comprehension of idioms. *Journal of Psycholinguistics Research, 12,* 429–442.

Gleitman, L. (1993). The structural sources of verb meanings. In P. Bloom (Ed.), *Language acquisition: Core readings.* Cambridge, MA: MIT Press.

Gleitman, L., Newport, E., & Gleitman, H. (1984). The current status of the motherese hypothesis. *Journal of Child Language, 11,* 43–79.

Gleitman, L., & Wanner, E. (1982). Language acquisition: The state of the state of the art. In E. Wanner and L. Gleitman (Eds.), *Language acquisition: The state of the art.* Cambridge: Cambridge University Press.

Glenn, C., & Stein, N. (1980). *Syntactic structures and real world themes in stories generated by children* (Technical report). Urbana: University of Illinois, Center for the Study of Reading.

Goffman, L., Schwartz, R. G., & Marton, K. (1996). Information level and young children's phonological accuracy. *Journal of Child Language, 23,* 337–347.

Goldfield, B. A. (1993). Noun bias in maternal speech to one-year-olds. *Journal of Child Language, 20*, 85–99.

Goldfield, B. A., & Reznick, J. (1990). Early lexical acquisitions: Rate, content, and the vocabulary spurt. *Journal of Child Language, 17*, 171–183.

Goldfield, B. A., & Snow, C. (1985). Individual differences in language acquisition. In J. Berko Gleason (Ed.), *The development of language*. Columbus, OH: Merrill.

Goldin-Meadow, S., & Morford, M. (1985). Gesture in early child language: Studies of deaf and hearing children. *Merrill-Palmer Quarterly, 31*, 145–176.

Goldman-Rakic, P. (1987). Development of cortical circuitry and cognitive function. *Child Development, 58*, 601–622.

Goldstein, B. A., & Iglesias, A. (1996). Phonological patterns in normally developing Spanish-speaking 3- and 4-year-olds of Puerto Rican descent. *Language, Speech, and Hearing Services in Schools, 27*, 82–89.

Golinkoff, R. M. (1993). When is communication a 'meeting of the minds'? *Journal of Child Language, 20*, 199–207.

Golinkoff, R. M., Hirsh-Pasek, K., Cauley, K., & Gordon, L. (1987). The eyes have it: Lexical and syntactic comprehension in a new paradigm. *Journal of Child Language, 14*, 23–46.

Golinkoff, R. M., & Markessini, J. (1980). "Mommy sock": The child's understanding of possession as expressed in two-noun phrases. *Journal of Child Language, 21*, 135–155.

Golinkoff, R. M., Mervis, C. B., & Hirsh-Pasek, K. (1994). Early object labels: The case for a developmental lexical principles framework. *Journal of Child Language, 21*, 135–155.

Gombert, J. E. (1992). *Metalinguistic development*. London: Harvester Wheatsheaf.

Goodglass, H., & Wingfield, A. (1998). The changing relationship between anatomic and cognitive explanation in the neuropsychology of language. *Journal of Psycholinguistic Research, 27*, 147–165.

Goodluck, H. (1986). Language acquisition and linguistic theory. In P. Fletcher & M. Garman (Eds.), *Language acquisition* (2nd ed.). New York: Cambridge University Press.

Goodman, K. (1976). Behind the eye: What happens in reading. In H. Singer & R. Ruddell (Eds.), *Theoretical models and processes of reading* (2nd ed.). Newark, DE: International Reading Association.

Goodman, Y. (1986). Children coming to know literacy. In W. Teale & E. Sulzby (Eds.), *Emergent literacy*. Norwood, NJ: Ablex.

Goodsitt, J. V., Morgan, J. L., & Kuhl, P. K. (1993). Perceptual strategies in prelingual speech segmentation. *Journal of Child Language, 20*, 229–252.

Goodwin, M. (1980). Directive-response speech sequences in girl's and boy's task activities. In S. McConnell-Ginet, R. Borker, & N. Furman (Eds.), *Women and language in liberation and society* (pp. 157–173). New York: Praeger.

Goossens, L. (1981). *On the development of the modals ands of the epistemic function of English*. Paper presented at the \ifth International Conference on Historical Linguistics, Galway, Ireland.

Gopnik, A., & Choi, S. (1990). Language and cognition. *First Language, 10*, 199–216.

Gopnik, A., Choi, S., & Baumberger, T. (1996). Cross-linguistic differences in early semantic and cognitive development. *Cognitive Development, 11*, 197–227.

Gopnik, A., & Meltzoff, A. (1984). Semantic and cognitive development in 15- to 21-month-old children. *Journal of Child Development, 11*, 495–513.

Gopnik, A., & Meltzoff, A. (1986). Relations between semantic and cognitive development in the one-word stage: The specificity hypothesis. *Child Development, 57*, 1040–1053.

Gopnik, A., & Meltzoff, A. (1987). The development of categorization in the second year and its relation to other cognitive and linguistic developments. *Child Development, 58*, 1523–1531.

Gordon, D., & Ervin-Tripp, S. (1984). The structure of children's requests. In R. Schiefelbusch & J. Pickar (Eds.), *The acquisition of communicative competence*. Baltimore: University Park Press.

Gordon, P. (1982). *The acquisition of syntactic categories: The case of the count/mass distinction*. Unpublished doctoral dissertation, Massachusetts Institute of Technology.

Gordon, P. (1988). Count/mass category acquisition: Distributional distinctions in children's speech. *Journal of Child Language, 15*, 109–128.

Gottfried, G. M. (1997). Using metaphors as modifiers: Children's production of metaphoric compounds. *Journal of Child Language, 24*, 567–601.

Gourley, J., Benedict, S., Gundersheim, S., & McClellan, J. (1983). *Learning about literacy from children: An ethnographic study in a kindergarten classroom.* Paper presented at the convention of the American Educational Research Association.

Gow, D. W., & Gordon, P. C. (1993). Coming to terms with stress: Effects of stress location in sentence processing. *Journal of Psycholinguistic Research, 22,* 545–578.

Greenberg, J., & Kuczaj, S. (1982). Towards a theory of substantive word-meaning acquisition. In S. Kuczaj (Ed.), *Language development: Vol. 1. Syntax and semantics.* Hillsdale, NJ: Erlbaum.

Greenfield, P. (1978). Informativeness, presupposition, and semantic choice in single-word utterances. In N. Waterson & C. Snow (Eds.), *The development of communication.* New York: Wiley.

Greenfield, P., & Smith, J. (1976). *The structure of communication in early language development.* New York: Academic Press.

Greenfield, P. A., & Savage-Rumbaugh, E. S. (1993). Comparing communicative competence in child and chimp: The pragmatics of repetition. *Journal of Child Language, 20,* 1–26.

Greenspan, S. (1988). Fostering emotional and social development in infants with disabilities. *Zero to Three, 8,* 8–18.

Greif, E., & Berko Gleason, J. (1980). Hi, thanks, and goodbye: Some more routine information. *Language and Society, 9,* 159–166.

Grice, H. (1975). Logic and conversation. In D. Davidson & G. Harmon (Eds.), *The logic of grammar.* Encina, CA: Dickenson Press.

Grieser, D. L., & Kuhl, P. (1988). Maternal speech to infants in a tonal language: Support for universal prosodic features in motherese. *Developmental Psychology, 24,* 14–20.

Griffiths, P. (1986). Early vocabulary. In P. Fletcher & M. Garman (Eds.), *Language acquisition (2nd ed.).* New York: Cambridge University Press.

Grimshaw, J. (1990). *Argument structure.* Cambridge, MA: MIT Press.

Grosjean, F. (1980). Spoken word recognition processes and the gating paradigm. *Perception and Psychophysics, 28,* 267–283.

Grosjean, F. (1982). *Life with two languages.* Cambridge: Harvard University Press.

Gruber, J. (1967). Topicalization of child language. *Foundations of Language, 3,* 37–65.

Grunwell, P. (1981). The development of phonology. *First Language, 2,* 161–191.

Gundloch, R. (1981). On the nature and development of children's writing. In C. Frederiksen & J. Dominic (Eds.), *Writing: The nature, development, and teaching of written communication* (Vol. 2). Hillsdale, NJ: Erlbaum.

Gutierrez-Clellen, V. F. (1998). Syntactic skills of Spanish-speaking children with low school achievement. *Language, Speech, and Hearing Services in Schools, 29,* 207–215.

Guttierrez-Clellan, V. F., & Heinrichs-Ramos, L. (1993). Referential cohesion in the narratives of Spanish-speaking children: A developmental study. *Journal of Speech and Hearing Research, 36,* 559–567.

Guttierrez-Clellan, V. F., & McGrath, A. (1991). *Syntactic complexity in Spanish narratives: A developmental study.* Paper presented at the annual convention of the American Speech-Language-Hearing Association, Atlanta, GA.

Haaf, W. L. (1996, March 11). Ohio researchers find better language skills in preschoolers from single parent homes. *Advance for Speech-Language Pathologists and Audiologists, 5.*

Haas, A. (1979). The acquisition of genderlect. *Annals of the New York Academy of Sciences, 327,* 101–113.

Haas, A., & Owens, R. (1985). *Preschoolers' pronoun strategies: You and me make us.* Paper presented at the annual convention of the American Speech-Language-Hearing Association.

Hadley, P. A. (1999). Validating a rate-based measure of early grammatical abilities: Unique syntactic types. *American Journal of Speech-Language Pathology, 8,* 261–272.

Haith, M. (1976). *Organization of visual behavior at birth.* Paper presented at the 22nd International Congress of Psychology.

Hakes, D. (1980). *The development of metalinguistic abilities in children.* Berlin: Springer-Verlag.

Hakes, D. (1982). The development of metalinguistic abilities: What develops? In S. Kuczaj (Ed.), *Language development: Vol. 2. Language, thought and culture.* Hillsdale, NJ: Erlbaum.

Hakuta, K., de Villiers, J., & Tager-Flusberg, H. (1982). Sentence coordination in Japanese and English. *Journal of Child Language, 9,* 193–207.

Hakuta, K. (1987). The second language learner in the context of the study of language acquisition. In P. Homel, M. Palij, & D. Aronson (Eds.), *Childhood*

bilingualism: Aspects in linguistic, cognitive, and social development (pp. 31–55) Hillsdale, NJ: Erlbaum.

Halliday, M. (1975a). Learning how to mean. In E. Lenneberg & E. Lenneberg (Eds.), *Foundations of language development: A multidisciplinary approach.* New York: Academic Press.

Halliday, M. (1975b). *Learning how to mean: Explorations in the development of language.* New York: Arnold.

Hamayan, E., & Damico, J. (1991). Developing and using a second language. In E. Hamayan & J. Damico (Eds.), *Limiting bias in the assessment of bilingual students* (pp. 40–75). Austin, TX: Pro-Ed.

Hammer, C. S., & Weiss, A. L. (1999). Guiding language development: How African American mothers and their infants structure play interactions. *Journal of Speech, Language, and Hearing Research, 42,* 1219–1233.

Hampson, J. (1989). *Elements of style: Maternal and child contributions to the referential and expressive styles of language acquisition.* Unpublished doctoral dissertation, City University of New York.

Hampson, J., & Nelson, K. (1993). The relation of maternal language to variation in rate and style of language acquisition. *Journal of Child Language, 20,* 313–342.

Hanzlik, J., & Stevenson, M. (1986). Interaction of mothers with their infants who are mentally retarded, retarded with cerebral palsy, or nonretarded. *American Journal on Mental Deficiency, 90,* 513–520.

Hardin, E. E., O'Connell, D. C., & Kowal, S. (1998). Reading aloud from logographic and alphabetic texts: Comparisons between Chinese and German. *Journal of Psycholinguistic Research, 27,* 413–439.

Harris, M., Barrett, M., Jones, D., & Brooks, S. (1988). Linguistic input and early word meanings. *Journal of Child Language, 15,* 77–94.

Harris, M., Jones, D., Brookes, S., & Grant, J. (1986). Relations between the non-verbal context of maternal speech and rate of language development. *British Journal of Developmental Psychology, 4,* 261–268.

Harris, M., Jones, D., & Grant, J. (1983). The nonverbal context of mothers' speech to infants. *First Language, 4,* 21–30.

Harris, M., Yeeles, C., Chasin, J., & Oakley, Y. (1995). Symmetries and asymmetries in early lexical comprehension and production. *Journal of Child Language, 22,* 1–18.

Harris, P., Kruithof, A., Terwogt, M., & Visser, T. (1981). Children's detection and awareness of textual anomaly. *Journal of Exceptional Child Psychology, 31,* 212–230.

Harste, J., Woodward, J., & Burke, C. (1984). *Language stories & literacy lessons.* Portsmouth, NH: Heineman.

Hart, B., & Risley, T. R. (1995). *Meaningful differences in the everyday experience of young American children.* Baltimore, MD: Paul H. Brookes.

Hartup, W. (1983). Peer relations. In E. M. Hetherington (Ed.), *Handbook of child psychology* (Vol. 4). New York: Wiley.

Hatch, E. (1971). The young child's comprehension of time connectives. *Child Development, 42,* 2111–2113.

Hayashi, R. (1988). Simultaneous talk—From the perspective of floor management of English and Japanese speakers. *World Englishes, 7,* 269–288.

Hayes, P. A., Norris, J., & Flaitz, J. R. (1998). A comparison of the oral narrative abilities of underachieving and high-achieving gifted adolescents: A preliminary investigation. *Language, Speech, and Hearing Services in Schools, 29,* 158–171.

Heath, S. (1983). *Ways with words: Language, life and work in communities and classrooms.* Cambridge: Cambridge University Press.

Heath, S. (1986a). Separating "things of the imagination" from life: Learning to read and write. In W. Teale & E. Sulzby (Eds.), *Emergent literacy.* Norwood, NJ: Ablex.

Heath, S. (1986b). Taking a cross-cultural look at narratives. *Topics in Language Disorders, 7(1),* 84–94.

Henderson, E. H., & Beers, J. W. (Eds.). (1980). *Developmental and cognitive aspects of learning to spell: A reflection of word knowledge.* Newark, DE: International Reading Association.

Hess, R. D., Kashiwagi, K., Azuma, H., Price, G. G., & Dickson, W. P. (1980). Maternal expectations for mastery of developmental tasks in Japan and the United States. *International Journal of Psychology, 15,* 259–271.

Hickey, T. (1993). Identifying formulas in first language acquisition. *Journal of Child Language, 20,* 27–41.

Hickman, M. (1986). Psychosocial aspects of language acquisition. In P. Fletcher & M. Garman (Eds.), *Language acquisition* (2nd ed.). New York: Cambridge University Press.

Hickman, M., Hendriks, H., Roland, F., & Liang, J. (1996). The marking of new information in children's narratives: A comparison of English, French, German, and Mandarin Chinese. *Journal of Child Language, 23*, 591–619.

Hickok, G. (1993). Parallel parsing: Evidence from reactivation in garden-path sentences. *Journal of Psycholinguistic Research, 22*, 239–250.

Hilke, D. (1988). Infant vocalizations and changes in experience. *Journal of Child Language, 15*, 1–15.

Hillenbrand, J. (1983). Perceptual organization of speech sounds by infants. *Journal of Speech and Hearing Research, 26*, 268–281.

Hirsh-Pasek, K., Kemler Nelson, D., Jusczyk, P., Cassidy, K., Druss, B., & Kennedy, L. (1987). Clauses are perceptual units for young infants. *Cognition, 26*, 269–286.

Hirsh-Pasek, K., Treiman, R., & Schneiderman, M. (1984). Brown and Hamlon revisited: Mother's sensitivity to ungrammatical forms. *Journal of Child Language, 11*, 81–88.

Hladik, E., & Edwards, H. (1984). A comparative analysis of mother-father speech in the naturalistic home environment. *Journal of Psycholinguistic Research, 13*, 321–332.

Hodgkinson, H. (1986). *Future search: A look at the present*. Washington, DC: National Education Association.

Hoff-Ginsberg, E. (1985). Some contributions of mothers' speech to their children's syntactic growth. *Journal of Child Language, 12*, 367–385.

Hoff-Ginsberg, E. (1986). Function and structure in maternal speech: Their relation to the child's development of syntax. *Developmental Psychology, 22*, 155–163.

Hoff-Ginsberg, E. (1990). Maternal speech and the child's development of syntax: A further look. *Journal of Child Language, 17*, 85–99.

Hoffman, P., & Norris, J. (1989). On the nature of phonological development evidence from normal children's spelling errors. *Journal of Speech and Hearing Research, 32*, 787–794.

Hoffner, C., Cantor, J., & Badzinski, D. (1990). Children's understanding of adverbs denoting degree of likelihood. *Journal of Child Language, 17*, 217–231.

Holdgrafer, G., & Sorenson, P. (1984). Informativeness and lexical learning. *Psychological Reports, 54*, 75–80.

Holzman, M. (1984). Evidence for a reciprocal model of language development. *Journal of Psycholinguistic Research, 13*, 119–146.

Horton, M., & Markman, E. (1980). Developmental differences in the acquisition of basic and superordinate categories. *Child Development, 51*, 708–719.

Howard, D. (1983). The effects of aging and degree of association on the semantic priming of lexical decisions. *Experimental Aging Research, 9*, 145–151.

Howlin, P., & Rutter, M. (1987). The consequences of language delay for other aspects of development. In W. Yule & M. Ritter (Eds.), *Language development and language disorders*. Philadelphia, PA: Lippincott.

Huerta-Macias, A. (1981). Codeswitching: All in the family. In R. Duran (Ed.), *Latino language and communicative behavior*. Norwood, NJ: Ablex.

Hummer, P., Wimmer, H., & Antes, G. (1993). On the origins of denial. *Journal of Child Language, 20*, 607–618.

Huttenlocher, J., Smiley, P., & Charney, R. (1983). Emergence of action categories in the child: Evidence from verb meaning. *Psychological Review, 90*, 72–93.

Huxley, R. (1970). The development of the correct use of subject personal pronouns in two children. In G. Flores d'Arcais & W. Levelt (Eds.), *Advances in psycholinguistics*. Amsterdam: North-Holland.

Iglesias, A. (1986, May 3). *The cultural-linguistic minority student in the classroom: Management decisions*. Workshop presented at the State University College at Buffalo, NY.

Ingram, D. (1976). *Phonological disability in children*. London: Arnold.

Ingram, D. (1986). Phonological development: Production. In P. Fletcher & M. Garman (Eds.), *Language acquisition* (2nd ed.). New York: Cambridge University Press.

Ingram, D. (1995). The cultural basis of prosodic modifications to infants and children: A response to Fernald's universalist theory. *Journal of Child Language, 22*, 223–233.

Irwin, J. W. (1980). The effects of linguistic cohesion on prose comprehension. *Journal of Reading Behavior, 12*, 325–332.

Isaacs, G. J. (1996). Persistence of non-standard dialect in school-age children. *Journal of Speech and Hearing Research, 39*, 434–441.

Jackendoff, R. (1990). *Semantic structures*. Cambridge, MA: MIT Press.

Jackson-Maldonado, D., Thal, D., Marchman, V., Bates, E., & Gutierrez-Clellan, V. (1993). Early lexical development in Spanish-speaking infants and toddlers. *Journal of Child Language, 20,* 523–549.

Jakobson, R., Fant, C., & Halle, M. (1951). *Preliminaries to speech analysis.* Cambridge: MIT Press.

James, S. (1980). *Language and sensorimotor cognitive development in the young child.* Paper presented at the annual convention of the New York Speech-Language-Hearing Association.

James, S., & Seebach, M. (1982). The pragmatic function of children's questions. *Journal of Speech and Hearing Research, 25,* 2–11.

Javier, R. A., Barroso, F., & Munoz, M. (1993). Autobiographical memory in bilinguals. *Journal of Psycholinguistic Research, 22,* 319–338.

Jenkins, J. (1969). Language and thought. In J. Voss (Ed.), *Approaches to thought.* Columbus, OH: Merrill.

Johnson, C. J., & Anglin, J. M. (1995). Qualitative developments in the content and form of children's definitions. *Journal of Speech and Hearing Research, 38,* 612–629.

Johnson, D., Toms-Bronowski, S., & Pittelman, S. (1982). Vocabulary development. *Volta Reviews, 84(5),* 11–24.

Johnson, H. (1975). The meaning of before and after for preschool children. *Journal of Exceptional Child Psychology, 19,* 88–99.

Johnson, H. & Chapman, R. (1980). Children's judgment and recall of causal connectives: A developmental study of "because," "so," and "and." *Journal of Psycholinguistic Research, 9,* 243–260.

Johnson, N. S. (1983). What do you do when you can't tell the whole story? The development of summarization skills. In K. E. Nelson (Ed.), *Children's Language* (Vol. 4) (pp. 315–383). Hillsdale, NJ: Erlbaum.

Johnston, J. (1982). Narratives: A new look at communication problems in older language disordered children. *Language, Speech, and Hearing Services in the Schools, 13,* 144–145.

Johnston, J. (1984). Acquisition of locative meanings: Behind and in front of. *Journal of Child Language, 11,* 407–422.

Joiner, C. (F. Supp. 1979). *Martin Luther King Junior Elementary School vs. Ann Arbor School District,* 1371–1391.

Juel, C. (1984). An evolving model of reading acquisition. In J. Niles & L. Harris (Eds.), *Changing perspectives on research in reading/language processing and instruction.* Newark, DE: National Reading Conference.

Jusczyk, P. W. (1999, Septerber 30). *Making sense of sounds: Foundations of language acquisition.* Presentation at State University of New York, Geneseo.

Kamhi, A. G., & Catts, H. W. (1999). Reading development. In H. W. Catts & A. G. Kamhi (Eds.), *Language basis of reading disabilities.* Boston: Allyn & Bacon.

Karmiloff-Smith, A. (1981). The grammatical marking of thematic structure in the development of language production. In W. Deutsch (Ed.), *The child's construction of language.* New York: Academic Press.

Karmiloff-Smith, A. (1986). Some fundamental aspects of language development after age 5. In P. Fletcher & M. Garman (Eds.), *Language acquisition* (2nd ed.). New York: Cambridge University Press.

Katz, R., Shankweiler, D., & Liberman, I. (1981). Memory for item order and phonetic recoding in the beginning reader. *Journal of Exceptional Child Psychology, 32,* 474–484.

Kaye, K. (1979). Thickening thin data: The maternal role in developing communication and language. In M. Bullowa (Ed.), *Before speech.* New York: Cambridge University Press.

Kaye, K. (1980). Why we don't talk "baby talk" to babies. *Journal of Child Language, 7,* 489–507.

Kaye, K., & Charney, R. (1981). Conversational asymmetry between mothers and children. *Journal of Child Language, 8,* 35–49.

Kearsley, R. (1973). The newborn's response to auditory stimulation: A demonstration of orienting and defense behavior. *Child Development, 44,* 582–590.

Keller-Cohen, D. (1987). Context and strategy in acquiring temporal connectives. *Journal of Psycholinguistic Research, 16,* 165–183.

Kelly, C., & Dale, P. (1989). Cognitive skills associated with the onset of multiword utterances. *Journal of Speech and Hearing Research, 32,* 645–656.

Kemper, R. (1985). *Metalinguistic correlates of reading ability in second grade children.* Unpublished doctoral dissertation, Kent State University.

Kemper, R. L., & Vernooy, A. R. (1993). Metalinguistic awareness in first graders: A qualitative perspective. *Journal of Psycholinguistic Research, 22,* 41–57.

Kemper, S. (1984). The development of narrative skills: Explanations and entertainments. In S. Kuczaj (Ed.), *Discourse development: Progress in cognitive development research*. New York: Springer-Verlag.

Kemper, S., & Edwards, L. (1986). Children's expression of causality and their construction of narratives. *Topics in Language Disorders, 7(1)*, 11–20.

Kessler, C. (1984). Language acquisition in bilingual children. In N. Miller (Ed.), *Bilingualism and language disability: Assessment and remediation* (pp. 26–54). San Diego, CA: College-Hill Press.

Kessler, C., & Quinn, M. E. (1987). Language minority children's linguistic and cognitive creativity. *Journal of Multilingual and Multicultural Development, 8*, 173–186.

Kinsbourne, M. (1981). The development of cerebral dominance. In S. D. Filskov & T. J. Boll (Eds.), *Handbook of clinical neuropsychology* (Vol. 2, pp. 399–417). New York: Wiley.

Klatsky, R. L. (1980). *Human memory: Structure and process*. San Francisco, CA: Freeman.

Klee, T. (1985). Role of inversion in children's question development. *Journal of Speech and Hearing Research, 28*, 225–232.

Klee, T., & Fitzgerald, M. (1985). The relation between grammatical development and mean length of utterance in morphemes. *Journal of Child Language, 12*, 251–269.

Klein, H. (1981). Early perceptual strategies for the replication of consonants from polysyllabic lexical models. *Journal of Speech and Hearing Research, 24*, 535–551.

Konefal, J., & Fokes, J. (1984). Linguistic analysis of children's conversational repairs. *Journal of Psycholinguistic Research, 13*, 1–11.

Konishi, T. (1993). The semantics of grammatical gender: A cross cultural study. *Journal of Psycholinguistic Research, 22*, 519–534.

Kroll, B. (1981). Developmental relationships between speaking and writing. In B. Kroll & R. Vann (Eds.), *Exploring speaking–writing relationships: Connections and contrasts*. Urbana, IL: National Council of Teachers of English.

Kuczaj, S. A. (1982). Language play and language acquisition. In H.W. Reese (Ed.), *Advances in child development and behavior* (Vol. 14). New York: Academic Press.

Kuczaj, S. A., & Maratsos, M. (1975). On the acquisition of front, back, and side. *Child Development, 46*, 202–358.

Kurland, B. F., & Snow, C. E. (1997). Longitudinal measurement of growth in definitional skill. *Journal of Child Language, 24*, 603–625.

Kyratzis, A., Lucariello, J., & Nelson, K. (1988). *Complementary slot filler and taxonomic relations as knowledge organizers for young children*. Unpublished manuscript, City University of New York.

Labov, W. (1972). *Language in the inner city*. Philadelphia: University of Pennsylvania Press.

Landberg, L., & Lundberg, L. (1989). Phonetic development in early infancy of four Swedish children during the first 18 months of life. *Journal of Child Language, 16*, 19–40.

Lanza, E. (1992). Can bilingual two-year-olds code-swtitch? *Journal of Child Language, 19*, 633–658.

Lashley, K. (1951). The problem of serial order in behavior. In L. Jeffress (Ed.), *Cerebral mechanisms in behavior*. New York: Wiley.

Lazar, R., Warr-Leeper, G., Nicholson, C., & Johnson, S. (1989). Elementary school teachers' use of multiple meaning expressions. *Language, Speech, and Hearing Services in Schools, 20*, 420–30.

Leap, W. L. (1993). *American Indian English*. Salt Lake City: University of Utah Press.

Lederberg, A., & Morales, C. (1985). Code switching by bilinguals: Evidence against a third grammar. *Journal of Psycholinguistic Research, 14*, 113–136.

Lee, V. (1981). Terminology and conceptual revision of the experimental analysis of language development: Why? *Behaviorism, 9*, 25–55.

Lemish, D., & Rice, M. (1986). Television as a talking picture book: A prop for language acquisition. *Journal of Child Language, 13*, 251–274.

Lemme, M., & Daves, N. (1982). Models of auditory linguistic processing. In N. Lass, L. McReynolds, J. Northern, & D. Yoder (Eds.), *Speech, language and hearing:* Vol. 1. *Normal processes*. Philadelphia: Saunders.

Lenneberg, E. (1964). A biological perspective of language. In E. Lenneberg (Ed.), *New directions in the study of language*. Cambridge: MIT Press.

Lenneberg, E. (1967). *Biological foundations of language*. New York: Wiley.

Leonard, L. (1976). *Meaning in child language*. New York: Grune & Stratton.

Leonard, L., & Loeb, D. (1988). Government-binding theory and some of its applications: A tutorial. *Journal of Speech and Hearing Research, 31*, 515–524.

Leonard, L., Newhoff, M., & Mesalam, L. (1980). Individual differences in early child phonology. *Applied Psycholinguistics, 1*, 7–30.

Leonard, L. B., Sabbadini, L., Volterra, V., & Leonard, J. S. (1988). Some influences of the grammar of English- and Italian-speaking children with specific language impairment. *Applied Psycholinguistics, 9*, 39–57.

Lerner, A., & Loewe, F. (1956). *My fair lady.* New York: Chappell.

Levin, B. (1993). *Emglish verb classes and alternatives: A preliminary investigation.* Chicago: University of Chicago Press.

Levin, E., & Rubin, K. (1982). Getting others to do what you want them to: The development of children's requestive strategies. In K. Nelson (Ed.), *Children's language* (Vol. 4). New York: Gardner Press.

Levitt, A. G., & Aydelott Utman, J. G. (1992). From babbling towards the sound system of English and French: A longitudinal two-case study. *Journal of Child Language, 19*, 19–49.

Levorato, M. C., & Cacciari, C. (1992). Children's comprehension of production of idioms: The role of context and familiarity. *Journal of Child Language, 19*, 415–433.

Levy, E., & Nelson, K. (1994). Words in discourse: A dialectal approach to the acquisition of meaning and use. *Journal of Child Language, 21*, 367–389.

Lewis, B. A., O'Donnell, B., Freebairn, L. A., & Taylor, H. G. (1998). Spoken language and written expression—Interplay of delays. *American Journal of Speech-Language Pathology, 7*, 77–84.

Lewis, D. J., & Windsor, J. (1996). Children's analysis of derivational suffix meaning. *Journal of Speech and Hearing Research, 39*, 209–216.

Lewis, M., & Freedle, R. (1973). Mother-infant dyad: The cradle of meaning. In P. Pilner, L. Kranes, & T. Alloway (Eds.), *Communication and affect: Language and thought.* New York: Academic Press.

Lewis, R. L. (1996). Interference in short-term memory: The magical number two (or three) in sentence processing. *Journal of Psycholinguistic Research, 25*, 93–121.

Liebergott, J., Ferrier, L., Chesnick, M., & Menyuk, P. (1981). *Prelinguistic conversation in normal and at risk infants.* Paper presented at the convention of the American Speech-Language-Hearing Association.

Lieven, E., & Pine, J. M. (1990). Review of E. Bates, I. Bretherton, & L. J. Snyder, From first words to grammar: Individual differences and dissociable mechanisms. *Journal of Child Language, 17*, 495–501.

Lieven, E. V. M., Pine, J. M., & Baldwin, G. (1997). Lexically based learning and early grammatical development. *Journal of Child Language, 24*, 187–219.

Lillo-Martin, D. (1991). *Universal grammar and American Sign Language: Setting the null argument parameters.* Dordrecht, The Netherlands: Kluwer Academic Publishers.

Lindsay, P., & Norman, D. (1977). *Human information processing* (2nd ed.). New York: Academic Press.

Lisker, L., & Abramson, A. (1965). Voice onset time in the production and perception of English stops. *Speech Research, Haskins Laboratories, 1.*

Lleo, C., & Prinz, M. (1996). Consonant clusters in child phonology and the directionality of syllable structure assignment. *Journal of Child Language, 23*, 31–56.

Lloyd, P., & Banham, L. (1997). Does drawing attention to the referent constrain the way in which children construct verbal messages? *Journal of Psycholinguistic Research, 26*, 509–518.

Locke, J. (1983). *Phonological acquisition and change.* New York: Academic Press.

Locke, J. (1986). Speech perception and the emergent lexicon: An ethological approach. In P. Fletcher & M. Garman (Eds.), *Language acquisition* (2nd ed.). New York: Cambridge University Press.

Locke, J. L. (1996). Why do infants begin to talk? Language as an unintended consequence. *Journal of Child Language, 23*, 251–268.

Loeb, D. F., & Leonard, L. B. (1991). Subject case marking and verb morphology in normally developing and specifically language-impaired children. *Journal of Speech and Hearing Research, 34*, 340–346.

Longacre, R. (1983). *The grammar of discourse.* New York: Plenum Press.

Love, R. (1981). The forgotten minority: The communicatively disabled. *Asha, 23*, 485–489.

Love, R., & Webb, W. (1986). *Neurology for the speech-language pathologist.* Boston: Butterworth's.

Lowe, R., Knutson, P. & Monson, M. (1985). Incidence of fronting in preschool children. *Language, Speech, and Hearing Services in the Schools, 16*, 119–123.

Lucariello, J. (1990). Freeing talk from the here-and-now: The role of event knowledge and maternal scaffolds. *Topics in Language Disorders, 10*(3), 14–29.

Lucariello, J., & Nelson, K. (1986). Context effects on lexical specificity in maternal and child discourse. *Journal of Child Language, 13*, 507–522.

Lueng, E. H., & Rheingold, H. L. (1981). Development of pointing as a social gesture. *Developmental Psychology, 17*, 215–220.

Luria, A. (1970). The functional organization of the brain. *Scientific American, 222*(3), 66–78.

Lust, B., & Mervis, C. (1980). Development of coordination in the natural speech of young children. *Journal of Child Language, 7*, 279–304.

MacLean, M., Bryant, P., & Bradley, L. (1987). Rhymes, nursery rhymes, and reading in early childhood. *Merrill-Palmer Quarterly, 33*(3), 255–281.

Macnamara, J. (1982). *Names for things: A study of human learning.* Cambridge, MA: MIT Press.

MacNeilage, P. (1970). Motor control of serial ordering in speech. *Psychological Review, 77*, 182–196.

MacWhinney, B. (1978). The acquisition of morphology. *Society for Research in Child Development Monograph, No. 43.*

MacWhinney, B. (1985). Acquisition of Hungarian. In D. Slobin (Ed.), *The crosslinguistic study of language acquisition.* Hillsdale, NJ: Erlbaum.

Maltz, D. N., & Borker, R. A. (1982). A cultural approach to male-female miscommunication. In J. J. Gumperz (Ed.), *Language and social identity.* Cambridge, UK: CUP.

Mandler, J. (1984). *Stories, scripts, and scenes.* Hillsdale, NJ: Erlbaum.

Mann, V., Shankweiler, D., & Smith, S. (1984). The association between comprehension of spoken sentences and early reading ability: The role of phonetic representations. *Journal of Child Language, 11*, 627–643.

Maratsos, M. (1983). Some current issues in the study of the acquisition of grammar. In P. Mussen (Ed.), *Carmichael's manual of child psychology* (Vol. III) (4th ed.). New York: Wiley.

Maratsos, M. (1988). The acquisition of formal word classes. In Y. Levy, I. Schlesinger, & M. Braine (Eds.), *Categories and processes in language acquisition.* Hillsdale, NJ: Erlbaum.

Marchman, V. A., & Bates, E. (1991). *Vocabulary size and composition as predictors of morphological development.* Technical Report No. 9103, Center for Research in Language, University of California, San Diego.

Marchman, V. A., & Bates, E. (1994). Continuity in lexical and morphological development: A test of the critical mass hypothesis. *Journal of Child Language, 21*, 339–366.

Marcos, H. (1987). Communicative function of pitch range and pitch direction in infants. *Journal of Child Language, 14*, 255–268.

Marcus, G. F. (1995). Children's overgeneralization of English plurals: A quantitative analysis. *Journal of Child Language, 22*, 447–459.

Marcus, G. F., Pinker, S., Ullman, M., Hollander, M., Rosen, T. J., & Xu, F. (1992). Overgeneralization in language acquisition. *Monographs of the Society for Research in Child Development, 57.*

Markman, E. M. (1992). The whole object, taxonomic, and mutual exclusivity assumptions as initial constraints on word meanings. In J. P. Byrnes & S. A. Gelman (Eds.), *Perspectives on language and cognition: Interrelations in development.* New York: Cambridge University Press.

Markman, E. M., & Hutchinson, J. E. (1984). Children's sensitivity to constraints on word meaning: Taxonomic versus thematic relations. *Cognitive Psychology, 16*, 1–27.

Markman, E. M., & Wachtel, G. (1988). Children's use of mutual exclusivity to constrain the meaning of words. *Cognitive Psychology, 20*, 121–157.

Marsh, G., Friedman, M., Welch, V., & Desberg, P. (1981). A cognitive-developmental theory of reading acquisition. In G. McKinnon & T. Weller (Eds.), *Reading research: Advances in theory and practice.* New York: Academic Press.

Martlew, M. (1980). Mothers' control strategies in dyadic mother/child conversations. *Journal of Psycholinguistic Research, 9*, 327–347.

Masar, F. (1989). Individual and dyadic patterns of imitation: Cognitive and social aspects. In G. E. Speidel & K. E. Nelson (Eds.), *The many faces of imitation in language learning.* New York: Springer-Verlag.

Masataka, N. (1992). Pitch characteristics of Japanese maternal speech to infants. *Journal of Child Language, 19*, 213–223.

Masataka, N. (1993). Effects of contingent and non-contingent maternal stimulation on the vocal behavior of three- to four-month-old Japanese infants. *Journal of Child Language, 20*, 303–312.

Masataka, N. (1995). The relation between index-finger extension and the acoustic quality of cooing in three-month-old infants. *Journal of Child Language, 22,* 247–257.

Maskarinec, A., Cairns, G., Butterfield, E., & Weamer, D. (1981). Longitudinal observations of individual infants' vocalizations. *Journal of Speech and Hearing Disorders, 46,* 267–273.

Masur, E. F. (1982). Mothers' responses to infants' object-related gestures: Influences on lexical development. *Journal of Child Language, 9,* 23–30.

Masur, E. F. (1983). Gestural development, dual-directional signaling, and the transition to words. *Journal of Psycholinguistic Research, 12,* 93–110.

Masur, E. F. (1997). Maternal labelling of novel and familiar objects: Implications for children's development of lexical constraints. *Journal of Child Language, 24,* 427–439.

Mateer, C. (1983). Motor and perceptual functions of the left hemisphere and their interaction. In S. Segalowitz (Ed.), *Language functions and brain organization.* New York: Academic Press.

Matthei, E. (1987). Subject and agent in emerging grammars: Evidence for a change in children's biases. *Journal of Child Language, 14,* 295–308.

Maxwell, D. (1984). The neurology of learning and language disabilities: Developmental considerations. In G. Wallach & K. Butler (Eds.), *Language learning disabilities in school age children.* Baltimore, MD: Williams & Wilkins.

Maxwell, S., & Wallach, G. (1984). The language-learning disabilities connection: Symptoms of early language disability change over time. In G. Wallach & K. Butler (Eds.), *Language learning disabilities in school-age children.* Baltimore: Williams & Wilkins.

Maynard, D. (1980). Placement of topic changes in conversation. *Semiotica, 30,* 263–290.

Maynard, S. K. (1986). On back channel behavior in Japanese and English casual conversation. *Linguistics, 24,* 1079–1108.

McCabe, A., & Peterson, C. (1985). A naturalistic study of the production of causal connectives by children. *Journal of Child Language, 12,* 145–159.

McCarthy, D. (1954). Language development in children. In L. Carmichael (Ed.), *Manual of child psychology.* New York: Wiley.

McCloskey, L. A. (1986). *Prosody and children's understanding of discourse.* Unpublished doctoral dissertation, University of Michigan, Ann Arbor.

McClure, F. (1981). Formal and functional aspects of the codeswitched discourse of bilingual children. In R. Duran (Ed.), *Latino language and communicative behavior.* Norwood, NJ: Ablex.

McCune-Nicolich, L. (1981). The cognitive bases of relational words in the single word period. *Journal of Child Language, 8,* 15–34.

McCune-Nicolich, L. (1986). Play-language relationships: Implications for a theory of symbol development. In A. Gottfried & C. C. Brown (Eds.), *Play interactions.* Lexington, MA: Lexington Books.

McCune-Nicolich, L., & Bruskin, C. (1982). Combinatorial competency in play and language. In K. Rubin & D. Pepler (Eds.), *The play of children: Current theory and research.* New York: Karger.

McKee, C., McDaniel, D., & Snedeker, J. (1998). Relatives children say. *Journal of Psycholinguistic Research, 27,* 573–596.

McLaughlin, B. (1978). *Second-language acquisition in children.* Hillsdale, NJ: Erlbaum.

McLean, J., & Snyder-McLean, L. (1978). *A transactional approach to early language training.* Columbus, OH: Merrill.

McMullen, L. M., & Pasloski, D. D. (1992). Effects of communication apprehension, familiarity of partner, and topic on selected "women's language" features. *Journal of Psycholinguistic Research, 21,* 17–30.

McNeill, D. (1970). *The acquisition of language: The study of developmental psycholinguistics.* New York: Harper & Row.

Meegaskumbura, P. B. (1980). Tondol: Sinhala baby talk. *Word, 31,* 287–309.

Menyuk, P., Menn, L., & Silber, R. (1986). Early strategies for the perception and production of words and sounds. In P. Fletcher & M. Garman (Eds.), *Language acquisition* (2nd ed.). New York: Cambridge University Press.

Merriman, W. E., & Bowman, L. L. (1989). The mutual exclusivity bias in children's word learning. *Monographs of the Society for Research in Child Development* (Serial No. 20, Vol. 54).

Mervis, C., & Mervis, C. (1988). Role of adult input in young children's category evolution: I. An observational study. *Journal of Child Language, 15,* 257–272

Mervis, C. B. (1987). Child-basic object categories and early lexical development. In U. Neisser (Ed.), *Concepts and conceptual development: Ecological and intellectual factors in categorization.* New York: Cambridge University Press.

Mervis, C. B. (1990). Operating principles, input, and early lexical development. *Communiczioni Scientifiche de Psicologia Generala, 4,* 31–48.

Mervis, C. B., & Bertrand, J. (1993). Acquisition of early object labels: The roles of operating principles and input. In A. P. Kaiser & D. B. Gray (Eds.), *Enhancing children's communication: Research foundations for intervention* (Vol. II). Baltimore, MD: Brookes.

Mervis, C. B., & Bertrand, J. (1995). Early lexical acquisition and the vocabulary spurt: A response to Goldfield & Reznick. *Journal of Child Language, 22,* 461–468.

Messer, D. (1980). The episodic structure of maternal speech to young children. *Journal of Child Language, 7,* 29–40.

Michaels, S. (1981). "Sharing time": Children's narrative styles and differential access to literacy. *Language and Society, 10,* 423–442.

Michaels, S. (1991). The dismantling of narrative. In A. McCabe & C. Peterson (Eds.), *Developing narrative structure* (pp. 303–352) Norwood, NJ: Ablex.

Millar, J., & Whitaker, H. (1983). The right hemisphere's contribution to language: A review of the evidence from brain-injured subjects. In S. Segalowitz (Ed.), *Language functions and brain organization.* New York: Academic Press.

Miller, G. A., & Gildea, P. M. (1987). How children learn words. *Scientific American, 257,* 94–99.

Miller, J. (1981). *Assessing language production in children.* Baltimore: University Park Press.

Miller, J. (1985, January 13). Beaucoons of words. *New York Times Magazine,* p. 9.

Miller, J., & Chapman, R. (1981). The relation between age and mean length of utterance in morphemes. *Journal of Speech and Hearing Research, 24,* 154–161.

Miller, J., Chapman, R., Branston, M., & Reichle, J. (1980). Language comprehension in sensorimotor stages 5 and 6. *Journal of Speech and Hearing Research, 4,* 1–12.

Miller, P., & Sperry, L. (1988). Early talk about the past: The origins of conversational stories of personal experience. *Journal of Child Language, 15,* 293–315.

Miller, W., & Ervin-Tripp, S. (1964). The development of grammar in child language. In U.Bellugi & R. Brown (Eds.), The acquisition of language. *Mono-*

graphs of the Society for Research in Child Development, 92.

Mills, A.E. (1981). It's easier in German, isn't it? The question of tag questions in a bilingual child. *Journal of Child Language, 8,* 641–647.

Minami, M., & McCabe, A. (1991). Haiku as a discourse regulation device: A stanza analysis of Japanese children's personal narratives. *Language and Society, 20,* 577–599.

Minami, M., & McCabe, A. (1995). Rice balls and bear hunts: Japanese and North American family narrative patterns. *Journal of Child Language, 22,* 423–445.

Mitchell, P., & Kent, R. (1990). Phonetic variation in multisyllabic babbling. *Journal of Child Language, 17,* 247–265.

Mithum, M. (1989). The acquisition of polysynthesis. *Journal of Child Language, 16,* 285–312.

Miura, I. (1993). Switching pauses in adult-adult and child-child turn takings: An initial study. *Journal of Psycholinguistic Research, 22,* 383–395.

Moerk, E. (1977). *Pragmatic and semantic aspects of early language development.* Baltimore: University Park Press.

Moerk, E. (1985). Analytic, synthetic, abstracting, and word-class-defining aspects of verbal mother-child interactions. *Journal of Psycholinguistic Research, 14,* 239–252.

Moerk, E. (1991). Positive evidence for negative evidence. *First Language, 11,* 219–251.

Moerman, M. (1988). *Talking culture: Ethnography and conversation analysis.* Philadelphia: University of Pennsylvania Press.

Molfese, V., Molfese, D., & Parsons, C. (1983). Hemisphere processing of phonological information. In S. Segalowitz (Ed.), *Language functions and brain organization.* New York: Academic Press.

Monson, D. (1982, May). *Effect of type and distance on comprehension of anaphoric relationships.* Paper presented at the International Reading Association WORD Research Conference, Seattle.

Moon, C., Bever, T. G., & Fifer, W. P. (1992). Canonical and non-canonical syllable discrimination by two-day-old infants. *Journal of Child Language, 19,* 1–17.

Moore, C., Harris, L., & Patriquin, M. (1993). Lexical and prosodic cues in the comprehension of relative certainty. *Journal of Child Language, 20,* 153–167.

Morehead, D., & Ingram, D. (1973). The development of base syntax in normal and linguistically deviant children. *Journal of Speech and Hearing Research, 16*, 330–352.

Morehead, D., & Morehead, A. (1974). A Piagetian view of thought and language during the first two years. In R. Schiefelbusch & L. Lloyd (Eds.), *Language perspectives—Acquisition, retardation, and intervention*. Baltimore: University Park Press.

Morford, M., & Goldin-Meadow, S. (1992). Comprehension and production of gesture in combination with speech in one-word speakers. *Journal of Child Language, 19*, 559–580.

Morgan, J., & Travis, L. (1989). Limits on negative information in language input. *Journal of Child Language, 16*, 531–552.

Morgan, J. E., Meier, R. P., & Newport, E. L. (1987). Structural packaging in the input to language learning: Contributions of prosodic and morphological marking of phrases to the acquisition of language. *Cognitive Psychology, 19*, 498–550.

Morgan, J. L. (1986). *From simple input to complex grammar*. Cambridge, MA: MIT Press.

Morikawa, H., Shand, N., & Kosawa, Y. (1988). Maternal speech to prelingual infants in Japan and the United States: Relationships among functions, forms and referents. *Journal of Child Language, 15*, 237–256.

Mowrer, O. (1954). The psychologist looks at language. *American Psychologist, 9*, 660–694.

Mulford, R. (1983). On the acquisition of derivational morphology in Icelandic: Learning about -ari. *Islenskt mal og almenn malfraedi, 5*.

Muma, J. (1978). *Language handbook*. Englewood Cliffs, NJ: Prentice Hall.

Muma, J., & Zwycewicz-Emory, C. (1979). Contextual priority: Verbal shift at seven? *Journal of Child Language, 6*, 301–311.

Murray, A., Johnson, J., & Peters, J. (1990). Fine-tuning of utterance length to preverbal infants: Effects on later language development. *Journal of Child Language, 17*, 511–525.

Myers, F., & Myers, R. (1983). Perception of stress contrasts in semantic and nonsemantic contexts by children. *Journal of Psycholinguistic Research, 12*, 327–338.

Myers, J., Jusczyk, P. W., Nelson, D. G. K., Charles-Luce, J., Wordward, A. L., & Hirsh-Pasek, K. (1996). Infants' sensitivity to word boundaries in fluent speech. *Journal of Child Language, 23*, 1-30.

Myers, N., & Perlmutter, M. (1978). Memory in the years from two to five. In P. Ornstein (Ed.), *Memory development in children*. Hillsdale, NJ: Erlbaum.

Myerson, R. (1975). *A developmental study of children's knowledge of complex derived words of English*. Paper presented to the International Reading Association.

Nagata, H. (1993). Unimmediate construction of syntactic structure for garden path sentences in Japanese. *Journal of Psycholinguistic Research, 22*, 365–381.

Nagel, H. N., Shapiro, L. P., Tuller, B., & Nawy, R. (1996). Prosodic influences on the resolution of temporary ambiguity during on-line sentence processing. *Journal of Psycholinguistic Research, 25*, 319-344.

Nagy, W. E., & Anderson, R. C. (1984). How many words are there in printed English? *Reading Research Quarterly, 24*, 262–282.

Nagy, W. E., Anderson, R. C., Schommer, M., Scott, J. A., & Stallman, A.C. (1989). Morphological families and word recognition. *Reading Research Quarterly, 24*, 262–283.

Nagy, W. E., Diakidoy, I. N., & Anderson, R. C. (1991). *The development of knowledge of derivational suffixes*. Technical Report N. 536, Center for the Study of Reading. Champaign: Univeristy of Illinois at Urbana-Champaign.

Naigles, L. (1990). Children use syntax to learn verb meanings. *Journal of Child Language, 17*, 357–374.

Nakayama, M. (1987). Performance factors in subject–auxiliary inversion by children. *Journal of Child Language, 14*, 113–125.

Namy, L. L., & Waxman, S. R. (1998). Words and gestures: Infants' interpretations of different forms of symbolic reference. *Child Development, 69*, 295–308.

National Center for Health Statistics (1983). *Births of Hispanic parentage, 1980. Monthly Vital Statistics Report*. Washington, DC.

National Center for Health Statistics (1985). *Advance report of final natality statistics, 1983. Monthly Vital Statistics Report, 34(6), Supplement* [DHHS Pub. No. (PHS) 85–1120]. Hyattsville, MD: Public Health.

Needham, W. P. (1992). Limits on literal processing during idiom interpretation. *Journal of Psycholinguistic Research, 21*, 1–16.

Nelson, D., Hirsh-Pasek, K., Jusczyk, P., & Cassidy, K. (1989). How the prosodic cues in motherese might assist language learning. *Journal of Child Language, 16*, 56–68.

Nelson, K. E. (1973). Structure and strategy in learning to talk. *Monographs of the Society for Research in Child Development, 38*.

Nelson, K. E. (1974). Concept, word, and sentence: Interrelations in acquisition and development. *Psychological Review, 81*, 267–285.

Nelson, K. E. (1977). The conceptual basis of naming. In J. Macnamara (Ed.), *Language learning and thought*. New York: Academic Press.

Nelson, K. E. (1981a). Individual differences in language development: Implications for acquisition and development. *Developmental Psychology, 17*, 170–187.

Nelson, K. E. (1981b). Social cognition in a script framework. In L. Ross & J. Flavell (Eds.), *The development of social cognition in children*. Cambridge: Cambridge University Press.

Nelson, K. E. (Ed.) (1986). *Event knowledge: Structure function in development*. Hillsdale, NJ: Erlbaum.

Nelson, K. E. (1991). The matter of time: Interdependencies between language and concepts. In S. A. Gelman & J. P. Byrnes (Eds.), *Perspectives on language and thought: Interrelations in development*. New York: Cambridge University Press.

Nelson, K. E., Fivush, R., Hudson, J., & Lucariello, J. (1983). Scripts and the development of memory. In M. T. Chi (Ed.), *Contributions to human development: Trends in memory development research* (Vol. 9). New York: Karger.

Nelson, K. E., Hampson, J., & Shaw, L. K. (1993). Nouns in early lexicons: Evidence, explanations, & implications. *Journal of Child Language, 20*, 61–84.

Nelson, L. K., & Bauer, H. R. (1991). Speech and language production at age 2: Evidence for tradeoffs between linguistic and phonetic processing. Journal of Speech and Hearing Research, 34, 879–892.

Newcomb, N., & Zaslow, M. (1981). Do 2½-year-olds hint? A study of directive forms in the speech of 2½-year-old children to adults. *Discourse Processes, 4*, 239–252.

Newport, E., Gleitman, A., & Gleitman, L. (1977). Mother I'd rather do it myself: Some effects and non-effects of maternal speech style. In C. Snow & C. Ferguson (Eds.), *Talking to children: Language input and acquisition*. New York: Cambridge University Press.

Nietupski, J., Scheutz, G., & Ockwood, L. (1980). The delivery of communication therapy services to severely handicapped students: A plan for change. *Journal for the Association of the Severely Handicapped, 5*, 13–23.

Ninio, A. (1980). Ostensive definition in vocabulary training. *Journal of Child Language, 7*, 565–573.

Ninio, A., & Snow, C. (1988). Language acquisition through language use: The functional sources of children's early utterances. In Y. Levy, I. Schlesinger, & M. Braine (Eds.), *Categories and processes in language acquisition*. Hillsdale, NJ: Erlbaum.

Nippold, M. A. (1991). Evaluating and enhancing idiom comprehension in language-disordered children. *Language, Speech, and Hearing Services in Schools, 22*, 100–106.

Nippold, M. A., & Haq, F. S. (1996). Proverb comprehension in youth: The role of concreteness and familiarity. *Journal of Speech, Language, and Hearing Research, 39*, 166–176.

Nippold, M. A., Hegel, S. L., Sohlberg, M. M., Schwarz, I. E. (1999). Defining abstract entities: Development in pre-adolescents, adolescents, and young adults. *Journal of Speech, Language, and Hearing Research, 42*, 473–481.

Nippold, M. A., & Martin, S. (1989). Idiom interpretation in isolation versus context: A developmental study with adolescents. *Journal of Speech and Hearing Research, 32*, 59–66.

Nippold, M. A., Martin S., & Erskine, B. (1988). Proverb comprehension in context: A developmental study with children and adolescents. *Journal of Speech and Hearing Research, 31*, 19–28.

Nippold, M. A., Schwarz, I. E., & Undlin, R. (1992). Use and understanding of adverbial conjuncts: A developmental study of adolescents and young adults. *Journal of Speech and Hearing Research, 35*, 108–118.

Nippold, M. A., & Sullivan, M. (1987). Verbal and perceptual analogical reasoning and proportional metaphor comprehension in young children. *Journal of Speech and Hearing Research, 30*, 367–376.

Nippold, M. A., & Taylor, C. L. (1995). Idiom understanding in youth: Further examination of familiarity and transparency. *Journal of Speech, Language, and Hearing Research, 38*, 426–433.

Nippold, M. A., Taylor, C. L., & Baker, J. M. (1995). Idiom understanding in Australian youth: A cross-cultural comparison. *Journal of Speech, Language, and Hearing Research, 39*, 442–447.

Nippold, M. A., Uhden, L. D., Schwarz, I. E. (1997). Proverb explanation through the lifespan: A developmental study of adolescents and adults. *Journal of Speech, Language, and Hearing Research, 40*, 245–253.

Nohara, M. (1992). Sex differences in interruption: An experimental reevaluation. *Journal of Psycholinguistic Research, 21*, 127–146.

Nohara, M. (1996). Preschool boys and girls use *no* differently. *Journal of Child Language, 23*, 417–429.

Nold, E. (1981). Revising. In C. Frederiksen & J. Dominic (Eds.), *Writing: The nature, development, and teaching of written communication* (Vol. 2). Hillsdale, NJ: Erlbaum.

Norris, J., & Bruning, R. (1988). Cohesion in the narratives of good and poor readers. *Journal of Speech and Hearing Disorders, 53*, 416–423.

Nugent, P., & Mosley, J. (1987). Mentally retarded and nonretarded individuals' attention allocation and capacity. *American Journal of Mental Deficiency, 91*, 598–605.

Obler, L. (1985). Language through the life-span. In J. Berko Gleason (Ed.), *The development of language*. Columbus, OH: Merrill.

O'Brien, M., & Nagle, K. (1987). Parents' speech to toddlers: The effect of play context. *Journal of Child Language, 14*, 269–279.

Ochs, E. (1982). Talking to children in Western Samoa. *Language and Society, 11*, 77–104.

Ochs, E., & Schieffelin, B. (1984). Language acquisition and socialization: Three developmental stories and their implications. In R. Shweder & R. LeVine (Eds.), *Culture and its acquisition*. New York: Cambridge University Press.

Ogura, T. (1991). A longitudinal study of the relationship between early language development and play development. *Journal of Child Language, 18*, 273–294.

Oller, D. (1978). Infant vocalization and the development of speech. *Allied Health and Behavior Sciences, 1*, 523–549.

Oller, D., & Eilers, R. (1982). Similarity of babbling in Spanish- and English-learning babies. *Journal of Child Language, 9*, 565–577.

Oller, D., & Eilers, R. (1983). Speech identification in Spanish and English-learning 2-year-olds. *Journal of Speech and Hearing Research, 26*, 50–53.

Oller, D., Eilers, R., Bull, D., & Carney, A. (1985). Prespeech vocalizations of a deaf infant: A comparison with normal metaphonological development. *Journal of Speech and Hearing Research, 28*, 47–62.

Oller, D., Eilers, R. E., Urbano, R., & Cobo-Lewis, A. B. (1997). Development of precursors to speech in infants exposed to two languages. *Journal of Child Language, 24*, 407–425.

Olmstead, D. (1971). *Out of the mouths of babes*. The Hague: Mouton.

Orsolini, M., Rossi, F., & Pontecorvo, C. (1996). Reintroduction of referents in Italian children's narratives. *Journal of Child Language, 23*, 465–486.

Osgood, C. (1963). On understanding and creating sentences. *American Psychologist, 18*, 735–751.

Oshima-Takane, Y. (1988). Children learn from speech not addressed to them: The case of personal pronouns. *Journal of Child Language, 15*, 95–108.

Otaki, M., Durrett, M., Richards, P., Nyquist, L., & Pennebaker, J. (1986). Maternal and infant behavior in Japan and America: A partial replication. *Journal of Cross-Cultural Psychology, 17*, 251–268.

Oviatt, S. (1982). Inferring what words mean: Early development in infants' comprehension of common object names. *Child Development, 53*, 274–277.

Owens, R. (1978). *Speech acts in the early language of non-delayed and retarded children: A taxonomy and distributional study*. Unpublished doctoral dissertation, The Ohio State University.

Owens, R. (1982). *Program for the acquisition of language with the severely impaired (PALS)*. Columbus, OH: Merrill.

Owens, R. (1986). Communication, language. and speech. In G. Shames & E. Wiig (Eds.), *Human communication disorders*. (p. 41) Columbus, OH: Merrill.

Owens, R. (1995). *Language disorders: A functional approach to assessment and intervention*. (Second edition) Boston, MA: Allyn & Bacon..

Owens, R., & MacDonald, J. (1982). Communicative uses of the early speech of nondelayed and Down syndrome children. *American Journal of Mental Deficiency, 86*, 503–511.

Ozyurek, A. (1996). How children talk about a conversation. *Journal of Child Language, 23*, 693–714.

Palermo, D. (1982). Theoretical issues in semantic development. In S. Kuczaj (Ed.), *Language development:* Vol. 1. *Syntax and semantics.* Hillsdale, NJ: Erlbaum.

Papousek, H. (1987, April). *Models and messages in the melodies of maternal speech in tonal and non-tonal languages.* Paper presented at the meeting of the Society for Research in Child Development, Baltimore, MD.

Papousek, M., Papousek, H., & Haekel, M. (1987). Didactic adjustments in fathers' and mothers' speech to their three-month-old infants. *Journal of Psycholinguistic Research, 16,* 491–516.

Parnell, M., Patterson, S., & Harding, M. (1984). Answers to wh- questions: A developmental study. *Journal of Speech and Hearing Research, 27,* 297–305.

Parsons, C. (1980). *The effect of speaker age and listener compliance and noncompliance on the politeness of children's request directives.* Unpublished doctoral dissertation, Southern Illinois University.

Paul, R. (1990). Comprehension strategies: Interactions between world knowledge and the development of sentence comprehension. *Topics in Language Disorders, 10(3),* 63–75.

Paulson, D. M. (1991). *Phonological systems of Spanish-speaking Texas preschoolers.* Thesis, Texas Christian University.

Pea, R. (1980). The development of negation in early child language. In D. Olson (Ed.), *The social foundations of language and thought: Essays in honor of Jerome S. Bruner.* New York: Norton.

Pea, R., & Mawby, R. (1981, August). *Semantics of modal auxiliary verb uses by preschool children.* Paper presented at the Second International Congress for the Study of Child Language, Vancouver, Canada.

Pearson, B. Z., Fernandez, S., & Oller, D. K. (1995). Cross-language synonyms in the lexicons of bilingual infants: One language or two? *Journal of Child Language, 22,* 345–368.

Pease, D., & Berko Gleason, J. (1985). Gaining meaning: Semantic development. In J. Berko Gleason (Ed.), *The development of language.* Columbus, OH: Merrill.

Pellegrini, A. D. (1985). Relations between symbolic play and literate behavior. In L. Galda & A. Pellegrini (Eds.), *Play, language and story: The development of children's literate behavior.* Norwood, NJ: Ablex.

Pellegrini, A. D., & Perlmutter, J. (1989). Classroom contextual effects on children's play. *Developmental Psychology, 25,* 289–296.

Penalosa, F. (1981). *Introduction to the sociology of language.* Rowley, MA: Newbury House.

Penman, R., Cross, T., Milgrom-Friedman, J., & Meares, R. (1983). Mothers' speech to prelingual infants: A pragmatic analysis. *Journal of Child Language, 10,* 17–34.

Penner, S. (1987). Parental responses to grammatical and ungrammatical child utterances. *Child Development, 58,* 376–384.

Perera, K. (1986). Language acquisition and writing. In P. Fletcher & M. Garman (Eds.), *Language acquisition* (2nd ed.). New York: Cambridge University Press.

Perera, K. (1994). Child language research: Building on the past, looking to the future. *Journal of Child Language, 21,* 1–8.

Perez-Pereira, M. (1994). Imitations, repetitions, routines, and the child's analysis of language: Insights from the blind. *Journal of Child Language, 21,* 317–337.

Perfetti, C. (1984). Reading acquisition and beyond: Decoding includes cognition. *American Journal of Education, 93,* 40–60.

Peters, A. M. (1983). *The units of language acquisition.* New York: Cambridge University Press.

Peters, A. M. (1985). Language segmentation: Operating principles for the perception and analysis of language. In D. I. Slobin (Ed.), *Crosslinguistic studies of child language.* Hillsdale, NJ: Erlbaum.

Peters, A. M. (1986). Early syntax. In P. Fletcher & M. Garman (Eds.), *Language acquisition* (2nd ed.). New York: Cambridge University Press.

Peterson, C. (1990). The who, when and where of early narratives. *Journal of Child Language, 17,* 433–455.

Peterson, C., & McCabe, A. (1983). *Developmental psycholinguistics: Three ways of looking at a child's narrative.* New York: Plenum Press.

Peterson, C., & McCabe, A. (1987). The connective "and": Do older children use it less as they learn other connectives? *Journal of Child Language, 14,* 375–381.

Petitto, L. A. (1984). *From gesture to symbol: The relationship between form and the meaning in the acquisition of personal pronouns in American Sign Language.* Unpublished doctoral dissertation, Harvard University, Cambridge, MA.

Petitto, L. A. (1985a, October). *On the use of prelinguistic gestures in hearing and deaf children.* Paper presented at the 10th Annual Boston University Conference on Language Development, Boston.

Petitto, L. A. (1985b). *"Language" in the pre-linguistic child* (Tech Rep. No. 4). Montreal: McGill University, Department of Psychology.

Petitto, L. A. (1986) *From gesture to symbol: The relationship between form and the meaning in the acquisition of personal pronouns in American Sign Language.* Bloomington: Indiana University Linguistics Club Press.

Petitto, L. A. (1987). On the autonomy of language and gesture: Evidence from the acquisition of personal pronouns in American Sign Language. *Cognition, 27(1)*, 1–52.

Petitto, L. A. (1988). "Language" in the pre-linguistic child. In F. Kessel (Ed.), *Development of language and language researchers: Essays in honor of Roger Brown* (pp. 187–221). Hillsdale, NJ: Erlbaum.

Petitto, L. A., & Marentette, P. F. (1990, October). *The timing of linguistic milestones in sign language acquisition: Are first signs acquired earlier than first words?* Paper presented at the 15th Annual Boston University Conference on Language Development, Boston, MA.

Petitto, L. A., & Marentette, P. F. (1991, April) The timing of linguistic milestones in sign and spoken language acquisition. In L. Petitto (Chair), *Are the linguistic milestones in signed and spoken language acquisition similar or different?* Symposium conducted at the Biennial Meeting of the Society for Research in Child Development, Seattle, WA.

Petrovich-Bartell, N., Cowan, N., & Morse, P. (1982). Mothers' perceptions of infant distress vocalizations. *Journal of Speech and Hearing Research, 25*, 371–376.

Pflaum, S. (1986). *The development of language and literacy in young children* (3rd ed.). Columbus, OH: Merrill.

Piaget, J. (1954). *The construction of reality in the child.* New York: Basic Books.

Pillon, A., Degauquier, C., & Duquesne, F. (1992). Males' and females' conversational behavior in cross-sex dyads: From gender differences to gender similarities. *Journal of Psycholinguistic Research, 21*, 147–172.

Pine, J. M. (1990). *Non-referential children: Slow or different?* Paper presented at the Fifth International Congress for the Study of Child Language, Budapest.

Pine, J. M., & Lieven, E. (1990). Referential style at thirteen months: Why age-defined cross sectional measures are inappropriate for the study of strategy differences in early language development. *Journal of Child Language, 17*, 625–631.

Pine, J. M., & Lieven, E. V. M. (1993). Reanalysing rote-learned phrases: Individual differences in the transition to multiword speech. *Journal of Child Language, 20*, 551–571.

Pinker, S. (1982). A theory of the acquisition of lexical interpretive grammars. In J. Bresnan (Ed.), *The mental representation of grammatical notions.* Cambridge, MA: MIT Press.

Pinker, S. (1984). *Language learnability and language development.* Cambridge, MA: Harvard University Press.

Pinker, S. (1989). Resolving a learnability paradox in the acquisition of the verb lexicon. In M. Rice & R. Schiefelbusch (Eds.), *The teachability of language.* Baltimore: Brookes.

Pinker, S. (1994). *Language and instinct.* New York: W. Morrow.

Pinsleur, P. (1980). *How to learn a foreign language.* Boston: Heinle and Heinle.

Plunkett, K. (1993). Lexical segmentation and vocabulary growth in early language acquisition. *Journal of Child Language, 20*, 43–60.

Plunkett, K., & Marchman, V. (1993). From rote learning to system building: The acquisition of morphology in children and connectionist nets. *Cognition, 48*, 21–69.

Poplack, S. (1981). Syntactic structure and social function of codeswitching. In R. Duran (Ed.), *Latino language and communicative behavior.* Norwood, NJ: Ablex.

Poulin-Dubois, D., Graham, S., & Sippola, L. (1995). Early lexical development: The contribution of parental labelling and infants' categorization abilities. *Journal of Child Language, 22*, 325–343.

Powers, S., & Lopez, R. (1985). Perceptual, motor, & verbal skills of monolingual and bilingual Hispanic children: A discrimination analysis. *Perceptual and Motor Skills, 60*, 1001–1109.

Preece, A. (1987). The range of narrative forms conversationally produced by young children. *Journal of Child Language, 14*, 353–373.

Preisser, D., Hodson, B., & Paden, E. (1988). Developmental phonology: 18–29 months. *Journal of Speech and Hearing Disorders, 53*, 125–130.

Premack, D. (1986). *Gavagai! or the future of the animal language controversy.* Cambridge: MIT Press.

Prescott, P. A. (1985). Differential reinforcing value of speech and heartbeats: A measure of functional lateralization in the neonate. *Dissertation Abstracts International, 48,* 286-B.

Prinz, P. (1983). The development of idiomatic meaning in children. *Language and Speech, 26,* 263–272.

Prutting, C. (1979). Process: The action of moving forward progressively from one point to another on the way to completion. *Journal of Speech and Hearing Disorders, 44,* 3–30.

Pye, C. (1988). *Precocious passives (and antipassives) in Quiche Mayan.* Paper presented at the Child Language Research Forum, Stanford University, Stanford, CA.

Pye, C., & Ratner, N. (1984). Higher pitch in BT is not universal: Acoustic evidence from Quiche Mayan. *Journal of Child Language, 11,* 515–522.

Pye, C., Wilcox, K., & Siren, K. (1988). Refining transcription: The significance of transcription "errors." *Journal of Child Language, 15,* 17–37.

Qualls, C. D., & Harris, J. L. (1999). Effects of familiarity on idiom comprehension in African American and European American fifth graders. *Language, Speech, and Hearing Services in Schools, 30,* 141–151.

Rabinowitz, M., & Glaser, R. (1985). Cognitive structure and process in highly competent performance. In F. D. Horowitz & M. O'Brien (Eds.), *The gifted and talented: Developmental perspectives* (pp. 75–98). Washington, DC: American Psychological Association.

Radford, A. (1988). Small children's small clauses. *Transactions of the Philosophical Society, 86,* 1–43.

Raghavendra, P., & Leonard, L. (1989). The acquisition of agglutinating languages: Converging evidence from Tamil. *Journal of Child Language, 16,* 313–322.

Raichle, M. E. (1994). Images of the mind: Studies with modern imaging techniques. *Annual Review of Psychology, 45,* 333–356.

Ratner, N. (1988). Patterns of parental vocabulary selection in speech to very young children. *Journal of Child Language, 15,* 481–492.

Read, C. (1981). Writing is not the inverse of reading for young children. In C. Frederiksen & J. Dominic (Eds.), *Writing: The nature, development, and teaching of written communication.* Hillsdale, NJ: Erlbaum.

Reber, A. (1973). On psycho-linguistic paradigms. *Journal of Psycholinguistic Research, 2,* 289–319.

Redlinger, W., & Park, T. (1980). Language mixing in young bilinguals. *Journal of Child Language, 7,* 337–352.

Rees, N., & Wollner, S. (1981). *An outline of children's pragmatic abilities.* Paper presented at the annual convention of the American Speech-Language-Hearing Association, Detroit.

Reich, P. (1986). *Language development.* Englewood Cliffs, NJ: Prentice Hall.

Reichle, J. (1990, April). *Intervention with presymbolic clients: Setting up an initial communication system.* Paper presented at the annual convention of the New York State Speech-Language-Hearing Association, Kiamesha Lake, New York.

Reilly, J. S., & Bellugi, U. (1996). Competition on the face: Affect and language in ASL motherese. *Journal of Child Language, 23,* 219–239.

Rembold, K. (1980). *An examination of the effects of verbal and non-verbal feedback in maternal speech to two-and-one-half-year-old children.* Unpublished manuscript, University of Wisconsin.

Rescorla, L. (1980). Overextension in early language development. *Journal of Child Language, 7,* 321–335.

Rescorla, L., & Fechnay, T. (1996). Mother-child synchrony and communicative reciprocity in late-talking toddlers. *Journal of Speech, Language, and Hearing Research, 39,* 200–208.

Reznick, J. S., & Goldfield, B. A. (1994). Diary vs. representative checklist assessment of productive vocabulary. *Journal of Child Language, 21,* 465–472.

Ricciardelli, L. A. (1992). Bilingualism and cognitive development in relation to threshold theory. *Journal of Psycholinguistic Research, 21,* 301–316.

Rice, M. L. (1984). Cognitive aspects of communicative development. In R. Schiefelbusch & J. Pickar (Eds.), *The acquisition of communicative competence.* Baltimore: University Park Press.

Richards, B. J. (1986). Yes/no questions in input and their relationship with rate of auxiliary verb development in young children. In R. A. Crawly, R. J. Stevens, & M. Tallerman (Eds.), *Proceedings of the Child Language Seminar.* Durham: University of Durham.

Richards, B. J. (1987). *Individual differences and the development of the auxiliary verb system in young children.* Unpublished doctoral dissertation, University of Bristol, UK.

Richards, B. J. (1988, March). *"Not wee-wee had he?": Individual differences and the development of tag questions in two- and three-year-olds.* Paper presented at the Child Language Seminar, University of Warwick, England.

Richards, B. J. (1990). *Language development and individual differences: A study of auxiliary verb learning.* New York: Cambridge University Press.

Richards, B. J., & Robinson, P. (1993). Environmental correlates of child copula verb growth. *Journal of Child Language, 20,* 343–362.

Richards, M. (1980). Adjective ordering in the language of young children: An experimental investigation. *Journal of Child Language, 6,* 253–277.

Ricks, D. (1979). Making sense of experience to make sensible sounds. In M. Bullowa (Ed.), *Before speech.* New York: Cambridge University Press.

Rispoli, M., (1994). Pronoun case overextension and paradigm building. *Journal of Child Language, 21,* 157–172.

Robb, M. P., Bauer, H. R., & Tyler, A. A. (1994). A quantitative analysis of the single-word stage. *First Language, 14,* 37–48.

Roberts, K. (1983). Comprehension and production of word order in stage I. *Child Development, 54,* 443–449.

Roberts, K., & Horowitz, F. (1986). Basic level categorization in seven- and nine-month-old infants. *Journal of Child Language, 13,* 191–208.

Robertson, S., & Suci, G. (1980). Event perception by children in the early stages of language production. *Child Development, 51,* 89–96.

Robey, B. (1985). America's Asians. *American Demographics, 53,* 22–29.

Robey, B. (1987). Locking up heaven's door. *American Demographics, 55,* 24–29.

Robinson, I. (1986). Blacks move back to the South. *American Demographics, 54,* 40–43.

Robinson-Zanatu, C. (1996). Serving Native American children and families: Considering cultural variables. *Language, Speech, and Hearing Services in Schools, 27,* 1996, 373–384.

Rogoff, B., & Chavajay, P. (1995). What's become of research on the cultural basis of cognitive development? *American Psychologist, 50,* 859–877.

Rome-Flanders, T., & Cronk, C. (1995). A longitudinal study of infant vocalizations during mother-infant games. *Journal of Child Language, 22,* 259–274.

Rondal, J. (1980). Fathers' and mothers' speech in early language development. *Journal of Child Language, 7,* 353–369.

Rondal, J., & Cession, A. (1990). Input evidence regarding the semantic bootstrapping hypothesis. *Journal of Child Language, 17,* 711–717.

Rondal, J., Ghiotto, M., Bredart, S., & Bachelet, J. (1987). Age-relation, reliability and grammatical validity of measures of utterance length. *Journal of Child Language, 14,* 433–446.

Ross, E. (1981). The aprosodias. *Archives of Neurology, 38,* 561–569.

Roth, F. (1986). Oral narrative abilities of learning-disabled students. *Topics in Language Disorders, 7(1),* 21–30.

Roth, F., & Davidge, N. (1985). Are early verbal communicative intentions universal? A preliminary investigation. *Journal of Psycholinguistic Research, 14,* 351–363.

Roth, F., & Spekman, N. (1985, June). *Story grammar analysis of narratives produced by learning disabled and normally achieving students.* Paper presented at the Symposium on Research in Child Language Disorders, Madison, WI.

Ruke-Dravina, V. (1981). In P. Dale & D. Ingram (Eds.), *Child language—An international perspective.* Baltimore: University Park Press.

Russell, C. (1982). Coming alive down South. *American Demographics, 50,* 19–23.

Russell, C. (1983). The news about Hispanics. *American Demographics, 51,* 14–25.

Rutter, M. (1987). The role of cognition in child development and disorder. *British Journal of Medical Psychology, 60,* 1–16.

Ryan, J. (1974). Early language development: Towards a communicational analysis. In P. Richards (Ed.), *The integration of a child into a social world.* London: Cambridge University Press.

Sachs, J. (1972). On the analyzability of stories by children. In J. Gumperz & D. Hymes (Eds.), *Directions in sociolinguistics: The ethnography of communication.* New York: Holt, Rinehart & Winston.

Sachs, J. (1983). Talking about the there and then: The emergence of displaced reference in parent-child discourse. In K. Nelson (Ed.), *Children's language* (Vol. 4). Hillsdale, NJ: Erlbaum.

Sachs, J. (1984). Children's play and communicative development. In R. Schiefelbusch & J. Pickar (Eds.), *The acquisition of communicative competence.* Baltimore: University Park Press.

Sachs, J. (1985). Prelinguistic development. In J. Berko Gleason (Ed.), *The development of language.* Columbus, OH: Merrill.

Sameroff, A., & Fiese, B. (1990). Transactional regulation and early intervention. In S, Meisels & J. Shonkoff (Eds.), *Early intervention: A handbook of theory, practice, and analysis.* New York: Cambridge University Press.

Sanchez, R. (1983). *Chicano discourse.* Rowley, MA: Newbury House.

Sander, E. (1972). When are speech sounds learned? *Journal of Speech and Hearing Disorders, 37,* 55–63.

Saville-Troike, M. (1988). Private speech: Evidence for second language learning strategies during the "silent" period. *Journal of Child Language, 15,* 567–590.

Saywitz, K., & Cherry-Wilkinson, L. (1982). Age-related differences in metalinguistic awareness. In S. Kuczaj (Ed.), *Language development: Vol. 2. Language, thought and culture.* Hillsdale: NJ: Erlbaum.

Scaife, M., & Bruner, J. (1975). The capacity of joint visual attention in the infant. *Nature, 253,* 265–266.

Scarborough, H., & Dobrich, W. (1990). Development of children with early language delay. *Journal of Speech and Hearing Research, 33,* 70–83.

Scarborough, H., Wyckoff, J., & Davidson, R. (1986). A reconsideration of the relationship between age and mean utterance length. *Journal of Speech and Hearing Research, 29,* 394–399.

Schaffer, H., Hepburn, A., & Collis, G. (1983). Verbal and nonverbal aspects of mothers' directives. *Journal of Child Language, 10,* 337–355.

Schaffer, R. (1977). *Mothering.* Cambridge: Harvard University Press.

Schane, S. (1973). *Generative phonology.* Englewood Cliffs, NJ: Prentice Hall.

Scherer, N., & Olswang, L. (1984). Role of mothers' expansions in stimulating children's language production. *Journal of Speech and Hearing Research, 27,* 387–396.

Schiefelbusch, R. (1978). Summary and interpretation. In R. Schiefelbusch (Ed.), *Bases of language intervention.* Baltimore: University Park Press.

Schieffelin, B. B. (1982). Cross-cultural perspectives on the transition: What differences do the differences make? In R. Golinkoff (Ed.), *The transition from prelinguistic communication: Issues and implications.* Hillsdale, NJ: Erlbaum.

Schieffelin, B. B., & Eisenberg, A. R. (1984). Cultural variation in children's conversations. In R. Schiefelbusch & J. Pickar (Eds.), *The acquisition of communicative competence.* Baltimore: University Park Press.

Schiff-Myers, N. (1992). Considering arrested language development and language loss in the assessment of second language learners. *Language, Speech, and Hearing Services in Schools, 23,* 28–33.

Schlesinger, I. (1971). Production of utterances and language acquisition. In D. Slobin (Ed.), *The ontogenesis of grammar.* New York: Academic Press.

Schlesinger, I. (1977). The role of cognitive development and linguistic input in language acquisition. *Journal of Child Language, 4,* 153–169.

Schmidt, C. L. (1996). Scrutinizing reference: How gesture and speech are coordinated in mother–child interaction. *Journal of Child Language, 23,* 279-305.

Schnur, E., & Shatz, M. (1984). The role of maternal gesturing in conversations with one-year-olds. *Journal of Child Language, 11,* 29–41.

Schober-Peterson, D., & Johnson, C. J. (1989). Conversational topics of 4-year-olds. *Journal of Speech and Hearing Research, 32,* 857–870.

Schober-Peterson, D., & Johnson, C. J. (1991). Non-dialogue speech during preschool interactions. *Journal of Child Language, 18,* 153–170.

Schwartz, J., & Tallal, P. (1980). Rate of acoustic change may underlie hemispheric specialization for speech perception. *Science, 207,* 1380–1381.

Schwartz, R., Chapman, K., Prelock, P., Terrell, B., & Rowan, L. (1985). Facilitation of early syntax through discourse structure. *Journal of Child Language, 12,* 13–25.

Schwartz, R., & Leonard, L. (1984). Words, objects, and actions in early lexical acquisition. *Journal of Speech and Hearing Research, 27,* 119–127.

Scollon, R., & Scollon, S. (1981). *Narrative, literacy and face in interethnic communication.* Norwood, NJ: Ablex.

Scopesi, A., & Pellegrino, M. (1990). Structure and function of baby talk in a day-care center. *Journal of Child Language, 17,* 101–114.

Scott, C. M. (1984a). Abverbial connectivity in conversations of children 6 to 12. *Journal of Child Language, 11,* 423–452.

Scott, C. M. (1984b, November). *What happened to that: Structural characteristics of school children's narratives.* Paper presented at the annual convention of the American Speech-Language-Hearing Association, San Francisco.

Scott, C. M. (1987). *Summarizing text: Context effects in language disordered children.* Paper presented at the First International Symposium, Specific Language Disorders in Children, University of Reading, England.

Scott, C. M. (1988). Producing complex sentences. *Topics in Language Disorders, 8*(2), 44–62.

Scott, C. M., Nippold, M. A., Norris, J. A., & Johnson, C. J. (1992, November). *School-age children and adolescents: Establishing language norms.* Paper presented at the annual convention of the American Speech-Language-Hearing Association, San Antonio.

Scoville, R. (1983). Development of the intention to communicate: The eye of the beholder. In L. Feagans, C. Garvey, & R. Golinkoff (Eds.), *The origins and growth of communication*. Norwood, NJ: Ablex.

Scribner, S., & Cole, M. (1981). *The psychology of literacy*. Cambridge, MA: Harvard University Press.

Scupin, E., & Scupin, G. (1907). *Bubi's erste kindheit. Ein tagebuch*. Leipzig: Grieben's Verlag.

Searle, J. (1965). What is a speech act? In M. Black (Ed.), *Philosophy in America*. New York: Allen & Unwin; Cornell University Press.

Sell, M. A. (1992). The development of children's knowledge structures: Events, slots, and taxonomies. *Journal of Child Language, 19*, 659–676.

Senechal, M. (1997). The differential effect of storybook reading on preschoolers' acquisition of expressive and receptive vocabulary. *Journal of Child Language, 24*, 123–138.

Sengoku, T. (1983). Mother–child relationship in Japan and the United States through behavioral observation. *Journal of Perinatal Medicine, 13*, 126–141.

Sexton, H. (1980). *The development of understanding of causality in infancy*. Paper presented at the International Conference on Infant Studies, New Haven.

Seymour, H., & Seymour, C. (1981). Black English and Standard American English contrasts in consonantal development of four and five-year old children. *Journal of Speech and Hearing Disorders, 46*, 274–280.

Shafer, V. L., Shucard, D. W., Shucard, J. L., & Gerken, L. (1998). An electrophysiological study of infants' sensitivity to the sound patterns of English speech. *Journal of Speech, Language, and Hearing Research, 41*, 874–886.

Shand, N., & Kosawa, Y. (1985). Japanese and American behavior types at three months: Infants and infant–mother dyads. *Infant Behavior and Development, 8*, 225–240.

Shannon, C., & Weaver, W. (1949). *The mathematical theory of communication*. Urbana: University of Illinois Press.

Shantz, C. U. (1983). Social cognition. In J. H. Flavell & E. M. Markman (Eds.), *Cognitive development* (pp. 1–156). New York: Wiley.

Shapiro, B., & Danley, M. (1985). The role of the right hemisphere in the control of speech prosody in propositional and affective contexts. *Brain and Language, 25*, 19–36.

Shapiro, L., Swinney, D., & Borsky, S. (1998). Online examination of language performance in normal and neurologically impaired adults. *American Journal of Speech-Language Pathology, 7*, 49–60.

Shapiro, L. P. (1997). Tutorial: An introduction to syntax. *Journal of Speech, Language, and Hearing Research, 40*, 254–272.

Shatz, M. (1987). Bootstrapping operations in child language. In K. Nelson & A. van Kleeck (Eds.), *Children's language* (Vol. 6). Hillsdale, NJ: Erlbaum.

Shatz, M., & Gelman, R. (1973). The development of communication skills: Modifications in the speech of young children as a function of the listener. *Monograph of Society for Research in Child Development, 38*.

Shatz, M., & O'Reilly, A. (1990). Conversational or communicative skill? A reassessment of two year-olds' behavior in miscommunication episodes. *Journal of Child Language, 17*, 131–146.

Shatz, M., Wellman, H., & Silber, F. (1983). The acquisition of mental verbs: A systematic investigation of the first reference to mental state. *Cognition, 14*, 301–321.

Shaw, G. (1916). *Pygmalion*. New York: Brentano's.

Shipley, K., & Banis, C. (1989). *Teaching morphology developmentally* (revised edition). Tucson, AZ: Communication Skill Builders.

Shipley, K., Maddox, M., & Driver, J. (1991). Children's development of irregular past tense verb forms. *Language, Speech, and Hearing Services in Schools, 22*, 115–122.

Shore, C. (1986). Combinatorial play: Conceptual development and early multiword speech. *Developmental Psychology, 22*, 184–190.

Shore, C., O'Connell, B., & Bates, E. (1984). First sentences in language and symbolic play. *Developmental Psychology, 20*, 872–880.

Shorr, D., & Dale, P. (1981). Prepositional marking of source-goal structure and children's comprehension of English passives. *Journal of Speech and Hearing Research, 24*, 179–184.

Short-Meyerson, K. J., & Abbeduto, L. J. (1997). Preschoolers' communication during scripted interactions. *Journal of Child Language, 24*, 469–493.

Shriberg, L. D. (1993). Four new speech and prosody voice measures for genetics research and other studies of developmental phonological disorders. *Journal of Speech and Hearing Research, 36*, 105–140.

Shute, B., & Wheldall, K. (1989). Pitch alteration in British motherese: Some preliminary acoustic data. *Journal of Child Language, 16*, 503–512.

Siedlecki, T., & Bonvillian, J. D. (1998). Homonymy in the lexicons of young children acquiring American Sign Language. *Journal of Psycholinguistic Research, 27*, 47–65.

Siegel-Causey, E., & Ernst, B. (1989). Theoretical orientation and research in nonsymbolic development. In E. Siegel-Causey & D. Guess (Eds.), *Enhancing nonsymbolic communication interactions among learners with severe disabilities* (pp. 15–47). Baltimore, MD: Brookes.

Singer, B. D., & Bashir, A. S. (1999). What are executive functions and self-regulation and what do they have to do with language-learning disorders? *Language, Speech, and Hearing Services in Schools, 30*, 265–273.

Singh, S., Woods, D., & Becker, G. (1972). Perceptual structure of 22 prevocalic English consonants. *Journal of the Acoustical Society of America, 52*, 1698–1713.

Skinner, B. F. (1957). *Verbal behavior.* New York: Appleton-Century-Crofts.

Slobin, D. (1973). Cognitive prerequisites for the development of grammar. In C. Ferguson & D. Slobin (Eds.), *Studies of child language development.* New York: Holt, Rinehart & Winston.

Slobin, D. (1978). Cognitive prerequisites for the development of grammar. In L. Bloom & M. Lahey (Eds.), *Readings in language development.* New York: Wiley.

Slobin, D. (1982). Universal and particular in the acquisition of language. In E. Wanner & L. Gleitman (Eds.), *Language acquisition: The state of the art.* New York: Cambridge University Press.

Slobin, D. (1985). *The crosslinguistic study of language acquisition.* Hillsdale, NJ: Erlbaum.

Slobin, D., & Aksu, A. (1982). Tense, aspect, and modality in the use of the Turkish evidential. In P. Hopper (Ed.), *Tense-aspect: Between semantics and pragmatics.* Amsterdam: Benjamins.

Smit, A. B., Hand, L. , Freilinger, J. J., Bernthal, J. E., & Bird, A. (1990). The Iowa articulation norms project and its Nebraska replication. *Journal of Speech and Hearing Disorders, 55*, 779–798.

Smith, M. (1933). Grammatical errors in the speech of preschool children. *Child Development, 4*, 183–190.

Smith, P. (1986). The development of reading: The acquisition of a cognitive skill. In P. Fletcher & M. Garman (Eds.), *Language acquisition* (2nd ed.). New York: Cambridge University Press.

Smith, P. M. (1985). *Language, sexes and society,* London: Blackwell.

Smitherman, G. (1994). *Black talk: Words and phrases from the hood to the amen corner.* New York: Houghton-Mifflin.

Smolak, L. (1987). Child character and maternal speech. *Journal of Child Language, 14*, 481–492.

Smolak, L. & Weinraub, M.(1983). Maternal speech: Strategy or response? *Journal of Child Language, 10*, 369–380.

Snow, C. (1981). Social interaction and language acquisition. In P. Dale & D. Ingram (Eds.), *Child language: An international perspective* (pp. 195–214). Baltimore, MD: University Park Press.

Snow, C. (1983). Literacy and language: Relationships during the preschool years. *Harvard Educational Review, 53*, 165–189.

Snow, C. (1984). Parent-child interaction and the development of communicative ability. In R. Schiefelbusch & J. Pickar (Eds.), *The acquisition of communicative competence.* Baltimore: University Park Press.

Snow, C. (1986). Conversations with children. In P. Fletcher & M. Garman (Eds.), *Language acquisition* (2nd ed.). New York: Cambridge University Press.

Snow, C., & Goldfield, B. (1983). Turn the page please: Situation-specific language acquisition. *Journal of Child Language, 10*, 551–569.

Snow, C., & Ninio, A. (1986). The contracts of literacy: What children learn from learning to read books. In W. Teale & E. Sulzby (Eds.), *Emergent literacy: Writing and reading.* Norwood, NJ: Ablex.

Snow, D. (1998). A prominence account of syllable reduction in early speech development: The child's prosodic phonology of *Tiger* and *Giraffe. Journal of Speech, Language, and Hearing Research, 41*, 1171–1184.

Snowling, M. J., Hulme, C., Smith, A., & Thomas, J. (1994). The effects of phoneme similarity and list length on children's sound categorization performance. *Journal of Experimental Child Psychology, 58*, 160–180.

Snyder, L., & Downey, D. (1983). Pragmatics and information processing. *Topics in Language Disorders, 4(1)*, 75–86.

So, L. K., & Dodd, B. J. (1995). The acquisition of phonology by Cantonese-speaking children. *Journal of Child Language, 22,* 473–495.

Spector, C. C. (1996). Children's comprehension of idioms in the context of humor. *Language, Speech, and Hearing Services in Schools, 27,* 307–315.

Speer, S. R., Kjelgaard, M. M., & Dobroth, K. M. (1996). The influence of prosodic structure on the resolution of temporary syntactic closure ambiguities. *Journal of Psycholinguistic Research, 25,* 249–272.

Speidel, G. E., & Herreshoff, M. J. (1989). Imitation and the construction of long utterances. In G. E. Speidel & K. E. Nelson (Eds.), *The many faces of imitation in children.* New York: Springer-Verlag.

Spencer, G. (1984). *Projections of the population of the United States by age, sex, and race: 1983–2080* [Current Population Reports, series P–25, No. 952]. Washington, DC: U.S. Department of Commerce, Bureau of the Census.

Sperling, M. T. (1990). Social-cognitive development of bilingual and monolingual children. *Dissertation Abstracts International, 50,* 5349B.

Spilich, G. (1983). Life-span components of text processing: Structural and procedural differences. *Journal of Verbal Learning and Verbal Behavior, 22,* 231–244.

Springer, S., & Deutsch, G. (1985). *Left brain, right brain.* New York: W. H. Freeman.

Sprott, R. A., & Kemper, S. (1987). The development of children's code-switching: A study of six bilingual children across two situations. In E. F. Pemberton, M. A. Sell, & G. B. Simpson (Eds.), *Working papers in language development: 1987, 2,* 116–134.

Staley, C. (1982). Sex-related differences in the style of children's language. *Journal of Psycholinguistic Research, 11,* 141–158.

Stanovich, K. (1980). Toward an interactive-compensatory model of individual differences in the development of reading fluency. *Reading Research Quarterly, 16,* 32–71.

Stark, R. (1979). Prespeech segmental feature development. In P. Fletcher & M. Garman (Eds.), *Language acquisition.* New York: Cambridge University Press.

Stark, R. (1986). Prespeech segmental feature development. In P. Fletcher & M. Garman (Eds.), *Language acquisition* (2nd ed.). New York: Cambridge University Press.

Stark, R. E., Bernstein, L. E., & Demorest, M. E. (1993). Vocal communication in the first 18 months of life *Journal of Speech and Hearing Research, 36,* 548–558.

Stein, N. (1982). What's in a story: Interpreting the interpretations of story grammar. *Discourse Processes, 5,* 319–335.

Stein, N., & Glenn, C. (1979). An analysis of story comprehension in elementary school children. In R. Freedle (Ed.), *New directions in discourse processing* (Vol. 2). Norwood, NJ: Ablex.

Stein, N., & Policastro, M. (1984). The concept of story: A comparison between children's and teachers' viewpoints. In H. Mandler, N. Stein, & T. Trabasso (Ed.), *Learning and comprehension of text.* Hillsdale, NJ: Erlbaum.

Stemberger, J. P. (1993). Vowel dominance in overregularizations. *Journal of Child Language, 20,* 503–521.

Stephany, U. (1986). Modality. In P. Fletcher & M. Garman (Eds.), *Language acquisition* (2nd ed.). New York: Cambridge University Press.

Stephens, M. I. (1988). Pragmatics. In M. A. Nippold (Ed.), *Later language development.* New York: College-Hill.

Stern, D. N. (1977). *The first relationship.* Cambridge: Harvard University Press.

Stern, D. N., Spieker, S., Barnett, R., & MacKain, K. (1983). The prosody of maternal speech: Infant age and context related changes. *Journal of Child Language, 10,* 1–15.

Stern, D. N., Spieker, S., & MacKain, K. (1982). Intonation contours as signals in maternal speech to prelinguistic infants. *Developmental Psychology, 18,* 727–735.

Stoel-Gammon, C. (1988). Prelinguistic vocalizations of hearing-impaired and normally hearing subjects: A comparison of consonantal inventories. *Journal of Speech and Hearing Disorders, 53,* 302–315.

Stoel-Gammon, C., & Dunn, C. (1985). *Normal and disordered phonology in children.* Austin, TX: Pro-Ed.

Stoel-Gammon, C., & Otomo, K. (1986). Babbling development of hearing-impaired and normally hearing subjects. *Journal of Speech and Hearing Disorders, 51,* 33–41.

Stone, L., Smith, H., & Murphy, L. (Eds.). (1973). *The competent infant: Research and commentary.* New York: Basic Books.

Sullivan, J. W., & Horowitz, F. D. (1983). The effects of intonation on infant attention: The role of rising contour. *Journal of Child Language, 10,* 521–534.

Sulzby, E. (1981). *Kindergartners begin to read their own compositions.* Final report to the Research Foundation of the National Council of Teachers of English.

Sulzby, E., & Zecker, L. B. (1991). The oral monologue as a form of emergent reading. In A. McCabe & C. Peterson (Eds.), *Developing narrative structure* (pp. 175–214). Hillsdale, NJ: Erlbaum.

Sussman, H., Franklin, P., & Simon, T. (1982). Bilingual speech: Bilateral control? *Brain and Language, 15,* 125–142.

Sutter, J., & Johnson, C. (1990). School-age children's metalinguistic awareness of grammaticality in verb form. *Journal of Speech and Hearing Research, 33,* 84–95.

Sutton-Smith, B. (1981). *The folkstories of children.* Philadelphia: University of Pennsylvania Press.

Sutton-Smith, B. (1986). The development of fictional narrative performances. *Topics in Language Disorders, 7(1),* 1–10.

Suzman, S. (1987). Passives and prototypes in Zulu children's speech. *African Studies, 46,* 241–254.

Swank, L. K. (1997). Linguistic influences on the emergence of written word decoding in first grade. *American Journal of Speech-Language Pathology, 6,* 62–66.

Tager-Flusberg, H. (1989). Putting words together: Morphology and syntax in the preschool years. In J. Gleason (Ed.), *Language Development* (pp. 139–171). Columbus: Macmillan.

Tannen, D. (1990). *You just don't understand: Talk between the sexes.* New York: Ballantine.

Tannen, D. (1994). *Gender and discourse.* New York: Oxford University Press.

Tanz, C. (1980). *Studies in the acquisition of deictic terms.* New York: Cambridge University Press.

Tao, L., & Healy, A. F. (1996). Cognitive strategies in discourse processing: A comparison of Chinese and English speakers. *Journal of Psycholinguistic Research, 25,* 597–616.

Tardif, T., Shatz, M., & Naigles, L. (1997). Caregiver speech and children's use of nouns versus verbs: A comparison of English, Italian, and Mandarin. *Journal of Child Language, 24,* 535–565.

Tarone, E. (1988). *Variation in interlanguage.* London: Edward Arnold.

Taylor, I. (1980). The Korean writing system: An alphabet? A syllabary? A logography? In P. Kolers, M. Wrolstad, & H. Bouma (Eds.), *Processing of visible language* (Vol. II). New York: Plenum Press.

Teale, W. (1984). Reading to young children: Its significance for literacy development. In H. Goelmann, A. Oberg, & F. Smith (Eds.), *Awakening to literacy.* Exeter, NH: Heinemann.

Temple, C., Nathan, R., & Burris, N. (1982). *The beginnings of writing.* Boston: Allyn and Bacon.

Templin, M. (1957). *Certain language skills in children.* Minneapolis: University of Minnesota Press.

Terrell, S. L., & Terrell, F. (1983). Effects of speaking Black English upon employment opportunities. *Asha, 25,* 27–29.

Terrell, S. L., & Terrell, F. (1993). African-American cultures. In D. E. Battles (Ed.), *Communication disorders in multicultural populations.* Stoneham, MA: Butterworth-Heinemann.

Tfouni, L., & Klatsky, R. (1983). A discourse analysis of deixis: Pragmatic, cognitive and semantic factors in the comprehension of "this," "that," "here," and "there." *Journal of Child Language, 10,* 123–133.

Thal, D., & Bates, E. (1988). Language and gesture in late talkers. *Journal of Speech and Hearing Research, 31,* 115–123.

Thal, D., Tobias, S., & Morrison, D. (1991). Language and gesture in late talkers: A one year follow-up. *Journal of Speech and Hearing Disorders, 34,* 604–612.

Thomson, J., & Chapman, R. (1977). Who is "Daddy" revisited: The status of two year olds' overextended words in use and comprehension. *Journal of Child Language, 4,* 359–375.

Thorne, B., Kramerae, C., & Henley, N. (Eds.) (1983). *Language, gender, and society.* Rowley, MA: Newbury House.

Thorum, A. (1980). *The Fullerton Language Test for Adolescents: Experimental Edition.* Palo Alto, CA: Consulting Psychologists Press.

Tibbits, D. (1980). Oral production of linguistically complex sentences with meaning relationships of time. *Journal of Psycholinguistic Research, 9,* 545–564.

Toda, S., Fogel, A., & Kawai, M. (1990). Maternal speech to three-month-old infants in the United States and Japan. *Journal of Child Language, 17,* 279–294.

Todd, P. (1982). Tagging after red herrings: Evidence against the processing capacity explanation in child language. *Journal of Child Language, 9,* 99–114.

Tognola, G., & Vignolo, L. (1980). Brain lesions associated with oral apraxia in stroke patients: A cliniconeuroradiological investigation with the CT scan. *Neuropsychologia, 18,* 257–272.

Tomasello, M., & Cale Kruger, A. (1992). Joint attention on actions: Acquiring verbs in ostensive and non-ostensive context. *Journal of Child Language, 19,* 311–333.

Tomasello, M., Conti-Ramsden, G., & Ewert, B. (1990). Young children's conversations with their mothers and fathers: Differences in breakdown and repair. *Journal of Child Language, 17,* 115–130.

Tomasello, M., & Farrar, J. (1984). Cognitive bases of lexical development: Object permanence and relational words. *Journal of Child Language, 11,* 477–493.

Tomasello, M., & Farrar, J. (1986). Joint attention and early language. *Child Development, 57,* 1454–1463.

Tomasello, M., & Mannle, S. (1985). Pragmatics of sibling speech to one-year-olds. *Child Development, 56,* 911–917.

Tomasello, M., Mannle, S., & Kruger, A. C. (1986). Linguistic environment of 1- to 2-year-old twins. *Developmental Psychology, 22,* 169–176.

Tomasello, M., Strosberg, R., & Akhtar, N. (1996). Eighteen-month-old children learn words in non-ostensive contexts. *Journal of Child Language, 23,* 157–176.

Tomasello, M., & Todd, J. (1983). Joint attention and lexical acquisition style. *First Language, 4,* 197–212.

Tompkins, C. A. (1998). Special forum on online measures of comprehension: Implications for speech-language pathologists. *American Journal of Speech-Language Pathology, 7,* 48.

Trevarthen, C. (1979). Communication and cooperation in early infancy: A description of primary intersubjectivity. In M. Bullowa (Ed.), *Before speech.* New York: Cambridge University Press.

Tronick, E., Als, H., & Adamson, L. (1979). Structure of early face-to-face communicative interactions. In M. Bullowa (Ed.), *Before speech.* New York: Cambridge University Press.

Trotter, R. (1983, August). Baby face. *Psychology Today, 17*(8), 14–20.

Trudeau, M., & Chadwick, A. (1997, February 7). *Language development.* National Public Radio.

Tuaycharoen, P. (1978). The babbling of a Thai baby: Echoes and responses to the sounds made by adults. In N. Waterson & C. Snow (Eds.), *Development of communication: Social and pragmatic factors in language acquisition.* New York: Wiley.

Tyack, D., & Gottsleben, R. (1986). Acquisition of complex sentences. *Language, Speech, and Hearing Services in Schools, 17,* 160–174.

Tyack, D., & Ingram, D. (1977). Children's production and comprehension of questions. *Journal of Child Language, 4,* 211–224.

Tyler, A., & Nagy, W. E. (1987). *The acquisition of English derivational morphology.* (Technical Report No. 407). Urbana, IL: Center for the Study of Reading.

U.S. Department of Health and Human Services. (1985). *Report of the Secretary's Task Force on Black and Minority Health,* Vol. I: *Executive Summary* [Pub. No. 491–313/44706]. Washington, DC.

U.S. Department of Health and Human Services. (1986). *Report of the Secretary's Task Force on Black and Minority Health,* Vol. IV: *Cardiovascular and Cerebrovascular Disease, Part I* [1986–62038:40716]. Washington, DC.

Vaid, J. (1983). Bilingualism and brain lateralization. In S. Segalowitz (Ed.), *Language functions and brain organization.* New York: Academic Press.

Vaidyanathan, R. (1988). Development of forms and functions of interrogatives in children: A language study of Tamil. *Journal of Child Language, 15,* 533–549.

Vaidyanathan, R. (1991). Development of forms and functions of negation in the early stages of language acquisition: A study in Tamil. *Journal of Child Language, 18,* 51–60.

Valian, V., & Eisenberg, Z. (1996). The development of syntactic subjects in Portuguese-speaking children. *Journal of Child Language, 23,* 103–128.

VanHekken, S., Vergeer, M., & Harris, P. (1980). Ambiguity of reference and listeners' reaction in a naturalistic setting. *Journal of Child Language, 7,* 555–563.

van Kleeck, A. (1982). The emergence of linguistic awareness: A cognitive framework. *Merrill-Palmer Quarterly, 28,* 237–265.

van Kleeck, A., & Schuele, C. M. (1987). Precursors to literacy: Normal development. *Topics in Language Disorders, 7,* 13–31.

van Kleeck, A., Gillam, R. B., Hamilton, L., & McGrath, C. (1997). The relationship between middle-class parents' book sharing discussion and their preschoolers' abstract language development. *Journal of Speech, Language, and Hearing Research, 40,* 1261–1271.

Veneziano, E., Sinclair, H., & Berthoud, I. (1990). From one word to two words: Repetition patterns on the way to structured speech. *Journal of Child Language, 17,* 633–650.

Vihman, M. (1985). Language differentiation by the bilingual infant. *Journal of Child Language, 12,* 297–324.

Vihman, M., & Greenlee, M. (1987). Individual differences in phonological development: Ages one and three years. *Journal of Speech and Hearing Research, 30*, 503–521.

Vygotsky, L. (1962). *Thought and language.* Cambridge: MIT Press. (Orig. pub. in 1934.)

Wales, R. (1986). Deixis. In P. Fletcher & M. Garman (Eds.), *Language acquisition* (2nd ed.). New York: Cambridge University Press.

Wallace, I. F., Roberts, J. E., & Lodder, D. E. (1998). Interactions of African American infants and their mothers: Relations with development at 1 year of age. *Journal of Speech, Language, and Hearing Research, 42*, 900–912.

Walley, A. (1993). The role of vocabulary development in children's spoken word recognition and segmentation ability. *Developmental Review, 13*, 286–350.

Wanska, S., & Bedrosian, J. (1985). Conversational structure and topic performance in mother-child interaction. *Journal of Speech and Hearing Research, 28*, 579–584.

Warren-Leubecker, A. (1982). *Sex differences in speech to children.* Unpublished master's thesis, Georgia Institute of Technology.

Washington, J. A., & Craig, H. K. (1998). Socioeconomic status and gender influences on children's dialectal variations. *Journal of Speech, Language, and Hearing Research, 41*, 618–626.

Waterman, P., & Schatz, M. (1982). The acquisition of personal pronouns and proper names by an identical twin pair. *Journal of Speech and Hearing Research, 25*, 149–154.

Watkins, O., & Watkins, M. (1980). The modality effect and echoic persistence. *Journal of Experimental Psychology: General, 109*, 251–278.

Weeks, L. A. (1992). Preschoolers' production of tag questions and adherence to the polarity-contrast principle. *Journal of Psycholinguistic Research, 21*, 31–40.

Wehren, A., DeLisi, R., & Arnold, M. (1981). The development of noun definition. *Journal of Child Language, 8*, 165–175.

Weiner, P. (1985). The value of follow-up studies. *Topics in Language Disorders, 5*(3), 78–92.

Weinstein, G. (1984). Literacy and second language acquisition: Issues and perspectives. *TESOL Quarterly, 18*, 471–484.

Weist, R. M. (1986). Tense and aspect. In P. Fletcher & M. Garman (Eds.), *Language acquisition* (2nd ed.). New York: Cambridge University Press.

Weist, R., Wysocka, H., & Lyytinen, P. (1991). Across-linguistic perspective on the development of temporal systems. *Journal of Child Language, 18*, 67–92.

Wellen, C. (1985). Effects of older siblings on the language young children hear and produce. *Journal of Speech and Hearing Disorders, 50*, 84–99.

Wells, G. (1979). Learning and using the auxiliary verb in English. In V. Lee (Ed.), *Language development.* New York: Wiley.

Wells, G. (1980). Adjustments in adult-child conversation: Some effects of interaction. In H. Giles, W. Robinson, & P. Smith (Eds.), *Language: Social psychological perspective.* Oxford: Pergamon Press.

Wells, G. (1985). *Language development in the pre-school years.* New York: Cambridge University Press.

Wells, G. (1986). Variation in child language. In P. Fletcher & M. Garman (Eds.), *Language acquisition: Studies in first language acquisition.* New York: Cambridge University Press.

Wells, G., Barnes, S., Gutfreund, M., & Satterly, D. (1983). Characteristics of adult speech which predict children's language development. *Journal of Child Language, 10*, 65–84.

Werker, J. F., & McLeod, P. J. (1989). Infant preference for both male and female infant-directed talk: A development study of attentional and affective responsiveness. *Canadian Journal of Psychology, 43*, 230–246.

Werner, E. E. (1984). *Child care: Kith, kin and hired hands.* Baltimore, MD: University Park Press.

Wertsch, J. V., & Tulviste, P. (1992). L.S. Vygotsky and contemporary developmental psychology. *Developmental Psychology, 28*, 548–557.

Westby, C. E. (1984). Development of narrative language abilities. In G. P. Wallach & K. Butler (Eds.), *Language disabilities in school-age children.* Baltimore: Williams & Wilkins.

Westby, C. E. (1986). Cultural differences affecting communication development. In L. Cole & V. Deal (Eds.), *Communication disorders in multicultural populations.* Washington, DC: American Speech-Language-Hearing Association.

Wetherby, A. M., Cain, D. H., Yonclas, D. G., & Walker, V. G. (1988). Analysis of intentional communication in normal children from the prelinguistic to the multiword stage. *Journal of Speech and Hearing Research, 31*, 240–252.

Wetherby, A. M., & Prizant, B. M. (1989). The expression of communicative intent: Assessment guidelines. *Seminars in Speech and Language, 10*, 77–91.

Whaley, J. (1981). Readers' expectation for story structure. *Reading Research Quarterly, 17*, 90–114.

Whitaker, J. H., Rueda, R. S., & Prieto, A. G. (1985). Cognitive performance as a function of bilingualism in students with mental retardation. *Mental Retardation, 6*, 302–307.

White, S. (1989). Back channels across cultures: A study of Americans and Japanese. *Language and Society, 18*, 59–76.

White, T. G., Power, M. A., & White, S. (1989). Morphological analsis: Implications for teaching and understanding vocabulary growth. *Reading Research Quarterly, 24*, 283–304.

Whitehurst, G. J., Kedesdy, J., & White, T. (1982). A functional analysis of meaning. In S. Kuczaj (Ed.), *Language development*: Vol. 1. *Syntax and semantics.* Hillsdale, NJ: Erlbaum.

Whitehurst, G. J., Smith, M., Fischel, J. E., Arnold, D. S., & Lonigan, C. J. (1991). The continuity of babble and speech in children with specific expressive language delay. *Journal of Speech, Language, and Hearing Research, 34*, 1121–1129.

Whorf, B. (1956). *Language, thought, and reality.* New York: Wiley.

Wiig, E., & Semel, E. (1984). *Language assessment and intervention for the learning disabled* (2nd ed.). Columbus, OH: Merrill.

Wilcox, M. J., Kouri, T., & Caswell, S. (1990). Partner sensitivity to communication behavior of young children with developmental disabilities. *Journal of Speech and Hearing Disorders, 55*, 679–693.

Wiley, A. R., Rose, A. J., Burger, L. K., Miller, P. J. (1998). Constructing autonomous selves through narrative practices: A comparative study of working-class and middle-class families. *Child Development, 69*, 833–847.

Wilkinson, L., Calculator, S., & Dollaghan, C. (1982). Ya wanna trade—just for awhile: Children's requests and responses to peers. *Discourse Processes, 5*, 161–176.

Wilkinson, L., Hiebert, E., & Rembold, K. (1981). Parents' and peers' communication to toddlers. *Journal of Speech, Language, and Hearing Research, 24*, 383–388.

Wilkinson, L., & Rembold, K. (1982). The communicative context of early-language development. In S. Kuczaj (Ed.), *Language development*: Vol. 2. *Language, thought and culture.* Hillsdale, NJ: Erlbaum.

Wing, C., & Scholnick, E. (1981). Children's comprehension of pragmatic concepts expressed in "because," "although," "if" and "unless." *Journal of Child Language, 8*, 347–365.

Winitz, H. (1983). Use and abuse of the developmental approach. In H. Winitz (Ed.), *Treating language disorders.* Baltimore: University Park Press.

Witelson, S. (1987). Neurobiological aspects of language in children. *Child Development, 58*, 653–688.

Wolf, M., Bally, H., & Morris, R. (1984). *Automaticity, retrieval processes, and reading: A longitudinal investigation of average and impaired readers.* Manuscript submitted for publication.

Wolff, P. (1963). Observations on the early development of smiling. In B. Foss (Ed.), *Determinants of infant behavior II.* New York: Wiley.

Worobey, J. (1989). Mother-infant interaction: Protocommunication in the developing dyad. In J. F. Nussbaum (Ed.), *Life-span communication: Normative processes.* Hillsdale, NJ: Erlbaum.

Wysocki, K., & Jenkins, J. R. (1987). Deriving word meanings through morphological generalization. *Reading Research Quarterly, 22*, 66–81.

Xu, F., & Pinker, S. (1995). Weird past tense forms. *Journal of Child Language, 22*, 531–556.

Yamada, J. (1992). Asymmetries of reading and writing kanji by Japanese children. *Journal of Psycholinguistic Research, 21*, 563–580.

Yeni-Komshian, G., & Rao, P. (1980). *Speech perception in right and left CVA patients.* Paper presented at the International Neuropsychological Society meeting.

Yoder, P., & Kaiser, A. (1989). Alternative explanations for the relationship between maternal verbal interaction style and child language development. *Journal of Child Language, 16*, 141–160.

Yopp, H. (1992). Developing phonological awareness in young children. *Journal of the Reading Teacher, 45*, 696–703.

Zinober, B., & Martlew, M. (1985). Developmental changes in four types of gestures in relation to acts and vocalizations from 10 to 21 months. *British Journal of Developmental Psychology, 3*, 293–306.

Author Index

Subject Index